CLINICAL NEUROLOGY FOR PSYCHIATRISTS

Third Edition

David Myland Kaufman, M.D.

Department of Neurology,
Montefiore Medical Center,
Albert Einstein College of Medicine,
Bronx, New York

1990

W. B. SAUNDERS COMPANY

Harcourt Brace Jovanovich, Inc.

Philadelphia, London, Toronto, Montreal, Sydney, Tokyo

W. B. SAUNDERS COMPANY
Harcourt Brace Jovanovich, Inc

The Curtis Center
Independence Square West
Philadelphia, PA 19106

Library of Congress Cataloging-in-Publication Data

Kaufman, David Myland.
    Clinical neurology for psychiatrists / David Myland Kaufman. —
3rd ed.
      p.   cm.
    Includes bibliographical references.
    ISBN 0-7216-3123-1
    1. Nervous System Diseases. 2. Neurology. 3. Psychiatrists.
I. Title.
    [DNLM: 1. Nervous System Diseases. 2. Psychiatry. WL 100 K205c]
RC346.K38 1990
616.8—dc20
DNLM/DLC
for Library of Congress   89-10682
                                            CIP

Acquisition Editor: Martin Wonsiewicz

Clinical Neurology for Psychiatrists   ISBN 0-7216-3123-1

Printed in the United States of America.

Last digit is the print number: 9   8   7   6   5   4   3   2   1

This is dedicated . . .
to the one I love:
My wife of 20 years,
Rita Gail Kaufman.

ACKNOWLEDGMENTS

Drs. Suzanne Gerber and Nancy Horowitz provided editorial assistance that was both critical and creative. Mr. Barry Morden and Ms. Meryl Ranzer were the artists who provided the wonderful illustrations. Ms. Louise Wolkis and her staff typed the manuscript diligently and thoughtfully.

Valuable suggestions and reviews have been made by my students and colleagues at Montefiore Medical Center, the Albert Einstein College of Medicine, and the course on which this book is based, "Clinical Neurology for Psychiatrists."

NOTE ABOUT THE
REFERENCES

Specific references are provided at the conclusion of most chapters, but some standard references might be consulted for information about many topics:

Adams RD, Victor M: *Principles of Neurology* (4 ed). New York, McGraw-Hill Book Co., 1989.

Cummings JL: *Clinical Neuropsychiatry*. Orlando, Grune & Stratton, 1985.

Heilman KM, Valenstein E: *Clinical Neuropsychology* (2 ed). New York, Oxford University Press, 1985.

Jefferson JW, Marshal JR: *Neuropsychiatric Features of Medical Disorders*. New York, Plenum Medical Book Co., 1981.

Joynt RJ (ed): *Clinical Neurology*. Philadelphia, J.B. Lippincott Co., 1988.

Kerson TS: *Understanding Chronic Illness: The Medical and Psychosocial Dimensions of Nine Diseases*. New York, The Free Press, 1985.

Menkes JH: *Textbook of Child Neurology* (3 ed). Philadelphia, Lea and Febiger, 1985.

Rowland L (ed): *Merritt's Textbook of Neurology* (8 ed). Philadelphia, Lea and Febiger, 1989.

Swaiman KF: *Pediatric Neurology: Principles and Practice*. St. Louis, The C.V. Mosby Co., 1989.

PREFACE

I have written *Clinical Neurology for Psychiatrists* from my perspective as a neurologist at a major teaching hospital to provide a straight-forward guide to the major areas of clinical neurology. In a format combining traditional neuroanatomic correlations with symptom-oriented discussions, the book emphasizes neurologic illnesses that are common, illustrate a principle, and cause or mimic psychiatric symptoms. Having evolved from the course by the same name that I founded in 1971, the book also serves as preparation for specialty qualifying examinations, particularly the one given by the American Board of Psychiatry and Neurology.

The first half of the book reviews classical anatomic neurology and describes how a physician might approach patients with a suspected neurologic disorder, identify central or peripheral nervous system disease, and correlate physical signs with psychiatric abnormalities. The second half discusses common neurologic symptoms, such as dementia, and broad clinical areas, such as multiple sclerosis. For each conditions, a chapter describes the relevant history and neurologic findings, easily performed office and bedside examinations, appropriate laboratory tests and their costs, differential diagnosis, and, for many conditions, suggestions for management. To further enhance the usefulness of the text, neurologic terminology is compared to the criteria in the *Diagnostic and Statistical Manual, Third Edition, Revised* (DSM-III-R).

Since the diagnosis of entire categories of illnesses, such as gait abnormalities, psychogenic neurologic deficits, facial dyskinesias, and other movement disorders, relies almost entirely on observation, and likewise since the most reliable tests, computed tomography (CT), magnetic resonance imaging (MRI), and electroencephalography (EEG), are visual records, each chapter includes abundant illustrations. Drawings of anatomic relationships, pictures of clinical cases and examinations, and reproductions of laboratory studies reinforce the text, graphically portray many illnesses, serve as the basis for test questions, and possibly offer many readers their first sight of several uncommon but important disorders.

Chapters are also supplemented with outlines for obtaining the relevant history; reproductions of standard tests, such as the Blessed Mental Status Test, Mini-mental Status, hand-held visual acuity card, and Abnormal Involuntary Movement Scale (AIMS) Revised; names, addresses, and telephone numbers of support groups; and references to recent articles, reviews, and classic studies. Most chapters and two review sections are followed by short-answer, essay, or illustration-based questions that enable readers to compare different conditions, apply the text to clinical situations, and prepare for examinations.

The first two editions of *Clinical Neurology for Psychiatrists* enjoyed success in the United States, Canada, and abroad. In the third edition, which has been rewritten five years since the previous edition, I have updated virtually all subjects to address advances in etiology, diagnosis, and treatment; added the comparisons of neurologic and DSM-III-R criteria; included numerous new illustrations; and introduced or greatly expanded the following topics:

- amnestic and frontal lobe syndromes, the persistent vegetative state and the locked-in syndrome, and other conditions that resemble dementia

- neurologic complications of aging and alcoholism

- AIDS-dementia complex and other complications of acquired immuno-deficiency syndrome (AIDS)

- peripheral nervous system diseases associated with mental status changes, including volatile substance abuse and Lyme disease

- complications of anticonvulsants used for psychiatric illnesses: carbamazepine (Tegretol), valproate (Depekote), and phenytoin (Dilantin)

- neurologic complications of psychotropic medications: seizures, neuroleptic malignant syndrome, hypertensive crises, and tardive dystonia

- specific psychogenic syndromes: pseudoseizures, hyperventilation with carpopedal spasm, and psychogenic movement disorders

- neurologic and psychiatric manifestations of brain tumors and metastatic cancer

- treatment of malignant and common nonmalignant pain syndromes, including postmastectomy pain, causalgia, and chronic back pain

- limbic system and the human Klüver-Bucy syndrome

- movement disorders particularly important to psychiatrists: facial dyskinesias and their treatment with botulinum toxin, AIMS test, dystonias, and tics and Tourette's syndrome

- uses of MRI and CT scanning

DAVID MYLAND KAUFMAN, M.D.

CONTENTS

CLASSICAL ANATOMIC NEUROLOGY

First Encounter with a Patient: Examination and Formulation

The neurologic examination, despite the ready availability of sophisticated tests, remains crucial. Beloved by neurologists, it is often a vivid portrayal of neurologic function and dysfunction. When neurologists say that they have seen a case of a particular disorder, they really mean that they have *seen* it.

Although many neurologic conditions may be suspected or diagnosed solely on the basis of the patient's history, psychiatrists should be familiar with the neurologic examination. Even if they themselves will not actually be examining patients, psychiatrists should know the significance of common neurologic symptoms and signs, be able to assess the conclusions of a neurologist, and interpret neurologic tests—all within the context of a psychiatric assessment.

Patients with suspected or known disease of the nervous system are examined in a systematic manner. Undeviating adherence to routine is vital to avoid omission, duplication, and ultimately confusion. Areas of interest are tested in detail, and the major components of the nervous system are examined sequentially. Despite obvious disease in one part of the nervous system, all areas are evaluated. An initial or screening neurologic examination can be completed in 20 minutes, after which detailed testing of areas of concern may be performed. The examiner, for example, might return to perform full mental status testing or to review inconsistent results.

EXAMINATION

The examiner should note the patient's age, sex, and handedness and then review the chief complaint, present illness, past medical history, family history, and social history. Some patients cannot relate the necessary information, but further evaluation of these patients may reveal that intellectual, language, or memory impairments were the reason that they were not able to comply. With the majority of patients who are able to relate a history, a brief series of standard questions is asked about their primary symptom, associated symptoms, and possible etiologic factors. Section 2 of this book, which deals with common symptoms, contains outlines for obtaining a pertinent history and making a general evaluation for each symptom.

While obtaining the history, the examiner should consider the possible types of neurologic deficits the patient may display during the subsequent physical examination. The examiner should be prepared, for instance, to look for disease primarily of the central nervous system (CNS), which includes the brain and spinal cord, or of the peripheral nervous system (PNS), which includes the nerve roots, plexuses, and peripheral nerves. In other words, without yielding to rigid preconceptions, some feeling for the problem at hand should be acquired after eliciting the patient's history.

The routine physical examination, outlined in Table 1-1, is a sequential evaluation of the functional anatomy of the nervous system: mental status, cranial nerves, motor system, reflexes, sensation, and cerebellar system. This format should be followed during every examination. Until this outline can be memorized, a copy should be taken to the patient's bedside, where it will serve both as a reminder and a place to record neurologic findings.

In the first part of the examination, during testing of the mental status, the examiner should assess the patient's general intellectual function and consider specific intellectual deficits, such as language impairment. These examinations are described in detail in Chapters 7 and 8. Tests of cranial nerves may reveal malfunctions of either individual nerves or groups of nerves, such as the *ocular motility nerves* (third, fourth, and sixth) and the *cerebellopontine angle* nerves (fifth, seventh, and eighth). The intricate tests and implications of abnormal findings are discussed in Chapter 4.

The examination of the motor system is usually performed to detect the severity and pattern of weakness. Mild to moderate weakness is called *paresis*, and severe weakness is called *plegia*. Any degree of weakness may be termed "paralysis."

More important than the severity of the weakness is its distribution. Whether paresis or plegia is present, either will be indicative of the origin of any motor

TABLE 1–1. NEUROLOGIC EXAMINATION

Mental Status
  Cooperation
  Orientation
  Language
  Memory for immediate, recent, and past events
  Higher intellectual functions, e.g., arithmetic, similarities/differences
Cranial Nerves
  I   Smell
  II   Visual acuity, visual fields, optic fundi
  III, IV, VI   Pupils' size and reactivity, extraocular motion
  V   Corneal reflex and facial sensation
  VII   Strength of upper and lower facial muscles, taste
  VIII   Hearing
  IX–XI   Articulation, palate movement, gag reflex
  XII   Tongue movement
Motor System
  Limb strength
  Spasticity, flaccidity, or fasciculations
  Abnormal movements, e.g., tremor, chorea
Reflexes
  Deep tendon reflexes (DTRs): biceps, triceps, brachioradialis, quadriceps, Achilles
  Pathologic reflexes: extensor plantar response (Babinski sign), frontal lobe release signs
Sensation
  Position, vibration, stereognosis
  Pain (pin)
Cerebellar system
  Finger-nose, heel-shin, and rapid alternating movements
  Gait

system impairment. If the lower face, the arm, and the leg on one side of the body are paretic, the pattern is called *hemiparesis*, and it indicates damage to the brain's contralateral cerebral hemisphere or brainstem. If both legs are weak, this pattern is called *paraparesis*, and it indicates damage to the spinal cord. In contrast, if the distal portions of the limbs are paretic, this pattern indicates damage of the PNS, rather than the CNS.

Two categories of reflexes are usually tested to assist in determining whether a problem is in the CNS or PNS and then for detailed localization. Deep tendon reflexes (DTRs) are normally present with uniform reactivity in all limbs. In neurologic disorders, their activity, symmetry, or both will be altered. Moreover, paresis is almost always associated with change in the DTRs. In general, with CNS injury (with corticospinal tract damage), DTRs are hyperactive, whereas with PNS injury they are hypoactive.

In contrast to DTRs, "pathologic" reflexes are not normally found in persons older than 1 year. If present, they are signs of damage to the CNS (Fig. 2-2). The most generally accepted indication of CNS injury is the *Babinski sign*. With this sign a clear understanding of terminology is important. Following plantar stimulation, the great toe normally moves downward, i.e., it has a flexor response. With damage of the brain or spinal cord, plantar stimulation typically causes the great toe to move upward, i.e., have an extensor response. The abnormal extensor response is a Babinski sign. This sign and others may be "present" or "elicited," but they are never "positive" or "negative." For example, a traffic stop sign is either present or not, but it is never positive or negative.

Other pathologic reflexes indicate impairment of the frontal lobes, e.g., "frontal release signs." As is discussed in Chapter 7, they are helpful in indicating an "organic" basis of a change in personality and, to a limited degree, are associated with intellectual impairment.

The examination of the sensory system is long and tedious. In addition, unlike abnormal DTRs and Babinski signs, which are reproducible, objective, and virtually impossible to mimic, the sensory examination relies almost entirely on the patient's report. The best approach under most circumstances is to perform tests of major modalities of sensation in a clear anatomic order and to accept the patient's report with reservations.

Sensation of position, vibration, and stereognosis (appreciation of an object's form by touching it), all of which are carried in the posterior columns of the spinal cord, are each routinely tested. Pain (pinprick) sensation, which is carried in the lateral columns, is usually tested with a pin.

Cerebellar function is evaluated by observing the patient for intention tremor and incoordination during several standard maneuvers that include the *finger-nose test* and rapid repetition of alternating movement test (Chapter 2). Finally, the patient's walk (*gait*) is observed for signs not only of incoordination (*ataxia*) but also for indications of paresis, involuntary movement disorders, and hydrocephalus (Table 2-4).

FORMULATION

The *formulation* is an appraisal of four problematic areas: the symptoms, signs, site of involvement (*localization*), and probable cause (*differential diagnosis*). A succinct and cogent formulation is the basis upon which neurologic problems are solved and cases are meaningfully presented to fellow physicians. Although somewhat ritualistic, this format encourages careful and critical review.

The clinician might have to support a conclusion that neurologic disease is present or, equally important, absent. For this step, psychologically induced (psychogenic) symptoms and signs must be separated, if only tentatively, from neurologic ones, but evidence must be demonstrable for either conclusion. Unlike psychiatrists, neurologists do not rely on a mental status examination to determine that a condition is psychogenic or neurologic. When the results of the mental status examination are in conflict with those of the physical examination, neurologists tend to invoke a Confucian attitude of "One Babinski sign is worth a thousand proverbs."

Likewise, neither a psychogenic nor neurologic etiology is a diagnosis of exclusion, and patients can have psychogenic conditions (Chapter 3) superimposed on neurologic ones. In practice, despite neurologists' inclinations, a diagnosis of a psychogenic disturbance is usually made only after exhaustive tests have excluded rare as well as common neurologic illnesses. During such an assessment, psychiatric evaluation might be performed concomitantly.

Localization of neurologic lesions requires the clinician to determine whether the illness affects the CNS or PNS (Chapters 2–6). Precise localization of lesions within those systems is possible and generally expected. The physician must also establish whether the nervous system is affected diffusely or only in a limited, discrete area. The site and extent of neurologic damage will indicate certain diseases. For example, cerebrovascular accidents and tumors generally involve only a single area of the brain, whereas degenerative conditions, (e.g., Alzheimer's disease) have a widespread and symmetric effect.

Finally, the differential diagnosis is offered as the most probable disease or diseases with which the symptoms, signs, and localization are consistent. When specific diseases cannot be determined, major categories of illnesses, such as "structural lesions," should be suggested.

A typical formulation might be: "Mr. Jones, a 56-year-old man, has had left-sided headaches for 2 months and a generalized seizure on the day before admission. He is lethargic and has papilledema, a right hemiparesis with hyperactive DTRs, and a Babinski sign. The lesion seems to be in the left cerebral hemisphere. Most likely he has a tumor, but a cerebrovascular accident (stroke) is a less likely possibility." In this formulation, the first sentence recounts the symptoms and an abbreviated relevant medical history, and the second sentence details the salient physical findings. The formulation tacitly assumes that neurologic disease is present because of the obvious, objective physical findings. The localization is based on the history of seizures and the right-sided hemiparesis and reflex abnormalities. The differential diagnosis is based on the probability that the patient has a lesion of the cerebral hemisphere.

To conclude, the physician should present a formulation that answers *The Four Questions of Neurology*:

- What are the *symptoms* of *neurologic* disease?
- What are the *signs* of *neurologic* disease?
- *Where* is the lesion?
- *What* is the lesion?

2

Central Nervous System Disorders

This chapter discusses physical and intellectual signs that accompany common lesions of the two components of the central nervous system (CNS), the brain and the spinal cord (Table 2-1). It describes signs of lesions in the major areas of the brain—the cerebral hemispheres, the basal ganglia, the brainstem (midbrain, pons, and medulla), and the cerebellum—and in the spinal cord. Chapter 3 contrasts signs of CNS lesions with those of psychogenic disturbances.

SIGNS OF CEREBRAL HEMISPHERE LESIONS

Signs indicating an injury of the cerebral hemisphere can be physical, intellectual, or, in the opinion of some, emotional (Table 2-2). Usually, the most prominent sign is *contralateral hemiparesis*, paresis of the opposite face, trunk, arm, and leg because of damage to the *corticospinal tract*. This tract originates in each cerebral cortex and terminates on motor neurons of the contralateral trunk and limbs (Fig. 2-1). Within the cerebral hemisphere, the corticospinal tract passes through the internal capsule. It then descends through the brainstem, but in the medulla crosses almost entirely within the *pyramids*. It descends in the spinal cord as the *lateral corticospinal tract*. Finally, it terminates by synapsing onto the *anterior horn cells* of the spinal cord.

During its course from the cerebral cortex to the anterior horn cells, the corticospinal tract is considered the upper motor neuron (UMN) (Fig. 2-2). The anterior horn cells of the spinal cord, which are the origin of the peripheral nerves, are considered the beginning of the lower motor neuron (LMN).

Thus, CNS lesions that damage the corticospinal tract are associated with *signs of UMN injuries* (Figs. 2-3, 2-4, and 2-5):

- paresis with muscle spasticity
- hyperactive deep tendon reflexes (DTRs)
- Babinski signs

In contrast, peripheral nerve lesions, including anterior horn cell or "motor neuron" diseases, are associated with *signs of LMN injuries*:

- paresis with muscle flaccidity
- hypoactive DTRs
- no Babinski signs

TABLE 2–1. SIGNS OF CNS LESIONS

Cerebral hemisphere*
  Hemiparesis with hyperactive DTRs and Babinski sign
  Hemisensory loss
  Homonymous hemianopsia
  Aphsias, hemi-inattention, and dementia
  Pseudobulbar palsy
Basal ganglia*
  Movement disorders: parkinsonism, athetosis, chorea, and hemiballismus
Brainstem
  Cranial nerve palsy with contralateral hemiparesis, hemisensory loss, or both; or ipsilateral or
    contralateral ataxia
  Internuclear ophthalmoplegia (MLF syndrome)
  Nystagmus
  Bulbar palsy
Cerebellum
  Tremor on intention
  Impaired rapid alternating movements (dysdiadochokinesia)
  Ataxic gait
  Scanning speech
Spinal cord
  Paraparesis or quadriparesis
  Sensory loss up to a "level"
  Bladder, bowel, sexual dysfunction

* Signs are contralateral to lesions.

Because the corticospinal tract has such a long course, hemiparesis and other signs of UMN damage may originate not only from lesions in the cerebral hemispheres but also from those in the brainstem or spinal cord. Localizing them depends on other features discovered during the examination. For example, signs of cerebral injury, such as aphasia, dementia, or homonymous hemianopsia, indicate that any hemiparesis probably originates in the cerebrum.

Sensory loss to certain modalities over one half of the body, (i.e., a *hemisensory* loss) is usually another indication of a contralateral cerebral lesion. Characteristically, a patient with a cerebral lesion loses position sensation, two-point discrimination, and the ability to identify objects by touch (stereognosis); however, pain sensation, which is "perceived" in the thalamus, is largely retained in almost all instances (Fig. 2-6).

TABLE 2–2. SIGNS OF CEREBRAL LESIONS

Either hemisphere*
  Hemiparesis with hyperactive DTRs and Babinski sign
  Hemisensory loss
  Homonymous hemianopsia
Nondominant hemisphere
  Hemi-inattention
  Anosognosia
  Constructional apraxia
Dominant hemisphere
  Aphasias
Both hemispheres
  Dementia
  Pseudobulbar palsy

* Signs are contralateral to lesions.

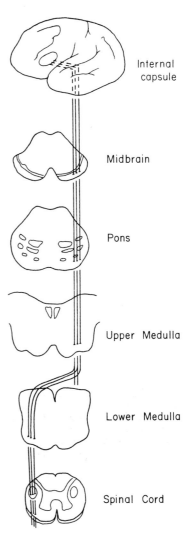

Internal capsule

Midbrain

Pons

Upper Medulla

Lower Medulla

Spinal Cord

FIGURE 2–1. The corticospinal tract originates in the cerebral cortex, passes through the internal capsule, and descends into the brainstem. It crosses in the pyramids, which are located in the medulla, to continue its descent as the contralateral corticospinal tract. Since the corticospinal tract crosses in the pyramids, it is referred to as the *pyramidal tract.* Its functions are modulated by the *extrapyramidal tract*, which originates in the basal ganglia (see below).

The pain-sensing role of the thalamus is clinically important. For example, a patient with a lesion of the cerebral cortex may be unable to locate or identify the painful area, but will still feel the intensity and discomfort of the pain. In particular, patients with common cerebral infarctions are still able to feel pain. Also, patients who had suffered from intractable pain did not obtain relief when they underwent experimental surgical resection of the cerebral cortex.

Loss of vision involving the same half of the visual field in each eye, *homonymous hemianopsia* (Fig. 2-7), is another reliable sign of a contralateral cerebral lesion. There are also characteristic patterns of visual loss associated with lesions involving the eye, the optic nerve, or the optic tract (Chapters 4 and 12). Of course, no visual loss accompanies brainstem, cerebellar, or spinal cord lesions.

Although hemiparesis, hemisensory loss, and homonymous hemianopsia are found with lesions of either cerebral hemisphere, several neurologic deficits are specifically referable either to the dominant or nondominant hemisphere. In approximately 95 percent of people, the left hemisphere is dominant because it governs the use of fine motor movements and language. Unless the physician

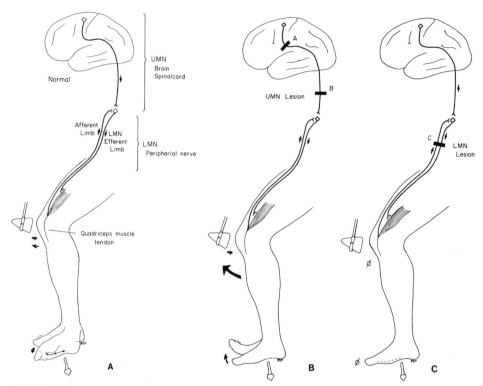

FIGURE 2–2. *A,* Normally, when the quadriceps tendon is percussed, a deep tendon reflex (DTR) is elicited. Also, when the sole of the foot is scratched in a certain manner to elicit a plantar reflex, the big toe bends downward (flexes). *B,* When brain or spinal cord lesions involve the corticospinal tract and cause UMN damage, the DTR is hyperactive and the plantar reflex is extensor, i.e., a Babinski sign is present. *C,* When peripheral nerve injury causes LMN damage, the DTR is hypoactive and the plantar reflex is absent.

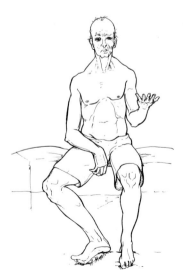

FIGURE 2–3. With severe right hemiparesis, the patient typically has weakness of the right lower face, the arm, and the leg. In the face, there is right-sided widening of the palpebral fissure and flattening of the nasolabial fold, but the forehead muscles appear normal. The right arm remains limply held; the elbow, wrist, and fingers are flexed. The right leg is externally rotated, and the hip and knee are also flexed.

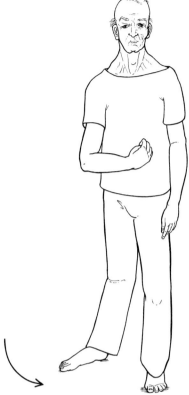

FIGURE 2–4. When the patient arises, the weakened arm retains its flexed position. The leg remains externally rotated, but the patient can walk by swinging the right leg in a circular path. This maneuver results in *circumduction* or a *hemiparetic* gait.

knows otherwise, he or she should assume that a patient is left hemisphere dominant, i.e., right-handed.

Disorders of the dominant hemisphere usually cause *aphasia*, which is impairment of verbal and written language (Chapter 8). Because language centers are adjacent to the motor cortex and descending corticospinal tract (see Fig. 8-1), lesions in the dominant hemisphere typically cause a combination of aphasia and right hemiparesis.

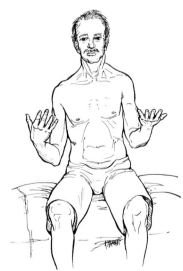

FIGURE 2–5. Mild hemiparesis may not be obvious. To exaggerate a subtle hemiparesis, the examiner should ask the patient to close his eyes and extend both arms with his palms held upright, as though he were holding a water glass on his outstretched hand. After 1 minute, the weakened arm will drift downward and the palm will turn inward (pronate). The imaginary water glass would spill inward, falling off the right palm. This arm's drift and pronation are a *forme fruste* of the posture that is seen with more severe paresis (Fig. 2-3).

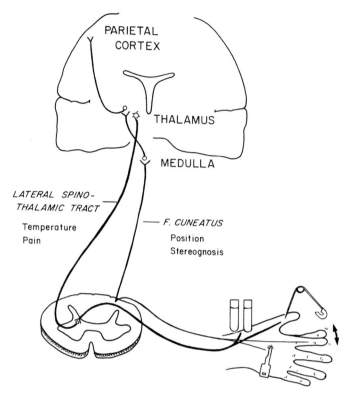

PARIETAL
CORTEX

THALAMUS

MEDULLA

LATERAL SPINO-
THALAMIC TRACT

Temperature
Pain

— *F. CUNEATUS*

Position
Stereognosis

FIGURE 2–6. Pain perception (tested by pinprick) and temperature sensation (tested by warm and cold test tubes) are carried to the spinal cord where, after a synapse, these sensations cross and ascend in the *contralateral* lateral spinothalamic tract. For practical purposes, they terminate in the thalamus. Position sense (tested by movement of the distal finger joint) and stereognosis (tested by tactile identification of common objects) are carried in the *ipsilateral* fasciculus cuneatus and f. gracilis, which together constitute the *posterior columns* (Fig. 2-14). These tracts cross and terminate in the cortex of the contralateral parietal lobe.

Disorders of the nondominant hemisphere usually cause more subtle and transient deficits. When the nondominant parietal lobe is injured, patients might have *hemi-inattention,* a constellation of psychologic abnormalities in which patients neglect left-sided visual perceptions, touch stimulation, and hemiparesis (Chapter 8). They may not even acknowledge their (left) hemiparesis, a condition known as *anosognosia.* These patients, who are said to have *constructional apraxia,* characteristically cannot copy simple forms (Fig. 2-8) or arrange matchsticks into certain patterns.

All signs discussed so far are referable to one cerebral hemisphere or the other. Bilateral cerebral hemisphere damage is suggested by *pseudobulbar palsy.* In this condition, best known for its psychiatric features, emotional lability and other mental aberrations are accompanied by dysarthria (speech impairment)

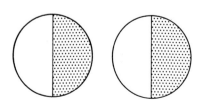

FIGURE 2–7. In homonymous hemianopsia, the same half of the visual field is lost in each eye. In this case, a right homonymous hemianopsia is attributable to damage of the left cerebral hemisphere.

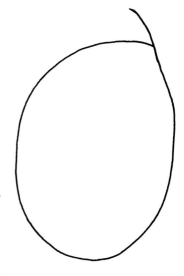

FIGURE 2-8. Constructional apraxia. The patient who drew these figures was a 68-year-old woman who had just developed a right parietal lobe infarction. On request, she was able to complete a circle (top figure). However, she could not draw a square on request (second highest figure) or even copy one (third highest figure). She spontaneously tried to draw a circle and attempted to retrace it (bottom figure). Note the characteristic rotation of the forms, the perseveration of certain lines, and the incompleteness of the second and lowest figures. Also note that the figures tend to move to the right-hand side of the page, suggesting that she is ignoring or "neglecting" the left-hand side of the page.

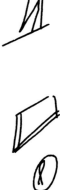

and reflex abnormalities. Pseudobulbar palsy must be distinguished from *bulbar palsy*, which does not result from cerebral damage (Chapter 4).

Dementia also indicates that both cerebral hemispheres are damaged. It is usually caused by Alzheimer's disease, multiple infarctions, alcohol-related damage, or by other *diffuse* structural or metabolic injury (Chapter 7). Since the CNS damage is usually extensive, dementia is associated with bilateral hyperactive DTRs, Babinski signs, and frontal lobe release reflexes, although not necessarily with hemiparesis or other lateralized findings. Whenever possible, a diagnosis of dementia or "organic mental syndrome" should be buttressed by a description of physical abnormalities.

The four conditions most likely to cause *discrete* unilateral or bilateral cerebral lesions are cerebral infarctions and other cerebrovascular accidents ("strokes"), primary or metastatic brain tumors, trauma, and multiple sclerosis. (A broader listing is offered in Table 2-3, and detailed discussions of strokes, tumors, and multiple sclerosis are presented in Section 2.)

TABLE 2–3. MOST COMMONLY OCCURRING CONDITIONS THAT DAMAGE THE CNS

Genetic
  Down's syndrome
  Wilson's disease
  Huntington's chorea
Congenital ("cerebral palsy," mental retardation, or both) Cerebral anoxia, kernicterus (jaundice), prematurity
Toxic
  Hepatic or renal failure
  Medications
  Illicit drugs
  Alcohol (and malnutrition)
Infectious
  Bacterial: Abscess* or meningitis
  Viral: Encephalitis or meningitis
  Acquired immune deficiency syndrome (AIDS)
Inflammatory*
  Multiple sclerosis
  Systemic lupus erythematosus (SLE)
Traumatic*
Neoplastic (tumors)*
  Primary: Glioblastoma, astrocytoma, meningioma
  Metastatic: Lung, breast
Vascular ("strokes")
  Infarction*
  Embolus*
  Hemorrhage*
  Anoxia from cardiopulmonary arrest
Degenerative (etiology unknown)
  Alzheimer's disease
  Creutzfeldt-Jakob disease
  Amyotrophic lateral sclerosis (ALS)

* Discrete cerebral damage.

SIGNS OF BASAL GANGLIA LESIONS

Since the corticospinal tract crosses in the pyramids, it is often called the *pyramidal* tract. The involuntary motor system that originates in the basal ganglia, in contrast, is called the *extrapyramidal* tract or extrapyramidal system. The extrapyramidal tract modulates motor tone and involuntary activity. Its major components are the caudate nucleus, the globus pallidus, the putamen, the substantia nigra, and the subthalamic nucleus (corpus of Luysii).

Basal ganglia injury often causes the dramatic, involuntary movement disorders discussed in detail in Chapter 18. They are described briefly below.

- *Parkinsonism* is the combination of resting tremor, rigidity, and bradykinesia (slowness of movement). Minor features include festinating gait (Table 2-4) and micrographia. Parkinsonism is associated with damage to the substantia nigra from degeneration (Parkinson's disease), antipsychotic medications, or toxins.

- *Athetosis* is the slow, continuous, writhing movement of the fingers, hands, face, and throat. It is usually caused by kernicterus or other perinatal brain injury.

- *Chorea* is intermittent jerking of limbs and trunk. The most important variety, *Huntington's* disease, the infamous hereditary condition, is associated with caudate nucleus atrophy.

TABLE 2–4. GAIT ABNORMALITIES

Gait	Associated Illness	Figure
Apraxia	Normal pressure hydrocephalus	7–7
Astasia-Abasia	Hysteria	3–2
Ataxia	Cerebellar damage	2–13
Festinating (marche à petits pas)	Parkinson's disease	18–9
Hemiparetic (circumduction)	Cerebrovascular accidents	2–4
(spastic hemiparesis)		13–2

• *Hemiballismus* is the intermittent flinging of the arm and leg on one side of the body. It is associated with small infarctions of the contralateral subthalamic nucleus.

Overall, when damage is restricted to the extrapyramidal tract, as in many cases of hemiballismus and athetosis, patients have no paresis, DTR abnormalities, or Babinski signs—the signs of corticospinal (pyramidal) tract damage. More important, in these cases patients have no intellectual abnormality.

On the other hand, several illnesses in which there is injury to the cerebral cortex as well as to the basal ganglia are characterized by a notorious association of mental abnormalities with involuntary movement disorders. The most noteworthy are Huntington's disease, Wilson's disease, and many cases of choreoathetotic cerebral palsy (Table 7-6).

Several features common to the movement disorders should be appreciated. Involuntary movements disappear during sleep. They are exacerbated by anxiety, fatigue, and stimulants. Finally, they may be suppressed for short periods of time by voluntary action. Unfortunately, these characteristics occasionally prompt physicians to diagnose patients with movement disorders as having a psychogenic disorder (Chapter 3).

Unlike illnesses that affect the cerebral hemispheres, basal ganglia diseases are slowly progressive and cause bilateral damage. They usually result from biochemical abnormalities. In contrast, discrete structural lesions, such as infarctions, tumors, or multiple sclerosis lesions ("plaques"), rarely injure the basal ganglia.

When there is unilateral basal ganglia damage, the signs are found contralateral to the lesion. One example ishemiballismus, which results from infarction of the contralateral subthalamic nucleus. Another is unilateral parkinsonism ("hemiparkinsonism") from degeneration of the contralateral substantia nigra.

SIGNS OF BRAINSTEM LESIONS

The brainstem contains the nuclei of the cranial nerves, the "long tracts" between the cerebral hemispheres and the extremities, and also several systems contained entirely within the brainstem itself (Fig. 2-9). Massive brainstem injuries, such as those resulting from extensive infarctions or barbiturate overdoses, cause coma. The commonly encountered small brainstem injuries, however, usually do not cause intellectual or personality impairment because mentation is an exclusive role of the cerebral cortex or at least the cerebral

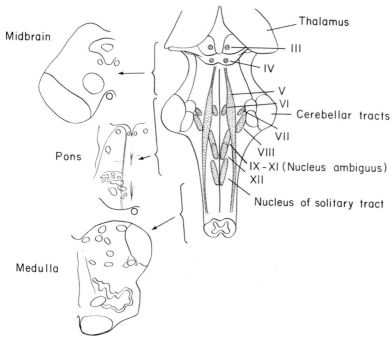

FIGURE 2–9. An overview of the brainstem (*right*) and the brainstem in cross-section (*left*). The midbrain contains the nuclei of cranial nerves III and IV. The pons contains nuclei V through VIII. The medulla contains nuclei IX through XII. The brainstem also contains important tracts that pass from the cerebellum and cerebral hemispheres to the brainstem and spinal cord. In addition, many other tracts, such as the medial longitudinal fasciculus, some cerebellar tracts, and the reticular activating system, are contained and act solely within the brainstem.

hemispheres. Similarly, as is explained later, diseases affecting the basal ganglia, cerebellum, or spinal cord are not associated with dementia unless the cerebral cortex is also affected.

Although brainstem injuries can cause *diplopia* (double vision) because of cranial nerve impairment, visual acuity in each eye remains normal. This is because the visual pathways, which pass from the chiasm to the cerebral hemispheres, do not travel within the brainstem (see Fig. 4-1).

Several syndromes are important because each illustrates critical anatomic relationships, such as the location of the different cranial nerve nuclei or the course of the corticospinal tract. Although each syndrome has an eponym, for practical purposes it is only necessary to identify each as the result of a lesion in the brainstem or, possibly, in a particular division of the brainstem— midbrain, pons, or medulla. Virtually all cases are caused by infarctions in branches of the basilar or vertebral arteries.

In the midbrain, where the oculomotor (third cranial) nerve passes through the descending corticospinal tract, both pathways can be damaged by a single small infarction. Patients with oculomotor nerve paralysis and contralateral hemiparesis typically have a midbrain lesion ipsilateral to the paretic eye (Fig. 4-8).

Likewise, patients with abducens (sixth cranial) nerve paralysis and contralateral hemiparesis typically have a pons lesion that is also ipsilateral to the paretic eye (Fig. 4-10).

Lateral medullary infarctions create a classic but complex picture. Patients

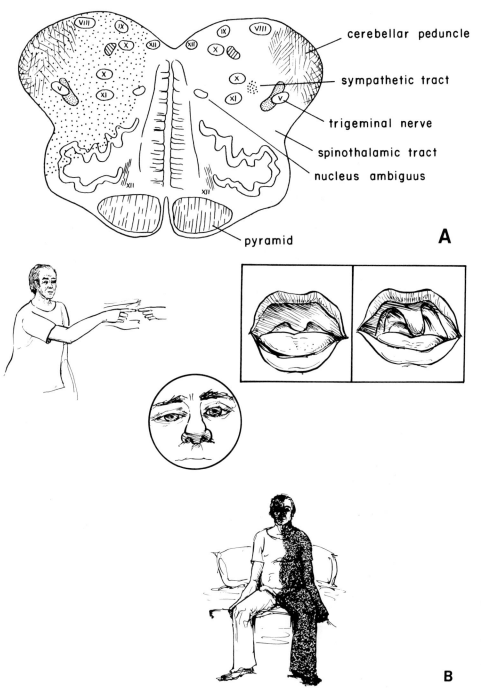

cerebellar peduncle

sympathetic tract

trigeminal nerve

spinothalamic tract

nucleus ambiguus

pyramid

A

B

FIGURE 2–10. *A*, Whenever the posterior inferior cerebellar artery (PICA) is occluded, the lateral portion of the medulla suffers infarction. This damages important structures: the cerebellar peduncle, the nucleus of the trigeminal nerve, the spinothalamic tract, the nucleus ambiguus (motor nuclei of cranial nerves IX–XI), and poorly delineated sympathetic fibers. Structures that escape damage are the corticospinal tract, the hypoglossal nerve, and the medial longitudinal fasciculus. The stippled area represents the region that would be infarcted when the right PICA or its parent artery, the vertebral artery, is occluded. *B*, This patient, who suffered an infarction of the right lateral medulla, has a right-sided Wallenberg syndrome. He has a right-sided Horner's syndrome (ptosis and miosis) because of damage to the sympathetic fibers and has right-sided ataxia because of damage to the ipsilateral cerebellar tracts. He has an alternating hypalgesia: diminished pain sensation on the *right* side of his face, accompanied by loss of pain sensation on the *left* trunk and extremities. Finally, he has hoarseness and paresis of the right soft palate because of damage to the right nucleus ambiguus: on voluntary phonation or in response to the gag reflex, the palate deviates upward toward his left because the right side of the palate is weak.

have paralysis of the ipsilateral palate because of damage to cranial nerves IX through XII; ipsilateral facial hypalgesia because of damage to cranial nerve V with contralateral anesthesia of the body (*alternating hypalgesia*) because of ascending spinothalamic tract damage; and ipsilateral ataxia because of ipsilateral cerebellar dysfunction. Fortunately, it is not necessary to recall all the features of this syndrome: good physicians only need to realize that those cranial nerve palsies and the alternating hypalgesia are characteristic of lower brainstem lesions (Fig. 2-10 A and B).

Although these particular brainstem syndromes are distinctive, the most frequently observed sign of brainstem dysfunction is *nystagmus* (repetitive, jerk-like eye movements). Resulting from any injury of the brainstem's large vestibular nuclei, nystagmus is usually a manifestation of one of the following disorders: multiple sclerosis; intoxications with alcohol, phenytoin (Dilantin), or barbiturates; Wernicke-Korsakoff syndrome; ischemia of the vertebrobasilar artery system; or merely viral labyrinthitis. It may also be associated with *internuclear ophthalmoplegia*, a disorder of ocular motility in which the brainstem's medial longitudinal fasciculus (MLF) is damaged by multiple sclerosis or infarction (Chapters 4 and 15).

SIGNS OF CEREBELLAR LESIONS

The cerebellum is composed of two hemispheres and a central portion, the *vermis*. Essentially, each hemisphere controls motor coordination of the ipsilateral limbs, and the vermis controls coordination of "midline structures," which are the head, neck, and trunk.

The control of coordination of the limbs on the *same side of the body* gives the cerebellum a unique quality captured by the aphorism, "Everything in the brain, except for the cerebellum, is backward." Another unique feature of the cerebellum is that, when one hemisphere is damaged, the other will eventually be able to perform almost all the functions for both. Thus, although loss of one cerebellar hemisphere will cause incapacitating dysfunction of the ipsilateral limbs, most patients regain function of the affected limbs within 1 year. Also, although acute cerebellar lesions cause impaired ipsilateral coordination, they do not cause paresis or significant reflex abnormality.

Since the cerebellum is isolated from the cerebral hemispheres, even its total destruction does not cause intellectual abnormalities. A good example of the lack of cognitive function in the cerebellum is the normal cognitive capacity of children who have undergone resection of a cerebellar hemisphere for treatment of trauma or a cerebellar astrocytoma (Chapter 19).

The primary sign of a cerebellar lesion is *intention tremor*. This characteristic tremor is elicited during the finger-nose test (Fig. 2-11) and heel-shin test (Fig. 2-12). It is present when the patient moves willfully and is absent when the patient rests. In contrast, parkinsonism causes a *resting tremor* that is typically present when the patient is sitting quietly at rest and reduced when the patient makes willful intentional movements (Chapter 18).

Another sign of a cerebellar lesion is impairment of the ability to perform rapid alternating movements, *dysdiadochokinesia*. When asked to slap the palm and then the back of the hand rapidly and alternately on his or her own knee, for example, a patient with dysdiadochokinesia will have uneven force, irregular rhythm, and breakdown of the alternating pattern.

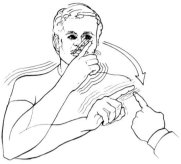

FIGURE 2–11. This young man, who has a multiple sclerosis plaque (lesion) in the right cerebellar hemisphere, has an *intention tremor*. During repetitive *finger-nose* movements, as his finger approaches his own nose and then the examiner's finger, it has a coarse and irregular path.

Damage of either the entire cerebellum or the vermis alone causes incoordination of the trunk, i.e., *truncal ataxia*. It forces the patient to place his or her feet widely apart when standing to produce a lurching, unsteady, and wide-based pattern of walking known as *ataxic gait* (Table 2-4 and Fig. 2-13). This gait abnormality is dramatically apparent in the staggering and reeling of people who are drunk.

With extensive cerebellar damage, voice production is beset by poor modulation, irregular cadence, inability to separate adjacent sounds, and prolonged pauses between syllables. Speaking as though reading a poem, patients with *scanning speech* can be distinguished by trained personnel from those with dysarthria found in bulbar and pseudobulbar palsy and other CNS conditions. More important, all these forms of dysarthria must be distinguished from aphasia (Chapter 8). Lastly, with cerebellar disease, DTRs have been described as being hypotonic or pendular; however, this is a subtle, rarely expected finding.

The disorders that are also responsible for most cerebral lesions—infarctions, multiple sclerosis, trauma, and tumors—cause almost all discrete cerebellar lesions. Their different clinical settings and associated signs make distinction among them relatively easy.

Generalized cerebellar dysfunction, in contrast, results more frequently from excessive intake of alcohol or certain medications, such as phenytoin (Dilantin), than from any discrete lesion. The most important situation is the Wernicke-

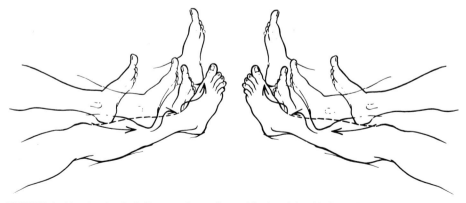

FIGURE 2–12. In the *heel-shin test*, the patient with the right-sided cerebellar lesion in Figure 2-11 displays limb *ataxia* or *tremor on intention* as his right heel wobbles when he moves it along the crest of his left shin.

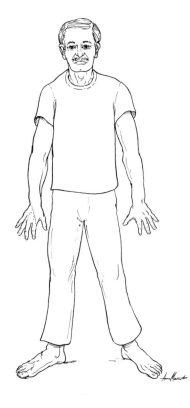

FIGURE 2–13. This man is a chronic alcoholic who suffers from diffuse cerebellar degeneration. His stance and his gait are broad-based and unsteady, i.e., he has an *ataxic gait*. He stands with his feet pointed outward to widen and thus steady his stance.

Korsakoff syndrome, in which excessive alcohol intake and poor nutrition lead to ataxia, nystagmus, peripheral neuropathy, and mental impairment characterized by memory loss. Any patient even suspected of having Wernicke-Korsakoff syndrome should immediately receive thiamine 50 mg IV to prevent serious brain injury.

SIGNS OF SPINAL CORD LESIONS

At the spinal cord's center is an H-shaped, gray matter structure composed largely of neurons that transmit nerve impulses in a horizontal plane. Surrounding it is white matter, composed of myelinated tracts conveying information in a vertical direction (Fig. 2-14). Curiously, this arrangement, gray matter on the inside with white outside, is the opposite of that found in the cerebral hemispheres.

The most important pathway of the white matter of the spinal cord is the descending voluntary motor tract, called the *lateral corticospinal tract*. Another important pathway is the ascending sensory tract system that includes the *posterior columns*, which carry position and vibration sensation; the *lateral spinothalamic tracts*, which carry temperature and pain; and the *anterior spinothalamic tracts*, which carry light touch. The white matter also contains the *spinocerebellar tract*, an ascending tract that conveys information required for coordination to the cerebellum.

A spinal cord lesion thus will interrupt descending motor and ascending sensory tracts. With a cervical spinal cord injury, for example, all motor function

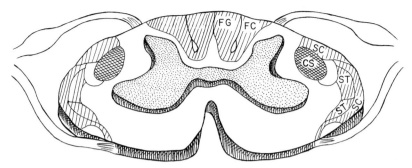

FIGURE 2–14. In this drawing of the spinal cord, the centrally located gray matter is stippled. The surrounding white matter contains myelin-coated tracts that ascend and descend within the spinal cord. Clinically important ascending tracts are the spinocerebellar tracts (SC), the lateral spinothalamic tract (ST), and the posterior columns [fasciculus cuneatus (FC) and fasciculus gracilis (FG)]. The most important descending tract is the lateral corticospinal tract (CS).

and sensation may be lost below the neck. The arms and legs, of course, will be paralyzed (*quadriparesis*). After 1 to 2 weeks, spasticity, hyperactive DTRs, and Babinski signs will develop. Also, there will be interruption of limb and trunk sensations, including those of bladder fullness and genital stimulation. With a midthoracic spinal cord injury, similarly, there will be leg paralysis (*paraparesis*), reflex changes, and sensory loss of the legs and trunk below the nipples (Fig. 2-15). With most spinal cord injuries there is sexual dysfunction (Chapter 16).

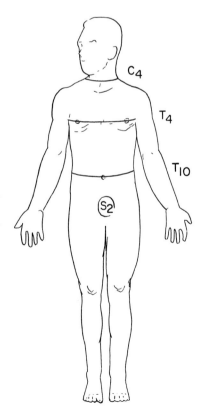

FIGURE 2–15. In a patient with a spinal cord injury, the "level" of hypalgesia will indicate the site of the damage: C–4 injuries cause hypalgesia below the neck; T–4, hypalgesia below the nipples; T–10, hypalgesia below the umbilicus.

A classic although rare disturbance, the *Brown-Séquard syndrome*, occurs when an injury transects the lateral half of the spinal cord (Fig. 2-16). In this condition, unilateral corticospinal tract damage causes paralysis of the ipsilateral limb(s), and lateral spinothalamic tract damage causes pain loss (*hypalgesia*) in the contralateral limb(s).

The position of the pain-carrying lateral spinothalamic tract offers an opportunity to alleviate unilateral pain. With a relatively simple neurosurgical procedure, *cordotomy*, surgeons produce considerable analgesia by selectively severing the lateral spinothalamic tract contralateral to the painful side.

With any discrete spinal cord lesion, of course, cerebral function is preserved. Patients with even a complete transection of the cervical spinal cord, although quadriplegic, retain intellectual, visual, and verbal facilities. Numerous veterans, for example, are paraplegic or quadriplegic from war wounds of their spinal cord, but nevertheless, their cognitive capacity is normal. It may appear to be impaired when various, strong psychologic processes predominate.

Most civilian spinal cord injuries result from automobile accidents, sports-related injuries, and other nonpenetrating injuries. In these cases, the spinal cord is usually crushed by dislocation of the cervical vertebrae.

Multiple sclerosis and metastatic cancer are the two illnesses in which the spinal cord is affected most often. Multiple sclerosis typically causes spinal cord damage alone or in combination with cerebellar, optic nerve, or brainstem damage (Chapter 15). Lung or breast tumors, which spread to the vertebral bodies, often compress the spinal cord.

With several illnesses, only specific tracts of the spinal cord may be affected (Fig. 2-17). In addition, in tabes dorsalis (syphilis) and combined-system disease (B_{12} deficiency), certain spinal cord tract damage is associated with cerebral injury. A dementia, which is at least partly reversible, is found in both conditions.

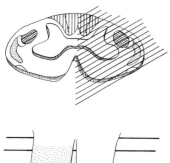

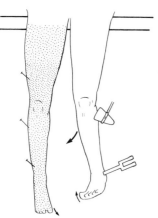

FIGURE 2–16. Hemitransection of the spinal cord (Brown-Séquard syndrome). In this case, the left side of the thoracic spinal cord has been transected, as by a knife wound. Injury to the left lateral corticospinal tract results in the combination of left-sided leg paresis, hyperactive DTRs, and a Babinski sign; injury to the left posterior column results in left leg vibration and position sense impairment; and, most striking, injury to the left spinothalamic tract causes loss of temperature and pain (pinprick) sensation in the right leg. The loss of pain sensation contralateral to the paresis is the hallmark of the Brown-Séquard syndrome.

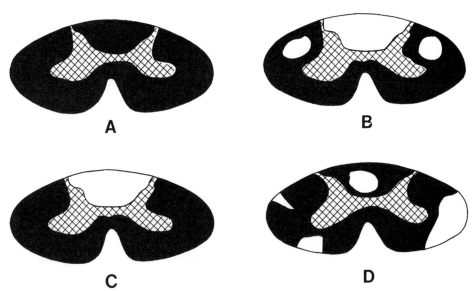

FIGURE 2–17. *A,* A standard spinal cord histologic preparation stains normal myelin ("white matter") black and leaves the central H-shaped column gray. *B,* In combined-system disease (vitamin B_{12} deficiency), damage to the posterior column and corticospinal tracts causes their demyelination and loss of stain. *C,* In tabes dorsalis (syphilis), damage to the posterior column causes loss of stain in that region. *D,* Multiple sclerosis, however, leads to scattered, irregular demyelination plaques.

Patients with multiple sclerosis have variable, irregular patches of spinal cord involvement and, unless the disease is advanced, usually no mental impairment. Also, in many cases of acquired immune deficiency syndrome (AIDS), spinal cord infection will cause damage (myelopathy). In these cases, patients usually also have cerebral infection that leads to dementia (Chapter 7).

SUMMARY

Physical abnormalities, sometimes in combination with intellectual ones, indicate the presence, location, and etiology of CNS injury. Signs that indicate that paresis is from CNS injury are hyperactive DTRs, spasticity, and Babinski signs. The signs of cerebral injury depend on whether the dominant hemisphere, nondominant hemisphere, or both hemispheres are injured.

Disorders that simultaneously affect the basal ganglia, as well as the cerebral hemispheres, and thus cause dementia are Huntington's disease and Wilson's disease. Those that simultaneously affect the spinal cord and cerebral hemispheres and cause dementia, are tabes dorsalis (syphilis), combined-system disease (B_{12} deficiency), and AIDS.

3

Psychogenic Neurologic Deficits

Classic studies of hysteria, conversion reactions, and related conditions included patients who had only rudimentary physical examinations and minimal, if any, laboratory testing. Studies that re-evaluated the same patients after many years found that as many as 20 percent of them eventually had specific neurologic diseases, such as movement disorders, multiple sclerosis, or seizures, that probably had been responsible for the symptoms. In addition, some patients had been suffering from systemic illnesses, such as anemia or congestive heart failure, that could have at least contributed to the symptoms. Another interesting aspect of those studies is that many conditions initially thought to be psychiatric are now considered to be neurologic, such as Tourette's syndrome, dystonia, migraine headache, and trigeminal neuralgia.

The misdiagnosis of psychogenic disorders is less frequent today because of more thorough clinical evaluations by physicians, a general tendency to rely on computed tomography (CT) and magnetic resonance imaging (MRI), and the development of specific psychiatric diagnostic criteria. On the other hand, the appropriate diagnosis may be more difficult because psychogenic deficits tend to be more subtle than in the past. For example, patients now rarely flail, suddenly become totally mute, or posture in the manner of the classic "grand hysterics." Patients are more realistic when they mimic neurologic illnesses possibly because they are exposed to accurate portrayals in the popular media. In many cases, patients embellish a physical impairment, creating a mixture of neurologic and psychogenic deficits. Typical problems are prolonged disability following apparently trivial injuries, such as minor automobile accidents, head trauma, and low back injuries, with impairments that require exhaustive, expensive evaluation for which no adequate physical explanation is found.

A psychiatrist can help clarify potentially psychogenic deficits by exploring the patient's perceptions, administering hypnosis, or conducting an amobarbital interview. Within the evaluation, the psychiatrist should delineate positive criteria for common psychiatric conditions associated with psychogenic neurologic deficits (Table 3-1): *conversion disorder, factitious disorder with physical symptoms,* and *malingering.* However, these conditions do not include *hypochondriasis* or *somatization disorder,* which are not associated with observable neurologic deficits. Their focus or preoccupation is on fear of serious illness—not on symptoms themselves. The multiplicity of complaints, in addition to the lack of physical signs, immediately suggests that the primary problem is psychogenic, rather than neurologic.

Although many patients may have a mixture of neurologic and psychogenic deficits, for a psychiatrist clearly to state a diagnosis of a psychiatric condition

TABLE 3–1. COMMONLY CITED CONDITIONS RESULTING IN PSYCHOGENIC NEUROLOGIC DEFICITS

Condition (DSM-III-R Code[1])	Consciousness Regarding Production of Deficit	Goal in Manifesting Deficit	Miscellaneous Features
Conversion disorder[2] (300.11)	Not conscious	Primary gain[3] Secondary gain[4]	*La belle indifference,* hysteric personality and symbolization have been poorly correlated with conversions
Factitious disorder with physical symptoms (301.51)	Conscious	To appear sick and receive medical care	Often has compulsive aspects. Patients typically fabricate medical problems, alter laboratory data, or induce illness.
Malingering (V65.20)	Conscious	Deception for specific incentive[5]	

[1] *Diagnostic and Statistical Manual of Mental Disorders, Third Edition, Revised.*
[2] A variety of somatiform disorder. Does not include only pain or sexual dysfunction.
[3] Keeping internal conflict unconscious.
[4] Being relieved of responsibility or given support.
[5] Avoid court date, military service, for example.

is very helpful. The primary physicians can then more confidently avoid or postpone invasive diagnostic procedures, surgery, and medications, especially ones that are habituating or otherwise dangerous. Sometimes, as long as serious, progressive physical illness has been excluded, physicians can consider some symptoms to be chronic illnesses. For example, low back injury or surgical incision pain can be treated as a "pain syndrome" with empiric combinations of antidepressant medications, analgesics, and psychotherapy, without expecting any of these modalities to cure the pain or determine its exact cause (Chapter 14).

Neurologists may have the cumbersome burden of attempting to show that a neurologic disease is *not* present. Even though the course of the illness is often the best test, neurologists may request many sophisticated procedures to exclude certain conditions. Their uncertainty about a diagnosis and their awareness of the current medicolegal climate often compel them to request many extensive, costly evaluations early in the course of apparently benign or psychogenic conditions. Once convinced of a deficit's psychogenic nature, neurologists can only offer patients reassurances and suggestions that the deficits will not be permanent. They often offer patients "face saving" exits by prescribing placebos, ineffective medications, or nonspecific treatment, such as physical therapy. Although these maneuvers are pragmatic, they are short term and possibly inappropriate. Another role of the psychiatrist would be to assist the neurologist managing the psychiatric aspects of the case.

PSYCHOGENIC SIGNS

Neurologists' usual initial guideline in determining whether a deficit is psychogenic is if it appears to violate the *Laws of Neuroanatomy*. For example, when temperature sensation is preserved while there is loss of pain perception, the deficit is considered to be nonanatomic and therefore psychogenic. Likewise, tunnel or tubular vision is considered to be a classic psychogenic disturbance (Fig. 12-8). Another general guideline is when a deficit is not constant. For example, a man with psychogenic paralysis might either walk when unaware of being observed, or he might reflexively employ his affected limbs to reposition himself. Likewise, hypnosis or an amobarbital interview might also transiently reverse psychogenic deficits.

Although the neurologist should be cautious, several motor deficits are justifiably considered psychogenic. Psychogenic paresis is often detected by a "give-way" effort in which the patient has normal exertion for only a brief (several second) period before returning to an apparent paretic position. It is also sometimes demonstrable using the *face-hand test*, in which a patient with psychogenic paresis momentarily exerts sufficient strength to deflect a falling hand from hitting the face (Fig. 3-1). Interestingly, psychogenic hemiparesis develops more often in the left than the right limbs. This predominance has been suggested to be a "punishment" of the sinister (left) hand or an effort to preserve function, by sparing the right hand, during a period of disability. Notably, a potentially misleading finding in patients with psychogenic hemiparesis is that their deep tendon reflexes, probably because of anxiety, are briskly reactive and their plantar reflexes appear to be extensor—as would occur in a cerebral lesion.

Another indication of psychogenic paresis, although exceptions are common, is a right hemiparesis that is unaccompanied by aphasia or right homonymous hemianopsia. One important exception would be, of course, if the patient were left-handed, and another is if an infarction were small and in the internal capsule, deep cerebrum, or upper brainstem, i.e., a "pure motor stroke."

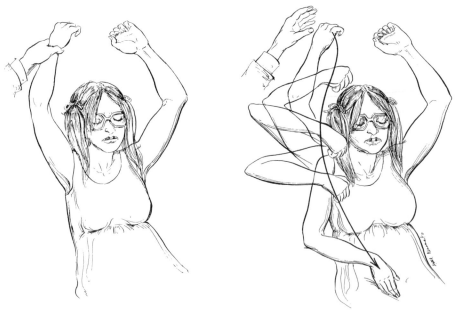

FIGURE 3–1. In the face-hand test, a young woman with psychogenic right hemiparesis inadvertently demonstrates her preserved strength by deflecting her falling "paretic" arm from striking her face as it is dropped by the examiner.

Psychogenic paresis is sometimes manifested by a characteristic gait disturbance, *astasia-abasia*, in which patients stagger, balance momentarily, and appear to be in great danger of falling. Instead, never seeming to fall, they grab hold of railings, furniture, and even the examiner (Fig. 3-2). This display of acrobatics is virtually diagnostic. Sometimes these patients appear to drag a weak leg, as though it were a totally lifeless object apart from their body: patients with hemiparesis swing their leg with a circular motion when walking (Fig. 2-4).

Several sensory abnormalities are also classic signs of a psychogenic deficit. Loss of sensation to pinprick that stops abruptly at the middle of the face and body, *splitting the midline*, is indicative of a psychogenic loss because the sensory nerve fibers of the skin normally spread across the midline (Fig. 3-3). Likewise, since vibrations naturally spread across bony structures, loss of vibration sensation over half of the forehead, jaw, sternum, or spine is psychogenic because this sensory loss is another example of splitting the midline.

As already mentioned, a classic psychogenic sensory loss is a discrepancy between pain and temperature sensations, which are normally carried together by the peripheral nerves and then the lateral spinothalamic tracts. (Discrepancy between pain and *position* sensations in the fingers, in contrast, is indicative of syringomyelia. In this condition the central fibers of the spinal cord, which carry pain sensation, are stretched by the expanding central canal.)

Intermittent blindness, tunnel vision, and inconsistent diplopia are also

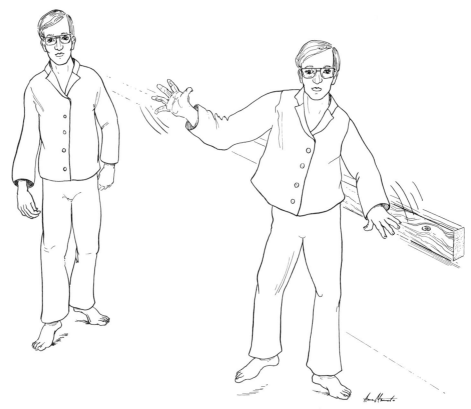

FIGURE 3–2. A young man with a psychogenic gait impairment demonstrates astasia-abasia by seeming to fall when walking, but catching himself by carefully balancing or grasping on to the railing. He actually displays good strength, balance and coordination through his series of acrobatics.

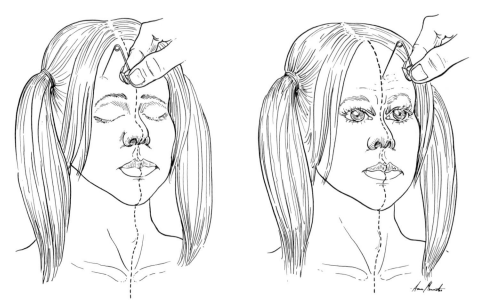

FIGURE 3–3.   A young woman with psychogenic left hemisensory loss appears not to feel a pinprick until the pin reaches the midline of her forehead, face, neck, or sternum, i.e., she splits the midline.

commonly cited psychogenic disturbances that are diagnosed because they violate the Laws of Neuroanatomy. (These visual disturbances are contrasted to neurologic visual disorders in Chapter 12.) Likewise, hearing loss in the ear ipsilateral to a hemiparesis is suggestive of a psychogenic etiology because auditory tract synapsing is so extensive in the CNS that some tracts are almost always preserved in CNS lesions (Fig. 4-15).

A distinct but common psychogenic disturbance is the *hyperventilation syndrome*. Patients, who might have underlying anxiety or panic attacks, develop light-headedness, paresthesias around their mouth and in their fingers and toes, and *carpopedal spasm* (Fig. 3-4). These symptoms, which might be confused with those of a partial complex seizure or a transient ischemic attack, are caused by a well-known physiologic mechanism. Overbreathing causes a fall in carbon dioxide tension, which leads to respiratory alkalosis. The associated rise in blood pH creates a relative hypocalcemia, which induces the tetany of muscles and the paresthesias. Although symptoms are reproducible by having a patient hyperventilate, this diagnostic maneuver may induce giddiness or even irra-

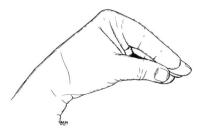

FIGURE 3–4.   Carpopedal spasm, which is the characteristic neurologic manifestation of hyperventilation, consists of flexion of the wrist and proximal thumb and finger joints. Also, although the thumb and fingers remain extended, they are drawn together and tend to overlap.

tionality. If so, the test may be aborted by having the patient continually rebreathe expired air from a paper bag cupped around the mouth.

PROBLEM CONDITIONS

Neurologists tend to misdiagnose several types of disturbances by considering disorders to be psychogenic when they are unique or bizarre, or when their severity is greater than expected. Such a conclusion may simply reflect an individual neurologist's lack of experience. Neurologists also misdiagnose disturbances as psychogenic when a patient has no accompanying objective physical abnormalities. This determination should likewise be accepted with some hesitancy because in many illnesses, such as multiple sclerosis, partial complex seizures, and small cerebrovascular accidents, objective signs are often transient, subtle, or easily overshadowed by psychic distress.

A common error is to fail to recognize cases of multiple sclerosis. The error occurs because, in the initial stages of multiple sclerosis, deficits may be evanescent, exclusively sensory, or so disparate as to appear to violate the Laws of Neuroanatomy. The correct diagnosis can now usually be made early and reliably with MRI scanning, visual evoked response testing, and cerebrospinal fluid analysis (Chapter 15). On the other hand, minor sensory or motor symptoms that are accompanied by variations in these highly sophisticated tests are likely to lead to some false-positive diagnoses of multiple sclerosis.

Another condition in which neurologists are prone to err is that of involuntary movement disorders. As noted previously (Chapter 2), these disorders in fact have stigmata of psychogenic illness. They can be bizarre, associated with mental abnormalities, and exacerbated by anxiety. Also, all movements will be reduced or even abolished during an amobarbital interview. Since laboratory tests are not practical or readily available, the diagnosis almost always rests on the neurologist's clinical evaluation. As a general rule, movement disorders should always first be considered neurologic (Chapter 18).

Seizures are often misdiagnosed in both directions. Many patients with psychogenic seizures actually have an underlying seizure disorder (epilepsy) upon which they elaborate (Chapter 10). In particular, many cases of "intractable" epilepsy are a mixture of psychogenic and neurologic seizures. In these individuals, either the psychogenic or epileptic seizures may be overshadowed by the other. Psychogenic seizures are usually only clonic and not accompanied by incontinence, tongue biting, or loss of body tone (Fig. 3-5). More telling, after a psychogenic seizure there is usually an immediate resumption of awareness and no retrograde amnesia. Unless monitoring is being done, an EEG cannot usually be obtained during any seizure episode, but one done after a psychogenic seizure would not show typical postictal electrical slowing or depression, and the characteristic postictal rise in the serum prolactin concentration would fail to occur.

Emotional and thought disorders that have been misdiagnosed in the past as being psychogenic have sometimes turned out to be the result of frontal lobe meningiomas and other brain tumors. The error has arisen because patients with these tumors often have had no overt intellectual or physical abnormalities. With the ready availability of the CT, MRI, and similar technology, physicians now rarely overlook any structural lesion.

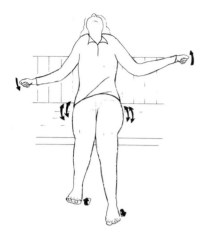

FIGURE 3–5. This young woman, who is screaming during an entire 30-second period, is having a psychogenic seizure. Its non-neurologic nature is revealed in several typical features. In addition to verbalizing throughout the period rather than only at its onset (as in an epileptic cry), she maintains her body tone which is required to keep her sitting upright, has alternating flailing limb movements rather than organized clonic jerks, and has subtle but suggestive pelvic thrusting. After such an episode, she would be fully alert, oriented, and able to recall events preceding and possibly during the episode, rather than being lethargic, dull, and amnestic.

REFERENCES

Baker JHE, Silver JR: Hysterical paraplegia. J Neurol Neurosurg Psychiatry 50:375, 1987

Caplan LR, Nadelson T: Multiple sclerosis and hysteria: Lessons learned from their association. JAMA 243:2418, 1980

Eisendrath SJ: Factitious illness: A clarification. Psychosomatics 25:110, 1984

Folks DG, Ford CV, Regan WM: Conversion symptoms in a general hospital. Psychosomatics 25:4:285, 1984

Ford CV, Folks DG: Conversion disorders: An overview. Psychosomatics 26:5:371, 1985

Galin D, Diamond R, Braff D: Lateralization of conversion symptoms: More frequent on the left. Am J Psychiatry 134:5:578, 1977

Gulick RA, Spinks IP, King DW: Pseudoseizures: Ictal phenomena. Neurology 32:24, 1982

Hurst LC: What was wrong with Anna O? J R Soc Med 75:129, 1982

King DW, Gallagher BB, Marvin AJ, et al: Pseudoseizures: Diagnostic evaluation. Neurology 32:18, 1982

Lazare A: Conversion symptoms. N Engl J Med 305:745, 1981

Mai FM, Nerskey H: Briquet's concept of hysteria: An historical perspective. Can J Psychiatry 26:57, 1981

Maloney MJ: Diagnosing hysterical conversion reactions in children. J Pediatr 97:1016, 1980

Reich P, Gottfried LA: Factitious disorders in a teaching hospital. Ann Intern Med 99:24, 1983

Roy A (ed): Hysteria. New York, John Wiley & Sons, 1982

Saint-Hilaire MH, Saint-Hilaire JM, Granger, L: Jumping Frenchmen of Maine. Neurology 36:1269, 1986

Weintraub MI: Hysterical Conversion Reactions. New York, SP Medical and Scientific Books, 1983

4

Cranial Nerve Impairments

The cranial nerves are numerous, and their functional neuroanatomy is complex. Individually, in pairs, or in groups, each might be impaired by various conditions. Moreover, even when a cranial nerve seems to be impaired, the problem might not be damage of the cranial nerve itself, but rather an underlying central nervous system (CNS) or psychogenic disturbance. Determining the presence and origin of an impairment of any particular cranial nerve depends upon knowing its function, interrelationships, and signs of damage.

This chapter reviews the the cranial nerves, discusses appropriate examinations, and describes deficits found in common physical and psychogenic disturbances. It concludes with an important detailed review of paresis of the lower cranial nerves, i.e., *bulbar palsy*, contrasted to the more commonly encountered condition, *pseudobulbar palsy*.

This chapter follows the customary practice of giving the Roman numeral designations to the 12 cranial nerves and presenting them in numerical order:

I	Olfactory	VII	Facial
II	Optic	VIII	Acoustic
III	Oculomotor	IX	Glossopharyngeal
IV	Trochlear	X	Vagus
V	Trigeminal	XI	Accessory
VI	Abducens	XII	Hypoglossal

An old mnemonic for this list is "On old Olympus's towering top, a Finn and German viewed some (spinal accessory) hops."

THE OLFACTORY NERVE (FIRST CRANIAL NERVE)

The function of the olfactory nerves is to transmit the sensation of smell to the brain. From sensory receptors within each nasal cavity, branches of the two olfactory nerves pass through the multiple holes of the cribriform plate of the skull to several areas of the brain. They terminate mostly in the frontal cortex, where olfactory sensory areas are located, and in the hypothalamus and amygdaloid complex, which are cornerstones of the limbic system. This input of olfactory sensation into the limbic system accounts for the influence of smell on psychosexual behavior.

When both olfactory nerves are totally impaired, patients have complete loss of smell, *anosmia*. To them, food is largely tasteless because aroma is lost.

To test the function of the olfactory nerve, the examiner asks the patient to smell substances through one nostril while the other is compressed. Testing must be done with such substances as tobacco and coffee, which are readily identifiable and not noxious. Irritative or volatile substances, such as ammonia and alcohol, are not suitable because they will stimulate the sensory endings of the trigeminal nerve, which are also within the nose, and elicit a reaction, thereby bypassing a (possibly damaged) olfactory nerve.

Anosmia is usually caused by trivial problems. It is found in many normal older people and in anyone with nasal congestion. Also, since the olfactory nerve can be sheared off as it passes through the cribriform plate, even minor head trauma can cause anosmia.

Unilateral anosmia, which is rare, may be the result of tumors adjacent to the olfactory nerve, such as olfactory groove meningiomas (Fig. 20-5). Anosmia caused by such tumors is associated with optic atrophy because the nearby optic nerve is also compressed. Most important, if these tumors involve the frontal lobe, personality changes, seizures, or hemiparesis typically accompany anosmia.

Anosmia may of course be a manifestation of a psychologic aberration. In such cases, patients are almost always unable to "smell" either irritative solutions, such as alcohol, or odorous substances, such as coffee. This complete loss would be possible only if the trigeminal as well as the olfactory nerve were impaired.

Olfactory hallucinations may be a manifestation of seizures that originate in the medial-inferior surface of the temporal lobe, the *uncus*. Such "uncinate seizures" are usually composed of discrete episodes, lasting several seconds, of ill-defined but often sweet smells associated with impaired consciousness and behavioral aberrations. Most important, they are usually the preliminary phase (*aura*) of partial complex seizures (Chapter 15).

Olfactory hallucinations, of course, can also be purely psychogenic. In contrast to those of uncinate seizures, psychogenic odors are almost always foul-smelling and continual.

THE OPTIC NERVE (SECOND CRANIAL NERVE)

The major function of the optic nerves is to transmit visual information from the eye to the brain. The optic *nerves*, which are heavily coated with CNS myelin, originate in the retina of each eye. Continuing toward the brain, they intersect at the optic chiasm, where their medial fibers cross, while their lateral fibers continue (Fig. 4-1). Thus, the optic *tracts* are formed from the temporal fibers of the ipsilateral eye and the nasal fibers of the contralateral eye. The optic tracts send a branch to the midbrain, then pass through the temporal and parietal lobes, and terminate in the occipital lobe cortex.

The complex system of optic nerves and tracts exemplifies an important and virtually unique feature of the optic nerves. The optic nerves and tracts are part of the CNS and subject to all illnesses, particularly multiple sclerosis (Chapter 15), that affect the brain and spinal cord. Therefore, visual impairments, more than other sign of any cranial injury, are most associated with mental impairments.

The optic nerves also regulate pupil size. Such pupillary adjustments are necessary both to focus the visual image on the retina (*accommodation reflex*) and also to permit the appropriate amount of light to fall on the retina (*light reflex*).

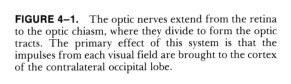

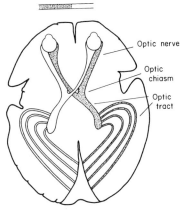

FIGURE 4–1. The optic nerves extend from the retina to the optic chiasm, where they divide to form the optic tracts. The primary effect of this system is that the impulses from each visual field are brought to the cortex of the contralateral occipital lobe.

Optic nerve

Optic chiasm

Optic tract

For these reflexes, the optic nerves form the afferent limb and carry information regarding an object's proximity and brightness. After synapsing in the midbrain, the oculomotor nerves (third cranial nerve) form the efferent limb and transmit impulses to the iris muscles of the pupils. Thus, the pupils constrict with either increased light or with a change in focus from a distant to a close object.

Routine testing of the optic nerve includes examination of (1) visual acuity (Fig. 12-2), (2) visual fields (Fig. 4-2), and (3) the ocular fundi (Fig. 4-3). However, the visual system is subject to numerous ocular, neurologic, iatrogenic, and psychogenic disturbances. Their complexity and importance have justified

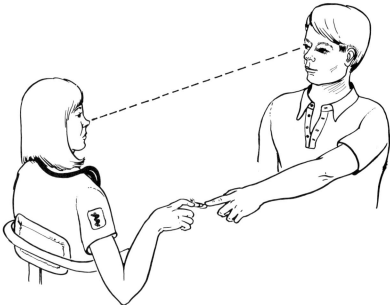

FIGURE 4–2. In testing visual fields by the confrontation method, this physician wiggles her index finger as the patient points to it without deviating his eyes from her nose. Each eye must be tested individually, and each of the four quadrants of each eye's field of vision must be tested. (Only in this way will bitemporal hemianopsias, which are associated with pituitary adenomas, be detected.) Young children and other patients unable to comply with this testing method may be examined in a more superficial but still meaningful manner by assessing their response to attention-catching objects brought into each field of vision from different directions. For example, a dollar bill, a toy, or a glass of water usually attracts notice. These objects' failure to catch the patient's attention when presented to one side suggests a hemianopsia.

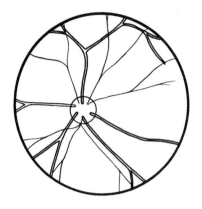

FIGURE 4–3. The normal optic fundus or disk is yellow, flat, and clearly demarcated from the surrounding red retina. The retinal veins, as everywhere else in the body, are larger than their corresponding arteries; however, the retinal veins can normally be seen to pulsate.

a separate discussion on visual disturbances relevant to a psychiatrist's practice (Chapter 12).

THE OCULOMOTOR, TROCHLEAR, AND ABDUCENS NERVES (THIRD, FOURTH, AND SIXTH CRANIAL NERVES)

The oculomotor, trochlear, and abducens nerves are considered as a group because they act together in a complementary manner to coordinate eye movement. The nerves and their heavily myelinated interconnecting brainstem circuit, the *medial longitudinal fasciculus (MLF)*, must be intact to permit depth perception and prevent diplopia (double vision). Unlike the optic nerve and the MLF, these cranial nerves are not part of the CNS.

The oculomotor nerves (third cranial nerves) originate in the midbrain. After passing through the red nucleus and corticospinal tract (Fig. 4-4), they leave the base of the brainstem and supply the pupil constrictor, the eyelid, and the adductor and elevator muscles of the eyeball (medial rectus, inferior oblique, inferior rectus, and superior rectus). Impairment of this nerve, which is a frequently occurring injury, leads to a common constellation of findings: diplopia when attempting to use the paretic muscle, pupillary dilation, ptosis, and outward deviation (abduction) of the eye downward and outward (Fig. 4-5).

Like the oculomotor nerves, the trochlear nerves (fourth cranial nerves)

MIDBRAIN

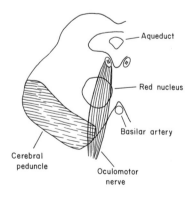

Aqueduct

Red nucleus

Basilar artery

Cerebral peduncle

Oculomotor nerve

FIGURE 4–4. The oculomotor nerve (third cranial nerve) arises as a pair of nerves from nuclei located in the dorsal portion of the midbrain. Each descends through the red nucleus, which carries contralateral cerebellar outflow fibers. Then they pass through the cerebral peduncle, which carries the corticospinal tract that will supply the contralateral trunk and limbs.

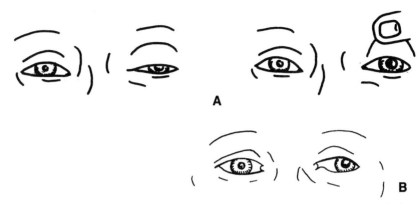

FIGURE 4–5. *A,* The patient with paresis of the *left oculomotor nerve* has ptosis and lateral deviation of the left eye, which has a dilated and unreactive pupil. *B,* In a milder case, close inspection reveals suble ptosis, lateral deviation of the eye, and dilation of the pupil. In both cases, patients have diplopia that increases when adducting the left eye, because gaze in that direction requires increased reliance on the paretic medial rectus muscle. Thus, these patients have diplopia on straight-ahead gaze that increases on rightward gaze (also see Fig. 12-13).

originate in the midbrain. They supply only the superior oblique muscle, which is responsible for depression of the eye when it is adducted (turned inward). However, since such complicated movements are difficult to assess and this nerve is rarely injured, only specialists are responsible for recognizing trochlear nerve injuries.

The abducens nerves (sixth cranial nerves), unlike the third and fourth cranial nerves, originate in the pons (Fig. 4-6). They pass through the brainstem near the facial nerve (seventh cranial nerve) and terminate entirely on the abductor (lateral rectus) muscle of the eyeball.

Abducens nerve impairment, which is relatively common, causes inturning (adduction) of the eye (Fig. 4-7), but no ptosis or pupillary changes. Diplopia also occurs on straight-ahead gaze and increases with greater reliance on the paretic lateral rectus muscle.

In summary, the lateral rectus muscle is innervated by the sixth cranial nerve, the superior oblique by the fourth, and all the rest by the third. A mnemonic captures this relationship: LR_6SO_4

In terms of ocular motility, the oculomotor nerve on one side is complementary to the abducens nerve on the other. Diplopia in one direction of gaze is explainable by a lesion in either the oculomotor nerve on one side or the abducens nerve on the other. For example, if a patient has diplopia when looking to the left, then either the left abducens nerve or the right oculomotor nerve may be paretic. Likewise, diplopia on right gaze suggests a paresis of either the right abducens nerve or left oculomotor nerve. Although elaborate diagnostic tests may be performed, the presence or absence of other signs of oculomotor nerve palsy (pupillary dilation and ptosis) usually indicates whether that nerve is responsible.

These ocular cranial nerves can be damaged in the midbrain or pons, in their course between the brainstem and eyeballs, or, as in myasthenia gravis, at their neuromuscular junctions (Fig. 6-1). When these nerves are damaged anywhere throughout their course, the cerebrum is rarely involved. Thus, in many common illnesses, such as myasthenia gravis, isolated nerve injuries, and the small brainstem strokes, patients typically do not have mental aberrations.

PONS

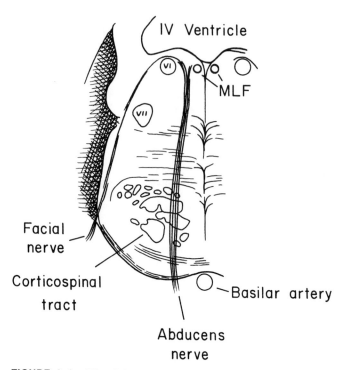

FIGURE 4–6. The abducens nerve (sixth cranial nerve) arises as a pair of nerves from nuclei located in the dorsal portion of the pons. At its origin, the abducens nerve is adjacent to the medial longitudinal fasciculus (MLF) (Chapter 15). As the nerve descends, it passes just medial to the facial nerve and its nucleus and then goes directly through the corticospinal tract.

However, one prominent exception is Wernicke's encephalopathy, in which memory impairments accompany damage to the oculomotor and abducens nerves and to the MLF. Another exception is *transtentorial herniation*, in which a cerebral mass lesion, such as a subdural hematoma, compresses the oculomotor nerve as it causes coma (Fig. 19-3).

Nevertheless, brainstem lesions are important though rare. They damage cranial nerves in combination with adjacent structures, such as the corticospinal tract, which carries motor function to the contralateral limbs, or the red nucleus, which carries cerebellar outflow to the contralateral limbs. These injuries lead to syndromes characterized by ocular motility paresis combined with contralateral hemiparesis or ataxia. Almost all these cases are the result of brainstem infarctions from an occlusion of a small branch of the basilar artery (Chapter 11). Despite the multiple, complex neurologic deficits, mental status is usually preserved.

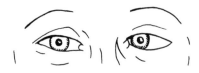

FIGURE 4–7. The patient with paresis of the *left abducens nerve* has medial deviation of the left eye. There will be diplopia on looking ahead and toward the left, but not when looking to the right (Fig. 12-14).

For example, a patient with a right-sided midbrain lesion might have right oculomotor nerve palsy, which would cause right ptosis and diplopia, and left hemiparesis (Fig. 4-8). Likewise, with a slightly different right-sided midbrain lesion, a patient might have right oculomotor nerve palsy and left tremor (Fig. 4-9). With a right-sided pontine lesion, a patient may have right abducens nerve paresis, causing diplopia, and left hemiparesis (Fig. 4-10). In each of these cases of brainstem injury, the mental status is normal.

The medial longitudinal fasciculus (MLF) links the nuclei of the oculomotor and abducens nerves in the brainstem (Figs. 4-10 and 15-3). Its interruption produces the *MLF syndrome*. This important condition causes a characteristic impairment of ocular motility closely associated with multiple sclerosis. This syndrome, also called *internuclear ophthalmoplegia*, consists of nystagmus of the abducting eye and failure of the adducting eye to cross the midline (Fig. 15-4).

The most common cause of an isolated oculomotor or abducens nerve palsy is diabetic infarction. Another frequently occurring cause is Wernicke's encephalopathy. Also, the oculomotor nerve is occasionally compressed by an aneurysm of the posterior communicating artery. The oculomotor nerve palsy, in such cases, is usually one component of a subarachnoid hemorrhage. In

MIDBRAIN

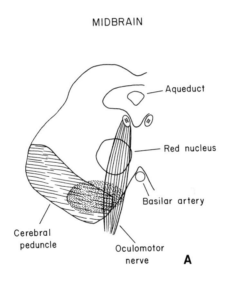

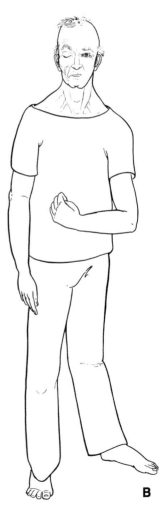

FIGURE 4–8. The syndrome of oculomotor nerve palsy and contralateral hemiparesis. *A*, A small right midbrain infarction may damage the oculomotor nerve that supplies the *ipsilateral eye* and the adjacent cerebral peduncle, which contains the corticospinal tract. That tract, which subsequently crosses in the medulla, supplies the *contralateral arm and leg*. *B*, This patient has right-sided ptosis from a right oculomotor nerve palsy, and left hemiparesis from right corticospinal tract injury.

MIDBRAIN

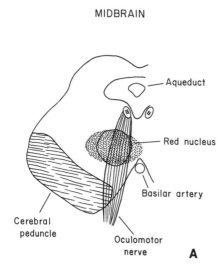

Aqueduct

Red nucleus

Basilar artery

Cerebral peduncle

Oculomotor nerve

A

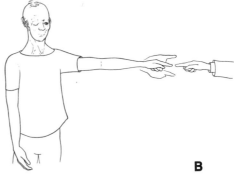

B

FIGURE 4–9. The syndrome of oculomotor nerve palsy and contralateral ataxia. *A*, A single small right midbrain infarction may damage the oculomotor nerve and the *red nucleus*, which conveys left cerebellar hemisphere outflow to the left arm and leg by a "double-cross." *B*, This patient has right ptosis from the oculomotor nerve palsy and left arm ataxia from the damage to the red nucleus.

PONS

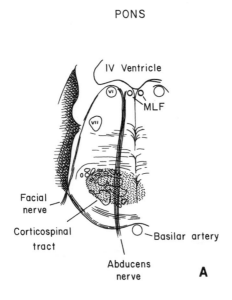

IV Ventricle

MLF

Facial nerve

Corticospinal tract

Basilar artery

Abducens nerve

A

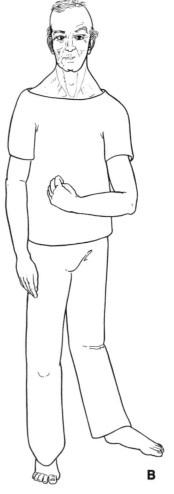

B

FIGURE 4–10. The syndrome of abducens nerve palsy and contralateral hemiparesis. *A*, A single small right pontine infarction may damage the abducens nerve, which supplies the *ipsilateral eye*, and the adjacent corticospinal tract, which supplies the *contralateral arm and leg*. (This is analogous to midbrain infarctions; see Fig. 4-8.) *B*, This patient has inward turning of the right eye from paresis of the right abducens nerve, and left hemiparesis from paresis of the right corticospinal tract damage.

contrast, in ALS and poliomyelitis, the oculomotor nerves are normal despite destruction of large numbers of motor neurons.

Some conditions in which frank ocular muscular paresis is evident curiously fail to produce diplopia. For example, intermittently dysconjugate, or "crossed," eyes are usually not associated with diplopia. If uncorrected in childhood, however, such muscle imbalances will lead to blindness of the deviated eye, *amblyopia*. Also, patients whose eyes are extremely divergent will not have diplopia because their brain somehow suppresses one of the images.

As for psychogenic disturbances, people can usually feign ocular muscle weakness only by staring inward, as if looking at the tip of their nose. Children often do this playfully; however, adults with their eyes in such a position are easily recognized as displaying voluntary, although bizarre, activity.

THE TRIGEMINAL NERVE (FIFTH CRANIAL NERVE)

The main functions of the trigeminal nerves are to provide sensory innervation to the face (Fig. 4-11) and motor supply to the jaw muscles. Also, the *corneal reflex* relies on the sensory innervation of the cornea by the trigeminal nerve. Stimulation of the cornea, as with a wisp of cotton, will trigger the synapse in the brainstem, excite both facial (seventh cranial) nerves, and make both eyes blink.*

The trigeminal nerve also supplies the large, powerful muscles that close and protrude the jaw. Since their main function is to assist in chewing, they are often called the "muscles of mastication." The *jaw jerk reflex*, another important reflex, is based on the motor function of the fifth nerve. Tapping the partially

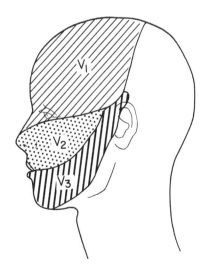

FIGURE 4–11. The three divisions of the trigeminal nerve provide the facial sensory innervation. The first division (V₁) supplies the forehead, the cornea, and the scalp up to the vertex; the second (V₂) supplies the malar area; and the third (V₃) supplies the skin of the lower jaw except for the angle.

---

* If the cotton tip is first applied to the right cornea and neither eye blinks, and then to the left cornea and both eyes blink, the interpretation would be that the right trigeminal nerve (the afferent sensory limb) is impaired. If application of cotton to the right cornea fails to provide a right eye blink, but succeeds in provoking a left eye blink, the interpretation here is that the right facial nerve (the efferent motor limb) is impaired.

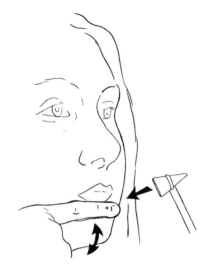

FIGURE 4–12. In the jaw jerk reflex, the jaw will move slightly downward and then rebound softly. Abnormalities are mostly a matter of the rapidity and strength of the rebound. In a hypoactive reflex, as found in bulbar palsy, there is little or no rebound. In a hyperactive reflex, as in pseudobulbar palsy, there is a quick and forceful rebound.

opened jaw will prompt its normal reflex closing (Fig. 4-12). Hyperactivity and other alterations of this reflex are discussed below (see Pseudobulbar Palsy).

Examination of the trigeminal nerve begins by testing sensation in its three sensory divisions. Cotton is brushed successively against each side of the forehead, cheek, and jaw. Areas of reduced sensation (i.e., *hypalgesia*) should conform to anatomic outlines. The corneal reflex is useful in assessing patients whose sensory loss is inconsistent.

Testing jaw muscle strength is done by asking the patient to clench and then protrude the jaw. In all patients with dysarthria, dysphagia, or emotional lability, the jaw jerk should be tested.

Injury of the trigeminal nerve causes facial hypalgesia, corneal reflex loss, jaw jerk hypoactivity, and weakness of the jaw muscles ipsilateral to the lesion. Such injuries, which are rare, may be caused by nasopharyngeal tumors, gunshot wounds, and tumors of the cerebellopontine angle, such as acoustic neuromas.

In *trigeminal neuralgia* (tic douloureux), which is usually caused by an aberrant vessel pressing on this nerve at its origin from the brainstem, people have bursts of lancinating pain, usually in the cheek or jaw, i.e., the V_2 or V_3 areas (Chapter 9). Another commonly encountered problem is *Herpes zoster* infection, which causes an excruciating pain in the nerve's V_1 division.

Finally, in psychogenic causes of "lost" facial sensation, the sensory loss will usually encompass the entire face or will be one aspect of sensory loss of one half of the body. In almost all cases, the following three nonanatomic features will be present: (1) The sensory loss will not involve the scalp (although its anterior portion is supplied by the trigeminal nerve); (2) despite the facial sensory loss, the corneal reflex will remain intact; and (3) when only one half of the face is affected, sensation will be lost sharply (rather than gradually) at the midline, i.e., the midline will be split.

THE FACIAL NERVE (SEVENTH CRANIAL NERVE)

The major functions of the facial nerves are to provide the sense of taste and the motor supply of facial muscles. As the trigeminal nerve supplies the muscles of mastication, the facial nerve supplies the "muscles of facial expression."

Cerebral impulses innervate the facial nerve motor nuclei of both the contralateral and ipsilateral pons. Consequently, the upper facial muscles are innervated by both cerebral hemispheres, whereas the lower ones are innervated only by the contralateral cerebral hemisphere (Fig. 4-13).

The facial nerve itself originates in the pons and leaves the brainstem at the cerebellopontine angle. It supplies the ipsilateral temporalis, orbicularis oculi, and orbicularis oris muscles, which are responsible for a person's smile, frown, grimace, or raised eyebrows.

Impulses from taste receptors of the anterior two thirds of the tongue are also conveyed in the facial nerve. (The glossopharyngeal nerve—the ninth cranial nerve—receives those from the posterior third.) Actually, taste sensation is limited in several important respects. Taste receptors detect only four fundamental sensations: bitter, sweet, sour, and salty. It is predominantly aroma, which is detected by the olfactory nerve, that gives food its flavor. Moreover, the olfactory nerve, not the facial nerve, has extensive connections with the cerebral cortex and limbic system.

Routine facial nerve testing involves examining the strength of the facial muscles and, occasionally, assessing taste. An examiner observes the patient's face, first at rest and then during a succession of maneuvers relying on various facial muscles, such as looking upward, closing one's eyes, and smiling. When weakness is detected, the examiner should try to ascertain if both the upper and lower, or only the lower, facial musculature is paretic. Upper and lower paresis suggests a lesion of the facial nerve itself. In this case, taste is also likely to be impaired. However, with unilateral or even bilateral facial nerve injuries, patients have no mental changes.

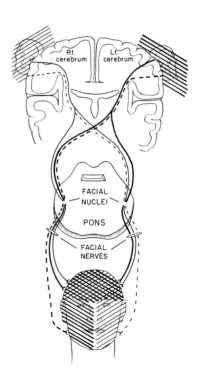

FIGURE 4–13. The facial nerve is derived, in almost a unique arrangement, from corticobulbar tracts originating in the ipsilateral as well as in the contralateral cerebral hemisphere. Each facial nerve supplies the muscles of facial expression, with the upper half of the face receiving cortical innervation from both hemispheres. As a result of cerebral injuries, only the lower half of the contralateral face is deprived of innervation. When facial nerve injuries occur, both the upper and lower half of the facial musculature are deprived of innervation.

Central   Peripheral

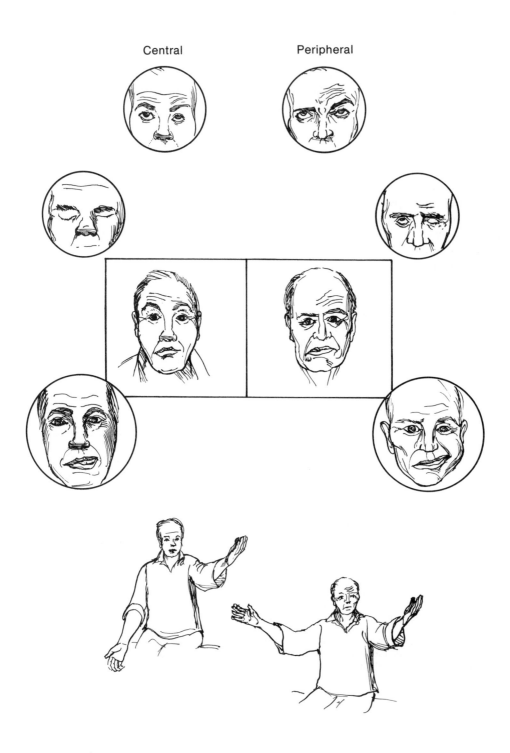

In contrast, paresis of only the lower facial musculature suggests a lesion of the contralateral cerebral hemisphere, which may be associated with mental changes. In such a case, paresis might affect the ipsilateral arm and leg, as well as the lower face. In addition, the deep tendon and plantar reflexes might be abnormal. With weakness of the right lower face, aphasia may be present. Taste sensation and other facial nerve functions will be preserved.

To test taste, the examiner applies either a dilute salt or sugar solution to the anterior portion of each side of the tongue, which must remain protruded to prevent the solution from spreading to its other parts. A patient will normally be able to identify the fundamental taste sensations but not those "tastes" that depend on aroma, such as onion and garlic.

Facial nerve damage results in paresis of ipsilateral upper and lower portions of the face with or without loss of taste sensation. *Bell's palsy*, an inflammatory injury, is probably the commonest facial nerve disorder (Fig. 4-14). Lacerations and tumors of the nerve or adjacent structures are also common causes of nerve injury. Cerebellopontine angle tumors, such as acoustic neuromas, affect the fifth, seventh, and eighth cranial nerves.

Patients with psychologic aberrations do not "develop" unilateral facial paresis, probably because such a posture is difficult to mimic. People who refuse to be examined, particularly children, might force their eyelids and mouth closed. The willful nature would be evident when the examiner finds resistance on opening the eyelids and jaw and the eyeballs tend to retrovert as the eyelids are pried open (Bell's phenomena).

FIGURE 4–14. Weakness of the face from cerebral and facial (seventh cranial) nerve injuries. The patient on the left has weakness of his lower right face from thrombosis of the left middle cerebral artery. He might be said to have a central (CNS) paralysis. In contrast, the patient on the right has right-sided weakness of both the upper and lower face from a right facial nerve injury (Bell's palsy). He might be said to have a peripheral (cranial nerve) paralysis.

In the *center boxed sketches*, the patients are pictured while at rest. The man with the central palsy, on the left, has flattening of the right nasolabial fold and sagging of the mouth downward to the right. This pattern of weakness indicates paresis of only the lower facial muscles. The man with the peripheral palsy on the right, however, has right-sided loss of the normal forehead furrows, in addition to flattening of the nasolabial fold. This pattern of weakness indicates paresis of the upper as well as the lower facial muscles.

In the *circled sketches at the top*, the patients have been asked to look upward—a maneuver that would exaggerate upper facial weakness. The man with central weakness has normal upward movement of the eyebrows and furrowing of the forehead. The man with peripheral weakness has no eyebrow or forehead movement, and the forehead skin remains flat.

In the *circled sketches second from the top*, the men have been asked to close their eyes—a maneuver that also would exaggerate upper facial weakness. The man with the central weakness has widening of the nasolabial fold, but he is able to close his eyelids and cover the eyeball. The man with the peripheral weakness is unable to close the affected eyelids, although his genuine effort is apparent by the retroversion of the eyeball (Bell's phenomenon).

In the *lowest circled sketches*, the men have been asked to smile—a maneuver that would exaggerate lower facial weakness. Both men have strength only of the left side of the mouth and thus it deviates to the left. If tested, the man with Bell's palsy would have loss of taste on the anterior two thirds of his tongue on the affected side.

The *bottom sketches* show the response when both men are asked to elevate their arms. The man with the central facial weakness also has paresis of the adjacent arm, but the man with the peripheral weakness has no arm paresis.

In summary, the man on the left with the left middle cerebral artery occlusion has paresis of his right lower face and arm. The man on the right with right Bell's palsy has paresis of his right upper and lower face and loss of taste.

THE ACOUSTIC NERVE (EIGHTH CRANIAL NERVE)

Each acoustic nerve is actually composed of two nerves with separate courses and different functions. The *cochlear nerve*, one of the two components, transmits auditory impulses from the ear to the superior temporal gyri of both cerebral hemispheres (Fig. 4-15). This bilateral cortical representation of sound means that, whereas damage to the acoustic nerve or ear itself may cause deafness in that ear, unilateral lesions of the brainstem or cerebral hemisphere will not cause hearing impairment. Since cerebral lesions do not impair hearing, patients with cerebrovascular accidents, tumors, and Alzheimer's disease typically have normal hearing.

During the routine examination, hearing is tested by the examiner whispering into one of the patient's ears while covering the other. Although this method does not permit an objective measure, the experienced physician can use this simple test to detect a gross hearing loss.

Hearing impairment may result from damage to the ear or the acoustic nerve. It is not, as already mentioned, usually a result of CNS injury. The auditory nerve may be damaged by medications, such as aspirin or streptomycin; by fractures of the skull; or by cerebellar angle tumors, such as acoustic neuromas associated with neurofibromatosis. Congenital acoustic nerve damage commonly results from in utero rubella infections or kernicterus (Chapter 13).

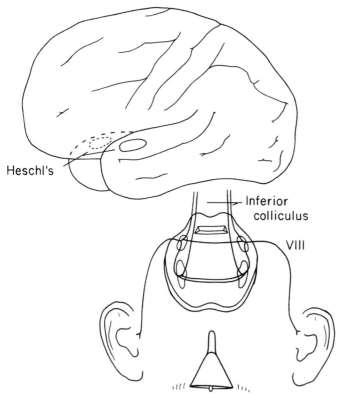

Heschl's

Inferior colliculus

VIII

FIGURE 4–15. The cochlear division of the acoustic nerve synapses extensively in the pons. Crossed and uncrossed fibers pass upward into the brainstem and terminate in the auditory (Heschl's) areas of both temporal lobes. In the dominant hemisphere, Heschl's area is adjacent to Wernicke's language area (Fig. 8-1).

Thus, children with mental retardation from these conditions often have marked hearing impairment.

When patients mimic deafness, the examiner may attempt to startle or awaken them from sleep with loud noises or have them look reflexly toward a noise (the *auditory-ocular reflex*). Factitious hearing loss may also be revealed by obtaining brainstem auditory evoked responses (BAERs) (Chapter 15).

Auditory investigations are necessary not only in diagnosing psychogenic disturbances but also in the full evaluation of people who cannot speak and of children with cerebral palsy, mental retardation, or autism.

Hearing loss may affect 25 percent of the elderly. In such cases, it can result from middle or inner ear degeneration or auditory nerve damage. With their vulnerability to sensory deprivations because of combinations of visual and hearing impairments, the elderly are prone to thought and emotional disturbances. Hearing aids should be dispensed readily and even on a trial basis. They may improve attentiveness and communication, and avert some mental aberrations.

A ringing or whistling sound in the ears, *tinnitus*, is another common problem among the elderly. Although it may be caused by medications that damage the inner ear, tinnitus is most often caused by ischemia resulting from atherosclerotic cerebrovascular disease. Likewise, a patient's audible heartbeat is often a manifestation of atherosclerotic cerebrovascular disease.

The other component of the acoustic nerve is the *vestibular nerve*. This nerve transmits labyrinth impulses that monitor equilibrium, orientation, and change in position.

The most characteristic symptom of vestibular nerve damage is *vertigo*, a sensation that one is spinning within the environment or that the environment is itself spinning. Dizziness, lightheadedness, giddiness, weakness, or unsteadiness are not equivalent to vertigo. Unfortunately, physicians mistakenly use these terms interchangeably. When vertigo is caused by vestibular dysfunction, then nystagmus, ataxia, and auditory changes are usually present. When vertigo is severe, nausea and vomiting develop.

Viral infections of the inner ear, *labyrinthitis*, affect the origin of the vestibular nerve and cause incapacitating vertigo with nausea. Traumatic injuries and ischemia cause similar symptoms. In addition, vestibular nerve damage may result from some of the medications that also cause cochlear nerve damage.

Ménière's disease, an important chronic vestibular nerve disorder of unknown etiology, causes episodes of vertigo, unilateral tinnitus, and nystagmus. Beginning in middle age and occurring in women more often than men, it leads to progressive hearing loss. In typical cases, attacks of Ménière's disease are readily identifiable; however, in the elderly they may be indistinguishable from basilar artery transient ischemic attacks. Many cases are justifiably confused with anxiety, but anxious patients do not have clear-cut vertigo, nystagmus, or progressive hearing loss.

THE GLOSSOPHARYNGEAL, VAGUS, ACCESSORY, AND HYPOGLOSSAL NERVES (NINTH THROUGH TWELFTH CRANIAL NERVES)

The ninth through twelfth cranial nerves are considered together because all arise from the lower brainstem, have certain common functions, such as production of speech, and are affected by the same disorders. For example, all these nerves are injured, along with cerebellar outflow fibers and other important tracts, in lateral medullary infarctions (Wallenberg syndrome, Fig. 2-10). Their impairment leads to another important clinical syndrome, bulbar palsy. This disorder, which itself merits special attention, is most notable because of its superficial resemblance to pseudobulbar palsy.

Bulbar Palsy

The *bulb*, or *medulla*,* contains the descending corticospinal tracts, the ascending sensory tracts, and the nuclei and initial portions of the ninth through the twelfth cranial nerves. These bulbar cranial nerves innervate the muscles of the soft palate, pharynx, larynx, and tongue. Their primary function is to implement cerebral commands to produce speech and to swallow food and saliva. They also control unconscious actions of the palate and pharynx, largely through swallowing and gag reflex mechanisms.

Injury to the bulbar cranial nerves, either within the brainstem or anywhere along their course, leads to bulbar palsy. This commonly occurring disorder is characterized by speech impairment (*dysarthria*), difficulty in swallowing (*dysphagia*), and unresponsiveness of the gag reflex. The salient clinical features are summarized and compared with those of pseudobulbar palsy in Table 4-1.

The examiner should listen to the patient's spontaneous speech during the history taking and then during repetition of phrases. Next, the patient should be asked to repeat single sounds that test speech production using lingual ("la"), labial ("pa"), and guttural ("ga") mechanisms. The examiner should note abnormalities in articulation, volume, cadence, and prosody (Chapter 8).

In most cases of bulbar palsy, patients have thickened speech with heavy nasal intonation. Some patients can be altogether mute. Even if a patient's speech is not strikingly abnormal during casual conversation, repetition of the guttural consonant, "ga . . . ga . . . ga . . . ," will usually evoke typically thickened, nasal sounds, uttered "gna . . . gna . . . gna . . . ."

In contrast to patients with aphasia, those with bulbar palsy, despite markedly impaired articulation, still employ normal syntax, express full meaning when speaking, and have normal understanding of verbal information. Moreover, their ability to express themselves in writing is preserved. People with bulbar palsy who are severely dysarthric, for example, would not be able to repeat the

TABLE 4–1. COMPARISON OF BULBAR AND PSEUDOBULBAR PALSY

	Bulbar	Pseudobulbar
Dysarthria	Yes	Yes
Dysphagia	Yes	Yes
Movement of palate		
Voluntary	No	No
Reflex	No	Yes
Jaw jerk	Hypoactive	Hyperactive
Emotional lability	No	Yes
Intellectual impairment	No	Yes

* For practical clinical purposes, however, the bulb is often considered to include the pons, as well as the medulla (Figs. 20-1 and 20-13).

phrase, "Please, pick up your hand." They would, however, be able to understand and follow the request and also be able to write the phrase correctly. Patients with aphasia, in contrast, typically would be unable to repeat the request and also would fail to understand or execute it. Moreover, they probably would not be able to write it (Aphasia, Chapter 8).

Normally, when saying "ah," a person's palate will contract and rise in a tentlike fashion, and the uvula will remain in the midline. A patient with bulbar palsy will characteristically have little or no palatal elevation because of the paresis induced by the nerve injury.

Another characteristic sign of bulbar palsy is dysphagia. Because of pharyngeal and palatal paresis, food tends to lodge in the trachea or be forced upward into the nasopharyngeal cavity. In fact, patients with advanced bulbar palsy nasally regurgitate liquids.

Though paucity of *voluntary* palatal movement and dysphagia are important characteristics of bulbar palsy, they do not by themselves distinguish bulbar from pseudobulbar palsy. Loss of the gag reflex, however, is distinctive (Fig. 4-16). In bulbar palsy, damage to the cranial nerves or their intramedullary connections nullifies stimulation of the posterior pharynx. In pseudobulbar palsy, as is discussed shortly, the gag reflex, far from being impaired, is hyperactive.

Depending on its cause, bulbar palsy is associated with still other physical findings. When the jaw muscles are involved, the jaw jerk reflex will be notably depressed (Fig. 4-12). When the brainstem is the site of neurologic disorder and the corticospinal tract is damaged, patients may have hyperactive DTRs and Babinski signs. However, as in other conditions with brainstem damage, bulbar palsy is usually not associated with mental aberrations.

Recognizing that a patient has bulbar palsy and determining whether the injury is within the brainstem or the cranial nerves in their course outside the brainstem will aid in establishing the neurologic illness. Conditions that commonly cause bulbar palsy by damaging the cranial nerves within the brainstem

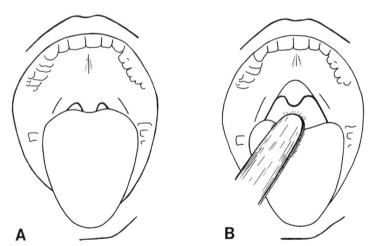

A   **B**

FIGURE 4–16. *A*, Normally, the soft palate forms an arch from which the uvula seems to hang. *B*, When the pharynx is stimulated, the normal gag reflex causes pharyngeal muscle contraction; the soft palate elevates straight upward, and the uvula remains in the midline. With impairment of the bulbar nerves (bulbar palsy), there may be little, no, or an asymmetric movement of the palate. With impairment of the corticobulbar tracts (pseudobulbar palsy), there is a brisk, overly forceful reaction that causes retching, coughing, or crying.

are amyotrophic lateral sclerosis (ALS) and thrombosis of a vertebral artery, although several decades ago, poliomyelitis was probably the most commonly encountered cause. Diseases likely to cause bulbar palsy by damaging the cranial nerves after they have exited the brainstem are Guillain-Barré syndrome, chronic meningitis, and tumors that grow along the base of the skull or within the adjacent meninges. Myasthenia gravis and botulism, which also cause bulbar palsy, do so by impairing the neuromuscular junction.

Pseudobulbar Palsy

Although dysarthria and dysphagia are present in both bulbar and pseudo-bulbar palsy, the two conditions differ in the sites of anatomic abnormality, quality of dysarthria and dysphagia, associated neurologic deficits, and spectrum of underlying causes. Pseudobulbar palsy is associated with damage to the frontal lobes and results from impairment of the corticobulbar tracts, which are upper motor neurons. Such damage is analogous to damage of the (adjacent) corticospinal tracts (Fig. 4-17).

In contrast, bulbar palsy results from damage to the lower brainstem or the bulbar cranial nerves along their course. This condition is caused by impairment of the nuclei of the nerves or of the nerves themselves, which are elements of lower motor neurons.

Clinical differences can be subtle. The speech of patients having pseudobulbar palsy is characterized by variable rhythm and intensity, and it is often said to have an "explosive" cadence. For example, when asked to repeat the consonant "ga," patients might blurt out "GA. GA.. GA . . ga . . . ga . . . ga." Their speech often has less of a nasal quality than is found with bulbar palsy. In general, the abnormal cadence is more striking than the abnormal articulation.

Although dysphagia is a characteristic manifestation of pseudobulbar palsy, liquids are swallowed relatively easily, and nasal regurgitation is uncommon. This less severe dysfunction in pseudobulbar palsy is the result of preservation of the swallowing and gag reflexes.

A major difference in the two conditions, however, is the reactivity of the gag reflex (Fig. 4-16). When tested, pseudobulbar palsy patients have brisk elevation of the palate and contraction of the pharynx, often overreacting with

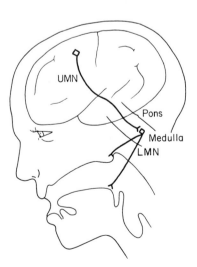

FIGURE 4–17. The corticobulbar tract is an upper motor neuron (UMN) tract that innervates the bulbar cranial nerves. These nerves are essentially lower motor neurons (LMNs). Damage to them, which causes bulbar palsy, abolishes the jaw jerk and gag reflexes: such areflexia is typical of LMN injury (Fig. 2-2C). Although mental changes may be the most prominent feature of pseudobulbar palsy, it is characterized by hyperactivity of these reflexes: such hyperactivity is typical of UMN injury (Fig. 2-2B).

coughing, crying, and retching. However, they have little or no palatal or pharyngeal movement in response to voluntary effort, as when attempting to say "ah."

Another major difference between the two conditions is that, although the jaw jerk reflex is depressed in bulbar palsy because the lower motor neurons of the cranial nerves are impaired, it is hyperactive in pseudobulbar palsy because the upper motor neurons of the corticobulbar tract are impaired. Also in pseudobulbar palsy, damage to the frontal lobes is so common that it almost always leads to signs of bilateral corticospinal tract damage, e.g., hyperactive DTRs and Babinski signs. Frontal lobe damage also leads to corticobulbar tract damage that causes subtle changes in the face (Fig. 4-18).

The notorious feature of pseudobulbar palsy is the accompanying alteration in the emotional state. Patients have inappropriate affect and fluctuation (*lability*) of emotions. In particular, they seem to cry or, less often, laugh in response to minimal provocation. Also as a manifestation of their emotional lability, they appear to switch readily between euphoria and depression.

The actual emotions of such patients are certainly not as expansive as the crying and laughing would suggest. Patients most often describe themselves as being awash with tearfulness. Amitriptyline, in relatively low doses (e.g., 75 mg or less daily) and apart from its antidepressant effect, may suppress the unwarranted *pathologic laughing* and *crying*.

A patient's tendency to cry or laugh is so dramatic that dysarthria and dysphagia may go unrecognized. Such emotionality is commonly and, in general, correctly attributed to pseudobulbar palsy, even without testing for dysarthria and dysphagia. Therefore, pseudobulbar palsy has become the commonly accepted explanation for unwarranted emotional states in people with brain damage,

On the other hand, the tendency toward tearfulness should not always be ascribed to brain damage. A great deal of true sadness can reasonably be expected under the circumstances of extensive and progressive incapacity.

Pseudobulbar palsy is associated with intellectual impairment (dementia) as well as with emotional lability because the extensive cerebral damage that underlies pseudobulbar palsy also causes dementia (Chapter 7). Likewise, when the left cerebral hemisphere is particularly damaged, pseudobulbar palsy may be associated with aphasia, usually of the nonfluent variety (Chapter 8). This

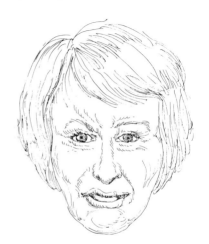

FIGURE 4–18. Patients with pseudobulbar palsy, such as this woman who has suffered multiple cerebral infarctions, often sit with a slack jaw, furrowed forehead, and vacant stare. The caricature of the mentally retarded person, with a deep voice (saying "dahh"), mouth open, and drooling, is the popular, implicit recognition of such extensive cerebral damage.

association, seen in reverse, might account for the tendency of some aphasic patients to appear tearful at any provocation. In any case, patients with pseudobulbar palsy should be carefully evaluated for dementia and aphasia.

The conditions causing pseudobulbar palsy are those that damage both frontal lobes or, more often, the entire cerebrum. Although a wide variety of degenerative, structural, or metabolic disturbances may be responsible, pseudobulbar palsy is most often the result of Alzheimer's disease, multiple cerebrovascular infarctions, or multiple sclerosis. Congenital cerebral damage (i.e., cerebral palsy) causes pseudobulbar palsy along with bilateral spasticity and choreoathetotic movement disorders. Finally, since ALS causes both upper and lower motor neuron damage, it causes a mixture of bulbar and pseudobulbar palsy. However, since ALS is a disorder of motor neurons exclusively, it is not associated with either dementia or aphasia (Chapter 5).

THE HYPOGLOSSAL NERVE (TWELFTH CRANIAL NERVE)

The hypoglossal nerves innervate the ipsilateral tongue muscles. They move the tongue within the mouth and protrude it when people eat and speak. The muscles tend to push the tongue contralaterally. Since the pressure on each side is balanced, the tongue protrudes in the midline.

The hypoglossal nerve originates from paired nuclei near the midline in the medulla. After the nerve leaves the base of the medulla, it passes through the base of the skull and travels through the neck to innervate the muscles of the tongue.

If one hypoglossal nerve were injured, that side of the tongue would be weakened, and in time, it would atrophy. When protruded, the tongue would deviate toward the weakened side because the normal, strong musculature would overpower the effort of the weakened side (Fig. 4-19). Such a finding illustrates the adage, "The tongue points toward the side of the lesion."

If both nerves were injured, as in bulbar palsy, the tongue would become immobile. In cases of ALS, fasciculations as well as atrophy might be observed (Fig. 5-4).

The most frequently occurring conditions in which one hypoglossal nerve is

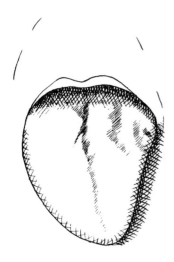

FIGURE 4–19. With (left) hypoglossal nerve damage, the tongue deviates toward the weaker side, i.e., turns toward the side of the lesion, and the affected (left) side atrophies.

damaged are brainstem infarctions, penetrating neck wounds, and nasopharyngeal tumors. Both hypoglossal and other bulbar cranial nerves are injured in Guillain-Barré syndrome, myasthenia gravis, and ALS.

SUMMARY

Identification of damage to the individual cranial nerves is helpful in localizing lesions and diagnosing particular neurologic illnesses. Cranial nerves are often damaged in combination with the corticospinal tracts in the brainstem. Important examples are cases of paresis of the oculomotor or abducens nerve combined with contralateral hemiparesis, and also the lateral medullary syndrome. Damage of the frontal lobes, which causes emotional lability with dysarthria and dysphagia (pseudobulbar palsy), mimics damage to the lower cranial nerves (bulbar palsy). When damage is restricted to cranial nerves or the brainstem, despite extensive motor and sensory impairment, patients generally do not have mental abnormalities.

QUESTIONS: CHAPTERS 1-4

1. A 68-year-old man has the sudden, painless onset of paresis of the right upper and lower face, inability to abduct the right eye, and paresis of the left arm and leg. Where is the lesion and what structures are involved?

2. What deficits would be produced with occlusion of the left internal carotid artery?

3. What symptoms and signs will a patient have with sudden occlusion of the right internal carotid artery?

4. A 20-year-old man has the subacute onset of complete loss of vision in the right eye, incoordination of the left hand, and moderate spastic paraparesis. What is the localization?

5. A 20-year-old woman complains of right eye "blindness," right hemiparesis, and right hemisensory loss. Pupillary and deep tendon reflexes are normal. She does not press down with her left leg while attempting to lift her right leg. What is her deficit and what is its origin?

6. What diseases with movement disorders are associated with dementia?

7. What physical abnormalities are frequently found with cerebral degenerative conditions such as Alzheimer's disease?

8. A 45-year-old woman, who was entirely well previously, has the sudden onset of jargon speech and hysteria. She is admitted to the psychiatric ward with a diagnosis of schizophrenia. The physical examination reveals only a right Babinski sign and an equivocal right hemiparesis. This common neurologic condition frequently mimics psychiatric disturbances. What is her deficit and what is its origin?

9. An elderly man has left ptosis, a dilated and unreactive left pupil, external deviation of the left eye, a right hemiparesis, right-sided hyperreflexia, and a right Babinski sign. He does not have either aphasia or hemianopsia. Where is (are) the lesion(s)?

10. A person is found to have a left superior homonymous quadrantanopsia. Where might the lesion be located?

11. A 60-year-old man has seizures that begin with clonic activity of the left hand

and spread to the left arm, then face, and then leg. Subsequently, he has transient paresis of the left arm. Where is the lesion?

12. A 50-year-old woman complains of gait difficulties and decreased hearing on the right for many years. The right corneal reflex is absent. The entire right side of her face is weak. Auditory acuity is diminished on the right. There is left-sided hyperreflexia with a Babinski sign and right-sided difficulty with rapid alternating movements. What structures are involved? Where is (are) the lesion(s)?

13. A 60-year-old man develops moderate interscapular back pain, paraparesis with hyperreflexia, loss of sensation below the umbilicus, and incontinence. Where exactly is the lesion?

14. A young man, having sustained an injury in a minor car accident, complains of being able to see an area of only 2 m^2, paralysis of the legs, and loss of sensation below the waist. On examination, he is found to have a constant visual loss of 2 m^2 at every distance, an inability to raise his legs or walk, brisk DTRs, and loss of pin and position sense in the legs and toes. Plantar responses are flexor, cremasteric and anal reflexes are present, and sensation of warm versus cold is intact. Formulate the case.

15. A 50-year-old man with mild dementia has absent reflexes, loss of position and vibration sensation, and ataxia. What nonstructural diseases must be considered?

16. A 55-year-old woman, thought to have depression, is then found to have right optic atrophy, papilledema on the left, and left hemiparesis. Where is the lesion?

17. A middle-aged man complains of impotence. He has been in excellent health except for hypertension. On examination, he has orthostatic hypotension and light-headedness, but the neurologic examination is otherwise normal. What neurologic condition(s) may be the cause or a contributing factor?

18. A 60-year-old man with right upper lobe pulmonary carcinoma has the rapid development of lumbar spine pain, paraparesis with areflexia, loss of sensation below the knees, and urinary and fecal incontinence. Where is the lesion?

19. Subsequently, the man in question 18 develops a flaccid, areflexic paresis of the right shoulder and arm and a right Horner's syndrome. Where is the lesion?

20. A 60-year-old man has developed stiffness of his left leg. Examination reveals that he has a spastic paraparesis, DTR hyperreflexia in all extremities, and bilateral extensor plantar response. Fasciculations are noted in the left leg, both arms, and tongue. Most muscle groups of the left arm are atrophied. All sensation, bladder and bowel function, and ocular movements are intact. What process is developing?

21. A 21-year-old woman has the mildly painful loss of vision in the left eye. She is found to have an acuity of 20/400 in the eye, a mild left hemiparesis with hyperreflexic DTRs and a Babinski sign, and right-sided ataxia. She had a similar episode 5 years before. Formulate the case.

22. A 40-year-old man has interscapular spine pain, paraparesis with hyperreflexia, bilateral Babinski signs, and a complete sensory loss below his nipples. Formulate the case and list the preliminary approach to the diagnosis.

23. Contralateral hemiparesis, hemisensory loss, and hemianopsia are found in lesions of either hemisphere. What higher cortical function deficits are specifically referable to the dominant or nondominant hemisphere?

24. An elderly man has vertigo, nausea, and vomiting. He has a right Horner's syndrome, loss of the right corneal reflex, and dysarthria because of paresis of the palate. What are the other features of this common eponymic syndrome? Which way does the palate deviate?

25. A 54-year-old woman complains of having experienced several episodes of shaking in her left leg beginning in the foot. There is hyperreflexia at the left knee and ankle and a left Babinski sign. What sensory abnormalities might be detected?

26. What area of the brain is the primary site of damage in Wilson's disease, Huntington's chorea, and choreiform cerebral palsy? What neurologic system is involved, and what are the traditional manifestations of abnormalities there?

27. Name the frontal lobe release reflexes. Are they always pathologic?

28–39. Define these symptoms or signs and specify the location of associated lesions.

28. Anosognosia

29. Aphasia

30. Astereognosis

31. Athetosis

32. Bradykinesia

33. Chorea

34. Dementia

35. Dysdiadochokinesia

36. Gerstmann's syndrome

37. Homonymous hemianopsia

38. Micrographia

39. Homonymous superior quadrantanopsia

40. Which of the following neurologic diseases are genetically transmitted and, if so, in what manner?
   a.   Alzheimer's disease
   b.   Amyotrophic lateral sclerosis
   c.   Cluster headaches
   d.   Creutzfeldt-Jakob disease
   e.   Down's syndrome
   f.   Duchenne's muscular dystrophy
   g.   Dystonia musculorum deformans
   h.   Familial amaurotic idiocy (Tay-Sachs)
   i.   Friedreich's ataxia
   j.   Guillain-Barré syndrome
   k.   Huntington's chorea
   l.   Migraine headaches
   m.   Sturge-Weber disease
   n.   Subacute sclerosing panencephalitis (SSPE)
   o.   Wilson's disease

41. A young man sustains closed head trauma. Afterward, he has insomnia, fatigue, and intellectual and personality changes and claims that food tastes differently. What might have happened?

42. A middle-aged woman has increasing blindness in the right eye, where the visual acuity is 20/400 and the disk is white. The right pupil does not react directly or consensually to light. The left pupil reacts directly, although not consensually. All motions of the right eye are impaired. Where is the lesion? What cranial nerve(s) is (are) involved?

43. In what condition do pupils accommodate but not react to light?

44. In what condition is a patient in an agitated, confused state with abnormally large pupils?

45. In what condition is a patient in coma with pinpoint-sized pupils?

46. What are the most common causes of asymptomatic miosis?

47. After sustaining a severe head injury, a comatose patient is admitted. The right pupil is dilated and unreactive. There is right hemiparesis and bilateral Babinski signs. What well-known catastrophe is happening?

48. On looking to the left, a patient has diplopia. What nerve(s) may be paretic?

49. On looking to the left, the left eye fails to abduct fully. Which nerve is probably involved?

50. If the right third cranial nerve were injured, how would the eyes appear? In what direction of gaze would diplopia occur?

51. Nystagmus is observed bilaterally, horizontally, and vertically in a 15-year-old girl who is lethargic and disoriented, walks with an ataxic gait, and has slurred speech. What is the most likely cause of her findings?

52. A young man complains of vertigo, nausea, vomiting, and left-sided tinnitus. He has nystagmus to the right. Where is the lesion?

53. A soldier has vertical and horizontal nystagmus, mild spastic paraparesis, and ataxia of finger-to-nose motion bilaterally. What process has occurred?

54. A man who has diplopia looks to the left, but the right eye fails to adduct across the midline and the left eye has nystagmus. Both eyes, however, are forward while looking ahead and converge while reading. What process has occurred?

55. A 35-year-old man, who has been shot in the back, has paresis of the right leg and loss of position and vibration sensation at the right ankle. Sensation of pinprick is lost in the left leg. Where is the lesion?

56. A 25-year-old man develops impotence. He has been found previously to have retrograde ejaculation during an evaluation for sterility. Since age 8, he has had diabetes mellitus. Examination of his fundi reveal hemorrhages and exudates. He has absent DTRs at the wrists and ankles, loss of position and vibration sensation at the ankles, and no demonstrable anal or cremasteric reflexes. Why is he impotent?

57. A 27-year-old man has a bitemporal hemianopsia. He has had loss of libido for 2 years and mild frontal headaches for the previous 3 months. Examination of the optic disks shows them to be white. The pupils are large but react to light. The right eye fails to abduct fully. Aside from a eunuchoid habitus, the routine physical examination reveals no abnormalities. What is the neurologic basis of his symptoms and signs?

58. An 8-year-old boy with increasing difficulty in athletic activities and with headaches, nausea, and vomiting is found to have papilledema, tremor on intention, ataxia of gait, bilateral hyperreflexia, and bilateral Babinski signs. Where is the lesion and what are the possible causes?

59. Gait abnormalities are important signs of neurologic diseases. Match the abnormality of the gait with its description.
   a. Short-stepped, narrow-based with a shuffle
   b. Impaired alternation of feet
   c. Broad-based and lurching
   d. Seeming to be extraordinarily unbalanced, but without falls
   e. Swinging one leg outward with excessive wear on the inner sole
      1. Apraxic
      2. Astasia-abasia
      3. Ataxic
      4. Festinating
      5. Hemiparetic

60. Match the descriptions of gait abnormalities with the associated neurologic illnesses.

a.	Cerebral infarction	1.	Apraxic
b.	Cerebellar degeneration	2.	Astasia-abasia
c.	Parkinsonism	3.	Ataxic
d.	Normal pressure hydrocephalus	4.	Festinating
e.	Hysteria	5.	Hemiparetic

61. Match the pictures (1,2,3) with the associated characteristics.
  a. Cerebral infarction
  b. Loss of taste on one side of tongue
  c. Idiopathic inflammation
  d. Normal
  e. Overexposure and drying of eye
  f. Loss of the corneal reflex

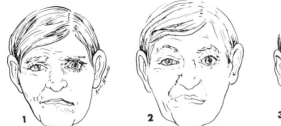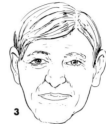

62–67. The patient who is pictured below is looking slightly to her right and attempting to raise both arms. Her left eye deviates across the midline to the right, but her right eye has no abduction.

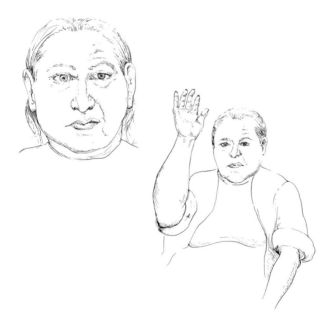

62. Paresis of which extraocular muscle prevents the affected eye from moving laterally?
  a. Right superior oblique
  b. Right abducens
  c. Left abducens
  d. Left lateral rectus
  e. Right lateral rectus

63. The left face does not seem to be involved by the left hemiparesis. Why might the left side of the face be uninvolved?
  a. It is. The left forehead and mouth are contorted.
  b. The problem is in the right cerebral hemisphere.
  c. The corticospinal tract is injured only after the corticobulbar tract has innervated the facial nerve.
  d. The problem is best explained by postulating two lesions.

64. On which side of the body would a Babinski sign be elicited?
    a. Right
    b. Left
    c. Both
    d. Neither

65. What is the most likely cause of this disorder?
    a. Bell's palsy
    b. Hysteria
    c. Cerebral infarction
    d. Medullary infarction
    e. Pontine infarction
    f. Midbrain infarction

66. With which conditions might such a lesion be associated?
    a. Homonymous hemianopsia
    b. Diplopia
    c. Impaired monocular visual acuity
    d. Intellectual impairment
    e. Aphasia if the patient were right cerebral dominant
    f. Various nondominant hemisphere syndromes

67. Sketch the region of the damaged brain, inserting the damaged structures and the area of damage.

ANSWERS

1. The damaged structures include the abducens and facial nerves on the right and the corticospinal tract that originates in the right cerebral hemisphere and passes through the right midbrain and pons before crossing in the medulla. Only a lesion on the right side of the pons could damage all these structures. Small infarctions are the most common cause of such lesions. (If the lesion pictured in Figure 4-10 extended more laterally, it would create these deficits.)

2. Unless anastomoses are present, occlusion of the left internal carotid artery will impair function of the left hemisphere and cause right-sided hemiparesis, hemisensory loss, homonymous hemianopsia, and aphasia.

3. As in the previous case, the patient will have contralateral hemiparesis, hemisensory loss, and homonymous hemianopsia. Notably, since such patients frequently have hemi-inattention, they may not describe their hemiparesis (anosognosia).

4. The patient probably has lesions in the right optic nerve, left cerebellum, and thoracic spinal cord. Such disseminated lesions are typically found in cases of multiple sclerosis.

5. The symptoms cannot be explained by a single lesion, cannot be confirmed by objective signs, and lack the usual accompanying symptoms, such as aphasia. Moreover, the patient fails to exert maximum effort voluntarily with one leg while "trying" to lift the other against resistance (Hoover's sign). Neurologic disease may not be present. Rather, she might have a psychogenic disturbance.

6. Dementia is part of Wilson's disease, Huntington's chorea, and Creutzfeldt-Jakob disease, but not necessarily part of Parkinson's disease, Sydenham's chorea, or choreoathetotic cerebral palsy.

7. Signs of frontal lobe dysfunction that are usually present with cerebral degenerative conditions include corticospinal tract abnormalities (hyperreflexic DTRs and Babinski signs), corticobulbar signs (dysarthria, hyperactive gag reflex, briskly reactive jaw jerk), and frontal lobe release signs (snout, suck, rooting, palmomental, and grasp reflexes).

8. Schizophrenia rarely develops in middle-aged individuals and almost never produces "word salad." More likely, the patient had a fluent aphasia and has subtle corticospinal tract signs from a left temporoparietal lesion.

9. The patient has a left oculomotor nerve palsy and right hemiparesis. Therefore, the lesion is in the left midbrain. As expected, he does not have a language or visual field deficit because the cerebrum is uninjured.

10. Such a defect is usually found with a lesion of the right temporal or inferior occipital lobes, but occasionally an optic tract lesion may be responsible.

11. The lesion is located in the right lateral cerebral cortex. It gives rise to focal motor seizures, which then have secondary generalization (a jacksonian march). Following the seizure, he has postictal (Todd's) paresis.

12. The right-sided corneal reflex loss, facial weakness, and hearing impairment all indicate damage to the trigeminal, facial, and acoustic cranial nerves, which emerge together from the brainstem at the right cerebellopontine angle. The right-sided dysdiadochokinesia, which indicates right-sided cerebellar damage, and the left-sided DTR abnormalities are also consistent with damage to the right cerebellopontine angle. Common lesions in this region are acoustic neuromas and meningiomas, which are often manifestations of neurofibromatosis.

13. The lesion is in the thoracic spinal cord at the T-10 level.

14. Many features of the examination indicate that the basis of his symptoms and signs is not neurologic. Hysteria or malingering is suggested by the following: (1) the constant area (2 m^2) of visual loss at all distances—tunnel vision—is contrary to the optics of vision, in which a greater area of vision is encompassed at greater distances from the eye; (2) the sensory loss to pain (pin) is inconsistent with preservation of thermal (warm versus cold) sensation because both sensory systems follow the identical anatomic pathways; and (3) despite his apparent paraparesis, the normal plantar response and intact anal and cremasteric reflexes indicate that both the upper and lower motor neuron systems are intact. The DTRs are typically brisk because of anxiety.

15. This patient has dysfunction of the posterior columns of the spinal cord and the cerebellar system. Conditions to be considered first are combined-system disease (pernicious anemia), tabes dorsalis, spinocerebellar degenerations, and heavy metal intoxication.

16. The patient has the classic Foster-Kennedy syndrome from a right frontal lobe tumor. The tumor compresses the underlying optic nerve, causing it to atrophy. The tumor also raises intracranial pressure, causing papilledema of the other optic nerve. Finally, the tumor causes contralateral hemiparesis because of the damage to the corticospinal tract of the frontal lobe.

17. Impotence, as well as orthostatic hypotension, may be the result of autonomic nervous system dysfunction. In this patient, antihypertensive medications may be responsible.

18. The paraparesis with absent DTRs, loss of sensation at the L-4 level, and lumbar spine pain suggest that the lesion is in the cauda equina.

19. This problem is from a brachial plexus injury that involves the nerve roots of C4-6 and the intrathoracic sympathetic chain. The patient has a Pancoast's tumor.

20. The patient has signs of corticospinal tract (upper motor neuron) disease in all extremities as evidenced by the generalized hyperreflexia, stiffness (spasticity) in the legs, and Babinski signs. In addition, he has disease of the anterior horn cells (lower motor neurons) as evidenced by the fasciculations and atrophy. Mentation, sensation, and sphincter and ocular muscles are typically uninvolved. He has the motor neuron disease, amyotrophic lateral sclerosis (ALS).

21. Several areas of the nervous system are involved: the left optic nerve, the right corticospinal tract, and the right cerebellar hemisphere. Moreover, this is the second episode. Since the patient has lesions that are disseminated in space and time, she most likely has multiple sclerosis. Although a single lesion in the midbrain might produce similar corticospinal tract and cerebellar (outflow tract) findings, vision would not have been affected.

22.   The lesion clearly affects the spinal cord at the T-4 level. Common causes include benign and malignant mass lesions (e.g., a herniated thoracic intervertebral disk or an epidural metastatic tumor); infections (e.g., abscess or tuberculoma); and inflammations, e.g., transverse myelitis or multiple sclerosis. A complete history, physical examination, routine laboratory tests, and thoracic spine and chest x-ray films should all be performed before a myelogram or spine CT or MRI scan is done.

23.   Aphasias and Gerstmann's syndrome are usually referable to dominant hemisphere lesions. Hemi-inattention, anosognosia, somatopagnosia, and constructional apraxia are found in nondominant hemisphere lesions. Perseverations, ideomotor apraxia, dementia, pseudobulbar palsy, and occasionally constructional apraxia and fluent aphasia result from bilateral or diffuse cerebral disease.

24.   The patient has a right-sided lateral medullary (Wallenberg's) syndrome. This includes crossed (right-facial and left-truncal) hypalgesia and right-sided ataxia. The palate will deviate to the left because of right-sided palatal weakness.

25.   The lesion, which is causing focal motor seizures, is located on the right medial cerebral cortex. There might be only loss of cortical sensation, e.g., stereognosis and two-point discrimination. Sensation of pain and temperature may be preserved because they are perceived in the thalamus. Most likely the lesion is a tumor (e.g., a parasagittal meningioma or glioblastoma), but a scar from a cerebral infarction is another possibility.

26.   These diseases, as does Parkinson's disease, affect the basal ganglia, which is the basis of the extrapyramidal (i.e., noncorticospinal) motor system. Basal ganglia dysfunction causes tremor, other movement disorders, rigidity, and bradykinesia. In contrast, corticospinal tract dysfunction causes spasticity, DTR hyperreflexia, and Babinski signs.

27.   The frontal release reflexes involve the face (snout, suck, and rooting reflex) and the palm (palmomental and grasp reflexes). Most neurologists include an increased jaw jerk. Almost all frontal release signs are normally present in infants, but in adults, none of them reliably indicates the presence of a pathologic condition. However, if several are detected, a frontal lobe lesion or cerebral degenerative condition is likely to be present.

28.   Anosognosia is failure to recognize a deficit or disease. The most common example is ignorance of a left hemiparesis from a right cerebral lesion that damages the parietal lobe.

29.   Aphasia is a language disorder in which verbal or written communication is impaired. It usually results from lesions in the dominant cerebral hemisphere.

30.   Astereognosis is inability to identify objects by touch. It is found with lesions of the contralateral parietal lobe.

31.   Athetosis is an involuntary movement disorder in which there is a slow writhing movement of the arm(s) or leg(s) that is more pronounced in the distal part of the extremity. Usually it is the result of basal ganglia damage from perinatal jaundice, anoxia, or prematurity.

32.   Bradykinesia (i.e., slowness of movement) is seen with many basal ganglia diseases and is characteristic of parkinsonism.

33.   Chorea is involuntary intermittent jerking of one or more extremities or of the trunk. It may be caused by tardive dyskinesia, several neurologic medications (e.g., L-dopa), and many basal ganglia diseases.

34.   Dementia is impairment of intellectual function. It usually results from diffuse cerebral damage or a single lesion, such as a frontal lobe meningioma, that creates a generalized effect.

35. Dysdiadochokinesia is impaired ability to perform rapid alternating movements. It is characteristic of cerebellar injury. When unilateral, it is due to lesions of the ipsilateral cerebellar hemisphere.

36. Gerstmann's syndrome is the combination of agraphia, finger agnosia, dyscalculia, and inability to distinguish right from left. It is found with lesions of the dominant hemisphere parietal lobe.

37. Homonymous hemianopsia is a visual field defect in which one half of each eye field is lost. The lesion is in the contralateral optic tract or intrahemispheric radiations. In a right homonymous hemianopsia, the right half of the field is lost:

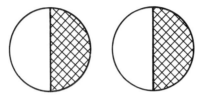

38. Micrographia is the writing of small letters. It is characteristic of parkinsonism.

39. Homonymous superior quadrantanopsia is the visual field defect in which the same top quarter is lost bilaterally:

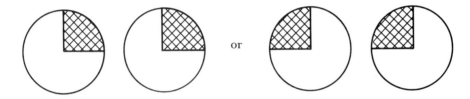

In bitemporal superior quadrantanopsia, neither eye appreciates the upper-outer quarter:

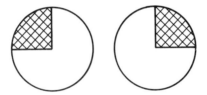

The former is found with lesions of the temporal or lower occipital lobe, whereas the latter is found with lesions of the optic chiasm.

40. a. Nongenetic, except autosomal dominant in certain families
   b. Nongenetic*
   c. Nongenetic
   d. Nongenetic*
   e. Nondysjunction (trisomy 21)
   f. Sex-linked recessive
   g. Autosomal recessive dominant or sporadic
   h. Autosomal recessive
   i. Autosomal recessive in typical cases
   j. Nongenetic*
   k. Autosomal dominant

---

* Probably infectious.

     l.   Frequently familial, especially in females, but not proven to be genetic

    m.   Autosomal dominant with variable penetration

    n.   Nongenetic*

    o.   Autosomal recessive

41.   The patient probably has had a contusion of both frontal lobes resulting in a postconcussive syndrome manifested by changes in mentation and personality. The anosmia results from shearing of the thin fibers of the olfactory nerve in their passage through the cribriform plate.

42.   The patient evidently has right-sided optic nerve damage because she has right-sided impaired visual acuity, optic atrophy, and loss of direct and indirect (consensual) light reaction. In addition, since there is complete extraocular muscle paresis, she probably has oculomotor, trochlear, and abducens nerve damage. Only a lesion located immediately behind the eye, such as a sphenoid wing meningioma, would be able to damage all these nerves.

43.   Tabes dorsalis with Argyll-Robertson pupils

44.   Atropine, scopolamine, and similar intoxications

45.   The combination of coma and miosis is commonly found in heroin, barbiturate, and other overdoses. Pontine infarctions and hemorrhages are infrequent causes.

46.   The most common causes of asymptomatic miosis are use of ocular medications for glaucoma and normal changes of old age.

47.   The patient probably has herniation of the right temporal lobe through the tentorial notch. This leads to compression of the ipsilateral third cranial nerve and the brainstem, i.e., the transtentorial herniation syndrome.

48.   Either the left sixth or right third cranial nerve is paretic.

49.   The left sixth cranial nerve is responsible.

50.   The right lid would be paretic, the right eye would be deviated laterally (abducted), and the pupil would be dilated. The patient would have diplopia on looking forward that would increase on looking to the left.

51.   The patient is probably intoxicated with alcohol, barbiturates, or other drugs of abuse. A cerebellar tumor is an unlikely possibility without signs of raised intracranial pressure or corticospinal tract damage. Multiple sclerosis is unlikely because of the patient's lethargy, disorientation, and young age.

52.   The unilateral nystagmus, hearing abnormality, nausea, and vomiting are most likely caused by left-sided inner ear disease, rather than neurologic dysfunction.

53.   This patient seems to have lesions in the brainstem producing nystagmus, in the cerebellum causing ataxia, and in the spinal cord causing paraparesis. The picture of disseminated lesions is typical of but not diagnostic of multiple sclerosis.

54.   The patient has internuclear ophthalmoplegia as the result of small lesions in the brainstem from multiple sclerosis, vascular infarctions, or inflammatory conditions.

55.   The patient suffers from a classical Brown-Séquard syndrome, i.e., hemitransection of the spinal cord. The lesion is at the right side of the thoracic spinal cord.

56.   The patient has a combination of peripheral and autonomic system neuropathy because of diabetes mellitus. A peripheral neuropathy is suggested by the distal sensory and reflex loss and the absent anal and cremasteric reflexes. Autonomic neuropathy is suggested by the retrograde ejaculation. Other manifestations of autonomic neuropathy that might be sought are urinary bladder hypotonicity, gastroenteropathy, and anhidrosis.

57. A lesion near the optic chiasm will cause optic atrophy and bitemporal hemianopsia. It might also damage the adjacent sixth cranial nerve by invading the cavernous sinus. Moreover, a eunuchoid appearance and the loss of libido may be referable to hypopituitarism or damage to the hypothalamus, which is directly above the optic chiasm. Therefore, this patient's symptoms and signs indicate that he has a tumor pressing against both the optic chiasm and adjacent endocrine structures. Such lesions are commonly chromophobe adenomas of the pituitary gland, craniopharyngiomas, and meningiomas. They are detectable with CT or MRI scans and by finding elevated serum prolactin levels.

58. The patient has increased intracranial pressure, compression of the corticospinal tracts, and cerebellar dysfunction. Most likely he has obstructive hydrocephalus from a cerebellar tumor—this is a relatively common pediatric condition. Lead intoxication, which causes diffuse neurologic dysfunction and cerebral swelling, can mimic a cerebellar tumor.

59. a-4; b-1; c-3; d-2; e-5.

60. a-5; b-3; c-4; d-1; e-2. Normal pressure hydrocephalus is characterized by dementia, incontinence, and, most strikingly, apraxia of gait. This gait disorder is typified by the inability to initiate alternating movements of the legs with appropriate shift of weight. The feet are often immobile because the weight is not shifted as the patient moves. The feet seem magnetized to the floor (Fig. 7-7). A pattern of walking in which the patient seems to alternate between a broad stance for stability and a narrow, tightrope-like stance, with contortions of the upper torso, is clearly psychogenic and termed astasia-abasia (Fig. 3-2). In cerebellar degeneration there is ataxia of the limbs and trunk that forces the patient to place his or her feet widely apart (in a broad base) to maintain stability. Since coordination is also impaired in cerebellar disease, the gait and other movements have an uneven, unsteady, lurching pattern (Fig. 2-13). A relatively minor feature of parkinsonism is the short-stepped gait with shuffling that is now called "festinating gait," but has been called *marche á petits pas* (Fig. 18-9). The hemiparesis and increased tone (spasticity) from cerebral infarctions force the patient to lift the paretic leg by swinging it from its hip. This motion, circumduction, permits walking despite the paresis if the hip and knee are extended. The weak ankle drags the inner front surface of the foot (Fig. 2-4).

61. a-2; b-1; c-1; d-3; e-1; f-1. Patient No. 1, who has weakness of his left upper and lower facial muscles, probably has Bell's palsy. With damage to the facial nerve, taste sensation is usually lost in the ipsilateral, anterior two thirds of the tongue. Paresis of the eyelid muscles does not permit spontaneous or reflex eyelid closure: dehydration and foreign body irritation can result. Patient No. 2 has weakness of his left lower facial muscles. This pattern of facial weakness is typical of contralateral cerebral injuries and is usually accompanied by arm and leg weakness, i.e., hemiparesis. Patient No. 3 is normal.

62–67. This patient has weakness of the right eye that prevents it from moving laterally, weakness of the right upper and lower face, and paresis of the left arm. She probably has damage of the right abducens (VI) and facial (VII) cranial nerves and the corticospinal tract before it crosses in the medulla. Such lesions are located in the base of the pons and are caused by occlusions of small branches of the basilar artery.

62. e. The right lateral rectus muscle is the extraocular muscle that has been damaged.

63. c.

64. b.

65. e. A right pontine infarction would produce this condition.

66. b. Diplopia would be present on right lateral gaze.

67.   PONS

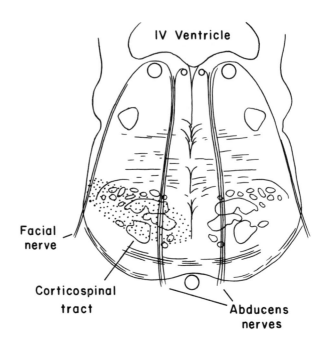

5

Peripheral Nerve Disorders

Clinical findings should distinguish peripheral nervous system (PNS) from central nervous system (CNS) disorders and should allow the PNS disorder to be localized. PNS disorders result from damage of the peripheral nerves singly, in groups, or entirely and are characterized by variable combinations of weakness, DTR loss, and sensory abnormalities.

These disorders are important because, besides causing neurologic deficits, some are associated with mental deterioration, systemic illness, or a fatal course.* This chapter describes the anatomy and clinical aspects of peripheral nerve injuries and presents details of several conditions, including some that are newly recognized. It then describes amyotrophic lateral sclerosis (ALS) and related motor neuron disorders. Last, it reviews the anatomy, signs, and treatment of nerve injury from herniated intervertebral disks and other orthopedic conditions.

ANATOMY

The corticospinal tracts, as discussed in Chapter 2, convey impulses from the motor cortex to the *anterior horn cells* of the spinal cord. These cells, the lower motor neurons (LMNs), give rise to the motor fibers of the peripheral nerves (Fig. 5-1).

Motor fibers exit the anterior spinal cord, and most mingle within the cervical or lumbosacral plexuses to form the major peripheral nerves, such as the femoral and radial nerves. Since many of these nerves are quite long, especially in the legs, they must conduct electrochemical impulses without diminution over considerable distances. *Myelin*, a lipid-based sheath surrounding the nerve fiber, acts as insulation for the transmission of these impulses.

When the nerve impulse reaches the terminal of the motor neurons, packets of acetylcholine (ACh) are released from storage vesicles. The ACh crosses the neuromuscular junction, binds to ACh receptors located on the muscle end plate, and thereby triggers muscle contraction (Chapter 6).

Sensory information is also transmitted along fibers within the peripheral

---

* Patients with Guillain-Barré syndrome may receive assistance from the Guillain-Barré Syndrome Support Group, P.O. Box 262, Wynnewood, PA 19096, (215) 649-7837. Those with ALS may receive assistance from the ALS and Neuromuscular Foundation, 2351 Clay, San Francisco, CA 94115, (415) 923-3604, The Amyotrophic Lateral Sclerosis Association, 15300 Ventura Boulevard, Sherman Oaks, CA 91403, (818) 990-2151, and The National A.L.S. Foundation, 185 Madison Avenue, New York, NY 10016.

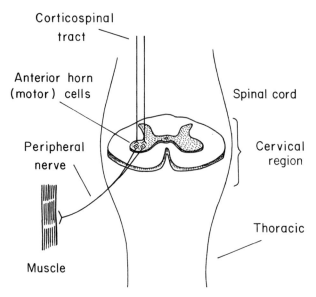

FIGURE 5–1. Within the spinal cord, the corticospinal tract synapses onto the *anterior horn cells*. The axons of these motor neurons join sensory fibers to form peripheral nerves.

nerves, but from the PNS to the CNS. Impulses from receptors in the skin, tendons, joints, and other areas flow toward the brain through peripheral nerves to the spinal cord. Virtually all major peripheral nerves carry both motor and sensory fibers.

CLINICAL CONDITIONS

Mononeuropathies are disorders of single peripheral nerves. Impairment of each major nerve causes a characteristic pattern of motor and sensory loss: paresis, DTR loss, and *hypalgesia* (loss of painful sensation) (Table 5-1).

The loss of an individual peripheral nerve often results from blunt trauma.

TABLE 5–1.   MAJOR PERIPHERAL MONONEUROPATHIES

	Major Associated Deficits		
Nerve	MOTOR PARESIS	DTR LOST	SENSORY LOSS
Median	Thumb and wrist flexor (thenar atrophy)	None	Thumb and index finger
Ulnar	Finger and thumb adduction ("claw hand")	None	Fourth and fifth fingers
Radial	Wrist and thumb extensors ("wrist drop")	Brachioradialis*	Dorsum of hand
Femoral	Knee extensors	Quandriceps (knee)	Anterior thigh
Sciatic	Ankle dorsi- and plantar flexors ("flail ankle")	Achilles (ankle)	Lateral calf and most of foot
Common peroneal	Ankle dorsiflexors and evertors ("foot drop")	None	Dorsum of foot and lateral calf

*When the radial nerve is damaged by compression in the spiral groove of the humerus, the triceps DTR is preserved.

Many nerves have long courses, during which they are protected in certain areas only by the overlying skin and subcutaneous tissue. These points are vulnerable to compression. For example, the radial nerve is subject to damage as it winds around the lateral humerus (Fig. 5-2), and the common peroneal nerve is apt to be injured as it winds around the lateral aspect of the fibula. Even leaning against the upper arm for several hours may therefore result in a "wrist drop," whereas pressure from continous crossing of the knees or wearing a tight lower leg cast may result in a "foot drop."

Likewise, some nerves pass through soft-tissue tunnels where they are in danger of being compressed. For example, because the median nerve passes through the cramped carpal tunnel of the wrist, minor trauma or fluid retention before menses or during pregnancy can entrap this nerve in the wrist. Median nerve damage within the carpal tunnel is called the *carpal tunnel syndrome*. This common condition causes painful paresthesias, especially at night, in the thumb and adjacent two fingers. In severe cases, pain develops in all the fingers and extends upward from the wrist toward the elbow, and thumb weakness develops. Typically, percussion on the flexor surface of the wrist elicits pain at the wrist that radiates to the palm (Tinel's sign).

Peripheral nerve damage can also result from diabetes mellitus, vasculitis (e.g., lupus, polyarteritis nodosa), lead intoxication, and other systemic illnesses. Mononeuropathies, which are occasionally the first clinical manifestation of these conditions, are often quite painful at their onset.

Mononeuritis multiplex is the injury of a combination of two or more, but not all, individual peripheral nerves. In addition, cranial nerve involvement might be found. For example, a patient with damage to the left radial, right sciatic, and right third cranial nerve would be said to have mononeuritis multiplex. This condition, which is less common than simple mononeuropathies, is usually the result of diabetes mellitus, vasculitis, or, in Africa and Asia, leprosy.

Polyneuropathy, or *neuropathy*, which does occur quite frequently, is the generalized, symmetric involvement of all peripheral nerves. It usually affects nerves in proportion to their length. Thus, the earliest symptoms are in the toes and feet, and then in the fingers and hands.

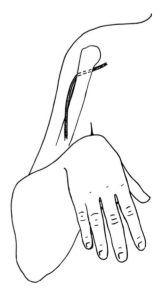

FIGURE 5–2. As the radial nerve winds around the humerus, it is liable to be compressed when an intoxicated person leans against the upper arm for several hours. When the radial nerve is damaged in this way, the wrist, finger, and thumb extensor muscles become paretic. Paralysis of extension of the wrist is called a "wrist drop."

Patients' symptoms usually reflect both sensory and motor impairment, although in some illnesses one or the other impairment may predominate. Patients generally have paresthesias in the distal part of their arms or legs. For example, they might describe "burning" or "tingling" in the fingers and toes. Sensory loss in the hands and feet, *stocking-glove hypalgesia* (Fig. 5-3), is another characteristic of neuropathy and a reflection of nerves being affected in proportion to their length.

As for motor impairment, patients will have weakness in the distal portions of their limbs and therefore difficulty using their fingers to perform fine, skilled movements, e.g., buttoning a shirt. Also, since their ankle and toe muscles will be much weaker than their hip muscles, patients will have difficulty raising their feet when they walk or climb stairs. Neuropathy usually leads to muscle atrophy and flaccidity and to loss of wrist and ankle DTRs because of interruption of the LMN (Fig. 2-2C).

Common Neuropathies

Guillain-Barré Syndrome

Neuropathy can be caused by many conditions; however, the most common causes are Guillain-Barré syndrome, diabetes mellitus, old age, nutritional problems including alcoholism, or exposure to a toxic substance (Table 5-2).

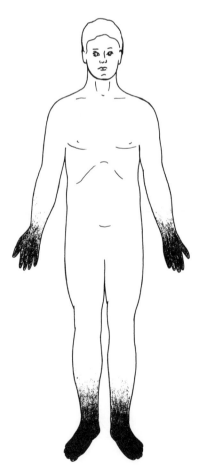

FIGURE 5–3. In cases of polyneuropathy, sensation is lost symmetrically and most severely in the distal portions of the limbs, and the legs are more severely involved than the arms. Since decreased pain sensation, hypalgesia, follows the pattern of someone wearing knee stockings and gloves, patients with this disturbance are said to have "stocking-glove hypalgesia."

TABLE 5–2.   IMPORTANT CAUSES OF NEUROPATHY

Endogenous toxins
    Diabetes mellitus
    Uremia*
    Acure intermittent and variegate porphyria*
Nutritional deficiencies
    Starvation: dieting, malabsorption, alcoholism*
    Combined-system disease/pernicious anemia*
Medicines
    Vitamin B_6 (pyridoxine)
    INH, nitrofurantoin, antineoplastic agents
Industrial or chemical toxins†
    Nitrous oxide (anesthesia)
    Metals: lead, organic and inorganic mercury
    Organic solvents: n-hexane and others (toluene*)
Infectious/inflammatory conditions
    Vasculitis: systemic lupus, polyarteritis*
    Infectious: mononucleosis, hepatitis, Lyme disease,* idiopathic (Guillain-Barré), leprosy, syphilis,*
        AIDS*
Familial (genetic) diseases
    Charcot-Marie-Tooth
    Friedreich's ataxia and other spinocerebellar degenerations
    Metachromatic leukodystrophy*

* Associated with mental status abnormalities.
† May be substances of abuse.

Idiopathic or "postinfectious demyelinating polyneuropathy," commonly known as the Guillain-Barré syndrome, is the quintessential PNS illness. It is a disorder of young and middle-aged adults in which patients first develop paresthesias and sensory loss of their fingers and toes, often after a viral respiratory illness. Over the next several days they develop areflexia, flaccid paresis in their limbs, initially in their feet and hands. The loss of motor function is much greater than the loss of sensation. Often patients become paraparetic. Sometimes they become quadriplegic and apneic (from paresis of the phrenic and intercostal nerves).

Their cerebrospinal fluid characteristically has a markedly elevated protein concentration (Table 20-1). The illness usually resolves spontaneously over 3 weeks to 3 months as the PNS myelin regenerates. Its severity and duration can be reduced with plasmapheresis. In this recently developed technique, which is also useful for myasthenia gravis, serum proteins, presumably including globulins that are toxic to myelin, are filtered from the blood. Attempting to remove substances toxic to the CNS has been attempted in schizophrenia, but plasmapheresis was not beneficial.

Guillain-Barré syndrome epitomizes the distinction between diseases of the PNS and CNS. Although paraparesis or quadriparesis with apnea might be a feature common to severe illness affecting either system, the patterns of muscle weakness, change in reflexes, and sensory distribution (Table 5-3) will implicate a brain or spinal cord injury (CNS damage) or a neuropathy (PNS damage). Also, in Guillain-Barré syndrome, as in most neuropathies other than diabetic neuropathy (see below), bladder, bowel, and sexual function are preserved. These pelvic organs might be spared in neuropathies because the nerves innervating them are relatively short fibers of the autonomic nervous system. With spinal cord disease, in contrast, patients usually have incontinence and impotence at the onset of the injury.

**TABLE 5-3.   CONTRAST OF CENTRAL AND
PERIPHERAL NERVOUS SYSTEM SIGNS**

	Central Nervous System	Peripheral Nervous System
Motor system	*Upper motor neuron*	*Lower motor neuron*
Paresis	Patterns*	Distral
Tone	Spastic†	Flaccid
Bulk	Normal	Atrophic
Fasciculations	No	Sometimes
Reflexes		
DTRs	Hyperactive	Hypoactive
Plantar	Babinski sign(s)	Absent
Sensation: areas	Patterns*	Hands and feet

* Examples: motor and sensory loss of one side or lower half of the body
(e.g., hemiparesis or paraparesis) and hemisensory loss.
† May be flaccid initially.

Another clinical consideration is the differences between demyelinating diseases of the CNS and PNS. Despite performing a similar insulating function, CNS and PNS myelin differ in their cells of origin (oligodendrocytes and Schwann cells, respectively), chemical composition, and antigenic capacity. Although damaged PNS myelin is regenerated and patients with Guillain-Barré syndrome recover, damaged CNS myelin is not regenerated, and clinical impairments are often permanent.

Demyelination of the CNS, in multiple sclerosis, for example, results in recurring, cumulative deficits referable to several discrete CNS areas, including the optic nerves (Chapter 15). The partial or even complete recovery that multiple sclerosis patients seem to achieve between episodes is probably from an inflammatory response subsiding, rather than regeneration of myelin. When the demyelination illness affects large areas of the cerebral CNS myelin, as often occurs in chronic progressively severe cases, it routinely results in dementia and other mental change.

From a psychiatric perspective, despite profound motor impairments, patients with uncomplicated cases of Guillain-Barré syndrome do not develop mental changes because it is a disease of the PNS. However, mental changes commonly occur when patients develop complications, such as cerebral anoxia from respiratory insufficiency, psychosis from high-dose steroids, hydrocephalus from retarded normal cerebrospinal fluid reabsorption, fluid and electrolyte imbalance, or ICU "psychosis" from days of being in a life-threatening situation with sleep deprivation. In other words, if patients with Guillain-Barré develop mental changes, serious medical complications may be the cause, and unless the patient is already on a respirator, sedatives and neuroleptics that might depress respirations should be avoided.

Diabetes

Diabetes mellitus, in contrast to Guillain-Barré syndrome, is associated with a neuropathy that is predominantly sensory. Unless the diabetes has led to brain damage, the neuropathy is not associated with mental aberrations. Almost all patients with diabetes for more than 10 years have loss of sensation and DTRs in the feet and ankles. Many suffer from painful paresthesias, which are especially distressing at night. Episodes of severe pain last for months and spontaneously subside. Although phenytoin (Dilantin) and carbamazepine (Tegretol) might be helpful in suppressing pain during a flare-up, tricyclic antidepressant medications taken at bedtime reduce the pain and also afford a restful night of sleep (Chapter 14).

In longstanding diabetic neuropathy, sensation in the fingertips is impaired, preventing those diabetics who are blind from "reading" Braille. For most patients, however, strength usually remains relatively normal.

Besides having neuropathy and mononeuritis multiplex, patients with long-standing diabetes can also have autonomic nervous system injury that includes impairment of gastrointestinal mobility, bladder muscle contraction, ejaculatory function, and impotence (Chapter 16). Unfortunately, fastidious control of blood glucose does not prevent diabetic neuropathy, but it does tend to postpone its onset or reduce its severity.

Aging Neuropathy

Elderly people have sensory losses attributable to peripheral nerve degeneration. This condition is not yet considered a neuropathy and has not yet been given a name, but it is an important entity. Almost all otherwise normal people who are 80 years of age or older have loss of some position and vibratory sensation in their toes and feet. Their sensory loss, which is accompanied by loss of ankle DTRs, prevents elderly persons from standing with their feet placed closely together. More important, it contributes to their falling.

Nutritional Neuropathies

Contrary to popular opinion, alcoholic neuropathy probably results not as much from alcohol as from the "starvation" that occurs when alcoholics subsist on alcohol and other carbohydrates devoid of thiamine (vitamin B_1). Likewise, although alcohol is directly toxic to the brain, starvation is important in the alcoholism associated with dementia and the Wernicke-Korsakoff syndrome. The neuropathy associated with alcoholism is predominantly, but not exclusively, sensory. Alcoholics with neuropathy usually have normal strength but mild loss of position perception and other sensations in their feet and ankles. The sensory loss is usually asymptomatic except when patients walk in the dark and must rely on position sense in their feet.

Starvation in other forms is also prone to cause neuropathy in a wide variety of clinical circumstances. Patients with anorexia nervosa occasionally develop a neuropathy that is predominantly sensory. However, possibly because these patients usually have some selective food intake and often scrupulously take vitamins, they have a low incidence of clinically significant impairment. Patients with metastatic cancer may develop a neuropathy that can be debilitating and, as is other nutritional neuropathies, is predominantly sensory. Another variety of nutritional neuropathy follows gastric bypass, gastric partitioning, and other gastrointestinal surgical procedures for obesity. These procedures create malabsorption. In many cases, the postoperative metabolic imbalance is so severe that cognitive and behavioral changes have also developed.

Not only does starvation lead directly to neuropathy but it also depletes the subcutaneous fat that normally wraps large nerves in a protective coat. Without this protection, nerves are susceptible to compression and other forms of minor trauma. Thus, people on "crash diets" quite commonly develop a foot drop from a peroneal nerve injury or a wrist drop from a radial nerve injury (Table 5-1 and Fig. 5-2).

Recently, food faddists have been found to have developed neuropathy when they have taken excessive quantities of vitamin B_6 (pyridoxine). Although the normal adult requirement of this vitamin is only 2 to 4 mg daily, many individuals who had been consuming several grams daily developed a profound sensory neuropathy.

Neuropathies Associated with Mental Status Abnormalities

Although finding mental status abnormalities in someone with brain injury would be entirely expectable, such abnormalities in a patient with a neuropathy, although rare, would indicate the presence of a neurologic condition rather than an exclusively psychogenic one, the co-existence of CNS and PNS involvement, or several specific illnesses (Table 5-2).

ACUTE INTERMITTENT PORPHYRIA (AIP). This classic illness, also called "Swedish porphyria," is an autosomal dominant genetic disorder of porphyrin metabolism. Patients with AIP experience attacks in which they develop combinations of colicky abdominal pain, mental disturbances that have been so bizarre as to be called "psychosis," and a neuropathy that can result in quadriplegia. During attacks the urine turns red. The Watson-Schwartz test and other tests for urinary porphyrins will be positive. Although attacks may be exacerbated if the patient is given barbiturates, phenothiazines may be given for psychosis. AIP and a related disorder, *variegate* or South African porphyria, which has similar manifestations, are both rare in the United States. Nevertheless, both conditions should be considered; either could be easily mistaken for a functional psychosis or a psychosomatic illness because of the nondescript, although often severe, abdominal pain and mental aberrations.

ALCOHOLISM. As noted before, neuropathy and dementia are frequent complications of alcoholism. In most casts, alcoholics have mental aberrations and peripheral neuropathy, but some have neuropathy without dementia or other aspects of Wernicke-Korsakoff syndrome (Chapter 2). Alcoholism can also cause degeneration of the cerebellum, damage to the pons (central pontine myelinolysis), and alcohol withdrawal seizures (Chapter 10).

COMBINED-SYSTEM DISEASE (PERNICIOUS ANEMIA OR B_{12} DEFICIENCY). Neuropathy is present in combined-system disease, although it is overshadowed by signs of spinal cord dysfunction and dementia. This disease is diagnosed by determining the serum B_{12} level or by performing a Schilling test and is treated with B_{12} injections. Since folic acid can reverse the anemia and other hematologic aspects of the disease, but permits the neurologic complications to worsen, folic acid can mask an important finding in patients with dementia.

LYME DISEASE. Named for the town in Connecticut where the disease was recently described as a form of arthritis, Lyme disease has become endemic in coastal New England, eastern Long Island, Wisconsin and Minnesota, and the Pacific Northwest. It is an infectious illness caused by a spirochete, *Borelia burgdorferi.* The most common vector is a tick that is carried by deer. The peak incidence for Lyme disease is June through September, when people are most likely to be bitten by the ticks as they walk in wooded areas.

Lyme disease is an indolent illness that affects several body systems in varying severity. Patients initially have systemic symptoms, typically including malaise, low grade fever, and arthralgias. They may also have a peculiar but poorly named skin lesion, *erythema chronicum migrans* (moving red rash), consisting of a red ring several inches in diameter that surrounds a red dot. This bull's-eye-shaped rash is often the site of the tick bite. A prominent feature of the illness, which may be its first manifestation, is arthritis that can mimic juvenile rheumatoid arthritis. Another common manifestation is cardiac arrhythmias. Lyme disease's tendency toward variable, multisystem manifestations is reminiscent of the more infamous spirochete infection, syphilis, which, because of its protean manifestations, was known as the "great imitator" of other illnesses.

Peripheral nervous system involvement is the most common nervous system manifestation of Lyme disease. In the initial phases of the illness, patients often have facial nerve palsy, unilaterally or bilaterally, that appears as Bell's palsy on one or both sides (Fig. 4-14). Other common symptoms are paresthesias and pain in the limbs as a result of nerve involvement. Sometimes PNS involvement is so extensive and severe that patients develop quadriparesis that mimics Guillain-Barré syndrome.

CNS involvement sometimes consists of headaches, meningeal signs, and, presumably because of encephalitis, mental aberrations that range from irritability to delirium. Dementia and psychosis have both been attributed to Lyme disease. At the onset of the illness, often when it is still undiagnosed, patients have persistent fatigue, continual dull headache, and similar nonspecific symptoms that are liable to be misinterpreted as depression or a psychosomatic illness. Occasionally, CNS signs of Lyme disease suggest multiple sclerosis.

The diagnosis of Lyme disease should be confirmed by serologic tests; however, since these tests have a significantly high false-negative rate, negative results should be repeated in suspected cases. Although the CSF will have variable degrees of pleocytosis and concentrations of protein and glucose, it will often test positive for Lyme disease. Treatment depends on the organs involved. Central nervous system involvement may require 2 weeks of intravenous antibiotics.

ACQUIRED IMMUNODEFICIENCY SYNDROME (AIDS). Among the many neurologic manifestations of AIDS, including dementia that affects 70 percent of patients (Chapter 7), a neuropathy can be detected when appropriate clinical and laboratory examinations, such as nerve conduction velocity studies, are performed. The neuropathy is probably caused by a direct viral infection of the peripheral nerve. The neuropathy accounts for some of the debility that eventually affects AIDS patients; however, unlike CNS involvement, it is usually a late manifestation of the illness.

An additional consideration is that AIDS predisposes patients to other nervous system infections. In particular, AIDS has been responsible for an increase in the incidence of syphilis. In patients with both illnesses, syphilis has usually been of the meningovascular variety, which is an acute meningitis or encephalitis condition, rather than the chronic varieties, such as dementia or tabes dorsalis.

Patients with *tabes dorsalis* often have signs of neuropathy. Their primary symptom is often lancinating, radicular pains that are accompanied by loss of the DTRs. Over 90 percent of patients also have Argyll-Robertson pupillary abnormalities. The clinical diagnosis can be confirmed by a positive FTA or VDRL test on the cerebrospinal fluid, but a negative result does not exclude a diagnosis (Chapter 7).

UREMIA. Uremic neuropathy is commonplace in patients undergoing maintenance hemodialysis. If uremia becomes pronounced, the neuropathy increases and the patient can develop an encephalopathy.

VASCULITIS.   Vascular inflammatory diseases, such as lupus or polyarteritis nodosa, often create infarctions in both the CNS and PNS arteries. When the arteries supplying the peripheral nerves are damaged, single or multiple mononeuropathies develop. Vascular inflammation in the brain, *cerebritis*, leads to the "3 S's of lupus": seizures, strokes, and psychosis.

METACHROMATIC LEUKODYSTROPHY (MLD).   MLD is a rare, autosomal recessive genetic disease in which both the CNS and PNS have extensive demyelination associated with accumulation of metachromatic granules in many organs. Thus, its symptoms reflect widespread neurologic and non-neurologic damage. Although MLD most often affects infants and children, it has been reported to have occurred in young and middle aged adults.

This illness notably causes dementia and peripheral neuropathy, and the dementia has been misdiagnosed as schizophrenia. In many cases, CNS involvement has caused only personality changes and other nonpsychotic mental changes. MLD also causes cerebellar dysfunction and peripheral neuropathy. Other organs, in addition to the nervous system, such as the gallbladder, testicles, and retina, are also damaged.

Peripheral nerves, which contain cytoplasmic inclusions, have slow conduction velocities. The activity of arylsulfatase A, a ubiquitous enzyme, is markedly decreased in the urine, leukocytes, serum, and amniotic fluid. The illness is diagnosed by demonstrating decreased activity of this enzyme in leukocytes and finding metachromatic lipid material in biopsies of peripheral nerves. No treatment is effective for MLD, and no cure is available for this or other genetic illnesses that cause dementia.

PSYCHIATRIC DISTURBANCES.   Such conditions as anorexia or alcoholism can cause nutritional deficiency neuropathy. Mononeuropathies result from unusual pressure against sensitive areas, as when patients remain in fixed positions during drug or alcohol intoxication or periods of catatonia.

VOLATILE SUBSTANCE ABUSE OR CHRONIC INDUSTRIAL EXPOSURE.   Recently, substance abuse or chronic exposure to certain vapors has been found to induce a profound neuropathy and, depending on the vapor, dementia. For example, nitrous oxide, a common gaseous anesthesia, has been repetitively inhaled by thrill-seekers, including dentists. Usually, after several minutes of euphoria and confusion, individuals return to their usual state. However, after several weeks of exposure, individuals often develop neuropathy although not dementia.

Another example is n-hexane, which is a common industrial solvent that is a major component of glue. Individuals who habitually "sniff glue" and workers who are chronically overexposed to n-hexane vapors develop neuropathy because a lipophilic property of n-hexane impairs PNS myelin. Toluene, which has one of the greatest potentials for abuse, is also a commonplace chemical and a component of solvents and glue. Like n-hexane, toluene is lipophilic, but it permeates CNS myelin and can therefore induce dementia. This dementia is usually accompanied by cerebellar signs, and it may be the first or most prominent manifestation of glue sniffing or other volatile substance abuse. Magnetic resonance imaging (MRI) can confirm CNS myelin injury with overexposure to toluene.

When ethylene oxide, carbon disulfide, and other industrial products, which have little potential for abuse, are inhaled in high enough concentrations for several months, they can attack both the CNS and PNS myelin and cause neuropathy and dementia. However, there is still controversy over whether industrial exposure to low concentrations of these substances on a chronic basis can lead to personality changes, subtle cognitive impairments, and fatigue.

Amyotrophic Lateral Sclerosis and Other Motor Neuron Disorders

Amyotrophic lateral sclerosis (ALS), a relatively uncommon disorder but one that merits special attention, is the best-known example of a *motor neuron disease*. In ALS, both upper and lower motor neurons degenerate, but sensory systems are unaffected. More important, despite the widespread CNS (motor neuron) destruction, mental faculties are preserved. The etiology of ALS remains an enigma, but recent work on similar diseases has shown that "slow virus" infections may cause this fearsome illness.

Amyotrophic lateral sclerosis is usually found only in people 45 years of age or older. One exception, however, was Lou Gehrig, the famous baseball player who developed ALS when he was about 37 years old and at the height of his career; thus, for decades ALS was known as "Lou Gehrig's disease."

Patients with ALS usually first notice weakness and subcutaneous muscular twitching, *fasciculations*, in a single limb. Initially, examination of the affected limb will alsoreveal paresis and atrophy—signs that together with the fasciculations reflect damage to the anterior horn cells of the spinal cord. In time, signs tend to spread in an asymmetric pattern to the other limbs (Fig. 5-4).

Characteristically, even atrophic muscles will have brisk DTRs. This surprising finding of hyperactive DTRs with muscle atrophy probably is the result of the

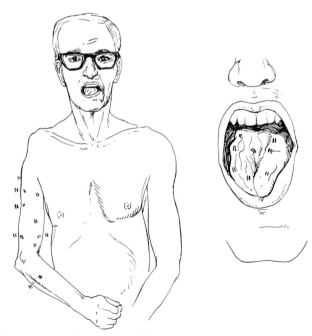

FIGURE 5–4. This elderly gentleman, who suffers from ALS, has typical (right arm) asymmetric limb atrophy, paresis, and fasciculations. His tongue also has fasciculations and atrophy, as indicated by clefts and furrows.

remaining lower motor neurons being supplied by damaged upper motor neurons. The hyperactive DTRs are naturally accompanied by Babinski signs, which are another manifestation of upper motor damage.

As ALS advances, atrophy and fasciculations will be recognized in the facial, pharyngeal, and tongue (bulbar) muscles, as well as in the limb muscles. Patients will then suffer from dysarthria and dysphagia, i.e., bulbar palsy. Pseudobulbar palsy usually will also be present. It will be indicated by a hyperactive gag reflex and jaw jerk. Being superimposed upon bulbar palsy, pseudobulbar palsy will eventually make speech unintelligible and swallowing impossible. Despite extensive motor impairment, ocular muscle control and bladder-bowel function remain entirely normal.

Patients remain tragically alert, mentally competent, and completely aware of their plight throughout the course of their disease, which is untreatable. Death usually occurs within 2 to 4 years from respiratory complications.

There are, unfortunately, other motor neuron diseases. These diseases, which also cause extensive loss of anterior horn cells, differ from ALS primarily in that upper motor neurons are not affected. Hereditary varieties of motor neuron diseases in infants (Werdnig-Hoffmann disease) and in adolescents (Kugelberg-Welander disease) are both characterized by flaccid quadriplegia with atrophic, areflexic muscles.

Poliomyelitis (polio) was the most frequently occurring motor neuron disease until development of the Salk vaccine. In this illness, viral infections damaged the anterior horn (motor neuron) cells of different regions of the spinal cord or lower brainstem (the bulb). Polio patients had paresis with muscle fasciculations and absent DTRs. When more than one limb was involved, the paralysis was typically asymmetric. Patients who suffered bulbar polio, and were said to have bulbar palsy (Chapter 4), had phrenic and intercostal nerve impairment that often caused respiratory muscle paralysis. Most of these patients had to be placed in the notorious "iron lung."

As in ALS, oculomotor, bladder, bowel, and sexual functions are normal in all forms of poliomyelitis (Chapters 12 and 16). Polio patients likewise retain normal mental function. Unfortunately, as recent studies have found, middle-age individuals who had poliomyelitis in childhood tend to develop an ALS-like condition, the *postpolio syndrome*, in which they develop further weakness accompanied by fasciculations.

Benign Fasciculations

Several innocent phenomena resemble motor neuron diseases. These conditions are transient and certainly not harbingers of neurologic disease. They are, nevertheless, frequently of great concern to medical students and others acquainted with ALS.

Many people have *benign fasciculations* in which muscle twitchings are not associated with weakness, atrophy, or reflex changes. They are usually precipitated by excessive physical exertion, psychologic stress, use of tobacco, excessive coffee intake, or exposure to some insecticides.

Myokymia, in which fasciculations are confined to the orbicularis oculi (eyelids), produces an annoying twitching or jerking movement around the eye. It also seems to be caused mostly by fatigue and anxiety. On the other hand, if the movements are forceful enough to close the eyelids and have a duration of 1 second, they may represent a facial dyskinesia (see blepharospasm, Chapter 18).

Orthopedic Disturbances

In cervical spondylosis, which can mimic ALS but is far more common, osteoarthritic changes of the vertebrae lead to encroachment on the foramina and narrowing of the spinal canal. Cervical nerve roots are pinched, and sometimes the spinal cord becomes compressed (Fig. 5-5). Because of the cervical nerve compression, patients might have neck pain with arm accompanied by hand paresis, atrophy, hypoactive DTRs, and fasciculations—signs of lower motor neuron injury. Depending on several factors, various sensory changes will be present. Patients with spinal cord compression will have lower extremity spasticity, hyperreflexia, and Babinski signs—signs of upper motor neuron injury.

Similarly, patients with *lumbar spondylosis* have lumbar nerve compression, and they will complain of low back pain. Although they could not have spinal cord compression (because the spinal cord terminates at the first lumbar vertebra [Fig. 16-1]), patients will have signs of damage to the lumbar peripheral nerves: leg and feet paresis, atrophy, fasciculations, sensory loss, and paresthesias. Most important, spondylosis, unlike ALS, is associated with spine pain; sensory loss in the limbs; and normal facial, pharyngeal, and tongue musculature.

Herniated intervertebral disks ("herniated disks") are one of several causes of low back pain, which is a ubiquitous condition and the most expensive American work-related injury. Each year, it disables over 5 million Americans and costs the public 16 billion dollars (Frymayer). Only a fraction of cases of low back pain are caused by herniated disks. Other causes are muscle and spine injury and retroperitoneal conditions, including endometriosis. As much as in any other neurologic condition, psychologic factors contribute to etiology, disability, and prognosis. Yet of all the potential causes, herniated disks are possibly the most important cause because they can injure nerve roots and because nerve root injury is the indication most commonly offered for surgery.

Herniated disks usually stem from prolonged pressure at the curve of the lower part of the spine. Strains, poor posture, or obesity squeeze the gelatinous intervertebral disk material that cushions adjacent vertebral bodies. Extruded (herniated) disk material presses against the adjacent nerve root. Over 90 percent of disk herniations involve the intervertebral disk at either the L4-5 or L5-S1 interspace (Fig. 5-6).

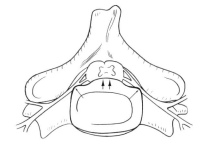

FIGURE 5–5. When cervical spondylosis occurs, both upper motor neurons (UMNs) and lower motor neurons (LMNs) may be damaged. The cervical spinal cord (UMNs) can be compressed by intervertebral ridges of bone (*double arrows*). The cervical nerve roots (LMNs) can be compressed by bony constrictions at the foramina (*single arrows*).

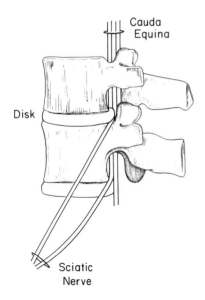

Cauda
Equina

Disk

Sciatic
Nerve

FIGURE 5–6. As the cauda equina branches to form the lumbar and sacral nerves, the nerve roots leave the spinal canal through foramina, where they might be compressed by herniations of the intervertebral disks. Patients with herniated disks will often feel pain radiating along the distribution of the sciatic nerve, as well as in their lower back. Their pains will be intensified by movements, such as coughing, sneezing, or straining at stool, that transiently further herniate the disk.

Patients with herniated lumbar disks usually complain mostly of low back pain and also of paresthesias that radiate to the buttocks and down the posterior or lateral aspect of the leg along the compressed nerve. Characteristically, buttock and leg pain, as well as the low back pain, is increased by coughing, sneezing, or elevating the straightened leg because these maneuvers press the herniated disk more strongly against the nerve root (Fig. 5-7). Pain that radiates in the distribution of the sciatic nerve, *sciatica*, is characteristic of a lumbar herniated disk and distinguishes it from other causes of low back pain.

If the herniation is large, it can lead to paresis and areflexia of ankle or toe muscles. Disk protrusions are occasionally so large that they affect the sacral nerve roots and cause bladder or sexual dysfunction. On the other hand, sexual dysfunction can rarely be legitimately attributed to low back pain or a herniated disk in the absence of paresis, areflexia, or previous spine surgery.

Cervical intervertebral disks will sometimes be herniated by trauma, such as a "whiplash" automobile injury. These patients will have neck pain that radiates down their arms and sometimes loss of a DTR. In this situation, as in low back pain, orthopedic and psychologic factors are very important.

Many patients with chronic low back pain are best approached by considering the pain itself as a chronic illness that the physician can ameliorate but not cure (Chapter 14). The goal might be improvement in function, rather than pain relief. In such cases, addictive analgesics and surgery must be avoided. Instead, physical therapy can become the mainstay of a treatment plan. A psychiatrist might prescribe antidepressant medications because they seem to have a particularly useful analgesic effect, even at doses that are smaller than those used for depression. Transcutaneous electrical nerve stimulation (TENS) also seems to be helpful, and this technique may be given as a short trial. Some patients respond to biofeedback and other predominantly psychologic approaches. Also, when patients involved in an accident assert that they have intractable pain and permanent disability, but have little or no objective impairments, they should be urged to conclude all litigation before physicians can be expected to relieve their pain.

Finally, the indications for surgery for herniated intervertebral disks must

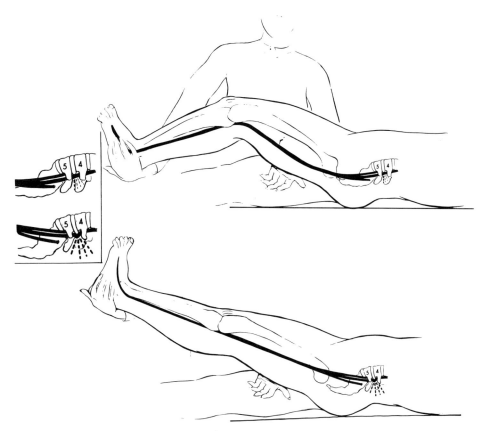

FIGURE 5–7. In cases of herniated disks, the low back pain will be intensified and often made to radiate to the buttocks if an examiner raises the patient's *straightened* leg (Lasègue's sign). In this maneuver the nerve root is compressed and irritated because it is drawn tautly against the edge of the herniated disk.

be strictly limited. Chronic pain alone is not a valid indication for surgery. Although a thorough psychologic assessment is necessary, the Minnesota Multiphasic Personality Inventory and other psychologic screening tests are unreliable in identifying those patients who will have a good surgical outcome.

REFERENCES

Abarbanel JM, Berginer VM, Osimani A, et al: Neurologic complications after gastric restriction surgery for morbid obesity. Neurology 37:196, 1987

Bailey RO, Baltch AL, Venkatesh R, et al: Sensory motor neuropathy associated with AIDS. Neurology 38:886, 1988

Crystal HA, Schaumburg HH, Grober E, et al: Cognitive impairment and sensory loss associated with chronic low-level ethylene oxide exposure. Neurology 38:567, 1988

Dalakas MC, Elder G, Hallett M, et al: A long-term follow-up study of patients with post-poliomyelitis neuromuscular symptoms. N Engl J Med 314:15, 1986

Eidelberg D, Sotrel A, Vogel H, et al: Progressive polyradiculopathy in acquired immune deficiency syndrome. Neurology 36:912, 1986

Ellenberg M: Diabetic neuropathy. In Ellenberg M, Rifkin H: Diabetes Mellitus: Theory and Practice, 3rd ed. New York, Medical Examination Publishing Co., 1983

Finelli PF: Metachromatic leukodystrophy manifesting as a schizophrenic disorder. Ann Neurol 18:94, 1985

Finkel MF: Lyme disease and its neurologic complications. Arch Neurol 45:99, 1988

Frymoyer JW: Back pain and sciatica. N Engl J Med *318*:291, 1988

Habicht GS, Beck G, Benach JL: Lyme disease. Sci Am *257*:78, 1987

Hormes JT, Filley CM, Rosenberg, NL: Neurologic sequelae of chronic solvent vapor abuse. Neurology *36*:698, 1986

Max MB, Culnane M, Schafer RNC, et al: Amitriptyline relieves diabetic neuropathy pain in patients with normal or depressed mood. Neurology *37*:589, 1987

Rosenberg NL, Kleinschmidt-DeMasters BK, Davis KA, et al: Toluene abuse causes diffuse central nervous system white matter changes. Ann Neurol *23*:611, 1988

Ryan CM, Morrow LA, Hodgson M: Cacosmia and neurobehavioral dysfunction associated with occupational exposure to mixtures of organic solvents. Am J Psychiatry *145*:1442, 1988

Sahenk Z, Mendell JR, Couri D, et al: Polyneuropathy from inhalation of N_2O cartridges through a whipped-cream dispenser. Neurology *28*:485, 1978

Schaumberg H, Kaplan J, Windebank A, et al: Sensory neuropathy from pyridoxine abuse: A new megavitamin syndrome. N Engl J Med *309*:445, 1983

Schaumburg HH, Spencer PS, Thomas PK: Disorders of Peripheral Nerves. Philadelphia, F. A. Davis Co., 1983

Seppalainen AM, Lindstrom K, Martelin T: Neurophysiological and psychological picture of solvent poisoning. Am J Ind Med *1*:31, 1980

So YT, Holtzman DM, Abrams DI, et al: Peripheral neuropathy associated with acquired immunodeficiency syndrome. Arch Neurol *45*:945, 1988

Waltz G, Harik SI, Kaufman B: Adult metachromatic leukodystrophy: Value of computed tomographic scanning and magnetic resonance imaging of the brain. Arch Neurol *44*:225, 1987

Westermeyer J: The psychiatrist and solvent-inhalant abuse: Recognition, assessment, and treatment. Am J Psychiatry *144*:903, 1987

QUESTIONS: CHAPTER 5

1. A 21-year-old heroin addict who overdoses awakens with an inability to extend his right wrist or fingers. All DTRs are intact except for the right brachioradialis DTR. Where is the lesion and what is its cause?

2. An 18-year-old woman has fatigue, a low grade fever, and "tingling" in her fingers and toes. On examination, she has splenomegaly; paresis of the ankle, knees, and wrists; absent DTRs; and hypalgesia in the feet. What process is evolving?

3. A 40-year-old obese man has the sudden onset of low back pain with inability to dorsiflex and evert his right ankle. Raising his straightened right leg produces back pain that radiates down the lateral leg. Sensation is diminished on the dorsum of the right foot. No alteration in DTRs is detectable. What is his problem?

4. A 54-year-old man with pulmonary carcinoma experiences 2 weeks of midthoracic back pain. He complains of the sudden onset of abnormal sensation in his legs and difficulty walking. Examination reveals marked weakness of both legs, areflexia of the legs, and hypalgesia from the toes to the umbilicus. What process is evolving?

5. A 27-year-old drug addict overdoses while sitting on a toilet. On awakening, he is unable to walk. Examination reveals paresis of the knee flexor (hamstring) muscles and all ankle and toe muscles. Although the knee DTRs are normal, the ankle DTRs and plantar reflexes are absent. Sensation is absent below the knees. Where is (are) the lesion(s) and what is the cause?

6. A 58-year-old carpenter complains of weakness of his right arm and hand. Examination reveals fasciculations and atrophy of the hand and triceps muscles with no elicitable triceps reflex. There is mild sensory loss along the medial surface of his right hand. What process is occurring?

7. A 30-year-old pregnant woman complains of tingling and numbness of the thumb and adjacent finger of both hands. She frequently drops objects. Examination reveals hypalgesia in the area she described as "numb" and mild paresis of some of the thumb flexor and opposition muscles. Percussion of the wrist recreates the paresthesias. Reflexes are normal. Where is (are) the lesion(s) and what is the cause?

8. A young woman has confusion and hallucinations, flaccid paresis, and abdominal pain. Her urine is red. What disease does she have? What test should be done immediately?

9. A 21-year-old woman has the sudden onset of inability to elevate and evert her right ankle. Although her DTR and plantar reflexes are normal, there is an area of hypalgesia on the lateral aspect of the calf and dorsum of the foot. Where is the lesion and what are possible causes?

10. Several workers in a chemical factory complain of tingling of their fingers and toes and weakness of the feet. Each worker has a stocking-glove hypalgesia and absent ankle DTRs. Which objective finding suggests that they suffer from a neuropathy? What are the common causes of industrial neuropathies?

11. A 29-year-old woman, recently found to have hypertension, rapidly develops a paresis of the dorsiflexors and evertors of the right foot, paresis of the extensors of the wrist and thumb of the left hand, and paresis of abduction of the right eye. Where is (are) the lesion(s) and what are the possible causes?

12. A 17-year-old man, after a (losing) fistfight, complains of inability to walk or feel anything below his waist. He has complete inability to move his legs, which have normally active DTRs and plantar responses. He has no response to noxious (pinprick) stimulation below his umbilicus, but sensation of position, vibration, and temperature is preserved. Where and what is the lesion?

13. A 68-year-old diabetic man has the sudden onset of pain in the anterior right thigh and difficulty walking. Examination reveals weakness of knee extension, an absent (quadriceps) knee DTR, and hypalgesia of the anterior thigh on the right. Where is the lesion and what is its cause?

14. A 34-year-old man with chronic low back pain has a sudden exacerbation while raking leaves. He has difficulty walking and pain that radiates from the low back down the left posterior thigh to the lateral ankle. He has paresis of plantar flexion of the left ankle and an absent ankle DTR. He has an area of hypalgesia along the left lateral foot. What has happened to him?

15. A 62-year-old man has the gradual onset of weakness of both arms and then the left leg. On examination he is alert and oriented, but has dysarthria. His jaw jerk is hyperactive and the gag reflex is absent. There are atrophy and fasciculations of the tongue and muscles of both arms and left leg. DTRs are hyperactive and Babinski signs are present. Sensation is intact. What disease process is occurring and how extensive is it?

16. A 47-year-old watchmaker is unable to move his thumbs and fingers. He has sensory loss of the medial three fingers but no change in reflexes. Where is (are) the lesion(s) and what is the cause?

17. An elderly man with chronic lumbar back pain radiating down both posterior thighs has paresis and atrophy of the calf muscles. Both ankle and plantar reflexes are absent. Fasciculations are observable in the calf muscles. The toes and dorsum of one foot are analgesic. Does he have ALS?

18. A 42-year-old schoolteacher has weight loss, burning dysesthesias of the feet, and a recent convulsion. Her sclerae are mildly icteric, and she has hepatosplenomegaly. She also has memory impairment, areflexia of the ankle and brachioradialis DTRs, and a stocking-glove hypalgesia. What areas of the nervous system are involved and what are the possible causes?

19. A 24-year-old man who makes and drinks moonshine develops a radial nerve palsy. What is the likely cause?

20. A 25-year-old man has a gait difficulty, from which his older sister also suffers. He has an ataxic gait and tremor on finger-nose and heel-shin movements. He has atrophy of the foot, calf, and hand muscles with areflexia of the plantar reflex and DTRs. He has diminished position and vibratory sensation at the ankles. His speech is scanning. What areas of the nervous system are involved? What type of disease is it?

21–25. Match the cause with the illness.

21. Acquired immunodeficiency syndrome (AIDS)

22. Lyme disease

23. Nitrous oxide neuropathy

24. N-Hexane neuropathy

25. Metachromatic leukodystrophy (MLD)
   a. Genetic abnormality
   b. Glue sniffing
   c. Spirochete infection
   d. Dental anesthetic abuse
   e. Viral infection

26–36. Which conditions are associated with fasciculations? (Yes or No)

26. Guillain-Barré

27. Spinal cord compression

28. Amyotrophic lateral sclerosis (ALS)

29. Insecticide poisoning

30. Werdnig-Hoffmann

31. Fatigue

32. Porphyria

33. Psychogenic stress

34. Cervical spondylosis

35. Lumbar spondylosis

36. Poliomyelitis

37. A 42-year-old man with onset of severe depression is brought to the hospital in coma with cyanosis, hypotension, and bradycardia. He has miosis, but full extraocular movements are observed on oculocephalic testing. There is flaccid, areflexic quadriplegia with fasciculations of the muscles. With what chemical has he attempted suicide? What medication is a relatively specific therapy?

38. Which of the following conditions are associated with sexual dysfunction?
   a. Peroneal nerve palsy
   b. Carpal tunnel syndrome
   c. Diabetes
   d. Poliomyelitis
   e. Multiple sclerosis
   f. Alcoholism
   g. ALS
   h. Myasthenia gravis

39. A 40-year-old man with rapidly advancing Guillain-Barré syndrome develops confusion, overwhelming anxiety, and then agitation. Which of the following statements are correct?
   a. He should be treated with sedation.
   b. He should be treated with tranquilizers.
   c. He may be developing hypoxia, hypercapnea, or both because of chest and diaphragm muscle paresis.
   d. He may have "ICU psychosis."
   e. Guillain-Barré syndrome is generally not associated with CNS complications early in its course.

40. A 43-year-old man admitted to the hospital for evaluation of several months of progressively severe polyneuropathy develops agitation, hallucinations, and disorientation. Of the various causes of neuropathy that are associated with mental status abnormalities, which one leads to mental changes after hospitalization?

41. Why is "glue sniffing" associated with neuropathy and occasionally with cognitive impairment?

42–45. A 60-year-old man who has had mitral valve stenosis and atrial fibrillation suddenly developed quadriplegia with impaired swallowing, breathing, and speaking. He required tracheostomy and a nasogastric feeding tube during the initial part of his hospitalization. Four weeks after the onset of the illness, examination reveals that he appears alert, establishes eye contact, and, although his eyes are immobile, he blinks appropriately to questions. His vision in both visual fields is intact. He remains quadriplegic with hyperactive DTRs and Babinski signs.

42. A preliminary evaluation should determine whether the neurologic condition is caused by CNS or PNS damage. What findings are helpful in this regard?

43. Is it possible to determine if the lesion is within the cerebral cortex or the brainstem?

44. Does the localization make a difference?

45. Which neurologic tests would help distinguish brainstem from extensive cerebral lesions?

46–60. Which conditions are associated with multiple sclerosis, Guillain-Barré syndrome, both, or neither?

46. Areflexic DTRs

47. Typically follows an upper respiratory tract infection

48. Unilateral visual loss

49. Paresthesias

50. Internuclear ophthalmoplegia

51. Paraparesis

52. Mental changes early in the course of the illness

53. Specific therapy available

54. Quadriparesis

55. Recovery through remyelination

56. Leads to pseudobulbar palsy

57. Leads to bulbar palsy

58. Where emotional lability of pseudobulbar palsy is frequently mistaken for "euphoria"

59. Typically a monophasic illness that lasts several weeks

60. Sexual dysfunction can be the only or primary persistent deficit
    a.   Multiple sclerosis
    b.   Guillain-Barré syndrome
    c.   Both
    d.   Neither

61. A 16-year-old woman has been subsisting on minimal quantities of food. She attributes her "good health" to megavitamin treatments. However, she develops symptoms and signs of a neuropathy. In what way can the neurologic picture be ascribed to her eating disorder?

62. Following gastric partitioning for morbid obesity, a 30-year-old man appears to be depressed. On examination, he is inattentive and has signs of a neuropathy. Before full consideration can be given to the change in affect, what evaluations ought to be performed?

63. A 29-year-old lifeguard, employed by a Cape Cod beach, developed profound malaise for 1 week and then bilateral facial weakness. Blood tests for mononucleosis, Lyme disease, AIDS, and other infective illnesses were negative. What should be the next step?

64. In which ways are CNS and PNS myelin similar?
    a.   Both derive from the same cells.
    b.   They are antigenically similar.
    c.   They insulate electrochemical transmissions.
    d.   They are affected by the same illnesses.

ANSWERS

1. The patient has a wrist drop from compression of the radial nerve as it winds around the humerus. This is a common problem in drug addicts and alcoholics who tend to lean against their arm while stuporous. Drug addicts are also liable to develop brain abscesses, AIDS, and cerebrovascular accidents—but these are all diseases of the CNS and would cause hyperactive DTRs, a different pattern of weakness, and probably, since the *right* arm is involved, aphasia.

2. The patient has symptoms and signs of peripheral neuropathy: paresthesias, distal weakness, areflexia, and sensory loss. In view of her systemic illness, the neuropathy may be due to mononucleosis.

3. The patient probably has a herniated intervertebral disk at L4-5 that compresses the L-5 nerve root. Identification of the particular root or disk, however, is not as important as recognizing this problem and its associated neurologic deficit.

4. The patient has an acute spinal cord compression from a metastatic tumor with paraparesis, sensory loss below T-12, and areflexia from "spinal shock." The absence of symptoms in the upper extremities, the presence of a sensory level, and localized back pain are inconsistent with polyneuropathy.

5. The patient has bilateral sciatic nerve injury resulting in paresis of the knee flexors and all foot muscles with loss of ankle reflexes. The sciatic nerves may be compressed while sitting on a toilet seat (toilet seat neuropathy). This is the lower extremity equivalent of the wrist drop, and it is also commonly encountered in drug addicts (see Question 1).

6. He has symptoms and signs of cervical spondylosis with nerve root compression. This condition is common among laborers. Cervical spondylosis resembles ALS because of the atrophy and fasciculations, but the sensory loss precludes that diagnosis. In cervical spondylosis, depending on the degree of foraminal compression, DTRs may be either hyperactive or hypoactive. In ALS, despite the loss of anterior horn cells, DTRs are almost always hyperactive.

7. The patient has bilateral carpal tunnel syndrome, i.e., median nerve compression at the wrist. She has the characteristic sensory and motor disturbances and Tinel's sign (percussion over an injured nerve creating a tingling sensation distally).
    The carpal tunnel syndrome frequently occurs when there is fluid accumulation in the carpal tunnel, e.g., during pregnancy, before menses, and following trauma to the wrist. Acromegaly and hypothyroidism are also conditions that also lead to tissue or fluid accumulation in the carpal tunnel.

8. She has acute intermittent porphyria. This condition may be diagnosed with a Watson-Schwartz test or determination of total urinary porphyrins. Phenothiazines may be used for the mental aberrations, but barbiturates are contraindicated.

9. She has the sudden, painless onset of a peroneal nerve injury. It commonly results from nerve compression by casts, crossing the legs, or leaning against furniture. The nerve is injured at the lateral aspect of the knee where it is covered only by skin and subcutaneous tissue. When patients lose weight, the nerve is vulnerable to compression because subcutaneous fat is depleted. Sometimes diabetes or a vasculitis causes an infarction of the nerve.

10. The loss of ankle DTRs is objective. Although the hypalgesia and other symptoms and signs can be mimicked, areflexia cannot. Heavy metals, organic solvents, N-hexane, and other hydrocarbons are industrial toxins that are frequently implicated as causes of neuropathies.

11. She has developed injuries to several different nerves: the right common peroneal, left radial, and right abducens nerves. This is a case of mononeuritis multiplex, which usually results from vasculitis, diabetes, or leprosy. Since she is hypertensive, vasculitis is a likely cause. Cerebral vasculitis may further complicate the illness.

12. Although many injuries may affect the spinal cord, there is no objective evidence of neurologic disease in this patient. The apparent paraplegia is not accompanied by reflex changes. More important, he is able to feel temperature changes but not pinpricks, although both sensations are carried by the same pathway. He probably has no neurologic injury.

13. He has had damage to the right femoral nerve. This injury has resulted in paresis of the quadriceps muscle and loss of its associated reflex. A diabetic infarction is the most likely cause.

14. He probably has a herniated L5-S1 intervertebral disk that compresses the S1 root on the left.

15. He has an obvious case of ALS with bulbar and pseudobulbar palsy and wasting of the limb muscles. The corticobulbar and corticospinal tracts, brainstem nuclei, and spinal anterior horn cells are all involved. However, in ALS there is no paresis of ocular movement, and mental faculties remain intact.

16. He has bilateral "tardy" (slowly developing) ulnar nerve palsies. This injury usually results from pressure on the ulnar nerves at the elbows. It is an occupational hazard of watchmakers, draftsmen, and other workers who must continuously lean on their elbows.

17. Clearly ALS should be considered because of the atrophy and fasciculations; however, the back pain and sensory loss are inconsistent with that diagnosis. Lumbar spondylosis, which is far more common than ALS, is the more likely disorder because of the back pain and hypalgesia.

18. The memory impairment and convulsion indicate that she has involvement of the cerebral cortex. She also has a neuropathy as indicated by the dysesthesia, distal sensory loss, and areflexia. The combination of CNS and PNS disease with organomegaly, jaundice, and a history of weight loss suggests a systemic illness. Malignancies, hepatitis, and toxins are possible, but alcoholism is the most common cause of this combination of CNS and PNS findings.

19. Lead pipes used in illegal distillation cause lead intoxication neuropathy. A compression neuropathy is also possible.

20. He has impairment of the cerebellum, peripheral nerves, and posterior columns of the spinal cord. This combination indicates a spinocerebellar degeneration, e.g., Friedreich's ataxia.

21.	e	**25.**	a
22.	c	**26.**	No
23.	d	**27.**	No
24.	b	**28.**	Yes

29.	Yes	**33.**	Yes
30.	Yes	**34.**	Yes
31.	Yes	**35.**	Yes
32.	No	**36.**	Yes

37.   He most likely has taken an insecticide that has marked anticholinesterase activity. He should be treated with atropine, 2 mg to 4 mg intravenously, and with additional doses at frequent intervals thereafter.

38.   a.   No
     b.   No
     c.   Yes
     d.   No
     e.   Yes
     f.   No
     g.   No
     h.   No

39.   c,d,e. Hypoxia, a common complication of Guillain-Barré syndrome, often causes anxiety and agitation as the first symptoms. Most patients who are thought to have an "ICU psychosis" actually have underlying cerebral dysfunction. Guillain-Barré syndrome is not directly associated with central nervous system dysfunction. (a and b are incorrect: sedatives and tranquilizers might depress respirations.)

40.   Alcoholic neuropathy is associated with delirium tremens (DTs) when hospitalized alcoholic patients are deprived of their usual alcohol. These patients also may develop alcohol withdrawal seizures, but the seizures usually precede the DTs.

41.   "Glue sniffing," chronic inhalation of vapors from cements, or abuse of paint thinners lead to neuropathy because these substances contain N-hexane and similar solvents. Since these chemical solvents are lipophilic, they damage the lipid-rich myelin coating of peripheral nerves. When toluene and certain other solvents are inhaled for periods of at least 2 months, dementia accompanied by cerebellar signs may develop.

42.   The hyperactive DTRs and Babinski signs indicate that there is CNS rather than PNS damage.

43.   A large single pontomedullary injury has caused oculomotor paresis, quadriparesis, and apnea. Nevertheless, his mental, visual, and upper brainstem functions should be intact. He can communicate by blinking his eyes. He has the well known "locked-in syndrome" (Chapter 11) and should not be mistaken for being comatose, demented, or vegetative.

44.   The localization of the lesion is important because if the damage is confined to the brainstem, as in this case, intellectual function is preserved. If the patient had suffered extensive cerebral damage, he would have had irreversible dementia. The presence or absence of mental function should determine the level of care and effort given to rehabilitation.

45.   Although a CT scan might be performed to detect or exclude a cerebral lesion, only an MRI might be sensitive enough to detect a brainstem lesion. An EEG in this case would be a valuable test because, since the cerebral hemispheres are intact, it would show a relatively normal pattern. Other suitable tests are electrophysiologic studies. Visually evoked responses (VERs) will determine the integrity of the entire visual system. Brainstem auditory evoked responses (BAERs) will determine the integrity of the auditory circuits that are predominantly brainstem functions.

46.	b	**49.**	c
47.	b	**50.**	a
48.	a	**51.**	c

52.	d	**57.**	b
53.	d	**58.**	a
54.	c	**59.**	b
55.	b	**60.**	a
56.	a		

61.   Teenagers develop a neuropathy from any of the usual causes (Table 5-2), but several causes might be given special consideration. Mononucleosis, a common condition of young adults, may be complicated by the development of a neuropathy in which there are more motor than sensory impairments. Other viral illnesses, such as hepatitis, may be complicated by the development of a neuropathy. Exposure to toxins used for thrill-seeking, including glue, paint thinners, alcohol, or nitrous oxide, should be considered, particularly when neuropathy develops concurrently in several teenagers. In anyone with an eating disorder or using megavitamin therapy, excessive consumption of pyridoxine (vitamin B_6) should be considered as a potential cause of neuropathy. In certain regions, Lyme disease is prevalent. Patients may have neuropathy and systemic symptoms, such as low grade fever and malaise.

62.   The various surgical procedures performed for either morbid obesity or ulcers, which remove part of the gastrointestinal tract, may be complicated by nutritional disorders, including Wernicke-Korsakoff syndrome (thiamine deficiency), combined-system disease (B_{12} deficiency), and fluid and electrolyte imbalance. Any change in mentation following these procedures requires immediate attention because it may be a manifestation of a potentially fatal metabolic aberration.

63.   The patient has a typical history and neurologic findings for Lyme disease. In many cases the blood test is negative early in the illness. Another possibility is that she has Guillain-Barré illness that began, as a small fraction of cases do, with paresis of the facial muscles. Myasthenia gravis is a possibility, but it is unlikely because of the absence of oculomotor paresis. The next step would be to perform a spinal tap to test the CSF for Lyme disease and look for the characteristic protein elevation of Guillain-Barré illness. If the diagnosis remains unclear, the best course would be to treat for Lyme disease.

64.   c

6

Muscle Disorders

Patients with muscle diseases,* including disorders of the neuromuscular junction, characteristically complain of weakness and may have findings that mimic CNS or PNS illness. These symptoms and signs, though relatively common, are easily overlooked or misinterpreted by the untrained examiner. This chapter discusses myasthenia gravis, which is the most important disease of the neuromuscular junction, and several common diseases of the muscles themselves, *myopathies*. It then reviews the relevant laboratory tests for diseases of nerve, neuromuscular junction, and muscle.

Muscle disorders are characterized by muscle weakness and hypoactive DTRs. Various disorders primarily affect combinations of ocular, facial, bulbar, and *proximal* limb muscles. The muscular sphincters of the bladder and bowel, however, are rarely affected.

Also, in most muscle diseases, in contrast to PNS disorders, the distal limb muscles are relatively normal, and there is no sensory loss. Most important, with several exceptions, muscular diseases are not associated with mental impairment. (The similarities and differences between CNS, PNS, and muscular diseases are outlined in Table 6-1.)

MYASTHENIA GRAVIS

Myasthenia gravis, the classic disorder of the neuromuscular junction, typically affects young women and older men. It is characterized by intermittent, asymmetric paresis of the facial, extraocular, and bulbar muscles. Although myasthenia usually occurs alone, it is sometimes associated with hyperthyroidism or mediastinal thymomas. The basic problem is an abnormal production of antibodies directed against muscle end-plate ACh receptors that block normal muscle contraction (Figs. 6-1 and 6-2).

Almost 90 percent of myasthenia patients first complain of diplopia and ptosis because of paresis of the ocular muscles. Characteristically, patients with myasthenia grimace when attempting to smile because of weakness of the facial muscle (Fig. 6-3). Their speech has a nasal quality because of nasopharyngeal muscle paresis. Ocular, facial, and vocal weakness are exaggerated when the patient makes a sustained effort either voluntarily or on the request of the examiner. For example, ocular weakness will worsen with prolonged upward gaze, and speech will sound even more nasal during long conversations. In

---

* Patients with myasthenia gravis may receive assistance from the Myasthenia Gravis Foundation, 7-11 South Broadway, White Plains, New York 10601, (914) 328-1717. Patients with muscular dystrophy and related disorders may receive assistance from the Muscular Dystrophy Association of America, 810 Seventh Avenue, New York, New York 10019, (212) 586-0808.

TABLE 6–1. SIGNS OF CNS, PNS, AND MUSCLE DISORDERS

	CNS	PNS	Muscle
Paresis	Pattern*	Distal	Proximal
Muscle tone	Spastic	Flaccid	Sometimes tender or dystrophic
DTRs	Hyperactive	Hypoactive	Normal or hypoactive
Babinski signs	Yes	No	No
Sensory loss	Hemisensorty	Stocking-glove	None

* Hemisparesis, paraparesis, etc.

moderately advanced cases, the neck, shoulder, and respiratory muscles become weak. In severe cases, apnea and quadriplegia develop, and patients can be so unable to communicate that they can be labeled "locked-in" (Chapter 11).

Several negative findings are important. Although extraocular muscles may be severely involved, intraocular muscles are spared. Therefore, despite paresis of the eyelids and eyeball motion, the pupils are equal, of normal size, round, and reactive to light. Even though there may be quadriparesis, the bladder and bowel sphincters will be unaffected. Of course, there is no sensory loss.

The physician's clinical diagnosis of myasthenia gravis can be confirmed by the Tensilon test in which 10 mg of edrophonium chloride (Tensilon) is administered intravenously. Saline is injected before or after as a control. Patients with myasthenia have a dramatic reversal of ocular and facial weakness that lasts for several minutes. This occurs because Tensilon inhibits degradation of ACh by acetylcholinesterase, causing increased neuromuscular junction ACh levels that react with remaining muscle ACh receptors to trigger contraction of the muscles.

Treatment of myasthenia gravis has been based on medicines that, like Tensilon, impede degradation of ACh. Recently, the administration of steroids and the use of plasmapheresis have been shown to be effective. Both presumably reduce antibodies to ACh receptors. Correction of hyperthyroidism or removal of mediastinal thymomas, if either condition is present, will improve or even eliminate myasthenia.

Several diseases resemble myasthenia gravis. One of the most commonly encountered is psychogenic "easy fatigability." Patients complain of dyspnea on exertion, an inability to walk, weakness of their arms, and even intermittent double vision. Manual muscle testing may elicit "weakness" of the arms and wrists. They do, however, have full functional ability and can walk, climb stairs, and dress. Moreover, they do not have asymmetric weakness or extraocular muscle palsy. Other causes of easy fatigability include Lyme disease, mononucleosis, and chronic EBV infection.

Lesions of the third cranial nerve, which result from midbrain infarctions or from compression by aneurysms of the posterior communicating artery, can

FIGURE 6–1. At the neuromuscular junction, the nerve ending contains vesicles of acetylcholine (ACh). When released across the junction, ACh binds to muscle ACh receptors, triggering a muscle contraction.

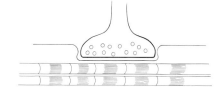

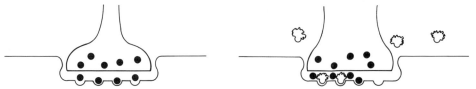

FIGURE 6–2. (*Left*) Normally, vesicles of acetylcholine (ACh) (*darkened circles*) cross the neuromuscular junction, bind onto ACh receptors, and initiate muscle contraction by depolarizing the membrane. The ACh is then entirely metabolized by the enzyme *acetylcholinesterase*. Unlike many neurotransmitters, such as dopamine, ACh is not taken back into the presynaptic neuron in either the CNS or PNS, i.e., there is no reuptake of ACh. (*Right*) In myasthenia gravis, abnormal antibodies (*tufted circles*) bind to many ACh receptors and prevent ACh binding.

ACh receptor activity can be enhanced by inhibiting ACh metabolism with *anticholinesterases*, such as edrophonium (Tensilon) and physostigmine. (Physostigmine has also been used experimentally to raise the abnormally low cerebral ACh concentrations in Alzheimer's disease [Chapter 7]).

Presynaptic neuron release of ACh can be impaired and muscle paresis induced by botulinum toxin (Fig. 18-24), which is an effective treatment for some facial dyskinesias characterized by muscle spasm (see blepharospasm, Chapter 18). Another medication that creates paresis is succinylcholine, which is a muscle relaxant used in conjunction with electroshock therapy. It directly depolarizes the neuromuscular junction membrane.

also cause extraocular muscle paresis. The difference, which is important but subtle, is that in these disorders, the pupil will be widely dilated and unreactive to light because the intraocular (pupillary) muscles are also affected. Facial or bulbar palsy can result from amyotrophic lateral sclerosis (ALS); inflammatory or infectious conditions, including Guillain-Barré syndrome, Lyme disease, and Bell's palsy; and low brainstem infarctions. In any case, of all these diseases that cause ocular, facial, bulbar, or systemic weakness, only myasthenia gravis responds to Tensilon.

MUSCLE DISEASES (MYOPATHIES)

Patients with a *myopathy*, as would be expected, usually complain primarily of weakness. In most myopathies, the shoulder and hip girdle muscles (i.e., the proximal muscles) are affected first, most severely, and often exclusively. These muscle groups, which have the greatest bulk, are indispensable for standing, climbing stairs, combing hair, and reaching upward; however, even when the weakness is extensive and severe, patients will have no oculomotor or sphincter

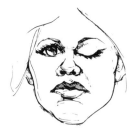
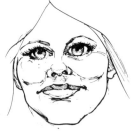

FIGURE 6–3. (*Left*) This young woman with myasthenia gravis developed a weakened left eyelid following several days of double vision. In addition to ptosis, she had generalized facial muscle weakness, especially evident in the loss of the contour of the right nasolabial fold and a sagging lower lip. (*Right*) After 10 mg of edrophonium (Tensilon) was administered intravenously, she had a brief but dramatic restoration of eyelid, ocular, and facial strength.

paresis, and they will still be able to use their hands. When myopathies lead to loss of muscle bulk, the muscle atrophy is called *dystrophy*.

The DTRs are hypoactive roughly in proportion to the degree of paresis of the muscle. Babinski signs, of course, would not be elicitable. Finally, with rare exceptions (two of which are described below), mental aberrations are not associated with myopathies.

Patients with inflammatory myopathies have muscle aches, *myalgias*, along with weakness. When affected muscles are palpated, patients usually have tenderness.

Clinically Important Myopathies

Although there are many causes of myopathies, the physician should be particularly aware of those that occur frequently, are associated with mental aberrations, or indicate a systemic illness.

Duchenne's dystrophy, which is called *muscular dystrophy* because it is the most frequently occurring variety, is a sex-linked genetic illness with expression in childhood. In other words, muscular dystrophy develops in boys whose mothers carried the abnormal gene. Gene mapping with DNA probes for "restriction fragment length polymorphisms (RFLPs)" has isolated the genetic defect to the short arm of the X chromosome and has permitted the diagnosis in utero and in (female) carriers. Although this technique is a major advance for detecting not only Duchenne's dystrophy but also myotonic dystrophy (see below), Huntington's chorea, familial Alzheimer's disease, and autosomal dominant manic-depressive disease, it is occasionally flawed by crossover of DNA and mutations. Duchenne's dystrophy has been associated with a virtual absence of a newly discovered protein, dystrophin. A variety of Duchenne's dystrophy, Becker's dystrophy, which has milder manifestations, is associated with abnormalities in the composition of dystrophin.

Muscular dystrophy begins with weakness in the boys' thighs and shoulders. It is first noticed as trouble with athletic activities, especially riding bicycles or climbing. The affected muscles are infiltrated with abnormal cells, and they appear bulky, *pseudohypertrophied*. Thus, the weakness appears paradoxical, occurring as it does in conjunction with apparently excellent muscular development (Fig. 6-4). By the end of childhood, however, as muscular dystrophy evolves, children become wheelchair-bound and have respiratory insufficiency. On careful evaluation, this illness has been found to be accompanied by mild mental retardation, making it one of the few myopathies associated with mental impairment. No treatment is available.

Myotonic dystrophy is another inherited myopathy, but it is an autosomal dominant genetic disorder carried on chromosome 19. Young adult men and women develop facial as well as proximal limb muscle weakness and dystrophy. More striking, affected muscles have prolonged contractions, *myotonia*, after voluntary effort or percussion. For example, patients are unable to release their grip for several seconds after opening a door or shaking hands, and their tongue and palm muscles have long-lasting ridges if struck with a reflex hammer.

Another unique feature of this illness is that various non-neurologic abnormalities are associated with the muscle abnormalities. Loss of temple hair, "frontal balding," is commonly combined with facial muscle atrophy. Patients

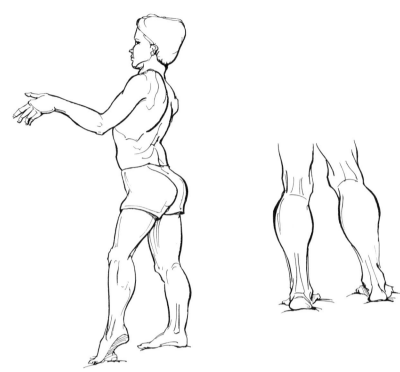

FIGURE 6–4. This 10-year-old boy with typical Duchenne's muscular dystrophy has a waddling gait and inability to raise his arms above his head because of weakness of the shoulder and pelvic girdle muscles. His calves and other weakened muscles are characteristically enlarged, *pseudohypertrophied*, because of cellular infiltration. There is also a typical exaggeration of the normal inward curve of the lumbar spine, *hyperlordosis*. These Duchenne's muscular dystrophy children are frequently pictured on fund-raising posters.

characteristically have a sunken and elongated face with prominent ptosis and a prominent forehead (Fig. 6-5). Other associated abnormalities include cataracts, cardiac conduction system disturbances, and endocrinologic abnormalities, such as testicular atrophy, diabetes, and infertility.

As with Duchenne's dystrophy, myotonic dystrophy is associated with mental status abnormalities. Patients are often described as having personality disorders, blunted affect, limited intelligence, and lack of initiative.

Polymyositis is a muscle inflammation or infection characterized by myalgias and tenderness. Weakness is usually mild, although occasionally it can be severe enough to be transiently debilitating. Unlike other myopathies, polymyositis is usually accompanied by signs of systemic illness, typically fever and malaise. Most often it is caused by a benign, self-limited systemic viral illness. In older adults, unlike children, polymyositis is often associated with underlying pulmonary or gastrointestinal malignancies.

Trichinosis is a special variety of polymyositis that is caused by *Trichinella* infection from eating undercooked pork or game. This illness is not confined to poor regions of the country, as it sometimes develops in affluent adventurous diners and hunters who eat their own kills. Finally, polymyalgia rheumatica, polyarteritis nodosa, and other systemic inflammatory diseases are routinely complicated by polymyositis.

Certain medications are another important cause of myopathies. They cause

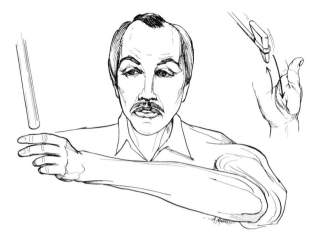

FIGURE 6–5. This young man with myotonic dystrophy has the typically elongated face caused by wasting of temporal and facial muscles, hairline recession, and ptosis. Because of myotonia, when his thenar eminence muscles are struck with a percussion hammer, they undergo a forceful, sustained contraction that pulls the thumb for 3 to 10 seconds, and he cannot release his grasp rapidly.

patients to become weak despite appropriate treatment of their primary illness. Thus, physicians may be confronted with the paradox of the patient deteriorating in strength or stamina while the initial illness is treated. The most frequent medication-induced muscle disorders are *steroid myopathy*, which is caused by the prolonged use of oral or parenteral steroid preparations, and *hypokalemic myopathy*, which is caused by taking diuretics without potassium supplements. Each of these myopathies is reversed when the medication is stopped.

Some rare naturally occurring myopathies are noteworthy. Patients with *periodic paralysis*, which is an inherited condition, suffer 1- to 8-hour episodes of quadriparesis because of transient hypokalemia. In *hyperthyroid myopathy*, weakness develops as part of an obvious systemic illness. Finally, muscle weakness and, frequently, cramps are hallmarks of Pompe's disease and McArdle's disease, which are rare inherited glycogen-storage diseases that are "important" biochemically, rather than clinically.

The Neuroleptic Malignant Syndrome

The neuroleptic malignant syndrome (NMS) is an iatrogenic disorder characterized by muscle rigidity so intense that it crushes muscles and leads to *rhabdomyolysis* (muscle necrosis), hyperpyrexia, and obtundation. Those patients who remain alert are mute and immobile. Most have tachycardia, diaphoresis, and other signs of autonomic dysfunction. Patients often have renal failure because of myoglobinemia, as well as cardiovascular collapse. The hyperpyrexia, with body temperatures often reaching 107°F, causes cerebral cortex damage. Not surprisingly, the mortality rate is 15 to 40 percent.

NMS has been repeatedly described in patients who have received dopamine-blocking or depleting medications. Most often these medications have been neuroleptics, but nonantipsychotic dopamine-blocking medications, such as metoclopramide (Reglan), have been implicated. Similarly, NMS has followed abrupt withdrawal of dopamine precursors, such as levodopa (Sinemet). Individuals who have been most susceptible have had pre-existing brain damage, physical exhaustion, dehydration, and acutely developing psychosis. In view of the context in which NMS cases develop, the underlying cause is postulated to be a reaction to sudden dopamine deficiency in the basal ganglia and hypothalamus. Presumably, the basal ganglia dysfunction produces the intense muscular rigidity, and the hypothalamus dysfunction results in impaired body heat dissipation. Alternatively, neuroleptics might interact with muscle cells and alter their calcium distribution.

Dehydration and renal failure cause an elevated blood urea nitrogen (BUN) concentration, and rhabdomyolysis causes a markedly elevated creatine phosphokinase (CPK) concentration. The EEG is normal or has only diffuse slowing, which is a mild and nonspecific abnormality indicative of either a toxic disorder or use of psychotropic medicines (Chapter 10). Recommended treatment has recently included electroshock therapy; L-dopa; bromocriptine (Parlodel), which may restore dopamine-like activity (Chapter 18); and dantrolene (Dantrium), which acts to restore intracellular calcium distribution.

Malignant Hyperthermia

Malignant hyperthermia (MH) is an inherited muscle disorder caused by general anesthesia or by the muscle relaxant, succinylcholine. As does NMS, it leads to muscle rigidity, rhabdomyolysis, hyperpyrexia, brain damage, and death. The immediate cause is thought to be an elevated calcium concentration in muscle cells. Dantrolene is reportedly an effective treatment. Since MH is an inherited condition, the family history of patients should be reviewed prior to electroshock treatment in which succinylcholine is to be administered. Other causes of the sequence of muscle necrosis, elevated CPK, fever, and altered mental states, but ones usually producing little diagnostic challenge and where muscle rigidity is not prominent, are hallucinogen ingestion, heat stroke, delirium tremens (DTs), and alcohol intoxication.

LABORATORY TESTS FOR NERVE AND MUSCLE DISEASE

Nerve Conduction Velocity (NCV) Studies

The NCV study can determine the site of nerve damage, confirm a clinical diagnosis of polyneuropathy, and distinguish polyneuropathy from myopathy. The NCV is normally 50–70 m/sec (Fig. 6-6). If a nerve is damaged, the NCV will be slowed at the point of injury, which can be located by proper placement of the electrodes, e.g., across the carpal tunnel. In a polyneuropathy, the NCV of all nerves will be slowed, typically to between 20 and 30 m/sec. In contrast, with a myopathy, the NCV will be normal. The cost of this test (1989) is about $50 for each nerve studied.

Electromyography (EMG)

Electromyographic studies are performed by inserting fine needles into selected muscles. The examiner observes the consequent electrical discharges

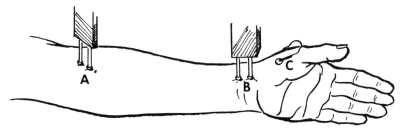

FIGURE 6–6. In determining nerve conduction velocity (NCV), a stimulating electrode that is placed at two points (*A* and *B*) along a nerve excites the appropriate muscle (*C*). The distances between the electrode and the responding muscle and the time intervals between nerve stimulation and muscle response are calculated to provide the NCV, which is normally 50–70 m/sec.

on an oscilloscope during complete muscle rest, voluntary contractions, and stimulation of the innervating peripheral nerve.

Electromyographic abnormalities almost always occur whenever a myopathy is present. Virtually all the muscles will have abnormal, *myopathic*, EMG patterns. In addition, with several diseases (e.g., myasthenia gravis, ALS, and myotonic dystrophy), distinctive patterns are observable.

Abnormal EMG patterns may also be found with mononeuropathies and peripheral neuropathy because muscles develop changes if their nerves are damaged. Thus, EMGs will assist in determining which peripheral nerve or nerve root, if any, is damaged. This test is particularly useful in cases of low back pain when attempting to document nerve damage from herniated disks. Electromyography studies cost between $250 and $500, depending on how many muscles are studied.

Serum Enzyme Determinations

Lactic dehydrogenase (LDH), serum glutamic-oxaloacetic transaminase (SGOT), and CPK are enzymes concentrated within muscle cells that escape into the bloodstream when muscles are damaged. Increases in their serum concentration are roughly proportional to the severity of muscle damage, being highest in neuroleptic malignant syndrome and similar disorders. Elevated CPK concentrations are characteristic of Duchenne's dystrophy patients and affected fetuses, and aid in the prenatal diagnosis of the disorder. Patients with peripheral neuropathy, of course, will have normal enzyme concentrations. Therefore, for patients with unexplained, ill-defined weakness, as well as ones with an apparent myopathy or neuroleptic malignant syndrome, the first specific laboratory test should be a determination of serum CPK, LDH, and SGOT concentrations. The cost is $15 to $50.

Muscle Biopsy

In expert hands, microscopic examination of muscle is useful when muscular atrophy might be the result of a neuropathy, ALS, or myopathy. Specific muscle disorders that might be diagnosed in this way include polymyositis, trichinosis, collagen-vascular diseases, and the rare glycogen-storage diseases. Nerve biopsy, on the other hand, is not performed routinely, since it is useful in uncovering only a few rare diseases.

REFERENCES

Abbott RJ, Loizou LA: Neuroleptic malignant syndrome. Br J Psychiatry *148*:47, 1986

Darras BT, Harper JF, Francke U: Prenatal diagnosis and detection of carriers with DNA probes in Duchenne's muscular dystrophy. N Engl J Med *316*:985, 1987

Guze BH, Baxter LR: Neuroleptic malignant syndrome. N Engl J Med *313*:163, 1985

Hoffman EP, Fischbeck KH, Brown RH, et al: Characterization of dystrophin in muscle-biopsy specimens from patients with Duchenne's or Becker's muscular dystrophy. N Engl J Med *318*:1363, 1988

Hyser CL, Griggs RC, Mendell JR, et al: Use of serum creatine kinase, pyruvate kinase, and genetic linkage for carrier detection in Duchenne and Becker dystrophy. Neurology *37*:4, 1987

Keck PE, Pope HG, McElroy SL: Frequency and presentation of neuroleptic malignant syndrome: A prospective study. Am J Psychiatry *144*:1344, 1987

Kellam AMP: The neuroleptic malignant syndrome, so-called: A survey of the world literature. Br J Psychiatry *150*:752, 1987

Martin JB: Genetic linkage in neurologic diseases. N Engl J Med *716*:1018, 1987

Rodriguez M, Gomez MR, Howard FM, et al: Myasthenia gravis in children: Long-term follow-up. Ann Neurol *13*:504, 1983

Yacoub OF, Morrow DH: Malignant hyperthermia and ECT. Am J Psychiatry *143*:1027, 1986

QUESTIONS: CHAPTER 6

1–3. A 17-year-old woman complains of occasional double vision when looking to the left. She denies headache and loss of visual acuity. She has right-sided ptosis and difficulty keeping her right eye adducted. Her pupils are 4 mm, round, and reactive. Her speech is nasal and her neck flexor muscles are weak. There is no paresis or reflex abnormalities of the limbs.

   1. Which diseases might explain the ocular abnormalities?
   a. Multiple sclerosis
   b. Psychogenic weakness
   c. Myasthenia gravis
   d. Right posterior communicating artery aneurysm

   2. Which test is likely to be most helpful?
   a. Electroencephalogram (EEG)
   b. Nerve conduction velocity (NCV)
   c. Electromyogram (EMG)
   d. Tensilon test
   e. Muscle enzymes: CPK, LDH, SGOT

   3. Which conditions may also be present?
   a. Hypothyroidism
   b. Hyperthyroidism
   c. Bell's palsy
   d. Thymoma

4–5. An 18-year-old woman, who is a dancer, develops progressive weakness of the toes and ankles. On examination she has loss of the ankle reflexes, unresponsive plantar reflexes, and decreased sensation in the toes and feet.

   4. Which diseases might explain her symptoms and signs?
   a. Myasthenia gravis
   b. Toxic polyneuropathy
   c. Polymyositis
   d. Guillain-Barré syndrome
   e. Thoracic spinal cord tumor

   5. Which tests would be most likely to be helpful in making a diagnosis?
   a. EEG
   b. NCV
   c. EMG

  d.   Tensilon test
  e.   Muscle enzymes: CPK, LDH, SGOT

6–11   A 6-year-old boy is beginning to have difficulty standing upright. He has to push himself up on his legs in order to stand. He has not been able to run since the age of 4 years. A cousin of the same age has a similar problem. The patient is well built and has a normal examination, except for paresis of his upper leg muscles and decreased quadriceps (knee) reflexes.

6.   What disease is the patient likely to have?
  a.   Porphyria
  b.   Peripheral neuropathy
  c.   Spinal cord tumor
  d.   Duchenne's muscular dystrophy
  e.   A psychogenic disorder

7.   What tests will help diagnose the case?
  a.   EEG
  b.   NCV
  c.   EMG
  d.   Tensilon test
  e.   Muscle enzymes

8.   What is the sex of the cousin?
  a.   Male
  b.   Female
  c.   Either

9.   Who is the carrier of the condition?
  a.   Father
  b.   Mother
  c.   Either

10.   How can a sister of the patient know if she is a carrier?

11.   What percentage of a carrier's children will also be carriers or have the disease?

12–15.   A 68-year-old man has aches and tenderness of the shoulder muscles. He is unable to lift his arms above his head. There is a blotchy red rash about his head, neck, and upper torso.

12.   What diseases should be considered?
  a.   Steroid myopathy
  b.   Dermatomyositis
  c.   Polyneuropathy
  d.   Periodic paralysis
  e.   Myasthenia
  f.   Trichinosis

13.   Which tests are most likely to confirm the diagnosis?
  a.   EEG
  b.   NCV
  c.   EMG
  d.   Tensilon test
  e.   Muscle enzymes
  f.   Skin and muscle biopsy
  g.   Nerve biopsy

14.   Which conditions are associated with dermatomyositis in the adult?
  a.   Dementia
  b.   Pulmonary malignancies
  c.   Diabetes mellitus
  d.   Gastrointestinal malignancies
  e.   Delirium
  f.   Polyarteritis nodosa

15. Which of the above conditions are associated with polymyositis in the child?

16–24. Which medications are associated with myopathies or neuropathies?

16. Prednisone

17. Chlorpromazine

18. Nitrofurantoin

19. Isoniazid (INH)

20. Hydrochlorothiazide

21. Amitriptyline

22. Thyroid extract

23. Lithium carbonate

24. Phenytoin (Dilantin)

a. Neuropathy
b. Myopathy
c. Neither
d. Both

25–27. A 50-year-old man has developed low back pain and difficulty walking. He has mild weakness in both legs, a distended bladder, diminished sensation to pinprick below the umbilicus, and equivocal plantar and DTRs. He has tenderness of the midthoracic spine.

25. With which conditions are his symptoms and signs most consistent?
a. Polymyositis
b. Herniated lumbar intervertebral disk
c. Idiopathic polyneuropathy
d. Thoracic spinal cord compression

26. If the routine history, physical examination, and laboratory tests, including a chest x-ray, were normal, which of the following tests should be performed next?
a. Computed tomography (CT) scan of the spine
b. X-ray studies of the lumbosacral spine
c. Myelogram
d. Tensilon test
e. Magnetic resonance imaging (MRI) of the spine

27. The diagnostic test confirms the clinical impression. If the condition does not receive prompt, effective treatment, which complications might ensue?
a. Sacral decubitus ulcers
b. Urinary incontinence
c. Permanent paraplegia
d. Hydronephrosis and urosepsis

28. Which of the following are complications of excessive or prolonged use of steroids?
a. Obesity, especially of the face and trunk
b. Steroid myopathy
c. Lumbar spine compression fractures causing severe low back pain
d. "Psychosis"
e. Opportunistic lung and CNS infections
f. Gastrointestinal bleeding
g. Easy bruisability

29. A 31-year-old woman, who has systemic lupus erythematosis (SLE), has been treated for 10 months with prednisone (40 mg daily). She has developed agitation, hallucinations, confusion, and a temperature of 100.5°F. Routine history, general physical examination, neurologic examination, and laboratory tests do not reveal the cause of the mental changes or a source of the fever. Which of the following tests or procedures should be attempted and in which order should they be performed?
a. Stop the steroids.
b. Begin haloperidol or another major tranquilizer.

    c. Do a CT scan of the head.
    d. Perform a lumbar puncture.
    e. Increase the steroid dosage

30. A 75-year-old woman is hospitalized for congestive heart failure, placed on a low salt diet, and given a potent diuretic. Although her congestive heart failure resolves, she develops somnolence, disorientation, and generalized weakness. What is the most likely explanation of her mental status change?
    a. Hypokalemia (low potassium)
    b. A cerebrovascular infarction
    c. A subdural hematoma
    d. Cerebral hypoxia from congestive heart failure
    e. Dehydration, hyponatremia, and hypokalemia

31. Which myopathies are associated with mental impairment?
    a. Polymyositis
    b. Duchenne's muscular dystrophy
    c. Carpal tunnel syndrome
    d. Myotonic dystrophy
    e. Periodic paralysis

32–37. Match the illness with its probable or usual cause:

32. Polymyositis in childhood	a.	Autosomal inheritance
33. Myotonic dystrophy	b.	Sex-linked recessive inheritance
	c.	Parasitic infection
34. Hypokalemic myopathy	d.	Viral illness
35. Trichinosis	e.	Underlying malignancy
	f.	ACh receptor antibodies
36. Duchenne's muscular	g.	Medications
37. Myasthenia gravis		

38–50. Match the illness or condition with the appropriate diagnostic test(s):

38. Carpal tunnel syndrome	a.	NCV
39. Spinal cord compression	b.	EMG
40. ALS	c.	CPK, LDH, and SGOT serum concentrations
41. Porphyria (acute intermittent)	d.	Myelogram
42. Polymyositis	e.	None of the above
43. Optic neuritis		

44. Herniated lumbar intervertebral disk

45. Left hemiparesis from a cerebrovascular accident

46. Uremic polyneuropathy

47. Myotonic dystrophy

48. Duchenne's muscular dystrophy

49. Guillain-Barré syndrome

50. Poliomyelitis

51–56. Match the phenomenon with the myopathy:

51. Unilateral ptosis	a.	Myasthenia gravis
52. Facial rash	b.	Duchenne's dystrophy
	c.	Myotonic dystrophy
53. Waddling gait	d.	Polymyositis

54. Inability to release a fist

55. Pseudohypertrophy of calf muscles

56. Premature balding and cataracts

57. Myasthenia gravis is a disorder in which antibodies damage the postsynaptic neuromuscular ACh receptor. Which of the following therapies are helpful?
   a. Giving steroids to reduce the abnormal immunologic reaction
   b. Performing plasmapheresis to draw ACh antibodies out of the bloodstream
   c. Giving medications that enhance the effectiveness of cholinesterase
   d. Giving medications that impair the effectiveness of cholinesterase
   e. Giving medications that cross the blood-brain barrier
   f. Performing a thymectomy if a thymoma is detected

58. A 50-year-old man complains of impotence. He had had poliomyelitis as a child, which caused a scoliosis and a weak and atrophied right leg and left arm. Deep tendon reflexes are absent in the affected limbs. What role do the polio-induced physical deficits play in his chief complaint?

59. A corporation's chief executive officer develops ALS. His left arm begins to weaken. Then a hostile takeover bid is initiated by a multinational conglomerate that claims the executive is losing his mental capabilities. Can this contention be supported by the facts known about ALS?

60. A 30-year-old woman with severe myasthenia gravis that is treated with high-dose anticholinesterase medications (e.g., Mestinon) is admitted to an intensive care unit for exacerbation of the myasthenia. Plasmapheresis and high-dose steroid treatment are begun. Nevertheless, on the day after admission, the patient becomes confused and agitated. What are the likely causes of her mental aberration?

61. Match the process with its terminology:
   a. Breakdown of muscle cells
   b. Determination of abnormal gene location
   c. Arising from lying position by pushing against one's own thighs

   1. Restriction fragment length polymorphisms (RFLPs)
   2. Rhabdomyolysis
   3. Gower's maneuver

62. Which of the following are *not* features common to neuroleptic malignant syndrome and malignant hyperthermia?
   a. Fever
   b. Muscle rigidity
   c. Brain damage
   d. Elevated CPK
   e. Tachycardia
   f. Familial tendency

ANSWERS

1. c. This is a classical case of myasthenia gravis with ocular, pharyngeal, and neck flexor paresis, but no pupil abnormality. In contrast, this pattern of neck flexor paresis, ocular muscle weakness, and ptosis does not occur in multiple sclerosis (MS). Although internuclear ophthalmoplegia does occur frequently in MS, it is manifested by nystagmus in the abducting eye, as well as paresis of the adducting eye. Patients cannot mimic paresis of one ocular muscle or ptosis. Aneurysmal compression of the third cranial nerve does produce ptosis and paresis of adduction, but it has a painful onset and the pupil becomes large and unreactive to light. Furthermore, the bulbar palsy could not be explained by an aneurysm.

2. d.

3. b,d.

4. b or d. She has distal lower extremity paresis, areflexia, and hypalgesia, which indicate a polyneuropathy. Common causes are alcohol, chemicals, and inflammation, e.g., Guillain-Barré syndrome. Myasthenia rarely affects the legs alone and does not cause a sensory loss. Likewise, the sensory loss and pattern of paresis preclude a diagnosis of muscle disease. A spinal cord tumor is unlikely because her ankle reflexes are not hyperactive, Babinski signs are not present, nor is there a "sensory level" or urinary incontinence.

5. b. NCV will probably confirm the presence of a peripheral neuropathy, but it will not suggest a particular cause.

6. d. This is a typical case of Duchenne's muscular dystrophy. The patient and his cousin have "Gower's sign"—in order to stand upright, they push against their own legs with their hands. Characteristically, the muscles are apparently hypertrophic in the early stages.

7. c and e. The affected muscle in muscular dystrophy will have abnormal (myopathic potential) patterns. Also, the CPK, LDH, and SGOT will be elevated.

8. a. It is a sex-linked trait.

9. b.

10. She can have the serum CPK level measured. An elevation will suggest she is a carrier. In the near future DNA analysis will be available.

11. One half of the boys and one half of the girls will inherit the disease-linked X chromosome. The boys who inherit it will develop the disease, but the girls who inherit it will only be carriers. Therefore, 25 percent of the children (one half of the boys) will have the disease, and 25 percent of the children (one half of the girls) will be asymptomatic carriers.

12. b and f. The muscle pain, tenderness, and paresis suggest an inflammatory myopathy. Steroid myopathy and most other metabolically induced myopathies are painless.

13. e and f. There will be a marked elevation in concentrations of serum CPK, LDH, and SGOT. A biopsy will confirm the diagnosis of dermatomyositis or identify vasculitis and *Trichinella* as possible causes.

14. b, d, f.

15. None. In children, polymyositis is associated only with viral illnesses.

16. b.

17. c.

18. a.

19. a.

20. b (via hypokalemia).

21. c.

22. b (hyperthyroid myopathy).

23. c.

24. a.

25. d. The patient has symptoms and signs of spinal cord compression at T-10. Metastatic tumors are the most frequent cause of spinal cord compression, but herniated thoracic intervertebral disks, multiple sclerosis, tuberculous abscesses, and trauma might be responsible. In contrast, polymyositis affects the arms as well as the legs and does not involve the bladder muscles, produce loss of sensation, or cause spine pain or tenderness.

26. a, c, or e, depending on the instituion. A myelogram would be performed to confirm spinal cord compression, determine its exact location, and indicate its nature. CT scanning or magnetic resonance imaging (MRI) of the spine will show a lesion, but emphasize different aspects.

27. a, b, c, d.

28. a–g.

29. b,c,d,e. The main diagnostic problem is determining whether the patient suffers from too much or too little steroids, i.e., steroid psychosis versus lupus cerebritis. Also, the use of steroids may have been complicated by the development of an opportunistic CNS infection, such as tuberculosis or cryptococcal meningitis. While diagnostic tests are being undertaken, psychosis must be controlled with major tranquilizers. The question of stopping or increasing steroids is best answered by increasing them because lupus cerebritis is more common than steroid psychosis and prednisone at only 40 mg daily is unlikely to cause steroid psychosis. Moreover, since the patient is under physical and psychiatric stress, she might develop adrenal crisis if chronically administered steroids were stopped abruptly.

A CT or MRI scan should be performed to exclude an intracranial mass lesion, such as an abscess or a subdural hematoma. If no mass lesion is detected, a lumbar puncture should be performed to examine the CSF, especially for evidence of infection.

30. e. Administration of potent diuretics to patients on low salt diets eventually leads to hyponatremia and dehydration. These conditions cause obtundation and confusion, especially in the elderly. Low potassium concentrations alone, however, do not cause mental abnormalities. The other possibilities are very unlikely.

31. b, d.

32. d.

33. a.

34. g.

35. c.

36. b.

37. f.

38. a. NCV studies will show a block of the median nerve at the affected wrist.

39. d.

40. b. EMG studies will reveal fibrillations that are roughly the electrical counterpart of fasciculations.

41. e. Although NCV studies might show slowed conduction, that finding is relatively nonspecific. The definitive test would be a Watson-Schwartz test or other test for urinary porphobilinogens.

42. c. Also, a muscle biopsy is frequently performed to confirm the diagnosis of polymyositis.

43. e. VERs (visual evoked responses) would be helpful.

44. b or d. Equivocal cases are studied with EMGs. CT or MRI scans are the best tests, but myelography is often needed.

45. e. None of these tests would be helpful. A CT or MRI scan of the head would be the best diagnostic test for a cerebrovascular accident.

46. a. NCV studies will reveal slowing of the nerves of the limbs.

47. b. EMGs will reveal characteristic electrical discharges associated with myotonia.

48. b and c. DNA studies will be available soon.

49. a. Guillain-Barré syndrome is a clinical diagnosis confirmed by an elevated CSF protein concentration, but NCV studies usually show slowing of velocities.

50. e. CSF examination would show lymphocytes, slightly raised protein, and depressed glucose.

51. a.

52. d.

53. b.

54. c.

55. b.

56. c.

57. a. Giving steroids in large doses is a powerful, effective treatment.
    b. Plasmapheresis can be effective even when all other modalities have failed.
    c. No. They would reduce neuromuscular junction ACh concentration.
    d. By reducing the effectiveness of cholinesterase, the quantity of ACh would increase. Muscle strength would increase as ACh receptors were stimulated by more ACh.
    e. Being a disorder of the neuromuscular junction, myasthenia gravis does not involve the brain. The anticholinesterases in common use, such as Mestinon (pyridostigmine), do not cross the blood-brain barrier and do not precipitate mental abnormalities.
    f. Removal of thymomas or even persistent thymus tissue improves the condition of patients with myasthenia gravis.

58. The polio-induced muscle weakness and atrophy are typically confined to the voluntary muscles of the trunk and limbs. Also, polio victims have no sensory loss, autonomic dysfunction, or sexual impairment. Although polio survivors sometimes develop a "postpolio" ALS-like syndrome in middle age, it does not cause sensory, autonomic, or sexual dysfunction. This patient's impotence must have another explanation.

59. ALS is strictly a motor neuron disease. No intellectual deterioration can be attributed to ALS. Although this illness can cause dysarthria and apparent loss of emotional control because of pseudobulbar palsy, ALS does not cause cognitive impairment.

60. Myasthenia gravis is basically a disorder of the ACh receptors of the voluntary muscles. These receptors are not present in the brain. Mental aberrations in myasthenia gravis are not attributable either to the illness or to anticholinesterase medications. However, in myasthenia patients, ventilatory failure could cause cerebral hypoxia, high-dose steroids could create psychotic behavior, or being confined to an intensive care unit may create a psychologically stressful situation that, superimposed upon medical illnesses, might precipitate "ICU psychosis."

61. a-2; b-1; c-3.

62. f.

SECTION 2

MAJOR NEUROLOGIC SYMPTOMS

INTRODUCTION

The second half of this book considers the most common neurologic symptoms encountered by psychiatrists. Although some are merely interesting conditions or minor annoyances for which patients only seek an explanation, many are an indication of a serious disease. Moreover, most symptoms that are discussed are associated with changes in mental status. Several are also included specifically because, possibly contrary to expectations, they are not associated with such changes. Familiarity with all of them should provide psychiatrists some expertise in neurologic illnesses, and also facilitate appropriate and reliable evaluations.

Each chapter is devoted to a single symptom and its clinical features, routine laboratory tests, and differential diagnosis. Discussions include the symptom's neuropsychologic aspects, related non-neurologic conditions, and underlying neuroanatomy. The neurologic viewpoint presented in this book occasionally differs with the diagnostic criteria in the *Diagnostic and Statistical Manual, Third Edition, Revised, (DSM-III-R)*. Whenever discrepancies occur, they are acknowledged. Although recommendations regarding medications and other treatments are provided, the physician must consult package inserts and other references for all indications, dosages, potential complications, and alternatives.

7

Dementia

The diagnostic criteria for *dementia* cited in the *Diagnostic and Statistical Manual, Third Edition, Revised, (DSM-III-R)* include an impairment in both short- and long-term memory and in at least one of the following: abstract thinking, judgment, or a higher cortical function, such as aphasia, apraxia, or agnosia. Furthermore, these disturbances must be sufficient to interfere with social activities or interpersonal relationships. This descriptive definition, which differentiates dementia, its related disorders, and normal aging, is generally accepted.

DISORDERS RELATED TO DEMENTIA

Mental Retardation

In contrast to dementia, mental retardation consists of intellectual impairments that result from congenital or early childhood brain injury. Moreover, in mental retardation, intellectual deficits are not progressive, and functional impairments are relatively stable. Mentally retarded individuals often have physical stigmata of cerebral injury, such as seizures and hemiparesis. They may have conditions that affect other organs, such as the neurocutaneous disorders (Chapter 13). The DSM-III-R classifies mental retardation and its several degrees—mild to profound (317.00–318.20)—within the *Developmental Disorders* (Axis II). Diagnostic criteria are a general intelligence quotient (IQ) of 70 or less; impairment of adaptive functions, such as social skills and personal independence; and onset before age 18 years. Of course, mentally retarded individuals may, in later life, develop dementia. One well-known example is that individuals who are mentally retarded as a result of Down's syndrome often develop dementia in middle age (see below).

Frontal Lobe Syndrome

Patients with damage to both frontal lobes have characteristic abnormalities in their mentation and behavior, loosely termed the *frontal lobe syndrome*. Since cognitive capacity is preserved, however, this condition is not strictly speaking a form of dementia. Although a syndrome and at least two varieties—the orbital syndrome and the dorsolateral syndrome—are described, most physicians identify only the general features of frontal lobe damage.

Patients with frontal lobe syndrome typically exhibit a slowness and lack of spontaneity in speech (abulia), thought, and emotion. When the normal

---

* Patients with dementia may receive assistance from the Alzheimer's Disease and Related Disorders Association, 360 North Michigan Avenue, Chicago, Illinois 60601, (312) 853-3060.

inhibitory function of the frontal lobes is damaged, patients are usually unrestrained in their emotions, behavior, and bladder control. In this vein, they sometimes manifest facetiousness, *witzelsucht*, comprised of uninhibited, superficially humorous, odd jocularity. Just as their mentation is viscous, their voluntary movements are slow or absent (bradykinesia or akinesia). They develop a slow, uncertain gait (frontal ataxia or gait apraxia [see below]). Frontal release signs may also be prominent (see below).

Conditions that usually cause the frontal lobe syndrome are discrete lesions, such as penetrating head wounds, a glioblastoma multiforme, and infarction of both anterior cerebral arteries. It is less frequently caused by Alzheimer's disease or multi-infarct dementia because these illnesses tend to affect the entire cerebral cortex. A modified version of the frontal lobe syndrome has been produced by the infamous *frontal lobotomy*, a neurosurgical procedure in which surgeons resect the frontal lobes or severe their large white matter tracts (Fig. 20-14).

Amnesia

Another distinct condition closely related to dementia is the *amnestic syndrome*, or simply *amnesia*, which is memory loss with otherwise preserved intellectual function. The distinction is based on the dictum that "memory loss alone is not dementia." The DSM-III-R and usual neurologic diagnostic criteria for amnesia require that patients be fully alert and have impairments only in both short- and long-term memory. The DSM-III-R also includes a third criterion: that no specific organic factor be related to the disturbance. Neurologists, however, find several distinct organic causes.

An amnestic syndrome that suddenly develops in previously healthy individuals and has a duration of several minutes to several hours is usually attributable to dysfunction of the temporal lobe or, more specifically, the limbic system (Fig. 16-5). The frequently cited causes of acutely occurring but short-lived amnesia are the Wernicke-Korsakoff syndrome, alcoholic blackouts and other complications of alcohol intoxication, partial complex seizures, transient global amnesia, and use of certain medications. Transient amnesia mayalso result from electroshock therapy.

Amnesia may persist for several weeks but may become permanent when the temporal lobes are physically injured. For example, as a major element of the postconcussive syndrome, amnesia often follows head trauma. In most cases of posttraumatic amnesia, the tips of the temporal lobes are contused when their anterior surfaces are thrown against the inner surface of the middle fossa (Fig. 20-1). Amnesia is a characteristic symptom of *Herpes simplex* encephalitis, a relatively common viral infection of the temporal lobes. In this condition, amnesia may be accompanied by other signs of temporal lobe damage, such as the Klüver-Bucy syndrome, personality changes, and partial complex seizures. In some cases of the Wernicke-Korsakoff syndrome or of head trauma, amnesia is permanent.

A certain degree of amnesia is a benign condition of the elderly, called *benign senescence* or *forgetfulness of old age*. This variety of amnesia is characterized by forgetfulness for the names of people; however, judgment, intellect, and language function remain normal.

In contrast to these neurologic causes of amnesia, one major study (Cummings) found that 66 percent of patients with amnestic episodes had had psychiatric disturbances, which were most often personality disorder, depression, or malingering. In this study, the essential diagnostic criterion for psychogenic amnesia was the inability to recall important personal information. Similarly, the DSM-III-R notes that, in patients having factitious disorder with psychological symptoms, memory testing often yields "inconsistent results."

Neuropsychologic Conditions

A feature accompanying memory impairment—and an interesting phenomenon that could be mistaken for dementia—is *confabulation*, in which patients, who do not recall or never knew certain information, invent answers that may be implausible in a sincere, forthcoming, and often jovial manner. Patients probably confabulate consciously to conceal impairments or unconsciously in denial of them. Confabulation is a well-known symptom of several unrelated conditions: Wernicke-Korsakoff's syndrome, Anton's syndrome (cortical blindness, Chapter 12), and the nondominant hemisphere syndrome (Chapter 8). Since it is associated with conditions referable to entirely different regions of the brain, confabulation does not have a consistent anatomic correlation.

Aphasia, anosognosia, apraxia, and several related disorders (Chapter 8) may impair mentation or communication, but their deficits are restricted to a single area of intellectual activity. Unlike dementia, they are caused by discrete lesions of the cerebral hemispheres. Skillful testing is therefore necessary to identify these disorders and to detect cases where they coexist with dementia.

NORMAL AGING

Dementia frequently must be distinguished from the cognitive and physiologic changes that accompany aging. Normal changes begin at age 65 years, when people are arbitrarily considered "old," and become pronounced after age 80 years. Studies have shown that, as people age, they develop impaired memory for both recent events and people's names. They also have a shorter attention span, slower learning speed (acquisition of new information), and decreased ability to perform complex tasks. Their general intelligence is slightly decreased, as measured by the *Wechsler Adult Intelligence Scale Revised (WAIS-R)*, and some information is relatively inaccessible. In contrast, normal older individuals have no loss of vocabulary, language ability, or general information, and they may remain well-spoken and knowledgeable.

Sleep is fragmented, sleep and awakening times are phase-advanced, and there is less stage 4 NREM sleep (Chapter 17). Older people usually lose deep tendon reflex (DTR) activity in their ankles, perception of vibration sensation in their legs, and some strength in their limbs. They also have impaired postural reflexes. These neurologic changes, combined with musculo-skeletal changes, lead to the common standing and walking pattern of elderly people known as "senile gait," an impairment characterized by increased flexion of the trunk and limbs, diminished arm swing, and short uncertain steps. Many older individuals can often compensate for their flexed posture and short steps by using a cane.

Other natural changes impair hearing and vision. These senses must be tested carefully in patients with mental aberrations because their loss can give the appearance of dementia, accentuate other physical disabilities, and, in the extreme case, lead to sensory deprivation and its complications, including hallucinations.

The electroencephalogram (EEG) typically has slowing of the background alpha activity. The dominant background rhythm in older individuals is frequently slower than the normal 8–12 Hz. Computed tomography (CT) and magnetic resonance imaging (MRI) may be normal, but often these studies reveal atrophy of the cerebral cortex, expansion of the sylvian fissure, and dilation of the lateral and third ventricles (Chapter 20).

Brain weight decreases with advancing age, and it eventually reaches about 85 percent of normal. Histologic changes include the loss of large cortical neurons and the presence of lipofuscin granules, granulovacuolar degeneration, neuritic (senile) plaques that contain amyloid, and neurofibrillary tangles. These age-related changes affect the frontal and temporal lobes more than the parietal lobe.

DEMENTIA

Causes

A seemingly endless number of illnesses can cause dementia. The traditional classification by etiology is only slightly more enlightening than grouping them alphabetically. Other classification systems are more informative. Based on their

TABLE 7–1. COMMONLY CITED CAUSES OF DEMENTIA AND THEIR INCIDENCE

Disease	Incidence (%)
Alzheimer's disease	50–60
Multiple infarctions	10–20
Alcoholism	6–11
Medications	0–8
Normal pressure hydrocephalus	4–12
Cerebral mass lesions	2–4
Pseudodementia*	7–12
AIDS-dementia complex°	
Rare causes	
Huntington's disease and related conditions†	
Infections	
Neurosyphilis	
Creutzfeldt-Jakob	
Encephalitis‡	
Metabolic abnormalities	
Hyper- or hypothyroidism	
Hepatic failure	
Pulmonary failure	
Combined-system disease	
Drug abuse	

* Depression and related conditions that cause cognitive impairment.
° The incidence is not yet determined, but it is probably the most frequent cause of dementia below age 50 years and in certain regions of the United States.
† Including Parkinson's and Wilson's disease (Chapter 18).
‡ Including subacute sclerosing panencephalitis (SSPE).

TABLE 7–2. COMMONLY CITED CAUSES OF DEMENTIA THAT AFFECT ADOLESCENTS

Metabolic abnormalities
    Wilson's disease
    Drug and alcohol abuse
Degenerative illnesses
    Huntington's disease
    Metachromatic leukodystrophy
    Other rare, usually genetically transmitted illnesses
Infections
    Subacute sclerosing panencephalitis (SSPE)
    AIDS-dementia complex

frequency, most cases of dementia are caused by Alzheimer's disease, multiple infarctions (multi-infarct dementia), and alcoholism (alcoholic dementia) (Table 7-1). Causes that affect adolescents should be differentiated (Table 7-2). Some causes are identifiable by their physical manifestations, such as peripheral neuropathy (Table 5-2) or involuntary movement disorders (Table 18-4). Dementia is genetic in several illnesses: Wilson's disease (autosomal recessive), Huntington's disease (autosomal dominant), some cases of Alzheimer's disease (autosomal dominant), and possibly Pick's disease. Physicians justifiably search first for reversible causes of dementia, even though only 8 percent of dementia cases are partially reversible and even less—3 percent—are fully reversible (Clarfield). Most reversible cases are associated with mild cognitive impairment lasting less than 2 years. The most common reversible causes are medications, depression, hypothyroidism, and other metabolic abnormalities. In some conditions, such as subdural hematomas and normal pressure hydrocephalus, dementia is theoretically reversible, but observable improvement is actually inconsistent.

Alternatively, certain mental status and neurologic abnormalities were purported to permit classification of dementias into "cortical" and "subcortical" groups. Once popular, this system is now losing credibility. Cortical dementias were accompanied by aphasia, agnosia, and apraxia, but patients remained alert, attentive, and ambulatory. The prime example of cortical dementia was Alzheimer's disease. In contrast, subcortical dementia was typified by less severe intellectual and memory dysfunction, but by the presence of apathy, slowed mental processing, and gait abnormalities. Its prime examples were Huntington's chorea, Parkinson's disease, normal pressure hydrocephalus, and multi-infarct dementia.

Mental Status Testing

Several screening tests, which can be administered in 5 to 10 minutes, are useful in detecting and estimating the severity of cognitive deficits. However, screening tests are coarse measurements that are limited in several respects: they tend to indicate dementia in people who have been isolated or poorly educated, and they are unreliable in distinguishing mild dementia from age-related memory impairments and depression. Since the screening tests and more detailed ones have been developed to detect the dementia associated with Alzheimer's disease, they may be unreliable in detecting dementia associated with other illnesses. Even when they indicate dementia from Alzheimer's disease,

Patient Initials [ ] [ ] [ ]
F   M   L

(1) Observation Date   (2) Patient Study Number
[ ] [ ] [ ]   [ ] [ ]
Month / Day / Year

Score each item 0 if correct, 1 if wrong.   Starting Time _____

[ ] Name _____

Correct Name, if wrong _____

[ ] Age _____ (D.O.B. _____

[ ] When born? _____ (Month, Year)

[ ] Where born? _____ Say: Some questions will be easy, some will be hard.

[ ] Name of this place _____

[ ] What street is it on? _____

[ ] How long are you here? _____ (How long today?)

[ ] Name of this city? _____

[ ] Today's date? _____ (Within a day)

[ ]   Month _____

[ ]   Year _____

[ ]   Day of Week _____

[ ]   Part of Day _____

[ ]   Time? (best guess) _____ (Time:) (Within 1 hour)

[ ]   Season _____

Something to remember (Score: immediate repetition-0; phrase by phrase-1; word by word-2; no repetition-3)

[ ] ____ John   ____ Brown   ____ 42   ____ Market St.   ____ Chicago   Repetition Score _____

[ ] Mother's first name _____ (Any sensible response)

[ ] How much schooling did you have? _____

[ ] Name of one specific school _____

[ ] What kind of work have you done? _____

[ ] Who is the president now? _____

[ ] Who was the last president? _____

[ ] Date of WW I (1914-18) _____ [ ] Date of WW II (1938-45) _____

Next 3 items: For uncorrected errors, score 2; for corrected errors, score 1.

[ ] Months of the year, backwards. Start with December . . . .

      D   N   O   S   A   Jl   Jn   M   Ap   Mch   F   Ja

[ ] Count 1–20

[ ] Count 20–1 (20 19 18 17 16 15 14 13 12 11 10 9 8 7 6 5 4 3 2 1)

[ ] Recall name & address ___ J ___ B ___ 42 ___ M ___ C (Cue with "John Brown" only. Score up to 5 errors.)

TOTAL BLESSED [ ]   Finishing Time _____

FIGURE 7–1. Blessed Mental Status Test. Each incorrect answer adds one point to the Blessed dementia score. The scores for normal middle-aged adults are 3 points or less. Studies have shown that older individuals with these scores have little probability of developing dementia. People with scores of 5 to 7 have approximately 50 percent chance of developing dementia within 2 years. People with dementia have scores of 8 points or higher. When they die, their brains have increased numbers of neuritic plaques. The critical questions are those requiring the repetition of the John Brown phrase, which requires recall of five items, and saying the months backward. Note that the dates of World Wars I and II are those of Britain's participation, and thus, with time and increasing cultural differences, the test will become less valid. [Reprinted from Blessed G, Tomlinson BE, Roth M: The association between quantitative measures of dementia and senile change in the cerebral gray matter of elderly subjects. Br J Psychiatry *114*:797, 1968. With permission of Dr. Blessed and The British Journal of Psychiatry.]

Patient . . . .
Examiner . . . .
Date . . . .

Maximum
Score   Score

ORIENTATION

5	( )	What is the (year)(season)(date)(day)(month)?
5	( )	Where are we: (state)(county)(town)(hospital)(floor).

REGISTRATION

3	( )	Name 3 objects: 1 second to say each. Then ask the patient all 3 after you have said them. Give 1 point for each correct answer. Then repeat then until he learns all 3. Count trials and record.
		Trials

ATTENTION AND CALCULATION

5	( )	Serial 7's. 1 point for each correct. Stop after 5 answers. Alternatively spell "world" backwards.

RECALL

3	( )	Ask for the 3 objects repeated above. Give 1 point for each correct.

LANGUAGE

9	( )	Name a pencil, and watch (2 points)

Repeat the following "No ifs, and, or buts." (1 point)
Follow a 3-stage command:
   "Take a paper in your right hand, fold it in half, and put it on the floor" (3 points)
Read and obey the following:

CLOSE YOUR EYES (1 point)

Write a sentence (1 point)
Copy design (1 point)
_____ Total score
ASSESS level of consciousness along a continuum _____

Alert   Drowsy   Stupor   Coma

INSTRUCTIONS FOR ADMINISTRATION OF MINI-MENTAL STATE EXAMINATION

ORIENTATION

1. Ask for the date. Then ask specifically for parts omitted, e.g., "Can you also tell me what season it is?" One point for each correct.
2. Ask in turn "Can you tell me the name of this hospital?" (town, county, etc.). One point for each correct.

REGISTRATION

Ask the patient if you may test his memory. Then say the names of 3 unrelated objects, clearly and slowly, about one second for each. After you have said 3, ask him to repeat them. This first repetition determines his score (0–3) but keep saying them until he can repeat all 3, up to 6 trials. If he does not eventually learn all 3, recall cannot be meaningfully tested.

ATTENTION AND CALCULATION

Ask the patient to begin with 100 and count backwards by 7. Stop after 5 subtractions (93, 86, 79, 72, 65). Score the total number of correct answers.

If the patient cannot or will not perform this task, ask him to spell the word "world" backwards. The score is the number of letters in correct order, e.g. dlrow = 5, dlorw = 3.

RECALL

Ask the patient if he can recall the 3 words you previously asked him to remember. Score 0–3.

LANGUAGE

Naming: Show the patient a wrist watch and ask him what it is. Repeat for pencil. Score 0–2.

Repetition: Ask the patient to repeat the sentence after you. Allow only one trial. Score 0 or 1.

3-State command: Give the patient a piece of plain blank paper and repeat the command. Score 1 point for each part correctly executed.

Reading: On a blank piece of paper print the sentence "Close your eyes" in letters large enough for the patient to see clearly. Ask him to read it and do what it says. Score 1 point only if he actually closes his eyes.

Writing: Give the patient a blank piece of paper and ask him to write a sentence for you. Do not dictate a sentence, it is to be written spontaneously. It must contain a subject and verb and be sensible. Correct grammar and punctuation are not necessary.

Copying: On a clean piece of paper, draw intersecting pentagons, each side about 1 in., and ask him to copy it exactly as it is. All 10 angles must be present and 2 must intersect to score 1 point. Tremor and rotation are ignored.

Estimate the patient's level of sensorium along a continuum, from alert on the left to coma on the right.

FIGURE 7–2. Mini-Mental State Examination. Points are assigned for correct answers. Scores of 20 points or lower indicate dementia, delirium, schizophrenia, or affective disorders alone or in combination. Such scores are not found in normal elderly people or those with neuroses or personality disorders. [Reprinted from Folstein MF, Folstein SE, McHugh PR; "Mini-mental state": A practical method for grading the cognitive state of patients for the clinician. J Psychiatr Res *12*:189, 1975, with permission.]

these tests are not sufficiently reliable as to make a thorough evaluation unnecessary.

One standard screening test is the *Blessed Mental Status Test* (Fig. 7-1). In this test, increased cognitive deficiency correlates with greater neuritic plaque concentration. Of the various screening tests available, this one has been the most definitively validated. A newer, more concise version, which is derived from the Blessed Test, is *The 6-Item Orientation-Memory-Concentration Test* (Blessed Orientation-Memory-Concentration Test [BOMC]) (Katzman, 1983).

Another standard screening test is the *Mini-Mental State* (Fig. 7-2). Unlike the others, this one tests visuospatial relationships and language function. Its results are consistent with those of the Blessed test and also correlate with neuritic plaques.

Extensive neuropsychologic test batteries are required when a diagnosis of dementia remains uncertain, a quantitative measure of the severity of dementia is required, or a coexisting aphasia or other neuropsychologic deficit is suspected. In early dementia, performance scales on the WAIS-R are lower than verbal scales, and intelligence is decreased from estimated premorbid levels. For patients who were unusually intelligent before the onset of their illness, sophisticated tests, such as the *Graduate Record Examination*, might be administered for comparison to prior test results. The *Boston Diagnostic Aphasia Examination* or the *Boston Naming Test* can be used to identify and categorize language impairments, so as not to mistake them for dementia. When a visuospatial disturbance is suspected, as is often the case, the *Benton Visual Retention Test* is recommended.

To achieve a diagnostic specificity of nearly 90 percent, a battery of neuropsychologic tests must be performed. One study claimed that giving the following four tests together takes relatively little time yet attains an accuracy of over 95 percent: the Logical Memory and Mental Control Subtests of the *Wechsler Memory Scale*, the *Trailmaking Test*, and Word Fluency for Letters S and P (Storandt, Tierney). On the other hand, the well-known *Halsted-Reitan Battery*, probably because of its comprehensive nature, is not used in its complete form. Only its Trailmaking test is incorporated into standard, clinically useful batteries.

TABLE 7–3. SCREENING LABORATORY TESTS FOR DEMENTIA

Routine tests
  Chest x-ray
  Electrocardiogram (EKG)
  Complex blood count
  Chemistry profile, e.g., SMA 6 and 12
  Urine analysis
Specific blood tests
  Thyroid function, e.g., T_4
  B_{12} level
  Syphilis test*
  Human immunodeficiency virus (HIV) antibodies†
Neurologic tests
  Electroencephalogram (EEG)
  Computed tomography (CT)
  Magnetic resonance imaging (MRI)

---

  * In testing for neurosyphilis, either the FTA-ABS or MHA-TP test is preferred to the VDRL (see text).
  † For individuals in risk groups.

For elderly people, the *Mattis Dementia Rating Scale*, which reliably measures six areas of cognitive function (Vitaliano), has been refined into the *Extended Scale for Dementia* (Hersch).

Although neurologists and psychiatrists traditionally rely on these neuropsychologic tests, a complementary format evaluates the *functional status* of patients in their performance of common activities that require judgment, memory, and attentiveness. No single functional status assessment is brief, generally accepted, or particularly suited to practice. However, Katz suggests that six apparently hierarchical activities offer a valid assessment of functional capacity: feeding, continence, transfer, toileting, dressing, and bathing. The critical items can be culled from various functional status assessments (Table 7-3). Alternatively, Reisberg and others have described the well-known *Global Deterioration Scale* that includes assessment of both functional and intellectual status. Whichever form is used, residual strengths should be identified and subsequently emphasized.

Laboratory Evaluation

When no cause of dementia is obvious, a series of screening laboratory tests is usually performed (Table 7-3). Compared to the annual cost of nursing home care ($25,000 to $65,000), the evaluation is cost-effective at about $1500.

Either a CT ($250) or MRI ($750) scan is usually the first specific test for the evaluation of dementia. Both are reliable in detecting brain tumors, subdural hematomas, and other mass lesions. Since the resolution of MRI is superior, it would be more helpful in diagnosing multiple infarctions and normal pressure hydrocephalus. However, neither scan can be diagnostic of Alzheimer's disease. Cerebral atrophy, which is the most common CT or MRI abnormality in dementia from Alzheimer's disease (Figs. 20-2 and 20-16), is also present in normal elderly persons, as well as in patients with Down's syndrome, alcoholic dementia, AIDS-dementia complex, some varieties of schizophrenia, and many other conditions.

A routine EEG ($175) will be abnormal in most cases of dementia. However, the EEG slowing characteristic of early Alzheimer's disease may be indistinguishable from that commonly seen in normal older age. A clearly abnormal EEG is rarely helpful in establishing the specific cause of dementia, but may be diagnostic of Creutzfeldt-Jakob disease and subacute sclerosing panencephalitis (SSPE)—conditions for which it shows "periodic complexes" (Fig. 10-6)—as well as valuable in diagnosing pseudodementia, where the EEG is normal or shows only slight background slowing.

A lumbar puncture ($250) should be performed to inspect the cerebrospinal fluid (CSF) when patients with dementia are suspected of having neurosyphilis, chronic meningitis, SSPE, or AIDS-dementia complex. It need not be performed routinely because of its low yield in the absence of fever, other signs of infection, or specific historical information. Many tests should be ordered only for particular indications. For instance, serum folate levels are not determined if anemia or suspected nutritional impairment is absent. If adolescents or young adults develop dementia, the evaluation might include testing for AIDS (see below), serum ceruloplasmin determination and slit-lamp examination for Wilson's disease, urine toxicology screens for drug abuse, and, rarely, urine analysis for metachromatic granules and arylsulfatase-A activity for metachro-

Functional Capacity Assessment
Fulfills professional/occupational responsibilities
Continues hobbies
Shops, keeps house, cooks
Maintains financial records: checkbook, credit accounts, etc.
Travels independently to work, friends, or relatives

FIGURE 7–3. The physician should assess whether the patient performs or at least tolerates these common activities. If an activity cannot be performed, the physician should determine if the reason is impaired intellectual ability, emotional disturbance, or physical incapacity. This is not a quantitative assessment, but a survey.

matic leukodystrophy (Chapter 5). Likewise, systemic lupus erythematosus (SLE) preparations, serum Lyme disease titer determinations, and other tests for systemic illness should be performed when there are clinical indications.

ALZHEIMER'S DISEASE

Since a "definite" diagnosis of Alzheimer's disease requires histologic examination of brain tissue, this criterion is rarely met in clinical practice. A diagnosis is considered "probable," acceptable for clinical purposes, and consistent with the criteria in DSM-III-R when (*a*) adults have the insidious onset of a progressively worsening dementia, and (*b*) clinical and laboratory evaluations (Table 7-3) have excluded other neurologic and systemic illnesses that could account for the dementia. These criteria yield a diagnostic accuracy of 90 percent.

Clinical Features

Although Alzheimer's disease typically runs a progressive course, its rate of progression and some clinical features can differ among individuals. Also, the course in about 10 percent of patients plateau for several years. Nevertheless, three progressive stages, based on the severity of intellectual deterioration, have been described. In the early stage, patients may be conversant, sociable, and physically intact, but testing reveals impaired judgment and memory. These individuals may be confused either at night or when they are moved to new surroundings. Their cognitive abnormalities must be elicited to be obvious. When casually seen, these impairments are liable to be misinterpreted as depression or benign senescence.

The middle stage of Alzheimer's disease is marked by overt memory loss accompanied by impairment in other intellectual functions. Language impairments, which appear in this stage, initially include a decrease in spontaneous verbal output and the onset of word-finding difficulties, e.g., *anomia* (Chapter 8). These impairments in expression are followed by a decline in comprehension of written and verbal communications. Since visuospatial abilities also become impaired, patients often develop constructional apraxia (Chapter 8). (Citing the language and contructional impairments, some neurologists continue to refer to Alzheimer's disease as a cortical dementia.) In addition, patients commonly suffer depression, hallucinations, and, in 20 to 40 percent of cases, prominent paranoid ideation that sometimes reaches psychotic proportions.

In the early and middle stages, a patient might have frontal release signs (Fig. 7-4), increased jaw jerk reflex (Fig. 4-12), and Babinski signs. Although dementia signifies extensive cerebral cortical destruction, patients typically have relatively few physical deficits. In particular, patients with Alzheimer's disease, unlike those with multi-infarct dementia, do not have lateralized signs, such as a hemiparesis or homonymous hemianopsia. Until the late stage of the illness, they are ambulatory: the common sight of an Alzheimer's disease patient wandering aimlessly but steadily through a neighborhood characterizes the disparity between intellectual and motor function.

In the late stage, physical as well as cognitive deficits become profound. Patients tend to be mute, unresponsive to verbal requests, and bedridden in a decorticate (fetal) posture. Although it is more indicative of Creutzfeldt-Jakob's disease, myoclonus (Chapter 18) may rarely be found in this stage of Alzheimer's disease.

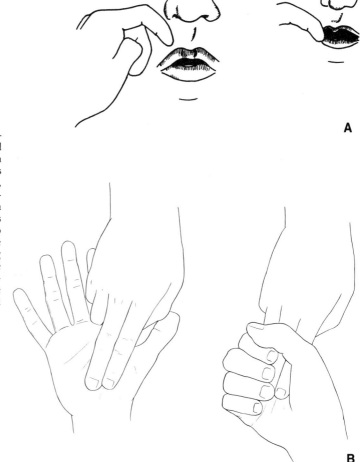

FIGURE 7–4. The frontal lobe release reflexes that have been found more frequently in demented than in nondemented elderly individuals are the snout and grasp reflexes. *A*, The snout reflex is elicited by tapping the patient's upper lip with a finger or a percussion hammer. This reflex causes the patient's lips to purse and the mouth to pout. *B*, The grasp reflex is elicited by stroking the patient's palm crosswise or the fingers lengthwise. The reflex consists of the patient's grasping the examiner's fingers and failing to let go despite requests.

Tests

The EEG can be normal in early Alzheimer's disease, when the clinical diagnosis is most difficult. Although over 80 percent of patients eventually have EEG background slowing, early EEG changes are difficult to distinguish from the slowing that normally occurs in the elderly. In the future, more sophisticated electrophysiologic testing, such as spectral frequency analysis and evoked responses (Chapter 15), might be able to pinpoint the onset of this disease.

Neither CT nor MRI scanning is definitive in diagnosing Alzheimer's disease at any stage of the illness. The classic changes on CT are atrophy of the cerebral cortex with widening of the third ventricle (Figs. 20-2 and 20-3). However, the implication of those findings is problematic. Many patients with Alzheimer's disease do not have them, and even when present, they are not conclusive because many normal or highly intelligent individuals, as well as those with any of a number of neurologic illnesses, have cerebral atrophy. Moreover, cerebral atrophy in Alzheimer's disease has no predictive value.

Compared to CT, MRI is the more sensitive in detecting cerebral atrophy and enlargement of the ventricles, and it is better at excluding small structural lesions. In addition, in Alzheimer's disease, MRI often shows nonspecific abnormalities in the white matter, *leuko-ariosis* (Fig. 20-16).

Positron emission tomography (PET) in the late stage of Alzheimer's disease, compared with age-matched controls, shows decreased cerebral oxygen and glucose metabolism in the frontal lobes, a pattern also seen in psychosis and depressive illness. PET remains a research technique that is impractical for routine clinical use (Chapter 20).

Since the histologic findings in Alzheimer's disease differ quantitatively rather than qualitatively from age-related changes, routine cerebral cortex biopsies may yield incorrect diagnoses. A cerebral cortical biopsy in cases of Alzheimer's disease is rarely indicated because a routine clinical evaluation is over 90 percent reliable, biopsy results are usually equivocal, and no effective treatment is available. However, a biopsy might be appropriate in patients suspected of having Creutzfeldt-Jakob disease, AIDS-dementia complex, or familial or otherwise atypical Alzheimer's disease.

Pathologic and Biochemical Abnormalities

Compared with age-matched controls, the brains of patients with Alzheimer's disease are more atrophic. The atrophy is pronounced in the association areas of the cerebral cortex but not in the areas subserving primary motor, sensory, or visual functions. Alzheimer's disease brains also have cortical neuron loss predominantly in the frontal and temporal lobes.

"Plaques and tangles" are commonly but incorrectly thought to be a diagnostic feature of Alzheimer's disease. Neurofibrillary tangles are paired helical protein filaments within neurons. In Alzheimer's disease, they are numerous and concentrated in the hippocampus. Although associated with Alzheimer's disease, neurofibrillary tangles do not correlate with the severity of dementia and are also found in other illnesses, such as dementia pugilistica and Parkinson's disease. The most reliable histologic feature is an increased concentration of neuritic plaques. Of the various histologic abnormalities of Alzheimer's disease, only the concentration of the plaques can be correlated with the severity of dementia.

A characteristic finding in Alzheimer's disease is that dementia is closely correlated with a pronounced loss of neurons in the *substantia innominata* (the *nucleus basalis Meynert*)—a group of large neurons located in the septal region beneath the globus pallidus (Fig. 18-1). Its neurons project upward to virtually the entire cerebral cortex, providing extensive cholinergic innervation. Their loss reduces cerebral cortex concentrations of *acetylcholine (ACh)* and the enzyme required for ACh synthesis, *choline acetyltransferase (CAT)*. Cerebral cholinergic activity is derived from acetylcholine, which is synthesized from acetylcoenzyme-A (acetylCoA) and choline:

$$\text{acetyl CoA} + \text{choline} \xrightarrow{\text{CAT}} \text{ACh}$$

Another biochemical abnormality in Alzheimer's disease is a pronounced reduction in the peptide neurotransmitter, *somatostatin*. Unlike the loss of acetylcholine, loss of somatostatin does not closely correlate with dementia. Other putative neurotransmitters that are depleted in Alzheimer's disease are Substance P, norepinephrine, vasopressin, and several polypeptides.

The severe reduction in acetylcholine that correlates with the severity of dementia has given rise to the "cholinergic hypothesis," which postulates that Alzheimer's disease dementia results from reduced cholinergic activity. It is supported by studies showing that scopolamine, which has central anticholinergic activity, induces brief Alzheimer-like cognitive impairments that can be reversed with physostigmine (Fig. 7-5) (Fuld). Even transdermal absorption of scopolamine from motion sickness patches has induced temporary amnesia in travelers.

Although the CAT deficiency is striking, it is not peculiar to Alzheimer's disease. Pronounced CAT deficiencies are also found in the cortex of brains from patients with Down's syndrome and Parkinson's disease that has resulted in dementia, although not in brains from patients with Huntington's disease (Chapter 18).

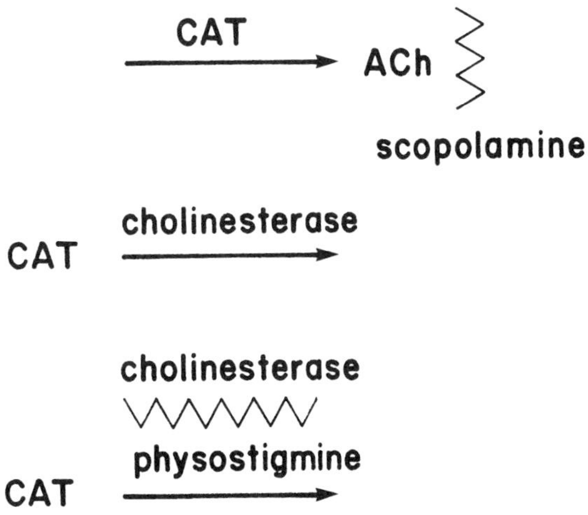

FIGURE 7–5. *Top*, Choline acetyltransferase (CAT) is the enzyme catalyzing acetylcholine (ACh) synthesis. Scopolamine, unlike most other anticholinergic substances, can cross the blood-brain barrier to block ACh. Atropine also blocks ACh, but unless large quantities are administered, it does not cross the blood-brain barrier. *Middle*, ACh is metabolized by cholinesterases. *Bottom*, Anticholinesterases, or cholinesterase inhibitors, preserve ACh concentrations. Anticholinesterases, such as edrophonium (Tensilon) and pyridostigmine (Mestinon), are used in treatment of myasthenia gravis where they preserve neuromuscular junction ACh (Fig. 6-2). For this reason, anticholinesterases are also widely used in insecticides, which cause paralysis by creating prolonged ACh activity at neuromuscular junctions. Physostigmine, which can cross the blood-brain barrier, is used in attempts to correct purported ACh deficits in tardive dyskinesia (Chapter 18) and Alzheimer's disease dementia. It is also used to counteract anticholinergic activity in cases of tricyclic antidepressant overdose.

Etiology

Many statistically significant associations—but not causal relationships—have been noted between Alzheimer's disease and other conditions. For example, head trauma, hyperthyroidism, and increased cerebral concentrations of aluminum silicate have been found significantly more frequently in Alzheimer's disease patients than in age-matched controls. Infectious organisms, including many virus-like agents, have also been proposed as etiologies.

Genetic abnormalities have received the most consideration as a possible etiology. The gene for amyloid has been detected in chromosome 21, and in cases of *familial Alzheimer's disease*, a gene has also been detected in chromosome 21. However, the genes for amyloid and Alzheimer's disease are not identical. In familial Alzheimer's disease, an autosomal dominant genetic inheritance pattern is evident. The illness begins in these patients in their fifth decade, and runs a fulminate course. The incidence among first-degree relatives of Alzheimer's disease patients eventually reaches 50 percent (Brietner).

Treatment

Despite compelling logic, treatments based on the cholinergic hypothesis have been disappointing. In attempting to restore normal ACh concentrations, researchers first gave ACh precursors, such as choline and lecithin (phosphatidyl choline). A complementary strategy to increase ACh concentrations has been to reduce its metabolism by administering centrally acting anticholinesterases, such as physostigmine and tetrahydroacridine (THA). These anticholinesterases, especially when administered with ACh precursors, may have improved memory, but only briefly and inconsistently. Moreover, serious flaws in the initial trial of THA, which is long acting and orally administered, have been exposed. Alternative strategies have been to provide ACh agonists, such as arecoline, oxotremorine, and bethanechol, by intraventricular as well as traditional administration. ACh release from cerebral neurons has been stimulated by using piracetam and praxilene.

Other approaches have been to replace somatostatin, vasopressin, and other polypeptides. Although reduced cerebral blood flow is a result, not a cause, of Alzheimer's disease, attempts have been made to restore normal blood flow. Investigators have prescribed vasodilators, such as cyclospasmol, and hydergine, which is an ergot alkaloid. The minimal improvement found with hydergine has been attributed to its antidepressant properties, but otherwise these medications have not been helpful.

Emotional and behavioral disorders associated with Alzheimer's disease and other illnesses that cause dementia do respond, albeit to a limited extent, to psychotropic medications. In view of the low ACh concentrations in Alzheimer's disease, recommended antidepressants—desipramine (Norpramin), trazodone (Desyrel), and nortriptyline (Pamelor)—have little anticholinergic activity. Also, as atrophied brains require less medication, reduced doses are indicated.

Anxiety, confusion, and insomnia can be treated with minor tranquilizers and sedatives. When these symptoms appear only at night, medications should be given pre-emptively in the late afternoon or early evening. Agitation, hallucinations, and thought disorders often require major tranquilizers. Although these medications entail a risk of inducing tardive dyskinesia and parkinsonism (Chapter 18), as well as urinary retention and other non-neurologic complications, they are indicated when psychotic mental aberrations endanger the patient and disrupt entire households.

Down's Syndrome

About 50 percent of Down's syndrome individuals who are older than 40 years develop an Alzheimer-like dementia superimposed on their mental retardation. Striking similarities between Down's syndrome and Alzheimer's disease suggest that Alzheimer's disease results from a genetic abnormality. Virtually all cases of Down's syndrome result from trisomy of chromosome 21. Abnormalities involving this chromosome are associated with Alzheimer's disease. Similar PET metabolic abnormalities are found in the two conditions. More strikingly, Alzheimer's disease and Down's syndrome have almost identical cholinergic depletion and histologic abnormalities, including the presence of neuritic plaques, neurofibrillary tangles, and loss of neurons in the nucleus basalis.

Pick's Disease

As does Alzheimer's disease, Pick's disease causes a progressive, untreatable dementia and many similar histologic changes in elderly individuals. Neuron loss occurs in the nucleus basalis Meynert as does a reduction in CAT in the cerebral cortex. Pick's disease, though rare, has a strong family tendency; however, a genetic etiology has not been established. Its histologic changes include atrophy of the frontal and anterior temporal lobes, but characteristically not the parietal lobes. As Alzheimer himself described, in Pick's disease the cytoplasm contains argentophilic (silver-staining) intraneuronal inclusions (Pick bodies). Subtle clinical differences exist between Pick's and Alzheimer's diseases. In Pick's disease, visuospatial ability is relatively preserved because the parietal lobe is spared, memory may be affected relatively late in the course, and temporal lobe atrophy produces prominent language impairments and elements of the Klüver-Bucy syndrome (Chapters 12 and 16).

NON-ALZHEIMER'S CAUSES OF DEMENTIA

Multi-Infarct Dementia

Unlike individuals with Alzheimer's disease, those who sustain multiple cerebrovascular accidents (CVAs) develop stepwise, progressive intellectual deterioration accompanied by prominent focal or lateralized signs. Spasticity, ataxia, pseudobulbar palsy, and hemiparesis are the most common signs, and patients usually have renal and cardiac disease as well. The neurologic community and the DSM-III-R diagnostic criteria for multi-infarct dementia are consistent in that both require dementia, a stepwise course, focal (lateralized) neurologic signs, and evidence of cerebrovascular disease.

CT and MRI scans usually show cerebral atrophy and often reveal cerebral infarctions. CT scans reveal multiple lucencies, and with even greater accuracy, MRI scans reveal distinctive white matter lesions. Although the EEG is almost always abnormal, changes are nonspecific. PET scans have been able to distinguish multi-infarct dementia from Alzheimer's disease by showing characteristic discrete hypometabolic areas.

Antihypertensive medications and possibly aspirin will diminish the likelihood of cerebral infarctions. However, antihypertensive medications can produce or exacerbate cognitive deficits, especially in the elderly.

Alcoholism

Chronic alcohol consumption is associated with a combination of intellectual deterioration, physical signs, and histologic changes. Although any one of these complications of alcohol abuse may predominate, they are all included in the rubric of the *Wernicke-Korsakoff syndrome*, a condition also found in people who have undergone starvation or dialysis. Thus, it is not always the result of alcohol toxicity. Nutritional deprivation, in particular a deficiency of thiamine (vitamin B$_1$)—an essential coenzyme in carbohydrate metabolism—may be responsible.

The outstanding clinical feature of the Wernicke-Korsakoff syndrome is an amnesia of previously known facts (retrograde amnesia) with an inability to learn new ones (antegrade amnesia). Although confabulation has often been considered a hallmark, it is rarely present. Most patients with Wernicke-Korsakoff syndrome also present with other mental impairments, such as poor judgment, apathy, and inattention. Physical signs of the Wernicke-Korsakoff syndrome are cerebellar dysfunction (Chapter 2), peripheral neuropathy (Chapter 5), and ocular motility abnormalities. In acute cases, ocular problems include conjugate gaze paresis, abducens nerve paresis, and nystagmus (Chapters 4 and 12).

CT and MRI scans may be normal or show only cerebral atrophy. The EEG is usually normal. Examination of the brain may show hemorrhage into the mammillary bodies and periaqueductal gray area. Since these structures are portions of the limbic system—the cornerstone of memory—damage to them results in the characteristic amnesia (Fig. 16-5).

Proper nutrition, especially thiamine administration, can partially reverse this dementia. However, only 25 percent of patients clinically recover, and pathologic changes are irreversible.

Alcoholics are also vulnerable to several other conditions that cause intellectual deterioration. Prone to trauma, they frequently harbor subdural hematomas, and those with Laënnec's cirrhosis are liable to develop hepatic encephalopathy from a high-protein meal or following gastrointestinal bleeding. Rarely, but interestingly, alcoholics have degeneration of the corpus callosum (Marchiafava-Bignami syndrome, Chapter 8). They can also have behavioral disturbances that include rage attacks, pathologic intoxication, and alcohol-withdrawal seizures. Since the seizures result from metabolic abnormalities, they are more likely to be generalized tonic-clonic seizures, rather than partial complex seizures.

Medication-Induced Dementia

Although medications often induce mental aberrations accompanied by lethargy, they sometimes cause intellectual impairments in patients who remain fully alert. Virtually every medication can be suspected. Some, such as reserpine and levodopa, routinely cause impairments, whereas others, such as cimetidine (Tagamet), do so infrequently and unpredictably. Ophthalmologic and trans-dermal medications, others not taken by pill or injection, and over-the-counter pills are often overlooked as culprits. In addition, nonpharmacologic treatments, such as cranial radiotherapy, may lead to iatrogenic mental changes.

The medicines most prone to induce mental aberrations are antidepressants, hypnotics, and antihypertensives. Of the antihypertensives, the "false neuro-transmitters," such as methyldopa (Aldomet), may be the most troublesome. In addition to inducing the aberrations, excessive use of antihypertensives can lead to orthostatic hypotension and syncope. Diuretics can cause dehydration, electrolyte imbalance, and toxic concentrations of other medications. The medications that neurologists frequently prescribe that can be responsible for inducing dementia are the anticonvulsants (Chapter 10), antiparkinson medi-cations (Chapter 18), and steroids (Chapter 15).

Normal Pressure Hydrocephalus

A cause of dementia that can be identified using clinical criteria is normal pressure hydrocephalus (NPH). Reversible by a relatively simple procedure, NPH is a clinical syndrome that consists of dementia, urinary incontinence, and *gait apraxia*. It is caused by meningitis, subarachnoid hemorrhage, or, most often, an unknown injury impeding CSF absorption through the arachnoid villi overlying the brain. Continued CSF production results in hydrocephalus (Fig. 7-6).

The NPH dementia is unusual—it is characterized as much by psychomotor retardation as by cognitive impairments. Moreover, it is accompanied or overshadowed by the physical features of the illness. Gait apraxia is usually the first and most prominent symptom of NPH (Fig. 7-7). Its severity is proportional to the degree of hydrocephalus, and with treatment, gait apraxia is the first and most likely symptom to improve. The urinary incontinence initially consists of urgency and frequency, but in severe cases, patients are totally incontinent.

CT and MRI scans show ventricular dilation with expansion of the temporal horns (hydrocephalus), minimal or no cerebral atrophy, and sometimes evidence of CSF reabsorption across ventricular surfaces (Figs. 20-4 and 20-15). Since this pattern resembles that of cerebral atrophy with resultant hydrocephalus, *hydrocephalus ex vacuo* (Fig. 20-3), the identification of NPH by CT and MRI scans is uncertain. The EEG is not diagnostically helpful, and CSF pressure and its protein and glucose concentrations are normal. The EEG is not diagnostically helpful.

Cisternography, which is a frequently used test, consists of injection of radio-active serum albumin (RASA), indium, or other substances into the subarachnoid space by a lumbar puncture and tracking the radioactive material as it diffuses upward toward the brain. Normally, and in most cases of Alzheimer's disease, the radioactive material can be followed as it diffuses over the cerebral hemispheres, where it is absorbed along with CSF through the arachnoid villi. In most cases of NPH, however, radioactive material accumulates within the cisterns at the base of the brain or within the ventricles and remains there for 72 hours or longer. Another test is a therapeutic trial of CSF withdrawal by repeated lumbar punctures to reduce the hydrocephalus. Clinical improvement after several lumbar punctures indicates NPH and predicts benefits from permanent CSF drainage.

Hydrocephalus can be permanently relieved by the placement of a thin plastic tube (shunt) into a lateral ventricle to divert CSF into the chest or abdominal cavity for absorption. A clinical response to shunt installation is generally found

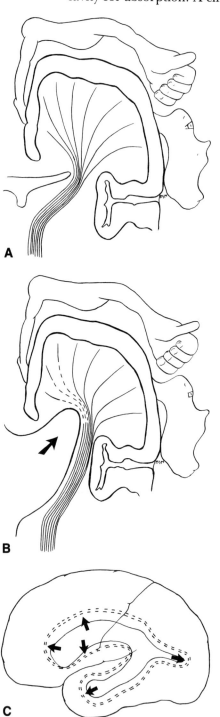

FIGURE 7–6. *A,B,* Ventricular expansion, as in normal pressure hydrocephalus, results in compression of brain parenchyma and stretching of the myelinated tracts of the internal capsule (Fig. 18-1). Since the tracts that govern the legs and the voluntary muscles of the bladder are most stretched, gait impairment (apraxia) and urinary incontinence are prominent symptoms. *C,* Also, since the CSF exerts force equally in all directions, the internal pressure on the frontal lobes leads to dementia and psychomotor retardation.

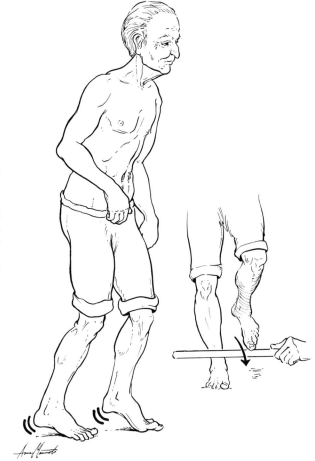

FIGURE 7–7.   Patients with gait apraxia fail to integrate the movements required to walk. Characteristically, they move their feet asynchronously and fail to place their weight on the forward foot. Their inability to shift their weight immobilizes their rear foot, which appears stuck or "magnetized" to the floor. Since their stepping reflex is relatively preserved, they can sometimes walk over a stick. Gait apraxia is one of several important characteristic gait abnormalities (Table 2-4).

in 40 to 60 percent of cases; however, when stringent diagnostic criteria are used, the improvement rate is as high as 80 percent. The neurosurgical complication rate ranges from 13 to 25 percent.

Although NPH is a reversible cause of dementia, the number of cases that are identified and then successfully treated are far fewer than would be expected. The problems are twofold: both the clinical and laboratory diagnosis are unreliable, and therapy is not consistently effective.

INFECTIONS

Neurosyphilis

Neurosyphilis, caused by persistent *Treponema pallidum* infection, has been largely of historic interest until the late 1980s when cases have been diagnosed in many AIDS patients. Neurosyphilis initially causes *acute syphilitic meningitis* or *meningovascular syphilis*, but only a small fraction of patients with these varieties of syphilis eventually develop dementia. The cognitive impairment of those who do is generally neither specific nor accompanied by prominent physical signs. Delusions of grandeur, despite their notoriety, occur rarely. In advanced neurosyphilis, patients have profound dementia, Babinski signs, dysarthria, tremulousness, and Argyll-Robertson pupils (Chapter 12), and their CT scans reveal cerebral atrophy. Dementia may be combined with other manifestations of neurosyphilis, such as tabes dorsalis, optic atrophy, and myelitis. Treatment with penicillin may improve cognitive impairments and reverse CSF abnormalities (see below); however, complete clinical recovery is rare.

A blood Venereal Disease Research Laboratory (VDRL) test (which costs $10 in 1989) is the standard screening test for syphilis. About 85 percent of neurosyphilis patients test positive. False-positive results, however, are commonly found in the "3 A's": old age, addiction, and autoimmune diseases. False-negative blood VDRL results may result from naturally occurring resolution of serologic abnormalities or from prior, sometimes inadequate, treatment. Tests that are more specific and more sensitive and are therefore called "confirmatory tests"—the blood *fluorescent treponemal antibody absorption (FTA-ABS) test* and the *treponema microhemagglutination assay (MHA-TP)* ($35)—are positive in more than 95 percent of neurosyphilis cases. A positive VDRL blood test should be confirmed with one of these tests. Likewise, whenever clinically warranted, despite a negative VDRL blood test, one of them should be ordered.

CSF testing should be done when asymptomatic individuals test positive on the FTA-ABS or MHA-TP, when individuals with intellectual deterioration or mental aberrations have a confirmatory blood test, or when patients with AIDS develop dementia. In about 60 percent of neurosyphilis cases, the CSF has an elevated protein concentration (45 to 100 mg/100 ml) and a lymphocytic pleocytosis (5 to 200 cells/ml); however, the CSF has 10 or fewer lymphocytes/ml in 90 percent of cases.

A positive CSF VDRL test, which can be found in the presence of a negative blood VDRL test, is highly specific and almost always diagnostic of neurosyphilis. Although the CSF VDRL test is rarely false-positive, it is false-negative in as many as 40 percent of neurosyphilis cases (Hooshmand). In these cases, neurosyphilis can still be diagnosed by the clinical situation, CSF protein elevation, and minimal pleocytosis. Overall, in equivocal cases, patients should be treated for neurosyphilis. Since for highly technical reasons, the FTA-ABS and MHA-TP tests cannot be applied to CSF, the VDRL remains the only currently available CSF test.

Subacute Sclerosing Panencephalitis

In subacute sclerosing panencephalitis (SSPE), children have an insidious onset of dementia, which may appear initially as behavioral disturbances, accompanied by myoclonus (Chapter 18). The average age of onset is 10 years, and patients tend to be from rural, low income families.

SSPE is diagnosed by an elevated CSF measles antibody titer and, during the initial stage of the illness, periodic complexes on the EEG (Fig. 10-6). CT scans show nonspecific ventricular dilation and cerebral atrophy that are more pronounced with longer duration and greater severity of the illness.

Although the infectious agent has not been identified, several observations point to a mutant measles virus: the CSF measles antibody titer is very high in SSPE patients and almost no children who have been vaccinated against measles have developed SSPE. Widespread immunization against measles in the United States has been credited with markedly reducing the incidence of SSPE.

Creutzfeldt-Jakob Disease

Creutzfeldt-Jakob disease, as does SSPE, causes dementia, myoclonus, and periodic EEG complexes. However, it usually affects people older than 65 years. Compared with Alzheimer's disease, Creutzfeldt-Jakob disease has a rapidly fatal course, lasting about 6 months. Cerebral cortex biopsy specimens, which are often required to diagnose this illness, reveal a characteristic *spongiform encephalopathy* and, less frequently, amyloid plaques.

The clinical and histologic features of Creutzfeldt-Jakob disease have been induced in animals by inoculation with brain tissue from human patients. Similarly, the disease has also been accidentally transferred to humans by corneal transplantation, intracerebral EEG electrodes, and biopsy specimens. Creutzfeldt-Jakob disease tragically developed in a group of children who received pituitary growth hormone extracted from human cadavers. This incident confirmed the infective nature of Creutzfeldt-Jakob disease and spurred the approval of genetically engineered human growth hormone. In contrast, Alzheimer's disease has not been transferred by any of these routes—a finding that supports a noninfectious etiology. The infectious agent in Creutzfeldt-Jakob disease is not measles or another common virus. It is believed to be a *prion*—an infective agent that contains protein but not DNA or RNA—which can be detected in human cerebral cortex biopsies using new stains.

Acquired Immunodeficiency Syndrome (AIDS)

Acquired immunodeficiency syndrome (AIDS) results from infection with the *human immunodeficiency virus (HIV)*. Previously called the human lymphotrophic virus Type III (HTLV III) or lymphadenopathy-associated virus (LAV), HIV is a *retrovirus*—a group of RNA viruses associated with immunodeficiency states and malignancies. Using *reverse transcriptase*, retroviruses reverse the usual sequence of genetic information so that it flows from RNA to DNA, and often becomes integrated into the host cell's DNA. From that point, viral DNA will be duplicated together with the host cell's genes.

HIV selectively infects and impairs T4 lymphocytes, often referred to as "helper" or "inducer" cells, that normally stimulate cytotoxic lymphocytes and antibody-producing B lymphocytes. The normal ratio of T4 to T8 lymphocytes is approximately 2; however, in AIDS patients, because of the loss of T4 cells, the T4:T8 ratio is less than 1. Destruction of the lymphocytes leaves AIDS patients vulnerable to opportunistic infections and neoplasms.

HIV also infects one or more cell types in the CNS, causing encephalitis, myelitis, meningitis, and other neurologic disturbances. Since the virus can be cultured from all parts of the CNS, including the CSF, these tissues as well as other bodily fluids are potentially infectious.

Within 6 months after HIV infection, antibodies to the virus are detectable in the serum by currently available tests. Before then, people are infectious, but these tests may not be sensitive enough for early detection. In other words, tests for HIV may be false-negative during the first 6 months of HIV infection. When antibodies are detectable, people are said to be "HIV positive." Although these individuals may appear healthy, they are infectious as well as susceptible to opportunistic infections diagnostic of AIDS. The reported rates of developing AIDS in HIV positive individuals vary considerably. One large study of HIV positive homosexual men found that 33 percent developed AIDS during a median follow-up of 15 months (Polk). However, as data accumulate, the incidence of AIDS among HIV positive individuals seems to be continuously revised upward.

The mean survival rate of AIDS patients is about 50 percent at 1 year and 15 percent at 5 years (Rothenberg). As might be expected, different groups had different survival rates. For example, the survival rate at 1 year for homoxexual men with Kaposi's sarcoma as the sole manifestation of AIDS was 80 percent, whereas for intravenous drug abusers with opportunistic infections it was 43 percent.

Among homosexual and bisexual males, the risk of HIV infection is associated with the number of sexual partners and having receptive anal intercourse. About 50 percent of these men studied in New York and as many as 70 percent in San Francisco are HIV positive; however, the incidence of new infections in this group is dramatically declining, largely due to public health education. In the other high-risk group, intravenous drug abusers and their sexual partners, the incidence of new infections is rising.

Babies born to women who are HIV positive are also at high risk. Infected in utero, during delivery, or through breast feeding, about 80 percent of babies and children with AIDS have a parent who is an intravenous drug abuser or the sexual partner of one. Since the baby of an HIV positive mother has a 50 to 75 percent chance of developing HIV infection, abortions are generally recommended to these women.

On the other hand, individuals who have close but nonsexual contact with AIDS patients generally do not become HIV positive, i.e., do not "seroconvert." In particular, members of the household and classmates of AIDS patients do not seroconvert. Also, of almost 1,000 health care workers who were exposed to blood from HIV infected patients, fewer than 0.5 percent seroconverted. The methods of exposure, which were preventable in one third of the cases, consisted of needle-stick injuries (80 percent), cuts with sharp objects (8 percent), open wound contamination (7 percent), and mucous membrane exposure (5 percent) (Marcus). Routine patient interviews and physical examinations, including pelvic and rectal examinations, have not been associated with seroconversion.

Aids-Dementia Complex

AIDS-dementia complex or simply *AIDS dementia* affects 50 to 70 percent of AIDS patients and is the most frequent neurologic complication of the illness. Moreover, dementia is sometimes the initial, most prominent, or only sign of AIDS. It can occur in HIV positive individuals with no other neurologic sign of AIDS. AIDS dementia also occurs in children with AIDS, although less frequently than in adults. Most cases of AIDS dementia are caused by direct HIV infection of the brain (i.e., HIV encephalitis), and virtually all patients are HIV positive.

The initial manifestations of AIDS dementia are poor memory, confusion, and impaired concentration. It then causes apathy, psychomotor retardation, and a flattened affect. Although some patients may have no physical impairments at the onset of AIDS dementia, most have problems with walking and fine motor movements, such as handwriting and closing buttons. Common findings are slow and clumsy movements, leg weakness and incoordination, and tremulousness of voice and limbs. As AIDS dementia worsens, patients frequently develop myoclonus or parkinsonism (Chapter 18). Also, they have systemic symptoms, such as weight loss and fevers, and develop characteristic purple plaques of Kaposi's sarcoma on the arms and face (Fig. 7-8).

Within 1 year of the onset of HIV encephalitis, 80 percent of patients develop florid dementia, frequently with psychotic features. Surviving patients eventually become incontinent, paraplegic, and uncommunicative. Although these signs of advanced AIDS dementia have been called "stereotyped" (Navia), they are similar to those of multi-infarct dementia and of the persistent vegetative state (Fig. 11-5).

The well-known fatal course of AIDS adds a strong emotional component that may overshadow cognitive impairments. The rate of suicide, perhaps precipitated by impetuous behavior and impaired judgment because of AIDS dementia, is greatly increased. The rate in men aged 20 to 59 who had AIDS was 36 times greater than that in men of the same age without AIDS (Marzuk).

CT and MRI scans reveal the cerebral atrophy characteristic of AIDS dementia, and MRI scans also show nonspecific scattered white matter abnormalities. Both scans usually detect the presence of opportunistic infections or neoplasms. The CSF shows an elevated protein content in most cases and pleocytosis and oligoclonal bands (Chapter 15) in a minority of cases.

At autopsy, the brain is atrophic. Histologic examination shows diffuse pallor of the white matter, perivascular infiltrates, gliosis of cerebral cortex, demyelination, microglial nodules, and multinucleated giant cells. HIV can be identified in brains of virtually all AIDS dementia patients. Although cytomegalovirus (CMV) can be identified in about 25 percent of brains, it is probably a superimposed infection and not the cause of the dementia.

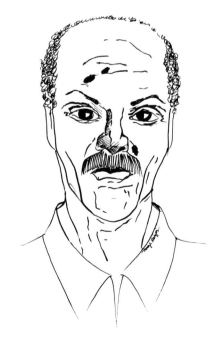

FIGURE 7–8. Although they may have no physical signs of neurologic involvement, patients with AIDS-dementia complex often have cachexia, easy fatigability, and readily recognizable Kaposi's sarcoma. These characteristic skin lesions are small, slightly raised, dry, and purple or red-brown patches.

Azidothymidine or AZT (Retrovir), an antiviral medication that acts by inhibiting reverse transcriptase, is virtually the only readily available medication that might be effective against AIDS. Although AZT may be helpful in slowing or possibly reversing AIDS dementia, its side effects include mental aberrations and bone marrow suppression, and it costs about $10,000 yearly.

Discrete Cerebral Lesions

Lateralized signs, such as focal seizures and hemiparesis, or evidence of increased intracranial pressure, such as severe headache and papilledema, indicates discrete cerebral lesions. In AIDS patients, the most common ones are certain CNS infections and lymphomas.

Cerebral infections cause lateralized signs and increased intracranial pressure, and can also exacerbate AIDS dementia. The protozoa, *Toxoplasmosis gandii*, is the most common CNS infection. Although a cerebral biopsy is required for definitive diagnosis, a working diagnosis is usually based on CT and MRI scans showing multiple ring-shaped lesions (Figs. 20-7 and 20-18) and an elevated serum toxoplasmosis antibody titer. Since antitoxoplasmosis medications are very effective and diagnostic testing is reliable, therapeutic trials of medications are often prescribed before subjecting a patient to cerebral biopsy.

The other organisms that cause discrete cerebral lesions are fungi, such as *Candida* and *Aspergillus*, *M. tuberculosis* (TB), and viruses, such as CMV and papovavirus. The last organism causes progressive multifocal leukoencephalopathy (PML). Neurosyphilis, which had almost been an extinct illness, has developed in some AIDS patients.

Cerebral neoplasms can mimic the clinical and radiographic features of cerebral toxoplasmosis; however, they usually cause only a single lesion that often requires a cerebral biopsy for diagnosis. The most common cerebral neoplasm that complicates AIDS is *primary cerebral lymphoma*. This tumor, which has a B-cell origin, is typically unifocal and poorly responsive to radiotherapy. Other cerebral malignancies are gliomas (Chapter 19) and metastatic Kaposi's sarcoma.

Other AIDS-Related Conditions

The spinal cord, as is the brain, is subject to various infections and neoplasms. In particular, HIV can infect the spinal cord and cause *vacuolar myelopathy*, a myelitis-like condition that results in paraparesis and other signs of spinal cord injury. Examination of the spinal cord shows a pattern of damage similar to combined-system disease, but vitamin B_{12} treatments have not been helpful.

Similarly, AIDS patients with or without dementia may develop meningitis from a variety of organisms. AIDS-related meningitis, which causes delirium, headache, and malaise, can mimic AIDS dementia, a discrete cerebral lesion, or depression. The most common variety of meningitis is probably acutely occurring, of several weeks' duration, relatively benign, and caused directly by HIV infection. Other common varieties are cryptococcal, bacterial, tuberculous, and syphilitic.

The peripheral nervous system (PNS) may be involved. Polyneuropathy, mimicking the Guillain-Barré syndrome (Chapter 5), and painful mononeuropathies occur frequently. Both are probably the result of an HIV infection of the PNS.

Preliminary Neurologic Evaluation

Since many neurologic problems can occur in AIDS patients or individuals at risk, psychiatrists must be able to distinguish among a debilitating emotional situation, depression, AIDS dementia, and a systemic illness. Despite public controversy, HIV testing should probably be performed routinely for individuals at risk. The enzyme-linked immunoassay (EIA) is the standard screening test; however, results may remain negative for 6 months after HIV infection and, since the EIA assay yields a small percent of false-positive results, positive tests must be repeated and confirmed with the Western blot or similar test. A test still in the experimental stage of development—the polymerase chain reaction (PCR)—detects minute quantities of viral DNA, rather than antibodies, in peripheral mononuclear cells. Since it does not require the presence of antibodies and is highly sensitive, the PCR may detect HIV infections earlier and with greater reliability than conventional tests.

Patients should also have serum toxoplasmosis titers determined and be tested for syphilis. Depending on the circumstances, tests might also be conducted for illnesses other than AIDS that are associated with the age or behavior of the patient, such as mononucleosis, hepatitis B, and subacute bacterial endocarditis.

A CT or preferably an MRI scan should be performed. An EEG would be of limited value, except in helping to distinguish dementia from depression. Unlike the evaluation for Alzheimer's disease, a lumbar puncture would usually be indicated for individuals who are at risk for AIDS and have dementia.

Pseudodementia

Pseudodementia, a condition in which psychiatric disturbances mimic dementia, is usually caused by depression, but schizophrenia, factitious disorder, or anxiety in the elderly may also be responsible. Unlike those with dementia from Alzheimer's disease, patients with pseudodementia associated with depression are typically middle-aged with previous episodes of depression, concerned about their situation, and beset with affective and vegetative disturbances. Moreover, their "cognitive impairments" are of shorter duration, fluctuate, and do not include disorientation. Indeed, many patients will perform normally on mental status examinations when actively encouraged and given additional time to complete the test. Mini-Mental State Tests may indicate depression. Their WAIS-R shows comparably abnormal performance and verbal scales; however, if psychomotor retardation is present, performance scales may be severely depressed. Allowing for age-related changes, the EEG is usually normal.

If typical cases of pseudodementia are readily identifiable, a psychiatrist's real problem would be to recognize this condition when it occurs in individuals older than 65 years. In them, pseudodementia might be overlooked because of prominent but inconsequential neurologic factors that may be associated with advanced age, such as benign forgetfulness, mild EEG slowing, and CT or MRI scans showing cerebral atrophy. Also, some patients have not had previous episodes of depression although they may have had other psychiatric conditions, and they may have no overt vegetative or affective disturbances. Although electroshock therapy and antidepressant medications have been recommended, both of these treatments may induce amnesia.

SERIOUS HEAD TRAUMA

Serious head trauma from penetrating wounds and closed injuries may be distinguished from minor head trauma by immediate posttraumatic unconsciousness lasting for more than 1 hour and permanent, prominent physical signs. In contrast, the postconcussive syndrome is a relatively minor variant considered under its most prominent symptom—headache (Chapter 9). The sequelae of serious head trauma have been attributed to more than just the nature and extent of the brain damage. Posttraumatic physical and mental deficits can be roughly correlated with the duration and depth of coma, as measured by the *Glasgow Coma Scale* (Jennett), and with the length of posttraumatic amnesia. Other prognostic factors are the premorbid intellectual and personality traits, non-neurologic complications of trauma, expectation of compensation, and unsettled litigation.

Common focal neurologic deficits—aphasia and hemiparesis—are usually attributable to structural lesions, such as intracerebral hematomas or contusions. Seizures, which are also the result of structural lesions, are usually of the partial complex or partial elementary variety. Seizures are particularly important because of their behavioral manifestations, tendency to cause further head injury, and association with cognitive impairments. Moreover, treatment with anticonvulsants may compound personality changes and cognitive impairments (Chapter 10). The duration of posttraumatic amnesia is associated with persistent personality changes, broad intellectual impairments, and, in severe cases, dementia. As noted previously, amnesia probably results from temporal lobe injury. Posttraumatic dementia is related to brainstem injury and intracerebral hematoma during coma and to focal neurologic deficits once consciousness has been restored. This variety of dementia is most evident in impaired concentration, information processing, and, particularly, memory. Head trauma can cause the *organic personality syndrome*, as well as dementia, as defined in DSM-III-R.

Relatively minor disturbances, such as personality changes, anxiety, depression, and behavioral disturbances, typically accompany or overshadow posttraumatic cognitive changes. Any psychiatric abnormalities can be exacerbated, and psychosis often occurs during the transition from coma to consciousness. Sometimes psychosis with aggressive aspects, severe depression, or, rarely, schizophrenia is permanent. As in the less pronounced psychiatric disturbances, contributing factors may be organically based emotional lability, speech and language impairments, and thought disorders.

Recovery of motor and language skills usually reaches a plateau within 6 months after the injury. Maximum intellectual recovery may be delayed until 12 to 24 months. In a typical case, following a period of coma of 1 to 3 days duration, and without brainstem injury or intracerebral hematoma, intellectual recovery will improve to at least a low normal level.

Dementia Pugilistica

The "punch drunk syndrome," or *dementia pugilistica*, results from repeated, relatively minor episodes of head trauma that routinely occur during boxing matches. Unlike the catastrophic head injury, this trauma usually leads to only momentary loss of consciousness and not to any immediately apparent mental or physical sequelae.

Dementia pugilistica is characterized by progressive intellectual deterioration that begins insidiously at the end of a boxing career and continues afterward. It is most likely to occur in lightweight boxers and alcoholics, and probably forces affected boxers to retire early. The dementia, which develops in proportion to the number of lost fights, is usually accompanied by corticospinal tract signs and parkinsonism (Chapter 18). The combination of physical and mental impairments makes the boxer vulnerable to additional head trauma that, unless interrupted, leads to further neurologic damage. The prevalence of dementia pugilistica has led to demands for regulations requiring protective headgear during all boxing matches.

TOXIC-METABOLIC ENCEPHALOPATHY

Patients with *toxic-metabolic encephalopathy* also have intellectual impairments; however, these have a different course, clinical features, and etiology than those found in dementia. Onset of the impairments in patients with this condition usually occurs during several hours to several days. If the underlying abnormality is corrected, symptoms resolve, but over a longer period. Despite

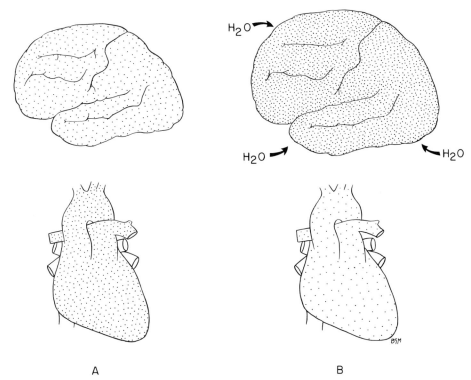

A   B

FIGURE 7–9. A perplexing clinical situation occurs when patients develop confusion, lethargy, and other mental symptoms following correction of certain metabolic abnormalities. For example, in cases of uremia or hyperglycemia, as portrayed in the sketches on the left, a roughly equal concentration of solute is present in the brain and blood. If there is overly vigorous treatment with dialysis or insulin, the solute concentration in the blood will be precipitously lowered. Since the solute is not cleared from the brain as rapidly as from the blood, the solute concentration in the brain will rise relative to that in the blood. The concentration gradient will cause free water to move into the brain, which will result in cerebral edema.

this apparent correction of underlying metabolic abnormalities, a patient's neurologic condition deteriorates (Fig. 7-9). Young children as well as old people, especially those with Alzheimer's disease, multi-infarct dementia, or other neurologic illness, are susceptible to toxic-metabolic encephalopathy from relatively minor disturbances. Common examples are febrile illnesses in young children and dehydration in elderly persons.

As in severe dementia, patients with toxic-metabolic encephalopathy are characteristically inattentive, confused, and beset by sensory misperceptions. Sometimes patients may have hypervigilant or manic periods. The clinical features that distinguish toxic-metabolic encephalopathy from dementia are a depression of the level of consciousness—from lethargy to stupor to coma—and mental aberrations that fluctuate on an hourly basis. Another distinguishing feature is autonomic system hyperactivity with sweating, tremulousness, and tachycardia.

As in Alzheimer's disease, focal neurologic deficits are usually absent, but characteristic signs may be elicited in several conditions: in Wernicke-Korsakoff syndrome, patients have oculomotor palsies, nystagmus, ataxia, and polyneuropathy (Chapters 5 and 12); patients with hepatic or uremic encephalopathy have *asterixis* (Fig. 7-10); and some patients with uremia, penicillin intoxication, and other conditions have myoclonus (Chapter 18).

Although patients with toxic-metabolic encephalopathy could be considered "delirious," they do not always meet the DSM-III-R criteria for *delirium*. Although requiring a similar course and clinical features, that diagnosis is broader than toxic-metabolic encephalopathy. For example, delirium would include postictal confusion and transient global amnesia (Chapters 10 and 11), which are conditions that neurologists classify under the basic mechanism, e.g., seizure or vascular disturbance. On the other hand, the DSM-III-R criteria exclude intoxications and withdrawal, which are conditions that neurologists almost always include in the category of toxic-metabolic encephalopathy.

Whatever the definition, hundreds of causes of toxic-metabolic encephalopathy are known, but only a few account for most cases seen in acute care hospitals (Table 7-4). The diagnosis of toxic-metabolic encephalopathy or delirium is usually evident in the patient's history, routine physical examination, or laboratory tests. EEG slowing and other abnormalities almost always coincide

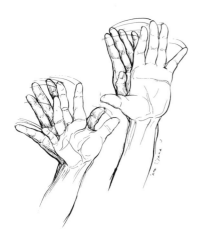

FIGURE 7–10. Asterixis is elicited by asking patients to extend their arms and hands, as though they were a policeman stopping traffic. The movements consist of the hands making a quick downward action and slow return to their extended position, as though someone were waving "goodbye." Asterixis indicates that patients have a toxic-metabolic encephalopathy.

TABLE 7–4. COMMONLY CITED FREQUENT CAUSES OF TOXIC-METABOLIC ENCEPHALOPATHY

Drug, alcohol, or medication intoxication
Hepatic or uremic encephalopathy
Fluid or electrolyte imbalance, especially dehydration
Pneumonia or other non-neurologic infection

with the onset of mental aberrations. In hepatic and uremic encephalopathy, the EEG may have characteristic triphasic waves (Fig. 10-5). CT and MRI scans are typically normal: they are really performed to exclude structural lesions that might mimic or coexist with toxic-metabolic encephalopathy. The CSF is tested when meningitis, encephalitis, or subarachnoid hemorrhage is suspected. Although treatment attempts to correct the underlying abnormality, routine medical care consists of providing fluids, electrolytes, and proper nutrition. Until the situation is rectified, minor or major tranquilizers might be necessary to make the patient safe, comfortable, and cooperative with testing and treatment.

REFERENCES

Dementia

American Psychiatric Association. Diagnostic and Statistical Manual of Mental Disorders, Third Edition—Revised, (DSM-III-R). Washington, DC, American Psychiatric Association, 1987
Becker PM, Feussner JR, Mulrow CD, et al: The role of lumbar puncture in the evaluation of dementia. J Am Geriatr Soc 33:392, 1985
Clarfield AM: The reversible dementias: Do they reverse? Ann Intern Med 109:476, 1988
Cummings JL: Dissociative states, depersonalization, multiple personality, and episodic memory lapses. In Cummings JL (ed): Clinical Neuropsychiatry. Orlando, FL, Grune & Stratton, 1985
George LK, Fillenbaum GG: OARS methodology: A decade of experience in geriatric assessment. J Am Geriatr Soc 33:607, 1985
Katz S: Assessing self-maintenance: Activities of daily living, mobility, and instrumental activities of daily living. J Am Geriatr Soc 39:721, 1983
Huber SJ, Shuttleworth EC, Paulson GW, et al: Cortical vs subcortical dementia: Neuropsychological differences. Arch Neurol 43:392, 1986
Jones EG: Neurotransmitters in the cerebral cortex. J Neurosurg 65:135, 1986
Kerson TS: Understanding Chronic Illness: The Medical and Psychosocial Dimensions of Nine Diseases. New York, The Free Press, 1985
Reisberg B, Ferris SH, De Leon MJ, et al: The global deterioration scale for assessment of primary degenerative dementia. Am J Psychiatry 139:1136, 1982
Stuss DT: The neuropsychology of the frontal lobes. BNI Quarterly 3:28, 1987
Terry RD, De Teresa R, Hansen LA: Neocortical cell counts in normal human adult aging. Ann Neurol 21:530, 1987
Tierney MC, Snow WG, Reid DW, et al: Psychometric differentiation of dementia: Replication and extension of the findings of Storandt and co-workers. Arch Neurol 44:720, 1987
Whitehouse PJ: The concept of subcortical and cortical dementia: Another look. Ann Neurol 19:1, 1986

Alzheimer's Disease

Berg L, Danziger WL, Storandt M, et al: Predictive features in mild senile dementia of the Alzheimer type. Neurology 34:563, 1984
Blessed G, Tomlinson BE, Roth M: The association between quantitative measures of dementia

and of senile change in the cerebral gray matter of elderly subjects. Br J Psychiatry *114*:797, 1968

Breitner JCS, Silverman JM, Mohs RC, et al: Familial aggregation in Alzheimer's disease. Neurology *38*:207, 1988

Cohen D, Eisdorfer C: The Loss of Self: A Family Resource for the Care of Alzheimer's Disease and Related Disorders. New York, W. W. Norton, 1986

Coyle T, Price DL, Delong MR: Alzheimer's disease: A disorder of cortical cholinergic innervation. Science *219*:1184, 1983

Cummings JL, Duchen LW: Klüver-Bucy syndrome in Pick disease: Clinical and pathologic correlations. Neurology *31*:1415, 1981

Cummings JL, Zarit JM: Probable Alzheimer's disease in an artist. JAMA *258*:2731, 1987

Cummings JL, Miller B, Hill MA, et al: Neuropsychiatric aspects of multi-infarct dementia and dementia of the Alzheimer type. Arch Neurol *44*:389, 1987

Dipple RL, Hutton JT (eds): Caring for the Alzheimer Patient: A Practical Guide. Buffalo, NY, Prometheus Books, 1988

Duara R, Grady C, Haxby J, et al: Positron emission tomography in Alzheimer's disease. Neurology *36*:879, 1986

Fillenbaum GG, Heyman A, Wilkinson WE, et al: Comparison of two screening tests in Alzheimer's disease: The correlation and reliability of the Mini-Mental State Examination and the Modified Blessed Test. Arch Neurol *44*:924, 1987

Folstein MR, Folstein SE, McHugh PR: "Mini-Mental State": A practical method for grading the cognitive state of patients for the clinician. J Psychiatr Res *12*:189, 1975

Fuld PA: Test profile of cholinergic dysfunction and of Alzheimer-type dementia. J Clin Neuropsychol *6*:380, 1984

Hersch EL: Development and application of the extended scale for dementia. J Geriatr Soc *27*:348, 1979

Hersch EL, Kral VA, Palmer RB: Clinical value of the London psychogeriatric rating scale. J Geriatr Soc *26*:348, 1978

Huff FJ, Becker JT, Belle SH, et al: Cognitive deficits and clinical diagnosis of Alzheimer's disease. Neurology *37*:1119, 1987

Hooshmand H, Escobar MR, Kopf SW: Neurosyphilis: A study of 241 patients. JAMA *219*:726, 1972

Hughes CP, Berg L, Danziger WL, et al: A new clinical scale for the staging of dementia. Br J Psychiatry *140*:566, 1982

Katzman, R: Alzheimer's disease. N Engl J Med *314*:964, 1986

Katzman, R, Terry R: The Neurology of Aging. Philadelphia, F.A. Davis Co., 1983

Koller WC, Glatt S, Wilson RS, et al: Primitive reflexes and cognitive function in the elderly. Ann Neurol *12*:302, 1982

Mace NL, Rabins PV: The 36-Hour Day: A Family Guide to Caring for Persons with Alzheimer's Disease, Related Dementing Illnesses, and Memory Loss in Later Life. Baltimore, The Johns Hopkins University Press, 1981

Mattis S: Mental status examination for organic mental syndrome in the elderly patient. In Bellak L, Karasu B: Geriatric Psychiatry: A Handbook for Psychiatrists and Primary Care Physicians. New York, Grune & Stratton, 1976, pp 77–121

McKann G, Drachman D, Folstein M, et al: Clinical diagnosis of Alzheimer's disease: Report of the NINCDS-ADRDA Work Group under the auspices of Department of Health and Human Services Task Force on Alzheimer's Disease. Neurology *34*:939, 1984

Schapiro MB, Ball MJ, Grady CL, et al: Dementia in Down's syndrome. Neurology *38*:938, 1988

Soininen B, Partanen JV, Puranen M, et al: EEG and computed tomography in the investigation of patients with senile dementia. J Neurol Neurosurg Psychiatry *45*:711, 1982

Volicer L, Fabiszenski KJ, Rheaume YL, et al (eds): Clinical Management of Alzheimer's Disease. Rockville, MD, Aspen, 1988

AIDS-Dementia Complex

Abramowicz M (ed): Diagnostic tests for AIDS. Med Letter *30*:73, 1988

Epstein LG, Sharer LR, Oleske JM, et al: Neurologic manifestations of human immunodeficiency virus infection in children. Pediatrics *78*:678, 1986

Friedland GH, Klein RS: Transmission of the human immunodeficiency virus. N Engl J Med *317*:1125, 1987

Gallo RC: The AIDS virus. Sci Am *256-1*,46, 1987

Marcus R, CDC Cooperative Needlestick Surveillance Group: Surveillance of health care workers exposed to blood from patients infected with the human immunodeficiency virus. N Engl J Med *319*:1118, 1988

Marzuk PM, Tierney H, Tardiff K, et al: Increased risk of suicide in persons with AIDS. JAMA *259*:1333, 1988

McArthur, JC: Neurologic manifestations of AIDS. Medicine *66*:407, 1987

Navia BA, Price RW: The acquired immunodeficiency syndrome dementia complex as the presenting or sole manifestation of human immunodeficiency virus infection. Arch Neurol *44*:65, 1987

Navia BA, Jordan BD, Price RW: The AIDS dementia complex. Ann Neurol *19*:517, 1986

Piel J (ed): What science knows about AIDS. Sci Am *259*:1988

Polk BF, Fox R, Brookmeyer R, et al: Predictors of the acquired immunodeficiency syndrome developing in a cohort of seropositive homosexual men. N Engl J Med *316*:61, 1987

Rosenblum ML, Levy RM, Bredesen DE (eds): AIDS and the Nervous System. New York, Raven Press, 1988

Rothenberg R, Woelfel M, Stoneburner R, et al: Survival with the acquired immunodeficiency syndrome: Experience with 5833 cases in New York City. N Engl J Med *317*:1297, 1987

Other Causes of Dementia

Black PM: Idiopathic normal-pressure hydrocephalus: Results of shunting in 62 patients. J Neurosurg *52*:371, 1980

Brown P, Cathala F, Castaigne P, et al: Creutzfeldt-Jakob disease. Ann Neurol *20*:597, 1986

Bulbena A, Berrios GE: Pseudodementia: Facts and figures. Br J Psychiatry *148*:87, 1986

Burke JM, Schaberg DR: Neurosyphilis in the antibiotic era. Neurology *35*:1368, 1985

Fisher CM: Hydrocephalus as a cause of disturbances of gait in the elderly. Neurology *32*:1358, 1982

Fisman M: Pseudodementia. Prog Neuro-Psychopharmacol Biol Psychiat *9*:481, 1985

Hershey LA, Modic MT, Greenough PG, et al: Magnetic resonance imaging in vascular dementia. Neurology *37*:29, 1987

Jennett B, Teasdale G, Galbraith S, et al: Severe head injuries in three countries. J Neurol Neurosurg Psychiat *40*:291, 1977

Jordan BD: Neurologic aspects of boxing. Arch Neurol *44*:453, 1987

Levin HS, Grafman J, Eisenberg HM: Neurobehavioral Recovery from Head Injury. New York, Oxford University Press, 1987

Marzewski DJ, Towfighi J, Harrington MG, et al: Creutzfeldt-Jakob disease following pituitary-derived human growth hormone therapy. Neurology *38*:1131, 1988

Prusiner SB: Prions and neurodegenerative diseases. N Engl J Med *317*:1571, 1987

Rappaport EB, Graham DJ: Pituitary growth hormone from human cadavers: Neurologic disease in ten recipients. Neurology *37*:1211, 1987

Reuler JB, Girard DE, Cooney TG: Wernicke's encephalopathy. N Engl J Med *312*:1035, 1985

Reynolds CF, Hoch CC, Kupfer DJ, et al: Bedside differentiation of depressive pseudodementia from dementia. Am J Psychiatry *145*:1099, 1988

Simon RP: Neurosyphilis. Arch Neurol *42*:606, 1985

Thomsen AM, Borgesen SE, Bruhn P, et al: Prognosis of dementia in normal-pressure hydrocephalus after a shunt operation. Ann Neurol *20*:304, 1986

Victor M: The Wernicke-Korsakoff Syndrome (2nd ed). Philadelphia, F. A. Davis Co., 1989

Winstead DK, Mielke DH: Differential diagnosis between dementia and depression in the elderly. In Green JB (ed): Borderland Between Neurology and Psychiatry. Neurology Clinics. Philadelphia, W.B. Saunders, 1984, pp 23–35

Zilber N, Rannon L, Alter M, et al: Measles, measles vaccination, and risk of subacute sclerosing panencephalitis (SSPE). Neurology *33*:1558, 1983

Toxic-Metabolic Encephalopathy

Abramowicz M (ed): Drugs that cause psychiatric symptoms. Med Letter *28*:81, 1986

Cummings JL: Organic psychosis. Psychosomatics *29*:16, 1988

Fraser CL, Arieff AI. Hepatic encephalopathy. N Engl J Med *313*:865, 1985

Stasiek C, Zetin M: Organic manic disorders. Psychosomatics *26*:394, 1985

Tishler PV, Woodward B, O'Connor J, et al: High prevalence of intermittent acute porphyria in a psychiatric patient population. Am J Psychiatry *142*:1430 1985

QUESTIONS: CHAPTER 7

1. What are the cardinal neurologic features of the following causes of dementia or delirium?

    a.   CNS lupus

    b.   Normal pressure hydrocephalus

     c.   Obstructive hydrocephalus
     d.   Wilson's disease
     e.   Huntington's disease
     f.   Bromism
     g.   Arsenic poisoning
     h.   Porphyria
     i.   Wernicke's encephalopathy
     j.   Myxedema madness
     k.   Tuberous sclerosis
     l.   Hepatic encephalopathy
     m.   SSPE
     n.   Creutzfeldt-Jakob disease

2. Name the single initial laboratory test that would indicate the following causes of dementia.

     a.   Myxedema
     b.   Combined-system disease
     c.   Porphyria
     d.   Arsenic poisoning
     e.   Lead poisoning
     f.   Tabes dorsalis
     g.   SSPE
     h.   Water intoxication
     i.   Bromism
     j.   Subarachnoid hemorrhage
     k.   Subdural hematomas
     l.   Creutzfeldt-Jakob disease
     m.   Wilson's disease
     n.   Sphenoid wing meningioma
     o.   Hepatic encephalopathy
     p.   Cryptococcal meningitis

3. In which causes of dementia is the EEG usually of diagnostic assistance?

     a.   Alzheimer's disease
     b.   SSPE
     c.   Olivopontocerebellar atrophy
     d.   Lead poisoning
     e.   Uremia
     f.   Hepatic encephalopathy
     g.   Creutzfeldt-Jakob disease
     h.   Neurosyphilis
     i.   Multi-infarct dementia
     j.   Frontal lobe tumors
     k.   Valium intoxication
     l.   Pseudodementia
     m.   Parkinson's disease
     n.   Herpes encephalitis
     o.   Subdural hematomas
     p.   AIDS dementia

4. The diagnosis of normal pressure hydrocephalus (NPH) has received much attention in the literature because installation of a ventricular-peritoneal shunt is said to correct the dementia.

     a.   What conditions predispose a patient to NPH?
     b.   What tests are used in an attempt to establish this diagnosis?

5. Is a cerebral cortex biopsy indicated in the routine diagnosis of Alzheimer's disease?

6. With which feature is Alzheimer's disease dementia most closely associated?

     a.   Large ventricles
     b.   Increased concentration of neuritic plaques

    c.   Increased concentration of neurifibrillary tangles
    d.   Degree of neuron loss

7. What medication or therapy (column B) is appropriate for severe intoxication of the following (column A)?

[A]		[B]	
1.	Lithium	a.	Physostigmine
2.	Bromide	b.	Hypertonic saline or water
3.	Heroin		restriction
4.	Methadone	c.	Atropine
5.	Phenobarbital	d.	Dialysis
6.	Imipramine (Tofranil)	e.	Saline, diuretics
7.	Valium	f.	Ethyl alcohol, 50 percent
8.	Water	g.	B_6
9.	Lead	h.	BAL (dimecaprol)
10.	Belladona alkaloids	i.	Penicillin
11.	Methanol	j.	Naloxone (Narcan)
12.	Arsenic	k.	Hypotonic saline
13.	Organic phosphates	l.	Glucose
14.	Phenothiazines	m.	Nonspecific supportive therapy
15.	Mercury		and possibly sedatives or
17.	Isoniazid (INH)		neuroleptics
18.	Scopolamine	n.	Propranolol (Inderal)
19.	L-dopa		
20.	Thyroxine		

8. What is the pattern of inheritance of the following diseases that cause dementia?
    1.   Wilson's disease
    2.   Huntington's disease
    3.   Porphyria, acute intermittent
    4.   Familial Alzheimer's disease
    a.   Sex-linked recessive
    b.   Autosomal recessive
    c.   Autosomal dominant

9. Which feature is *not* common to Alzheimer's disease and Down's syndrome?
    a.   An abnormality on chromosome 21
    b.   Dementia
    c.   Presence of cerebral plaques and tangles
    d.   Low concentrations of cerebral acetylcholine
    e.   Abnormalities in the nucleus basilis of Meynert
    f.   High incidence of leukemia

10. With which condition has Alzheimer's disease *not* been associated?
    a.   History of hyperthyroidism
    b.   Increased brain aluminum silicate concentration
    c.   Other family members with the illness
    d.   Down's syndrome
    e.   Creutzfeldt-Jakob disease

11. Which of the following conditions are reversible forms of dementia?
    a.   AIDS dementia
    b.   Cerebral toxoplasmosis
    c.   Postanoxic encephalopathy
    d.   Serious head injury
    e.   Normal pressure hydrocephalus
    f.   Acute intermittent porphyria
    g.   Myxedema
    h.   Kernicterus
    i.   Combined-system disease
    j.   Dementia pugilistica
    k.   Lead poisoning

l.   Wernicke-Korsakoff syndrome
m.   Pellagra
n.   Cryptococcal meningitis
o.   SSPE
p.   Down's syndrome
q.   Cerebral syphilis
r.   AIDS-associated cerebral lymphoma
s.   Multi-infarct dementia
t.   Subdural hematomas
u.   Alzheimer's disease
v.   Pick's disease
w.   Creutzfeldt-Jakob
x.   Wilson's disease
y   Parkinson's disease

12.   Match the histologic finding in Alzheimer's disease with its description.

1.   Paired helical filament
2.   Cluster of degenerating nerve terminals with an amyloid core
3.   Group of neurons beneath the globus pallidus

a.   Neurofibrillary tangles
b.   Neuritic plaque
c.   Substantia innominata or nucleus basalis of Meynert

13.   What is the most common form of dementia accompanied by a peripheral neuropathy?

14.   Which is the most common EEG finding in patients with early Alzheimer's disease?

a.   Theta and delta activity
b.   Periodic complexes
c.   High-voltage fast activity
d.   Normal or slight slowing of the background activity

15.   In which conditions is cerebral atrophy found on MRI or CT scans?

a.   Alzheimer's disease
b.   Down's syndrome
c.   Normal aging
d.   Normal pressure hydrocephalus
e.   Encephalitis
f.   Pseudotumor cerebri
g.   AIDS dementia
h.   Cerebral toxoplasmosis

16.   With which condition is cerebral atrophy, as detected by CT or MRI, most closely associated?

a.   Alzheimer's disease
b.   Intellectual impairment
c.   Old age

17.   Positron emission tomography (PET) and other studies have demonstrated decreased cerebral glucose metabolism and decreased oxygen consumption in Alzheimer's disease. Nevertheless, how is it known that Alzheimer's disease does not result from cellular hypoxia?

18.   From which area of the brain do the majority of cerebral cortex cholinergic fibers originate?

a.   Hippocampus
b.   Basal ganglia
c.   Frontal lobe
d.   Nucleus basalis of Meynert

19–22.   Choline acetyltransferase (CAT) is the fundamental enzyme in synthesis of acetylcholine (ACh). What is the effect of the following substances on ACh activity?

19. Neostigmine

20. Scopolamine

21. Organic phosphate insecticides

22. Physostigmine

a. Increases ACh activity
b. Decreases ACh activity
c. Does not change ACh activity

23. What are the features of multi-infarct dementia that are *not* present in Alzheimer's disease?
   a. Prominent physical impairments, e.g., spasticity
   b. History of hypertension and cerebrovascular infarctions
   c. Helpfulness of EEG in diagnosis
   d. A CT or MRI scan showing multiple lucencies
   e. Improvement in symptoms with antihypertensive treatment

24. Which are frequently found features of Wernicke-Korsakoff syndrome?
   a. A CT or MRI scan that is normal or shows atrophy
   b. Confabulation
   c. Hemorrhage in portions of the limbic system
   d. Full recovery after treatment

25. Why do some patients with active neurosyphilis have negative blood VDRL tests?
   a. Autoimmune diseases often cause false-negative tests.
   b. After years, the VDRL tends to revert to being negative.
   c. Small doses of antibiotics, given for unrelated reasons, partially but inadequately treat syphilis. The VDRL reverts to being negative, but neurosyphilis persists.
   d. Very high antibody levels interfere with standard test.

26. Possibly 40 percent of patients with neurosyphilis have negative CSF VDRL tests. How should the clinician evaluate the CSF in cases where neurosyphilis is suspected?
   a. Do a lumbar puncture. If there is CSF pleocytosis or increased protein concentration, treatment for neurosyphilis should be given despite a negative CSF VDRL.
   b. Perform a lumbar puncture and treat if the CSF FTA-ABS test is positive.
   c. Do a lumbar puncture on all patients with dementia.
   d. Do a lumbar puncture on all patients with a positive blood VDRL.
   e. Do a lumbar puncture if there is a history of syphilis that was untreated, physical signs indicate neurosyphilis, or a positive VDRL test is confimred by a more specific test.

27. Of the following, which is the most specific blood test for syphilis?
   a. VDRL
   b. Microhemagglutination assay (MHA-TP)
   c. Wasserman
   d. Colloidal gold curve

28. Which are characteristics of Pick's disease?
   a. Relatively preserved visuospatial ability
   b. Familial tendency
   c. Preserved parietal lobe despite otherwise generalized cerebral atrophy
   d. Argentophilic intraneuronal bodies
   e. Transmissibility to monkeys
   f. Ready clinical identification

29. What are neurologic complications of professional boxing?
   a. Dementia pugilistica
   b. Intracranial hemorrhage
   c. Parkinsonism
   d. Slowed reaction times
   e. Progression of dementia after retirement

30. Which forms of intellectual deterioration are associated with peripheral neuropathy?

a. Alzheimer's disease
b. Wernicke-Korsakoff syndrome
c. Metachromatic leukodystrophy
d. Uremia
e. Nitrous oxide abuse
f. Acute intermittent porphyria
g. Combined system disease (B_{12} deficiency)
h. Polyarteritis
i. AIDS dementia

31. Which movement disorders are associated with incapacitating cognitive impairments?

a. Choreoathetosis
b. Lesch-Nyhan syndrome
c. Dystonia musculorum deformans
d. Tourette's syndrome
e. Essential tremor
f. Rigid form of Huntington's disease

32. A 65-year-old man was brought to the Emergency Room by his family who said that he suddenly became "confused." On examination, he was fully alert and attentive but distraught. He was unable to recall recent or prior events, the date, or any of three objects after a 3-minute delay. His language was normal, and at least grossly, his judgment was intact. The symptoms resolved after 2 hours. Which of the following conditions was this episode most likely to represent?

a. Hysteria
b. Dementia
c. Nondominant hemisphere ischemia
d. Transient global amnesia

33–35. Each of the following conditions is associated with confabulation. Where is the usual primary site of brain damage?

33. Wernicke-Korsakoff syndrome

34. Anton's syndrome

35. Nondominant hemisphere syndrome

a. Right parietal lobe
b. Periventricular gray matter, mamillary bodies
c. Occipital lobes, bilaterally

36. Which of the following traits is characteristic of normal individuals who are older than 65 years?

a. Shorter attention span
b. Slower acquisition of new information
c. Decreased ability to perform new tasks
d. Slight decrease in intelligence, as measured by the WAIS-R.
e. Significant loss of vocabularity
f. Impairments in language ability
g. Decreased general information

37. A 68-year-old man has the onset of dementia. His blood VDRL test is positive at a 1:8 dilution, but no other test indicates a specific cause. Should he be treated for syphilis?

a. Yes, and at doses of penicillin suitable for neurosyphilis.
b. No.
c. Not until a further blood test, such as the FTA-ABS or MHA-TP, confirms the diagnosis. The VDRL test result may be a biologic false-positive result.
d. Perhaps. If the clinical suspicion is high or if a confirmatory blood test is positive, then examination of the CSF is indicated (see Question 26). Of course, he may require treatment for syphilis that has not involved the nervous system.

38. A 30-year-old homosexual man is found to have a positive HIV test. He has no physical or mental symptoms. What are the implications of the test result?

a. He has AIDS.

b. He is infective and should not donate blood.

c. He has at least a 50 percent probability of having the AIDS-dementia complex.

d. He has an unknown probability of developing AIDS, but a reasonable estimate would be 10 percent yearly.

39. Which is the skin malignancy characteristically associated with AIDS?

a. Lymphoma

b. Herpes

c. Kaposi's sarcoma

d. Chancre

40. If a pregnant woman is HIV positive, what is the probability that the infant will develop AIDS?

a. 10 percent

b. 50 percent

c. More than 50 percent

d. Unknown

41. What is the cause of AIDS-dementia complex?

a. HIV encephalitis

b. Toxoplasmosis

c. Cerebral lymphoma

d. Unknown

42. What is the most common cause of multiple discrete cerebral lesions in AIDS patients?

a. Cerebral lymphoma

b. Kaposi's sarcoma

c. Cryptococcal meningitis

d. Toxoplasmosis

ANSWERS

1. a. Seizures, strokes, and psychosis (the three S's)

b. Dementia, incontinence, and gait apraxia

c. Headache, papilledema, and bilateral Babinski signs

d. Dementia, tremor, rigidity, and Kayser-Fleischer corneal rings

e. Dementia, chorea, and, in young adults, rigidity

f. Dementia with psychotic appearance, acneiform skin rash, headache, and lethargy

g. Nonspecific mental dullness and peripheral neuropathy

h. Recurrent episodes of delirium, seizures, peripheral neuropathy, and abdominal pain with dark red urine (acute intermittent porphyria only)

i. Amnesia with nystagmus, ocular paresis, ataxia, and peripheral neuropathy

j. Rarely occurring, excited, confusional state

k. Adenoma of face, seizures, and dementia, usually beginning in childhood

l. Lethargy, confusion, and asterixis

m. Dementia and myoclonus, usually in rural boys

n. Rapidly developing dementia, pyramidal and extrapyramidal motor findings, and myoclonus

2. a. Serum T_4 level

b. Serum B_{12} level

c. Watson-Schwartz test or urine porphyrin levels

d. Serum heavy metal tests or fingernail analysis

e. Serum heavy metal tests

f. CSF-VDRL, if positive (see text)

g. EEG (periodic complexes) and CSF measles antibody

  h. Serum electrolytes
  i. Serum electrolytes
  j. Bloody or xanthochromic CSF from a lumbar puncture, or a CT or MRI scan showing blood
  k. CT or MRI scan
  l. EEG (periodic complexes) and brain biopsy (spongiform encephalopathy)
  m. Serum ceruloplasmin level and slit-lamp examination
  n. CT or MRI scan
  o. EEG (triphasic waves) and liver function tests; blood ammonia levels are inconsistent
  p. Cryptococcal antigen test of the CSF

3. b, e, f, g, j, k, l, n.

4. a. Subarachnoid hemorrhage, chronic meningitis, but mostly unknown causes
  b. CT or MRI scan and cisternography

5. No. Since neuritic plaques and neurofibrillary tangles are found in normal aged brains, routine histologic examination cannot be diagnostic. However, if appropriate studies can be performed, a lowered acetylcholine or choline acetyltransferase level would be virtually diagnostic.

6. b.

7. 1–e; 2–e; 3–j; 4–j; 5–d; 6–a; 7–m; 8–b; 9–h; 10–m; 11–f; 12–h; 13–c; 14–m; 15–h; 16–m; 17–g; 18–m; 19–m, g; 20–n.

8. 1–b; 2–c; 3–c; 4–c.

9. f.

10. e.

11.

a.	No		n.	Yes
b.	Yes		o.	No
c.	No		p.	No
d.	Yes		q.	Yes
e.	Yes		r.	No
f.	Yes		s.	No
g.	Yes		t.	Yes
h.	No		u.	No
i.	Yes		v.	No
j.	No		w.	No
k.	No		x.	Yes
l.	Yes		y.	No
m.	Yes			

12. 1–a; 2–b; 3–c.

13 Wernicke-Korsakoff syndrome

14. d.

15. a, b, c, g.

16. c.

17. Since several studies have demonstrated that oxygen *extraction* is normal, the O_2 consumption is low because cerebral requirements are low. In Alzheimer's disease and other conditions in which cerebral metabolism is lowered, the oxygen consumption is secondarily lowered. As a practical point, giving oxygen to Alzheimer's disease patients will not reverse the dementia.

18. d.   **20.** b.

19. a. (but not in the brain) **21.** a. (but not in the brain)

22. a.   **23.** a, b, d.

24. a, c. (The mamillary bodies are part of the limbic system.)

25. b, c, d. (A positive VDRL should be confirmed before doing a lumbar puncture.)

26. a, e. Also many clinicians would treat for neurosyphilis, if there were a confirmatory blood test, even if the CSF were entirely normal.

27. b.

28. a, b, c, d.

29. a, b, c, d, e.

30. b, c, d, e, f, g, h, i (see Table 5-2).

31. a (but not always), b, f.

32. d. The patient had a 2-hour episode of memory impairment with preservation of consciousness, perception, and judgement. Any disturbance in which memory is selectively impaired is called an *amnestic syndrome*. Most are caused by temporal lobe dysfunction produced by ischemia, infarction, epilepsy, or hemorrhage. In this case, the memory impairment is called *transient global amnesia*, which is believed to result from ischemia of the posterior cerebral arteries that supply the temporal lobe. It is most common in individuals older than 65 years, and it may be precipitated by sexual intercourse, physical stress, or strong emotions. Other causes of transient amnesia are partial complex seizures, Wernicke-Korsakoff syndrome, and the use of certain medications, such as scopolamine. Psychiatric disturbances cause transient amnesia as often as do neurologic disorders.

33. b.   **38.** b, d.

34. c.   **39.** c.

35. a.   **40.** c.

36. a, b, c, d.   **41.** a.

37. c, d.   **42.** d.

8

Aphasia and Related Disorders

Language impairment, or *aphasia,** differs from dementia (Chapter 7) both in its circumscribed neuropsychologic characteristics and in its origin, which is usually a single, discrete cerebral lesion, such as a cerebrovascular accident (CVA) (Chapter 11). Unlike dementia, aphasia usually results from damage to certain areas of the *dominant hemisphere*, the cerebral hemisphere that governs language function. Language function includes verbal language (speaking and listening), written language (reading and writing), and even sign language.

In addition to governing language function, the dominant hemisphere integrates language with intellect, emotion, and the sensory modalities (such as the tactile, auditory, and visual systems). Thus it provides the primary avenue for conscious communication of thoughts and emotions.

However, the dominant hemisphere does not necessarily govern languages that are learned as adults, including "second languages," writing that is based on pictures (e.g., hieroglyphics), or use of obscenities, i.e., cursing, which is usually a distillation of strong emotions. The dominant hemisphere also plays a minimal role in imparting that combination of inflection, rhythm, and tone that comprises the *prosody* of speech. Musicians have been shown to process music, as language, in the dominant hemisphere; however, the nondominant hemisphere usually has more influence in people who have no particular creative or interpretive musical skill.

Cerebral hemisphere dominance for normal language is accompanied by control of fine, rapid hand movements ("handedness") and, to a lesser degree, reception of vision and hearing. For example, right-handed people, who have left cerebral hemisphere dominance, not only rely on their right hand for writing and throwing a ball but also their right foot for kicking, right eye when peering through a telescope, and right ear for *dichotic listening*, listening to words spoken simultaneously in both ears.

Autopsy and radiologic studies have shown that the superior surface of the dominant temporal lobe has significantly greater cortex area than that of the nondominant lobe because it has more gyri and deeper sulci. This region, the *planum temporale*, contains important elements of the language pathway. Notably, according to some reports, the normal cortical asymmetry between the dominant and nondominant temporal lobes is lacking in some patients with autism and chronic schizophrenia—two conditions with prominent language abnormalities.

About 90 percent of all people are left hemisphere dominant for language and are right-handed. Of the others, many are also left hemisphere dominant

---

* Patients with aphasia and related disorders may receive assistance from the American Speech-Language-Hearing Association, 10801 Rockville Pike, Rockville, Maryland 20852, (301) 897-5700.

or are mixed-dominant, but appear to be ambidextrous or even left-handed. Many people who are truly ambidextrous excel in playing certain sports and performing on musical instruments. These people appear to have been endowed with language, music, and motor skill function in their right as well as left hemispheres.

In contrast, left-handed people may have naturally occurring right hemisphere dominance, or instead, their right hemisphere may have become dominant as a consequence of congenital injury to the left cerebral hemisphere (Chapter 13). Left-handed people are found in disproportionate numbers among those who excel in various skilled endeavors but, as might be expected, are also among those who are mentally or physically impaired. For example, a greater than expected number of left-handed people are musicians, artists, mathematicians, and athletes.* However, left-handedness is also over-represented among children with dyslexia and other learning disabilities, stuttering, and general clumsiness, as well as among people with major impairments—mental retardation, epilepsy, and certain major psychiatric disorders, including autism and some forms of schizophrenia.

Left-handed people with mixed or predominantly right hemisphere dominance may become aphasic if either hemisphere is injured by a CVA. Their site of cerebral injury is less clearly related to the variety of aphasia and the associated physical deficits than in right-handed individuals. However, the prognosis for their recovery is better.

Although the left hemisphere is usually dominant (the rest of this chapter assumes that it always is), sometimes dominance must be established with certainty. For example, when the temporal lobe must be partially resected because of intractable partial complex epilepsy (Chapter 10), only a limited resection of the dominant temporal lobe would be permissible to avoid creating aphasia. Cerebral dominance can be established with the *Wada test* in which sodium amobarbital is injected directly into each carotid artery: when the dominant hemisphere is perfused, the patient becomes briefly aphasic.

APHASIA

Functional Neuroanatomy

Impulses conveying speech, music, and uncomplicated sound travel from the ears along the acoustic (eighth cranial) nerves into the brainstem. Crossed and uncrossed brainstem tracts bring them to the primary auditory cortex, *Heschl's gyri*, in each temporal lobe (Fig. 4-15). Most musical and some other impulses remain in the nondominant hemisphere. Those conveying language are transmitted to *Wernicke's* area, which is in the dominant temporal lobe, and travel in an arc within the *arcuate fasciculus* through the temporal and parietal lobes to *Broca's area* (Fig. 8-1). Within this pathway, words are perceived as language

---

* Closely examining this general rule about athletes, Hemenway found that left-handed athletes tend to be more successful than right-handed ones only in those sports that involve direct confrontation and have active defenses, such as baseball, tennis, fencing, and boxing. In these sports, left-handed athletes have a tactical advantage, such as a left-handed batter's greater closeness to first base. In sports that do not have direct confrontation, such as swimming, golf, and pole vaulting, Hemenway found little difference between right- and left-handed athletes. Thus he doubts that left-handedness confers an intrinsic advantage for athletes.

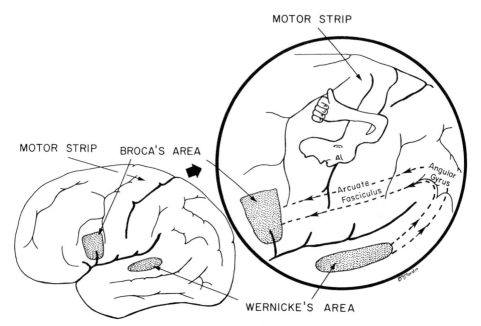

MOTOR STRIP

MOTOR STRIP   BROCA'S AREA

Arcuate Fasciculus

Angular Gyrus

WERNICKE'S AREA

FIGURE 8–1. The left cerebral hemisphere contains Wernicke's area in the temporal lobe and Broca's area in the frontal lobe. The arcuate fasciculus, which connects Wernicke's and Broca's areas, travels from the temporal lobe back to the parietal lobe, where it passes through the angular gyrus, and then arcs forward to the frontal lobe. The cerebral cortex motor area for the right hand and face is adjacent to Broca's area.

and integrated with psychologic information and various sensory modalities. Broca's area, which is immediately anterior to motor centers for the right arm, face, larynx, and pharynx, receives the processed, integrated language and in turn governs the articulation of spoken language.

Using this model, several normal language patterns and important clinico-pathologic correlations have been postulated. For example, when people repeat aloud what they hear, impulses go to Wernicke's area, pass through the arcuate fasciculus, and arrive at Broca's area for speech production (Fig. 8-2). Also, when people read aloud, impulses are initially received by the visual cortex in the left and right occipital lobes (Fig. 4-1). Those impulses from the left visual field are received by the right occipital cortex and must travel through the posterior corpus callosum to reach the left (dominant) cerebral hemisphere. There, the combined impulses from the left and right visual cortices travel through the arcuate fasciculus to Broca's area (Fig. 8-3).

Patients with lesions almost anywhere in the arc made by Wernicke's area,

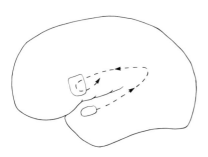

FIGURE 8–2. When patients repeat aloud, language is received in Wernicke's area and transmitted through the parietal lobe by the arcuate fasciculus to Broca's area. This area innervates the adjacent cerebral cortex for the tongue, lips, larynx, and pharynx, as well as for the right face and arm.

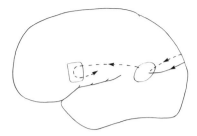

FIGURE 8–3. When patients read aloud, visual impulses are received by the left and right occipital visual cortex regions. Both regions send impulses to the left parietal region. Those from the left visual field, which are received in the right cortex, must first pass through the posterior corpus callosum (see Fig. 8-4).

the arcuate fasciculus, and Broca's area cannot repeat phrases. Conversely, this arc may be isolated by anoxia from the surrounding cerebral cortex so that patients can only repeat but not initiate conversation (see below, Isolation or Transcortical Aphasia).

Lesions such as CVAs that damage Broca's area are also apt to damage the adjacent motor cortex and thus cause dysarthria and right hemiparesis, as well as aphasia. In contrast, lesions that damage Wernicke's area or the arcuate fasciculus are not apt to cause dysarthria or hemiparesis. Lesions that damage the posterior corpus callosum interrupt the path for written information received by the left visual field as it travels from the visual cortex of the right hemisphere to the language centers of the left hemisphere; as a result, written material cannot be read.

Clinical Evaluation

In previous years, aphasia was divided according to various systems. One of the most widely used systems classified aphasia as *receptive (sensory)* or *expressive (motor)* on the basis of the relative impairment of verbal reception or expression; however, this nomenclature is not practical because most aphasic patients have mixtures of receptive and expressive impairments. The neurologic community has now adopted a division of aphasia into *nonfluent* and *fluent* based on the quality of a patient's verbal output (Table 8-1).

TABLE 8–1. THE SALIENT FEATURES OF MAJOR APHASIAS

Feature	Nonfluent Aphasia	Fluent Aphasia
Previous descriptions	Expressive	Receptive
	Motor	Sensory
	Broca's	Wernicke's
Spontaneous speech	Nonverbal	Verbal
Content	Paucity of words, mostly nouns and verbs	Complete sentences with normal syntax
Articulation	Dysarthric, slow, stuttering	Good
Errors	Telegraphic speech	Paraphasic errors, nonspecific phrases, circumlocutions
Response on testing		
Comprehension	Preserved	Impaired
Repetition	Impaired	Impaired
Naming	Impaired	Impaired
Associated deficits	Right hemiparesis (arm, face > leg)	Hemianopia, hemisensory loss
Localization of lesion	Frontal lobe	Temporal or parietal lobe (occasionally diffuse)

Fluent and nonfluent aphasias are usually evident during conversation, history taking, or mental status examination. Although neuropsychologists often use sophisticated tests, such as the *Boston Naming Test* and the *Boston Diagnostic Aphasia Examination* (Goodglass and Kaplan), clinicians can administer a standard series of simple verbal tests. This entire sequence can be repeated with written requests and responses; however, with rare exceptions (described below), written deficits will parallel verbal deficits. The standard aphasia tests evaluate three basic language functions:

- *Comprehension*, tested by asking the patient to follow simple requests, such as picking up one hand.
- *Naming*, tested by asking the patient to say his or her own name and that of common objects, such as a pen or key.
- *Repeating*, tested by asking the patient to recite several short phrases, such as, "The boy went to the store."

Nonfluent Aphasia

Nonfluent aphasia is characterized by a paucity of speech. Whatever speech is produced consists almost exclusively of single words and short phrases, with preferential use of highly meaningful words, such as nouns and verbs. Speech is typically at a rate of less than 50 words per minute—much slower than the normal rate of 100 to 250 words per minute. Moreover, articulation is poor and the cadence so irregular that the speech pattern is sometimes called "telegraphic." For example, in response to a question about food, a patient might stammer ". . . fork . . . steak . . . eat . . ."

Patients with nonfluent aphasia are unable to say their own name or the names of common objects, and cannot repeat simple phrases. However, they have relatively normal comprehension, which can be illustrated by their ability to follow verbal requests, such as "Close your eyes" or "Raise your left hand." Nonfluent aphasia was originally designated "expressive" because of this combination of speech impairment and preserved comprehension.

The lesion responsible for nonfluent aphasia is located in or near Broca's area and is almost always a discrete structural injury, such as a middle cerebral artery occlusion. Diffuse cerebral injuries, such as metabolic disturbances or Alzheimer's disease, are practically never the cause.

Nonfluent aphasia, since it stems from a Broca's area lesion, is characteristically associated with paresis of the right arm and lower face. It is also associated with *buccofacial apraxia*, which is not actually a paresis but an inability to execute normal facial, lip, and tongue movements voluntarily, although the muscles themselves are not paretic. Buccofacial apraxia causes some of the aphasic patients to have difficulty speaking distinctly. In severe cases, it can lead to virtual mutism, so-called *aphemia*. To evaluate buccofacial apraxia, the examiner asks the patient to say "La . . Pa . . La . . Pa . . La . . Pa . . ," blow out an imagined match, or protrude the tongue in different directions. Patients will not be able to follow these abstract requests, but yet can use the same muscles reflexly, unconsciously, or automatically, i.e., they will be able to blurt out a few words, sing, eat, or blow out an actual match.

Nonfluent aphasia patients so often become frustrated, tearful, and distraught that emotional disturbances have been considered characteristic. Although purely emotional disturbances with aphasia may be understandable, there is actually an organic basis in many cases. Many patients, particularly those who have had several CVAs, may actually be revealing signs of either dementia, pseudobulbar palsy (Chapter 4), or both. Nonfluent aphasia, dementia, and pseudobulbar palsy can be confused with each other, but in fact, because all three can originate in frontal lobe injury, they may occur together.

An extreme form of nonfluent aphasia is *global aphasia*, which is characterized by virtually complete loss of language function. Aside from uttering some unintelligible sounds and following an occasional gestured command, patients with global aphasia are mute and unresponsive. Their devastating language impairment is accompanied by right hemiplegia, a comparably severe motor deficit. Responsible lesions are so extensive that most of the left hemisphere, including both Broca's and Wernicke's areas, is injured. Internal carotid artery occlusions and penetrating head wounds are two of the most frequent causes.

Fluent Aphasia

Fluent aphasia consists of plentiful, articulate speech that contains complete, grammatically correct sentences spoken at a relatively normal rate. However, many of the words are incorrect or nonsensical. These errors, which are called *paraphasic errors* or *paraphasias*, may make conversation unintelligible.

Paraphasias include word substitution, such as "clock" for "watch" (a related paraphasia), or "glove" for "knife" (an unrelated paraphasia). Words may be altered, such as "breat" for "bread" (a literal paraphasia). Most striking are strings of nonsensical coinages (*neologisms*), such as "I want to fin gunt in the fark," and use of words that rhyme (*clang associations*).

Patients may speak in *circumlocutions*, as though they were trying to avoid dealing with their word-finding difficulty. They may also tend toward *tangential discussions*, as though once the wrong word was chosen, they pursue the idea triggered by their error.

Nevertheless, speech prosody is true to patients' emotions. When patients' words fail them, they can reveal their emotions by voice tone, facial and body movements, and occasionally cursing. Also, most patients will still be able to produce a melody even though they may be unable to say lyrics. For example, patients can hum a tune, such as "Jingle Bells," but if they attempt to sing, their lyrics will be strewn with paraphasias.

In contrast to nonfluent aphasia, fluent aphasia is associated with minimal physical deficits (Table 8-1). Significant hemiparesis is generally lacking. Usually, right-sided hyperactive deep tendon reflexes (DTRs) and a Babinski sign are the only motor signs present. However, right-sided sensory impairment and homonymous hemianopsia may be present because of interruptions of the sensory and visual cerebral pathways.

Lesions that cause fluent aphasia are usually discrete structural ones, such as small CVAs, in the temporoparietal region that damage Wernicke's area or the arcuate fasciculus. However, unlike nonfluent aphasia, fluent aphasia is sometimes caused by diffuse cerebral injury, including Alzheimer's disease.

Varieties of fluent aphasia have been described, but their distinctions tend to turn on subtle and complex points. Moreover, their clinicopathologic correlations are unreliable because of individual variations in anatomy, language lateralization, and speech production. Nevertheless, several varieties are recognizable and are important because they may be confused with nonaphasic conditions, particularly dementia and psychologic aberrations. One variety of fluent aphasia is *anomia* or *anomic aphasia*, which is simply an inability to name common objects. Anomia is associated with Alzheimer's disease, in which case it may be found along with dementia; however, in many patients, anomia is the only manifestation of a variety of aphasia.

Another classification scheme rests on a variety of aphasia called *transcortical aphasia* or *isolation aphasia*. It results from isolation of the Wernicke-Broca arc caused by damage to the surrounding perisylvian or "watershed" cortex by hypotension, anoxia, carbon monoxide poisoning, or occasionally Alzheimer's disease. Since the language system itself remains intact, although no longer in communication with the rest of the cerebrum, patients can repeat whatever they hear, but they cannot participate in meaningful conversation, follow requests, or name objects. Depending on the injury, a right hemiparesis may be present. The salient feature of transcortical aphasia is a remarkable disparity between patients seeming to be mute, yet being easily able to repeat long and complex sentences. Patients often repeat readily, involuntarily, and apparently compulsively. A cursory examination could understandably confuse their speech with irrational jargon. Transcortical aphasia and its varieties (sensory and motor) hold great theoretical importance because in these conditions portions of the language arc may be studied apart from others.

In this scheme, transcortical aphasia must also be directly contrasted to *conduction aphasia*. In this condition, a discrete lesion located in the arcuate fasciculus interrupts or *disconnects* the language arc. Thus, although patients are fluent and have good comprehension, their language impairment is characterized by loss of the ability to repeat.

MENTAL ABNORMALITIES WITH LANGUAGE IMPAIRMENTS

Distinguishing aphasia from dementia and recognizing when they coexist are more than academic exercises. A diagnosis of aphasia almost always suggests that a patient has had a discrete dominant cerebral hemisphere injury. Since a CVA or other structural lesion would be the most likely cause, the appropriate evaluation would include a CT or MRI scan (Chapter 20). In contrast, a diagnosis of dementia suggests that the most likely cause would be Alzheimer's disease or another diffuse process, and the evaluation might include an EEG, CSF analysis, and various blood tests, as well as a scan.

Aphasia and dementia have several distinguishing features. Patients with aphasia usually have had the sudden onset of their language impairment, and those with nonfluent aphasia usually also have dysarthria and a prominent right hemiparesis. Dementia takes months or more to develop and typically has no associated hemiparesis or dysarthria. Patients with fluent aphasia may appear demented because they might have trouble recounting the date and place, repeating a series of numbers, and following requests. However, their language will almost always be strewn with paraphasias.

The most reliable distinguishing feature is that both fluent and nonfluent aphasia patients have difficulty with one or more of the three standard language function tests: comprehension, naming, and repeating. Although patients with dementia in its early stages may have some naming and memory problems, they are usually fully verbal, articulate, and able to perform reasonably well on the standard language function tests. However, an important exception is the association of anomia with dementia. This impairment probably results because people's naming ability, unlike the other basic language functions, is heavily dependent on memory and probably particularly vulnerable to intellectual decline.

Patients with severe dementia have a paucity of speech and a limited vocabulary. When these patients do speak, they tend to *perseverate*, or repeat thoughts and words. Two forms of perseveration are *echolalia*, the parrot-like echoing of other people's words, and *palilalia*, which is repetition of the patient's own words.

Sometimes patients might be found to have both aphasia and dementia. This combination might occur in cases of multi-infarct dementia or when a person with Alzheimer's disease sustains a CVA. These cases are notoriously difficult to diagnose because aphasia invalidates all but the most sophisticated tests of intellectual function.

Although the distinction between aphasia and dementia may be difficult, that between fluent aphasia and *schizophrenic speech* can be even more troublesome. These two conditions are confused because of common language abnormalities that include circumlocutions, tangentialities, and neologisms. Moreover, as the thought disorder of schizophrenic patients becomes more pronounced, their language abnormalities increase in frequency and become more similar to those of fluent aphasia. Also, aphasia itself may be emotionally disturbing: to be suddenly unable to communicate may be as bewildering as suddenly finding that everyone speaks a foreign language.

Despite these similarities, many differences can be discerned. Schizophrenic speech usually develops in patients who are in their third decade and have had longstanding mental disturbances. In schizophrenic speech, neologisms and other paraphasias are usually neither frequent nor conspicuous. Moreover, comprehension, naming, and repetition are almost always preserved.

In contrast, people who develop aphasia are usually in their sixth or seventh decade. Although they may be distraught, they are often aware that they cannot communicate and request help. Possibly because of self-monitoring, their responses are shorter and more pointed. If a right homonymous hemianopsia or other lateralized finding can be elicited, aphasia from a cerebral lesion is indicated; however, such physical deficits unfortunately are sometimes not found because they may be subtle or because the patient's excitement or inability to cooperate precludes a proper examination.

Language usage abnormalities, but not aphasia, are also a prominent aspect of *childhood autism*. Autistic children begin to speak later than normal and often remain mute until they do so. Their grammar is poor, incorrect pronouns are assigned ("pronoun reversal"), and echolalia is common. Also, they have limited prosody and generally do not use gestures meaningfully. On the other hand, autistic children do not display several of the cardinal features of aphasia: paraphasias, anomias, and comprehension impairment.

Mutism and apparent language abnormalities can also be associated with psychogenic disturbances. In these situations, the language impairment is usually transient, inconsistent, and amenable to suggestion. The examiner should ask the patient to communicate in writing. In this way, patients with psychogenic mutism will reveal intact language function. If this does not work, an amobarbital interview might be attempted.

TABLE 8–2.   CLINICAL EVALUATION FOR APHASIA

Spontaneous speech: fluent versus nonfluent
Verbalization tests
  Comprehension (ability to follow requests)
  Naming (common objects: tie, keys, pen)
  Repetition (simple phrases, complex phrases)
Specific abnormalities
  Circumlocutions, tangents
  Nonspecific phrases
  Paraphasic errors
    Related ("spoon" for "fork")
    Unrelated ("football" for "fork")
    Literal ("fark" for "fork")
    Neologistic ("neible" for "fork")
Reading and writing (repeat above tests)
Associated physical signs
  Corticospinal tract
    Hemiparesis (especially lower face and arm)
    Babinski sign
  Motor skills
    Buccolingual apraxia
    Limb apraxia
  Sensory system
    Loss of cortical modalities (position, stereognosis)
  Visual tracts
    Homonymous hemianopsia
    Superior quadrantanopsia (with temporal lobe lesions)

Perhaps the most common aphasia-like psychogenic condition is simple word-finding or name-recalling difficulties attributable to psychodynamic processes. "Blocking," for example, is so close to a transient anomic aphasia that it may be thought of neurologically as the result of diffuse cerebral cortex physiologic dysfunction precipitated by psychologic factors. Another aphasia-like condition is the Freudian slip. Examples that are found in everyday conversation can be interpreted as paraphasias, as well as revelations of the unconscious. A newscaster's reference to the former "Treachery Secretary Regan" might be entirely psychologic; however, when a physician's former secretary, who is being evaluated for a left temporal lobe tumor, says that she has been Dr. So-and-so's "medical cemetery," one can interpret the slip as an indication of the patient's fears of death, a comment on the competence of her former employer, or a manifestation of a lesion involving the language centers of the brain.

RELATED DISORDERS: ALEXIA, AGRAPHIA, AGNOSIA, AND APRAXIA

Although aphasia is the most frequently occurring language disorder, several others are important and also stem from injury of the dominant hemisphere. *Alexia*, reading inability, and *agraphia*, writing inability, are almost always found together; however, an important exception is *alexia without agraphia*.

This is a rare condition in which people cannot read but can transcribe dictation or write their thoughts, and then are unable to read their own writing.

Alexia without agraphia results from a destructive lesion encompassing the dominant (left) occipital lobe and adjacent posterior corpus callosum (Fig. 8-4).

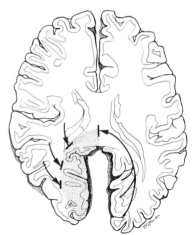

FIGURE 8–4. *Alexia without agraphia* is caused by lesions that damage the left occipital lobe and the posterior corpus callosum. Visual impulses are not received by the damaged left occipital cortex. Those that do reach the right cortex cannot be transmitted across the damaged corpus callosum to the left cerebral language centers. Thus, written language is incomprehensible; however, since the language and motor centers themselves remain intact, writing is still possible.

Patients are unable to see anything in their right visual field because of the left occipital cortex lesion. In addition, left visual impulses that reach the right occipital cortex cannot be conveyed to the language centers of the left hemisphere. Thus, patients cannot comprehend written material presented to either visual field. However, they can still write full sentences from memory, imagination, or dictation because these forms of information reach the language centers through intact pathways that can communicate with the necessary motor areas. In pure cases, despite the right homonymous hemianopsia and alexia, other language and physical abilities of patients remain intact.

Agraphia may also occur in the controversial *Gerstmann's syndrome*. In this condition, which has been attributed to lesions in the *angular gyrus* of the dominant parietal lobe (Fig. 8-1), agraphia is accompanied by three other abnormalities: *acalculia* (impairment of arithmetic skills), *finger agnosia* (inability to identify fingers), and *left/right confusion*. The status of Gerstmann's syndrome as a distinct clinical entity has been questioned because patients rarely display all four components simultaneously, and those who do have most components usually also have fluent aphasia. Nevertheless, the constellation of Gerstmann's signs, even if they do not constitute a syndrome, is useful. The signs may be sought in adults with CVAs. In evaluating children for learning disabilities, children with dyscalculia are frequently also found to have poor handwriting (agraphia), and left/right confusion accompanied by physical signs of dominant hemisphere injury, such as right-sided hyperactive DTRs or a Babinski sign (Chapter 13).

Another neuropsychologic disturbance that can be the result of dominant hemisphere injury is *agnosia*. This is a perceptual disorder in which patients cannot recognize objects despite intact sensory systems, intellectual capabilities, and language function. It should not be confused with either dementia or aphasia—other conditions in which patients might not be able to say the names of objects but can recognize them. For example, if a man with agnosia were shown a stop sign, he could name it and describe it, but he would be unable to explain its meaning. Another perceptual disturbance, *prosopagnosia*, is the inability to identify familiar faces, such as those of historical figures or family members. It is often found with inability to identify objects out of their usual (visual) context, such as a shirt pocket cut from a shirt. Unlike aphasia, prosopagnosia is often the result of bilateral occipitotemporal lesions. In contrast, identification of unknown faces, which probably relies more on spatial concepts than simple memory, is primarily a function of the nondominant hemisphere.

Color agnosia or *anomia*, a variety of agnosia, is the inability to recognize color correctly that is not a manifestation of color blindness, dementia, or aphasia. It supposedly results from damage to the dominant occipitotemoral region. Patients with color agnosia are unable to name the colors of painted cards or other colored objects; however, in striking contrast, they are able to match cards of the same color and also recite from memory the colors of common objects, such as the sky (see Agnosia, Chapter 12, Visual Disturbances).

Apraxia, which is the motor system's equivalent of aphasia, is the inability to execute learned actions despite normal strength, sensation, coordination, and, more important, comprehension. This impairment is thought to result from either faulty integration, or "disconnection," of motor with sensory and language centers.

Typically, patients with apraxia cannot perform a particular movement at the request of the examiner, but they might still be able to do it as an automatic or unconscious action if they are provided with sufficient cues, such as might be obtained by using the actual objects or by seeing the examiner performing the movement. Although several clinically useful varieties of apraxia have been described (Table 8-3), the most important ones are the two varieties of *ideomotor apraxia*: *buccofacial* and *limb apraxia*. Both are associated with aphasia, attributable to injury of the dominant frontal or parietal lobe (Fig. 8-5), and are usually the result of a localized CNS lesion, such as a middle cerebral artery infarction.

Buccofacial apraxia, which was discussed in detail previously, is associated with nonfluent aphasia. It is characterized by patients' inability to move their cheeks, lips, or tongue in response to specific requests.

In limb apraxia, which is associated with both fluent and nonfluent aphasia,

TABLE 8–3. COMMON APRAXIAS

Apraxia	Tests	Lesion's Usual Location	Associated Deficits
Constructional	Copy figure or arrange matchsticks	Nondominant parietal lobe	Left hemi-inattention
Ideational	Pretend to take a cigarette from a pack and light it, or to fold and mail a letter, i.e., a complex sequential action	Both frontal lobes or entire cerebrum	Dementia
Ideomotor		Dominant posterior frontal or anterior parietal lobe	Aphasia
Buccofacial	Pretend to blow out a match or to use a straw, or repeat syllables		
Limb	Pretend to brush teeth, unlock a door, or pick up a ball, i.e., a simple action		
Gait	Walk, start-stop-start, turn	Entire cerebrum, especially normal pressure hydrocephalus	Dementia

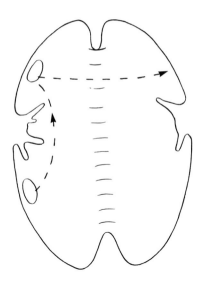

FIGURE 8–5. In a schematic overview of the brain, commands for purposeful, skilled movements are received by Wernicke's area in the posterior dominant (left) cerebral hemisphere. They are transmitted anteriorly to the motor regions of that hemisphere and then, through the anterior corpus callosum, to the contralateral motor strip. Interruptions of the path within the left cerebral hemisphere result in ideomotor apraxia of both arms. Lesions in the anterior corpus callosum will interrupt only those impulses destined to control the left arm and leg.

patients are not able to use the limbs on either side of their body to execute simple actions. Patients cannot pretend to brush their teeth, comb their hair, or kick a ball. They cannot salute or move their hands in certain patterns. Characteristically, when asked to pretend to use an object, these patients will use their hand as though it were the actual object. A commonly cited example is that they will brush their teeth with a forefinger instead of pretending to hold a toothbrush. However, as in the other apraxias, patients will be able to perform commands if supplied with cues or by imitating the examiner.

In *ideational apraxia*, still another form of apraxia, patients cannot perform motor activities that require several sequential steps. For example, patients cannot pretend to remove a cigarette from a pack and then light it, or pretend to fold a letter, place it into an envelope, and then affix a stamp. Although patients might complete segments of these tasks, they cannot complete the entire sequence in order.

Ideational apraxia is usually found to result from either diffuse cerebral disease or injuries of both frontal lobes. It is often a manifestation of dementia. Actually, ideational apraxia is not surprising in Alzheimer's disease or multi-infarct dementia because patients with dementia have trouble with organization, planning, and conceptualizing.

These neuropsychologic disorders hold great interest for neurologists. Some are clinically helpful in recognizing a neurologic basis for intellectual or perceptual problems. Many indicate how the normal brain functions. Most are dramatic when properly demonstrated. Virtually all appeal to the examiner's own sense of linguistics and curiosity about the process of thinking.

From a practical viewpoint, however, the clinical features and pathologic correlations of apraxia, alexia, and related neuropsychologic disorders are relatively inconsistent and have limited usefulness. Many patients have multiple CVAs or extensive damage from Alzheimer's disease, and thus they have combinations of these neuropsychologic disorders or an inextricable mixture of them with aphasia or dementia. Rare patients have an isolated nonaphasic neuropsychologic disorder. Pathologic studies are far from being uniform in showing that a particular area of the brain is responsible for these isolated disorders. Since individuals tend to have different cognitive "styles," some people being highly verbal and others not, lesions in the same area of the brain are apt to produce somewhat different manifestations, and individuals with the same lesion are apt to compensate differently.

NONDOMINANT HEMISPHERE SYNDROMES

Hemi-Inattention

Although aphasia and the other disturbances discussed so far, such as agraphia and apraxia, are attributable in large measure to injuries of the dominant hemisphere, several important psychologic disturbances are attributable to nondominant hemisphere injury. The most important disorder associated with nondominant injury is *hemi-inattention* (*hemispatial neglect*). It originates in injury of the nondominant parietal lobe cortex and the underlying structures, including the thalamus, reticular activating system, and other structures that govern arousal and direct attention.

Patients with right parietal lobe infarction characteristically ignore visual, tactile, and other stimuli that originate from their left side. Typically, they will disregard or fail to perceive objects in their left visual field despite suggestions that important things can be seen there (Fig. 8-6). Also, when both sides of their body are touched, patients neglect the left-sided stimulation (*extinction on double simultaneous stimulation* [*DSS*]) and report that only their right side was touched. Sometimes patients even fail to shave the left side of their face and leave their left side undressed (*dressing apraxia*).

Anosognosia, which is the refusal to accept any associated physical deficit (usually a left hemiparesis), is a crucial aspect of hemi-inattention. Patients typically cannot identify the affected part of their body (*somatopagnosia* or *autotopagnosia*), and occasionally claim that the examiner's (normal) left hand, rather than their own paretic left hand, is theirs. Sometimes they say that the weakened hand belongs to yet a third person. Whatever mechanism they may employ to ignore the hand's paresis, they fail to use the hand, which usually lies motionless (*akinetic*).

Since patients with left hemiparesis tend to deny, rationalize, confabulate, and employ other defense mechanisms, they often refuse to accept physical therapy and hospital routine in the initial phase of a nondominant parietal lobe CVA. Thus, patients with left hemiparesis should be checked for anosognosia to forestall management problems. In several days to several weeks, patients begin to accept their loss.

Denial and confabulation, of course, are not restricted to nondominant hemisphere injury. Both are prominent signs in suddenly occurring cortical blindness (Anton's syndrome, Chapter 12), and confabulation is found in Wernicke-Korsakoff syndrome (Chapter 7).

Another manifestation of nondominant hemisphere injury is *constructional apraxia*, in which patients lose their ability to integrate visual information with fine motor skills (Table 8-3). In particular, *visuospatial* perceptual impairments often prevent them from copying simple figures or arranging matchsticks in patterns (Fig. 8-7). The primary problem in what is sometimes called *visuocon-structive disability* is that patients cannot organize spatial information. The

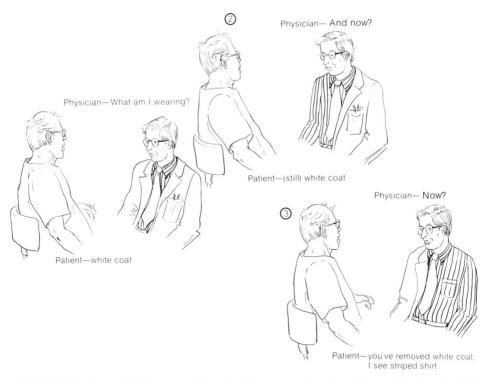

FIGURE 8–6. In a classic demonstration of left *hemi-inattention*, the patient, neglecting left-sided stimulation, perceives only that the examiner is wearing whatever he sees in his own right visual field. Even if the patient's problem were simply a left homonymous hemianopsia, he still would have explored and discovered, with his intact right visual field, that the examiner was half-dressed.

FIGURE 8–7. When asked to draw a clock, a patient with *constructional apraxia* drew an incomplete circle, repeated (perseverated) the numerals, and placed them asymmetrically. When attempting to copy the figure on the upper left, the patient repeated several lines, failing to draw any figure. The patient also misplaced and rotated the position of the lower left figure (also see Fig. 2-8).

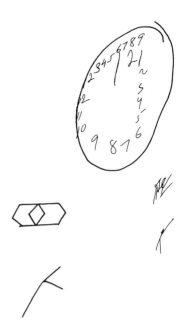

disability, however, cannot always be ascribed entirely to a nondominant lesion. It can also be found in patients with diffuse cerebral dysfunction and sometimes in patients with left hemisphere damage.

Aprosody

Several authors have recently described how patients with nondominant hemisphere lesions cannot appreciate emotional aspects of speech. These patients are said to have *aprosody*. For example, a patient would be unable to discern the contrasting implications of the question, "Are you going to the dance?" asked first by a gleeful mother, then by a jealous friend. Not only are the patients unable to discern other people's emotional tone but they themselves also speak in a monotone, being unable to convey affective nuance in their speech. They are also unable to sing because, although they can repeat the lyrics to a song, they cannot convey its melody.

Aprosody tends to be accompanied by loss of nonverbal forms of communication, or the *paralinguistic components* of speech, such as facial expression and limb gesture. These are physical aspects of communication that, as does prosody, lend credence, emphasis, and affect to spoken words. They are popularly recognized as "body language." Indeed, gestured communication seems different and somewhat more fundamental than spoken communication—people disbelieve someone who smiles excessively when making promises.

An examiner testing for aprosody and the loss of paralinguistic components of speech must first ascertain that they are not caused by neurologic conditions other than nondominant hemisphere injuries, such as parkinsonism. The examiner should request that the patient ask a question, such as "May I have the ball?," in the manner of a cute child, a friend, and an angry schoolteacher. The question should be asked with appropriate vocal and facial expressions. Then the examiner should ask the question, impersonating the same characters while the patient tries to identify them. An alternative but less demanding test is to ask the patient to identify emotions in expressive pictures of people.

Extending the concept that the nondominant hemisphere confers affect on language, several authors have suggested that the nondominant hemisphere is also responsible for general affect, complex nonverbal processes, a holistic cognitive approach, and impulsiveness. The dominant hemisphere, they suggest, is responsible for verbal, sequential, and analytic cognitive processes and for reflectiveness.

DISCONNECTION SYNDROMES

Although many psychologic functions are governed almost entirely by either one hemisphere or the other, the multitude of human endeavors, including learning and expression of emotion, require communication between both hemispheres. Appropriate interhemispheric connections are the myelin-coated axonal (white matter) bundles, *commissures*, of which the most conspicuous is the *corpus callosum*. Others are the massa intermedia and the anterior, posterior, and hippocampal commissures.

Injuries that damage the commissures deprive each hemisphere of some of the other's information and thus lead to a group of interesting psychologic disturbances called *disconnection syndromes*. One disturbance that has already been discussed is alexia without agraphia (Fig. 8-4). Conduction aphasia is also a disconnection syndrome, but one that results from an intrahemispheric disruption.

The *anterior cerebral artery syndrome*, a classic example, is an injury to the corpus callosum produced by infarction of the anterior cerebral arteries. In this condition, not only are both frontal lobes damaged but also information cannot pass from the left hemisphere language centers to the appropriate right hemisphere motor center. Thus, although the patient's left arm and leg will have normal spontaneous movement, these limbs will not respond to an examiner's verbal or written requests, i.e., the patient will have unilateral (left-sided) limb apraxia (Fig. 8-5).

The corpus callosum also occasionally fails to develop in utero (*congenital absence*), and sometimes it is damaged by excessive consumption of red wine (*Marchiafava-Bignami syndrome*). Disconnection signs may be present in these cases, but they are subtle and variable.

Split Brain

The most important disconnection syndrome is the "split brain," which is the result of surgical sectioning of the corpus callosum usually performed for control of intractable epilepsy (Chapter 10). In split brain cases, since the cerebral hemispheres are virtually isolated from each other, examiners may present certain information exclusively to one of the patient's hemispheres. For example, by showing the patient pictures, writing, and other visual information within one visual field, only the contralateral hemisphere will receive the information (Fig. 8-8). Likewise, tactile information can be presented to only one hemisphere by having a blindfolded patient touch objects with the contra-lateral hand. However, since auditory pathways are duplicated in the brainstem (Fig. 4-15), sounds that are heard in only one ear are received to a certain extent by both hemispheres. A variety of striking abnormalities can be demonstrated by such testing largely because visual, other sensory, and emotional data from the right hemisphere cannot be transmitted to the language centers of the left hemisphere.

In testing a patient's left cerebral hemisphere function, written questions or requests are presented to the right visual field, and objects to identify are placed in the right hand. The patient can respond correctly by speaking and by writing with the right hand. To written and verbal requests for particular right arm and leg movements, the patient also responds correctly; however, the left limbs are unable to follow the same requests because of left limb apraxia (Figs. 8-5 and 8-8).

In testing right hemisphere function, visual information is shown in the patient's left visual field. Since impulses cannot travel to the language centers, the patient cannot read, respond to written requests, or name objects. Nevertheless, the patient is able to use the left hand to copy complex figures, and is also able to perform well on tests of mathematical ability, pattern discrimination, facial recognition, and perception of emotion.

Sophisticated testing has shown that not only can each hemisphere experience emotion but also each hemisphere might simultaneously experience a different, sometimes conflicting, emotion. For example, a picture that evokes humor can

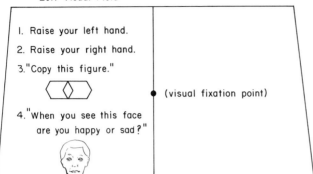

I. Raise your left hand.

2. Raise your right hand.

3."Copy this figure."

4."When you see this face
   are you happy or sad?"

● (visual fixation point)

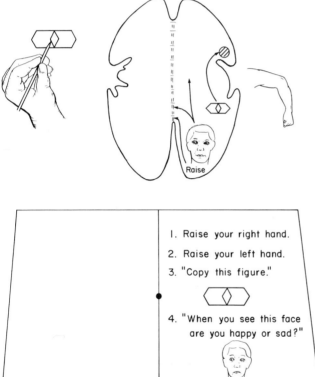

FIGURE 8–8. In patients who have the split brain syndrome following a commissurotomy, each hemisphere can be tested individually by showing requests, objects, and pictures in the contralateral visual field. *A*, The right hemisphere may receive written requests shown in the left visual field.However, since this hemisphere is unable to transmit written messages through the corpus callosum to the left cerebral hemisphere, patients cannot read. Since connections to the ipsilateral motor area are intact, the *left* hand can copy figures. Also, although patients cannot verbalize the feelings that emotionally laden pictures evoke, patients typically have sympathetic nonverbal responses. *B*, The left hemisphere can receive and read written requests shown in the right visual field and, with the right hand, comply with them; however, since the language areas cannot send information through the corpus callosum, the left hand cannot comply. Figures shown to the left hemisphere can be copied only to a crude resemblance. Patient can describe the emotional tone of a picture, but they are devoid of the accompanying affect.

I. Raise your right hand.

2. Raise your left hand.

3. "Copy this figure."

4. "When you see this face
   are you happy or sad?"

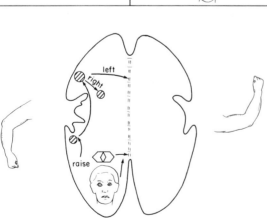

be shown in one visual field and one that evokes sadness in the other. In this case, tests of each hemisphere will reveal a different emotion.

In addition, each hemisphere also has been shown to reason independently by nonverbal, if not verbal, processes and to learn properly presented facts, sequences, and ideas. However, some information obtained by one hemisphere cannot be shared with the other. In particular, since patients cannot describe information that is presented to the right hemisphere, many of their experiences do not reach conscious expression or cannot be verbalized.

Split brain studies have suggested that in normal persons the two hemispheres of the brain might have independent memory, thought processes, and emotions. Indeed, many mental processing systems may be operating simultaneously, in parallel, and without requiring language. Although the systems may complement each other, they might occasionally conflict. Studies clearly indicate that emotions in the right hemisphere may be less accessible to verbal description, and that the behavior that would be initiated by one hemisphere is sometimes in conflict with the behavior that would be initiated by the other.

REFERENCES

Albert ML, Helm-Estabrooks N: Diagnosis and treatment of aphasia. JAMA *259*:1205, 1988

Bear DM: Hemispheric specialization and the neurology of emotion. Arch Neurol *40*:195, 1983

Bryden MP, Ley RG: Right-hemisphere involvement in the perception and expression of emotion in normal humans. In Heilman KH, Satz P (eds): Neuropsychology of Human Emotion. New York, The Guilford Press, 1983, pp 6–44

Cranberg LD, Filley CM, Hart EJ, et al: Acquired aphasia in childhood. Neurology *37*:1165, 1987

Critchley M, Henson RA (eds): Music and the Brain: Studies in the Neurology of Music. London, William Heinemann Medical Books Ltd, 1977

Damasio AR, Damasio H: The anatomic basis of pure alexia. Neurology *33*:1573, 1983

Damasio AR, Damasio H, Hoesen GWV: Prosopagnosia: Anatomic basis and behavior mechanisms. Neurology *32*:331, 1982

Faber R, Abrams R, Taylor MA, et al: Comparison of schizophrenic patients with formal thought disorder and neurologically impaired patients with aphasia. Am J Psychiatry *140*:1348, 1983

Ferro JM, Martins IP, Tavora L: Neglect in children. Ann Neurol *15*:281, 1984

Gazzaniga MS, Risse GL, Springer SP, et al: Psychologic and neurologic consequences of partial and complete cerebral commissurotomy. Neurology *25*:10, 1975

Gerson SN, Benson DF, Frazier SH: Diagnosis: Schizophrenia versus posterior aphasia. Am J Psychiatry *134*:966, 1977

Geschwind N: Specializations of the human brain. In Flanagan D (ed): The Brain: A Scientific American Book. San Francisco, W. H. Freeman Co, 1979, pp 6-44

Goodglass H, Kaplan E: The Assessment of Aphasia and Related Disorders, 2nd ed. Philadelphia, Lea & Febiger, 1983

Graff-Radford NR, Welsh K, Godersky J: Callosal apraxia. Neurology *37*:100, 1987

Geiger G, Lettvin JY: Peripheral vision in persons with dyslexia. N Engl J Med *316*:1238, 1987

Heilman KM, Valenstein E (eds): Clinical Neuropsychology, 2nd Ed. New York, Oxford University Press, 1985

Hemenway D: Bimanual dexterity in baseball players. N Engl J Med *309*:1587, 1983

Hier DB, Mondlock J, Caplan LR: Behavioral abnormalities after right hemisphere stroke. Neurology *33*:337, 1983

Homan RW, Criswell E, Wada JA, et al: Hemispheric contributions to manual communication (signing and finger-spelling). Neurology *32*:1020, 1982

Kertesz A, Nicholson I, Cancelliere A, et al: Motor impersistence: A right-hemisphere syndrome. Neurology *35*:662, 1985

Levine DN, Warach JD, Benowitz L, et al: Left spatial neglect. Neurology *36*:362, 1986

Motley MT: Slips of the tongue. Sci Am *253*:116, 1985

Naeser MA, Borod JC: Aphasia in left-handers. Neurology *36*:471, 1986

PeBenito R, Fisch CB, Fisch ML: Developmental Gerstmann's syndrome. Arch Neurol *45*:977, 1988

Portal JM, Romano PE: Patterns of eye-hand dominance in baseball players. N Engl J Med *319*:655, 1988

Ross ED, Harney JH, Utamsing C, et al: How the brain integrates affective and propositional language into a unified behavior function. Arch Neurol *38*:745, 1981

Shaywitz BA, Waxman SG: Dyslexia. N Engl J Med *316*:1268, 1987

Weinstein EA, Friedland RP (eds): Advances in Neurology: Hemi-Inattention and Hemisphere Specialization. New York, Raven Press, 1977

Weintraub S, Mesulam MM, Kramer L: Disturbance in prosody. A right-hemisphere contribution to language. Arch Neurol *38*:742, 1981

QUESTIONS: CHAPTER 8

1–5. Formulate the following cases:

CASE 1

A 68-year-old man suddenly develops right hemiparesis. He only utters "Oh, Oh!" when stimulated. He makes no response to questions or requests. His right lower face is paretic, and both the right arm and leg are flaccid and immobile. He is inattentive to objects in his right visual field.

CASE 2

A 70-year-old man has been unable to speak fully or use his right arm since suffering a cerebrovascular accident (CVA) the previous year. He can only say "weak, arm," "go away," and "give . . . supper me" with slurring. On request, he can raise his left arm, protrude his tongue, and close his eyes. He can name several objects, but he cannot repeat phrases. His right arm is paretic, but he can walk.

CASE 3

Over a period of 6 weeks, a previously healthy 64-year-old woman has developed headaches, progressively severe difficulty finding words, and apparent confusion. She speaks continuously and incoherently: "Go to the warb," "I can't hear," "My heat hurts." She is unable to follow commands, name objects, or repeat phrases. On examination, there is pronation of the outstretched right arm, a right Babinski sign, and papilledema. Visual fields cannot be tested.

CASE 4

A 34-year-old man with mitral stenosis has the sudden onset of language difficulty after a transient left-sided headache. Although fully articulate and able to follow requests and repeat phrases, he has difficulty in naming objects. For example, when a pen, pin, and penny are held up in succession, he frequently uses the name of one for the other and repeats the name of the preceding object; however, he can point to the "money," "sharp object," and "writing instrument" when these objects are placed in front of him. No abnormal physical signs are detected on neurologic examination.

CASE 5

A 54-year-old man complains of several months of difficulty in thinking and being unable to remember the word he desires. Although his voice quivers, he is fully conversant and articulate. He is able to write the correct responses to questions; however, his answers are slow and poorly written. He is able to name six objects, follow double requests, and repeat complex phrases. On further testing, he has difficulty recalling six digits, three objects after 3 minutes, and both recent and past events. Judgment seems intact. The remainder of the neurologic examination is normal.

6.–10. Match the lesions that are pictured schematically with those expected in cases 1–5.

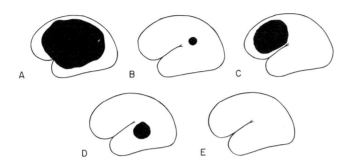

11–26. Match the lesion with the expected associated finding(s).

11. Paresis of one recurrent laryngeal nerve

12. Pseudobulbar palsy

13. Bulbar palsy

14. Dominant hemisphere temporal lobe lesion

15. Lateral medullary syndrome

16. Laryngitis

17. Dominant hemisphere angular gyrus lesion

18. Dominant hemisphere parietal lobe lesion

19. Nondominant hemisphere disorientation parietal lobe lesion

20. Bilateral frontal lobe tumor

21. Bilateral anterior cerebral artery infarction

22. Streptomycin toxicity

23. Alcohol intoxication

24. Periaqueductal hemorrhagic necrosis (Wernicke's encephalopathy)

25. Dilantin toxicity

26. Infarction of left posterior cerebral artery

a. Dysarthria, including hoarseness
b. Dysphagia
c. Dementia
d. Dyscalculia
e. Fluent aphasia
f. Constructional apraxia
g. Dyslexia
h. Deafness
i. Mutism
j. Left-right parietal lobe lesion
k. Finger agnosia
l. Hyperactivity
m. Sixth cranial nerve palsy
n. Alexia
o. Ataxia
p. Dressing apraxia
q. Anosognosia
r. Hemi-inattention
s. Left limb apraxia

27. A 34-year-old man was found and revived after he attempted suicide by sitting in a car that was parked in a garage with the motor running. During the next week, he only sat in bed and looked out of the window. He displayed no emotion and did not speak or respond to requests. When evaluating his mental status, the examiner also found that the man was virtually mute. However, he seemed to repeat in intricate detail whatever he was asked and occasionally whatever was said on television. His deep tendon reflexes were brisk, and he had bilateral palmomental reflexes. His plantar reflexes were equivocal.

The examiner was uncertain if the patient had depression, dementia, or other neuropsychologic abnormality. Please discuss the case and suggest further evaluation.

28.   A left-handed 64-year-old male schoolteacher sustained a cerebral thrombosis of the right middle cerebral artery. What might be predicted regarding language function?
   a.   He will certainly develop aphasia.
   b.   He will have left hemiparesis if he has aphasia.
   c.   If he develops aphasia, his prognosis is relatively good.
   d.   If he has aphasia, he will have a homonymous hemianopsia.

29.   If the patient in the previous question were believed to have a tumor in the right temporal lobe that could be resected, how could the language function of the right cerebral hemisphere be established preoperatively?
   a.   An MRI scan could be performed.
   b.   A CT scan could show differences in the *planum temporale*.
   c.   Barbiturates infused into the carotid artery of the dominant hemisphere would cause aphasia.
   d.   A PET study would indicate cerebral dominance for language.

30.   In which conditions are confabulations *not* found?
   a.   Anton's syndrome
   b.   Gerstmann's syndrome
   c.   Anosognosia
   d.   Wernicke-Korsakoff syndrome

31.   Match the speech abnormality (dysarthria) with the illness:
   a.   Hypophonia   1.   Myasthenia gravis
   b.   Scanning speech   2.   Parkinsonism
   c.   Nasal speech   3.   Multiple sclerosis

32.   Which conditions *usually* cause aphasia?
   a.   Chronic subdural hematomas
   b.   Myasthenia gravis
   c.   Multiple sclerosis
   d.   Parkinsonism

33.   A 40-year-old nurse describes that when she awoke earlier in the morning, for about 5 minutes she had "expressive aphasia," by which she meant that she was unable to speak or gesture, but she understood most of the news on the radio. During that time she had no other symptoms and she stayed in bed.
   Which of the following conditions are reasonable explanations for her episode?
   a.   Seizure
   b.   Transient ischemic attack (TIA)
   c.   Migraine
   d.   Sleep disorder

34.   A 70-year-old man complains of the sudden inability to read. Although he can write his name and many sentences that are dictated to him, he cannot read aloud or copy written material. His speech is fluent and contains no paraphasic errors. On further examination, it is found that he can see objects only in his left visual field. What is this man's difficulty and where is the responsible lesion(s)?

35.   A 68-year-old man has a car accident in which he drifted into oncoming traffic. When questioned by police, he was unaware of a weak left arm. On examination by a physician, the patient was shown to have a left homonymous hemianopsia, a mild left hemiparesis (which the patient denied), and failure to recognize his weak left arm. What intellectual processes are present?

36.   A 60-year-old woman with longstanding depression has agitation, a language disturbance, and dysarthria. Initially misdiagnosed as having an exacerbation of her psychiatric disorder, she was recognized as suffering from an aphasia that was characterized by a paucity of words and impaired ability to express herself. She was also shown to have a mild right hemiparesis. An MRI scan indicated an occlusion of the left middle cerebral artery. In planning her rehabilitation management, which additional associated findings should be sought?

  a. Constructional apraxia
  b. Gait apraxia
  c. Limb apraxia
  d. Left homonymous hemianopsia
  e. Buccofacial apraxia
  f. Ideational apraxia

37. Patients with nondominant hemisphere lesions are reported to have loss of the normal inflections of speech and diminished associated facial and limb gestures. What are the technical terms used to describe these findings?

38. A man, who has undergone a corpus callosum commissurotomy for intractable seizures, is shown a typewritten request to raise both arms. What will be his response when the request is shown in his left visual field? In the right visual field?

39–44. With which other conditions are the various forms of apraxia associated?

39. Gait	a. Aphasia
	b. Hemi-inattention
40. Constructional	c. Dementia
	d. Dysarthria
41. Ideational	e. Incontinence
	f. Left homonymous hemianopsia
42. Limb	g. Right homonymous hemianopsia
	h. Aprosody
43. Buccofacial	
44. Ideomotor	

ANSWERS

1–5.

Case 1. This is a case of complete loss of language function, global aphasia, with right hemiplegia and homonymous hemianopsia. The cause is probably an occlusion of the left internal carotid artery creating a large infarction of the left hemisphere.

Case 2. Since he can manage only a few phrases or words in a telegraphic pattern, this patient has nonfluent aphasia, which is typically accompanied by right hemiparesis in which the arm is more paretic than the leg. The lesion encompasses Broca's area and the adjacent cortical motor region. It was probably caused by an occlusion of the left middle cerebral artery.

Case 3. The patient has fluent aphasia characterized by a normal quantity of speech beset by paraphasic errors and only subtle right-sided corticospinal tract abnormalities. There is probably a lesion in the left parietal or posterior temporal lobe. The headaches and papilledema, given her age, previous good health, and the course of the illness, suggest that it is a mass lesion, such as a glioblastoma multiforme (Chapter 19).

Case 4. This is a case of anomic aphasia, which is a variety of fluent aphasia where language impairment is restricted to the improper identification of objects, i.e., a naming impairment. Although its origin may be Alzheimer's disease, since this patient has mitral stenosis and the illness began suddenly with a headache, it was probably caused by a small embolic CVA (Chapter 11).

Case 5. The patient does not have any sign of aphasia. His difficulty with memory might be either early dementia or psychogenic inattention. Further evaluation that might be performed could include neuropsychologic studies or laboratory tests that might reveal an origin of the dementia, such as an EEG and a CT or MRI scan.

6. *Case 1*, drawing a.	**8.** *Case 3*, drawing d.
7. *Case 2*, drawing c.	**9.** *Case 4*, drawing b or d.

10. *Case 5*, drawing e.

11. a.

12. a, b, d, l.

13. a, b.

14. e.

15. a, b, o.

16. a.

17. d, j, k (Gerstmann's syndrome).

18. d, e, g, j, k.

19. f, p, q, r.

20. c, possibly also a, b, and i.

21. s and possibly c and i.

22. h, o.

23. a, d, o.

24. c, m, o.

25. o.

26. n.

27.   The patient was probably exposed to excessive carbon monoxide. As in cases of cardiac arrest and strangulation where patients survive, any form of cerebral anoxia creates cerebral cortex damage. When patients permanently lose all intellectual and voluntary motor function, they are said to be in the *persistent vegetative state* (Chapter 11).

In this case, the cerebral damage was incomplete. It probably isolated the arc of cerebral cortex comprised of Wernicke's area, the arcuate fasciculus, and Broca's area. Isolation of this crucial region from the rest of the cerebral cortex causes *transcortical aphasia* that permits repetition of words and phrases, no matter how complex; however, since language information cannot interact with the rest of the brain's language system, patients with this variety of aphasia cannot name objects or follow requests. Since a large portion of the cerebral cortex is damaged, patients usually also have cognitive impairments, paresis, and frontal release signs.

In cases where cerebral cortex damage is superimposed on depressive illness or other psychologic aberration, the clinical picture is unpredictable. In such patients, detailed testing of language function must be part of the mental status examination.

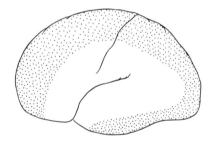

Fig. (above) In transcortical aphasia, which is usually induced by hypoperfusion-induced hypoxia, the most vulnerable portions of the cerebral cortex are damaged, and the Wernicke's area-Broca's area arc is often spared. Language processes may continue within this region, but they receive no input from other regions of the cerebral cortex.

28.   c. Left-handed individuals who have normal intelligence are often still predominantly left-hemisphere dominant or they have mixed cerebral dominance. Moreover, language centers in the right hemisphere are not arranged consistently with respect to each other or to the motor and visual tracts within the hemisphere. If left-handed individuals suffer an infarction of the right cerebral hemisphere, they do not necessarily develop aphasia or the usual associated deficits. They may develop aphasia if they have infarction in the left cerebral hemisphere. However, left-handed individuals, compared to right-handed individuals, have a better prognosis regarding resolution of aphasia presumably because of some degree of mixed dominance in most left-handed individuals.

29.   c. Infusion of barbiturates directly into the carotid artery produces aphasia if it perfuses the cerebral hemisphere that is prominantly or exclusively dominant for language function. This test, the *Wada Test*, is the standard procedure to determine if a cerebral hemisphere is dominant before removal of cerebral neoplasms or an epilepsy scar focus.

PET scans are difficult to perform because of the need for short-lived cyclotron-generated substrates and the PET scan's relatively poor resolution of metabolic function. Although the *planum temporale* (the superior surface of the temporal lobe cortex) has a greater area in the dominant than nondominant temporal lobe, the difference is not always present and, even when present, cannot be reliably visualized with CT or MRI scans.

30. b. Gerstmann's syndrome is a controversial entity that consists of the combination of right and left confusion, dyslexia, dyscalculia, and finger agnosia. It is usually attributed to lesions in the angular gyrus of the parietal lobe of the dominant hemisphere. Denial of blindness (Anton's syndrome) typically involves blind patients confabulating or fantasizing about the appearance of objects presented to them. It occurs most often in elderly people who undergo ophthalmologic surgical procedures and cannot temporarily see out of either eye. Failure to acknowledge a left hemiparesis or similar deficit (anosognosia) is often accompanied by confabulation, denial, and other defense mechanisms. Although confabulations are described in the Wernicke-Korsakoff's syndrome, they are rare. When they do occur, the patients usually also have marked memory impairments.

31. a-2; b-3; c-1.

32. None. Subdural hematomas are extra-axial. Although chronic subdural hematomas typically cause headaches and dementia, they usually do not cause aphasia or other localized neurologic symptoms. Myasthenia gravis is a disorder of the neuromuscular junction and therefore does not cause dementia, aphasia, or other sign of a central nervous system dysfunction. Multiple sclerosis affects the cerebral white matter to a large extent only late in its course. Although it may then cause dementia, it practically never causes aphasia. Parkinsonism may cause dysarthria (hypophonia and tremulousness) and, late in the illness, dementia; however, it rarely causes aphasia.

33. All. She might have had a partial seizure originating in the left frontal lobe. During a postictal period, she might have had aphasia and a right hemiparesis that prevented her from gesturing. A TIA in the distribution of the left carotid artery might also have caused aphasia, with or without right hemiparesis. Hemiplegic migraines, which can cause speech impairment, can occasionally affect adults. An episode of "sleep paralysis," such as hypnopompic cataplexy, may cause virtual quadriparesis and mutism. Overall, transient aphasia is similar to transient hemiparesis (see Hemiplegic Migraines, Chapter 9, and Carotid Artery TIAs, Chapter 11).

34. He clearly has alexia, as demonstrated by his inability to read, and also a right homonymous hemianopsia. He does not have agraphia because he can transcribe dictation and write words from memory. Nor does he have aphasia. Thus, he has the syndrome of alexia without agraphia. This syndrome is caused by a lesion in the left occipital lobe and posterior corpus callosum. The left occipital lesion would explain the failure of visual information to pass from the intact right visual cortex through the corpus callosum to the left (dominant) hemisphere for integration (Fig. 8-4). Since memory and auditory circuits, as well as the corticospinal system, are intact, he can write words that he hears or remembers. Such lesions are usually caused by infarctions of the left posterior cerebral artery or by infiltrating brain tumors, such as a glioblastoma multiforme.

35. He probably had the accident because a left homonymous hemianopsia prevented him from seeing oncoming traffic. More important, he has anosognosia (failure to recognize one's illness). As in this man, these perceptual distortions characteristically are found in patients with parietal lobe lesions.

36. c,e. Limb and buccofacial apraxias are associated with dominant hemisphere lesions. Their identification is important because these impediments are potentially major obstacles in speech and physical therapies.

37. Aprosody and loss of paralinguistic components of speech.

38. When the request is shown in his left visual field, he will raise neither arm because the written information will not reach the left hemisphere language centers. When the request is shown in his right visual field, the information will reach the language centers and he will raise his right hand; however, the command to move his left hand may not reach the right hemisphere's motor center (Fig. 8-8).

39. c, e.

40. b, f, h.

41. c.

42. a, g.

43. a, d, g.

44. a, g.

9

Headaches

Headaches can be a chronic and recurrently incapacitating illness, symptoms of serious disease, or barometers of emotional stress. Their clinical importance lies also in their association with unusual symptoms, such as visual hallucinations, and in the contributing role, which is usually exaggerated, of psychologic factors. Almost three quarters of Americans have at least occasional headaches. Headaches together with backache and other benign pain disorders (Chapter 14) cause $55 billion in lost time every year.

Several varieties of chronic headache have distinctive patterns, are associated with unusual symptoms, and are affected by psychologic factors. These are *muscle contraction* (or *tension*) headaches, *migraines,** *cluster* headaches, *postconcussive* headaches, and *trigeminal neuralgia* (tic douloureux). Diagnosis in most cases is based not on physical or laboratory findings, which are usually normal, but on the patient's description of the headache and of its response to particular medicines.

On the other hand, acute or steadily progressive but otherwise nonspecific headaches may be manifestations of an underlying disease that can lead to permanent neurologic injury or death. These diseases are *temporal arteritis, intracranial mass lesions, pseudotumor cerebri, meningitis,* and *subarachnoid hemorrhage.* In these headaches, the patient's description is not as distinctive as in the preceding group, but abnormalities in the neurologic examination and laboratory tests usually allow the physician to make an accurate and possibly life-saving diagnosis.

MUSCLE CONTRACTION (TENSION) HEADACHES

Despite recent evidence that implicates cranial vascular dysfunction, tension headaches are still generally attributed to achy contraction (tension) of the scalp, neck, and face muscles (Fig. 9-1). Tension headaches typically develop in the afternoon and may be produced by physical fatigue, cervical spondylosis, bright light, or loud noise, as well as by emotional stress (Table 9-1). They are found almost exclusively in adults, more frequently in women than in men, and, probably because of psychologic rather than genetic reasons, in successive family members.

Therapy

Ideally a clearcut psychologic or physical origin should be demonstrated; however, the relief of a headache with simple measures not only indicates the

---

* Patients who have migraines may receive assistance from The National Headache Foundation, 5252 North Western Avenue, Chicago, Illinois 60625, (312) 878-7715.

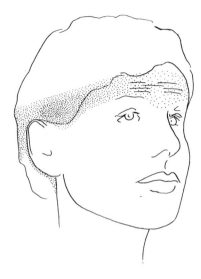

FIGURE 9–1.   Patients with muscle contraction (tension) headaches usually complain of a band-like squeezing, symmetric pressure at their neck, temples, or forehead.

headache's benign origin but also provides the cure. Several successful therapies have been empirically established. Although practice may differ, certain steps are usually followed by neurologists:

- **Step 1**. In *abortive* therapy, simple analgesics should be taken at the very start of a headache (or any pain) to prevent its full development. Thus, medicine should be kept in the car, at work, and in pocketbooks: it should be taken at the first inkling of a headache. Patients should first try common analgesics, such as aspirin, acetaminophen (e.g., Tylenol), or combinations of caffeine with aspirin, e.g., APC or Excedrin (Table 9-2). Non-narcotic prescription medications, such as Fiorinal, may elicit a better response, but this is mostly because of a physician's implicit endorsement.

- **Step 2**. Preventive, or *prophylactic*, therapy should be given if abortive therapy is ineffective or requires excessive medicine. Minor tranquilizers

TABLE 9–1.   IMPORTANT ITEMS IN A HEADACHE HISTORY

WHAT IS ITS NATURE?
  Severity: mild, moderate, severe
  Type: throbbing,* aching, sharp
  Location: unilateral (hemicranial),* bilateral, frontal, periorbital*
  Precipitants: stress, relief from stress,* menses,* missing meals,* too much or too little sleep,*
    glare,* alcohol,* chocolate,* medications (vasodilators, birth control pills)*
  Relief: rest, sleep,* alcohol, coffee, vasoconstrictors*
WHAT SYMPTOMS ARE ASSOCIATED WITH THE HEADACHE?
  Aura*: visual, personality change
  Autonomic dysfunction*: nausea, vomiting, polyuria, polydipsia
  Photophobia (light),* hyperacusis (noise)*
WHAT ARE ITS TEMPORAL CHARACTERISTICS?
  Were they present in childhood?
  What is their duration?
  Do they begin in the morning?
  Do they occur during sleep?*
  Are they most frequent on weekends?
  Do they occur in clusters?
IS THERE A HISTORY OF CAR-SICKNESS AS A CHILD?*
IS THERE A PARENT OR SIBLING WITH SIMILAR HEADACHES?

* Symptoms that indicate migraines.

TABLE 9–2. MEDICATIONS FOR MUSCLE CONTRACTION, MIGRAINE, OR
OTHER HEADACHES*

Medicine	Composition
APC	Aspirin, phenacetin, caffeine
Bellergal-S	Phenobarbital, ergotamine, belladonna
Bufferin	Aspirin, aluminum glycinate, magnesium carbonate
Cafergot†	Ergotamine, caffeine
Cafergot P-B†	Ergotamine, caffeine, belladonna, pentobarbital
Calcium channel blockers‡§	Diltiazem, nifedipine, verapamil
Elavil	Amitriptyline
Excedrin	Aspirin, acetaminophen, salicylamide, caffeine
Fiorinal	Butalbital, caffeine, aspirin
Inderal‡	Propranolol
Lithium	Lithium
Midrin	Isometheptene, dichloraphenazone, acetaminophen
Steroids	Prednisone, dexamethasone
Sansert‡	Methysergide
Wigraine†	Ergotamine, caffeine

* Consult package insert for indications, dosage, contraindications, precautions, and side effects.
† Available in both suppository and tablet form for abortive therapy of migraines.
‡ Prophylactic therapy of migraines.
§ Examples.

(e.g., diazepam) or combinations of sedative and vasoactive medicines (e.g., Bellergal-S) are often helpful if taken daily. Especially effective are amitriptyline (Elavil) and other antidepressants in small doses administered mostly at night, even in patients who are not overtly depressed (Chapter 14, Pain).

Step 3. Insight-oriented psychotherapy and classic psychoanalysis directed toward headaches have not proved significantly beneficial. Whether such modalities help the headache patient by providing insight or reduction in anxiety is a different but also unanswered question. Alternate non-pharmacologic approaches are biofeedback training, relaxation, and stress coping training. Studies have shown that biofeedback is effective in reducing headaches and decreasing medicine intake for about 6 months in about 50 percent of carefully selected patients. Its results are similar whether monitoring is by an electroencephalogram (EEG), electromyogram (EMG), skin temperature, blood pressure, or pulse. Also, preliminary studies have indicated that transcutaneous electrical nerve stimulation (TENS) may be helpful for tension headache.

MIGRAINES

According to the time-honored theory, migraines result from brief constriction of cerebral arteries, usually in the carotid artery system (Fig. 11-1), followed by prolonged, flaccid dilation that allows unsuppressed pulsations to stretch the arterioles. The pulsatile distentions, it is suggested, release bradykinin-like substances that give rise to the headache. A new theory is that migraines are caused by "neuronal depression," i.e., impaired metabolism of cerebral neurons. Decreased cerebral metabolic requirements rather than vasoconstriction lead to decreased cerebral blood flow.

Migraine and its varieties are thought by some investigators to be a genetic illness expressed through serotonin metabolism abnormalities. Studies have shown that plasma serotonin falls during the attack of migraine; that serotonin antagonists, such as methysergide (Sansert), prevent migraines; and that reserpine, which depletes serotonin, induces migraines. However, hormonal fluctuations and actions of a myriad of other substances have also been implicated.

Whatever the cause of migraines, the most important feature is that any migraine headache is virtually always accompanied by sensory, psychologic, and autonomic nervous system dysfunction. In many cases of migraine, the nonheadache symptoms may overshadow the headache or even occur without any headache whatsoever.

In the *classic variety* of migraine, which affects only about 20 percent of patients, the headache is preceded by an *aura*. Auras can be almost any symptom of brain dysfunction, but for almost all individuals with classic migraine, the aura is a particular visual hallucination (Table 9-3). This usually involves a partial graying of the visual field (*scotoma*) (Fig. 9-2A), flashing zigzag lines (*scintillating scotomata*) (Fig. 9-2B), crescents of brilliant colors (Fig. 9-2C), tubular vision, or distortion of objects (*metamorphosia*). Although olfactory hallucinations can be a migraine aura, they are more likely a manifestation of a partial complex seizure (Chapter 10). In children, auras can be recurrent colicky or "cyclic abdominal pain" with nausea and vomiting.

The *common variety*, which affects about 75 to 80 percent of migraine patients, has no preceding aura. The headache characteristically lasts 4 to 24 hours, is throbbing at its onset, and is initially felt on one side of the head (hemicranially) and mostly behind or around only eye (retro- or periorbitally). Although typically hemicranial initially, in about 50 percent of patients the headaches move to the opposite side or become generalized (Fig. 9-3). After the first one-half to 1 hour, the pain usually becomes dull, symmetric, and continual—not unlike the pain of a severe tension headache.

Accompanying physical symptoms, including nausea, vomiting, photophobia, and hyperacusis (sensitivity to noise), often lead to prostration. In most cases, migraines are preceded or accompanied by mood changes and minor behavioral disturbances. They are an important cause of transient mental status changes that can mimic psychiatric disorders (Table 9-4). Patients may become depressed or dysphoric. They tend to withdraw and seek dark quiet places to escape from people, as well as from light and noise. If unable to find solitude, they may become distraught. At the beginning of a headache, many patients become feverishly active and work excessively. They also may drink large quantities of water and crave food or sweets, particularly chocolate. Children can appear confused and also often become overly active. When children can rest, they

TABLE 9–3. CAUSES OF VISUAL HALLUCINATIONS*

Delirium tremens (DTs)
Intoxications
  Alcoholic hallucinosis
  Illicit: LSD and other hallucinogens
  Medicinal: L-dopa, scopolamine, and others
Migraines, classic variety
Narcolepsy (hypnopompic and hypnogogic hallucinations) (Chapter 17)
Sudden blindness, e.g., Anton's syndrome (Chapter 12)
Seizures (Chapter 10)
  Elementary (visual)
  Complex partial

* Commonly cited neurologic conditions.

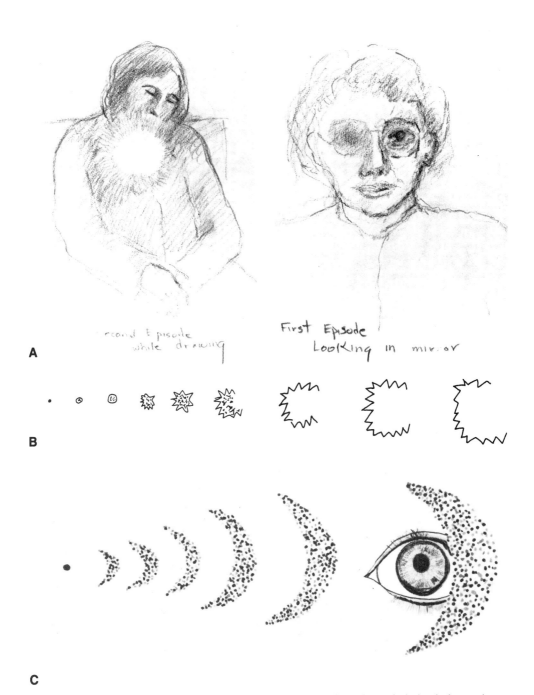

A. rcond Episode while drawing

First Episode Looking in mirror

B

C

FIGURE 9–2. *A.* These drawings, by a migraine patient, show the typical visual obscuration, a *scotoma*, that precedes her classic migraine. In both cases, a small circular area near the center of vision is lost entirely or reduced in clarity. *B.* The patient who drew this aura, a *scintillating scotoma* that she sees prior to her classic migraine, wrote, "In the early stages, the area within the lights is somewhat shaded. Later, as the figure widens, you can sort of peer right through the area. Eventually, it gets so wide that it disappears." Typically, this scotoma has an angulated margin, which is brightly lit, and an opaque interior that begins as a star and expands into a crescent. Patients, particularly children, may provide valuable diagnostic information if they are asked to draw what they "see" before a headache. *C.* A 30-year-old female artist in her first trimester of pregnancy had several classic migraine headaches that were almost always heralded by this scotoma. It began as a blue dot and, over 20 minutes, enlarged to a crescent of brightly shimmering, multicolored dots. When the crescent's intensity was at its peak, she was so dazzledthat she lost her ability to see and think clearly. On the day after delivery, the aura and headache returned for the final time.

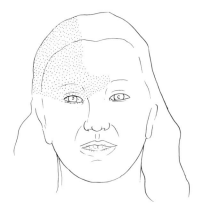

FIGURE 9–3.   Patients with migraines have throbbing, hemicranial headaches that, in about 50 percent of cases, either move to the other side of the head or become generalized.

may be so unable or unwilling to respond that they are said to be in a "stupor." After a migraine clears, especially when it ends with sleep, patients sometimes experience a remarkable calm euphoria.

Classic and common migraines, even more than tension headaches, occur more frequently in women than in men and tend to affect more than one family member. In contrast to tension headaches, migraines occur in children and adolescents, as well as adults, and they begin in the early morning rather than the afternoon. In women, migraines often start at menarche, recur premenstrually, and may be aggravated by birth control pills. Reports conflict as to whether migraines are worse during pregnancy, but they clearly return in the first postpartum week or with resumption of menses. In men and women, migraines may occur during REM sleep (Chapter 17), sometimes exclusively (*nocturnal migraines*).

Another important characteristic of migraines is that they can be precipitated by certain physical factors, such as hypoglycemia caused by skipping meals, excessive sleep, menses, alcohol, and stress. The alcoholic drinks most likely to precipitate a migraine are red wine and brandy, and the least likely, vodka and white wine. Alcoholic drinks can also provoke cluster headaches. In contrast to their effect on these vascular headaches, alcoholic drinks do ameliorate tension headaches.

The role of stress is particularly interesting. Stress can precipitate migraines, as it probably does tension headaches, but in many patients *relief* of stress is

TABLE 9–4.   CAUSES OF TRANSIENT, RECURRENT ALTERED MENTAL STATUS*

Drugs
  Illicit
  Medicinal
Metabolic aberrations, e.g., hypoglycemia
Migraines
Seizures (Chapter 10)
  Absence
  Partial complex
Sleep attacks, e.g., narcolepsy, sleep apnea naps (Chapter 17)
Transient global amnesia (Chapter 11)
Transient ischemic attacks (TIAs) (Chapter 11)

* Commonly cited neurologic conditions.

also associated with migraine. For example, a woman who may have a difficult job might awaken on Saturday or Sunday mornings with migraines. Likewise, at the start of a vacation, especially after examinations, students often develop migraines. However, contrary to popular belief, migraines affect people in all socioeconomic groups and all personality types. Obsessive persons, although probably more disturbed by having migraines, may not be particularly susceptible to them.

Other Migraine Varieties

Migraines that occur in children, *childhood migraines*, are similar to the migraines of adults except that more boys than girls are affected, visual auras occur more often, and autonomic symptoms, particularly nausea and vomiting, are even more troublesome. Behavioral disturbances are more common, with abnormal activity ranging from hyperactivity to a stuporous unresponsiveness. Children often develop an acute confusional episode, in which they are virtually incoherent and distraught.

In *basilar migraines*, headaches and mental changes, which include confusion and unresponsiveness, are accompanied by symptoms that reflect cerebellum and brainstem dysfunction, such as ataxia, vertigo, and diplopia. This variety of migraine, which particularly affects children, is believed to arise from changes in the vertebrobasilar, rather than the carotid, artery system (Fig. 11-2).

Hemiplegic migraines, which may occur in both children and adults, are characterized by combinations of hemiparesis, hemiparesthesia, and aphasia preceding or accompanying otherwise typical hemicranial migraine headaches. Sometimes the hemiparesis may even develop without an associated headache. Thus, in evaluating a patient who has had transient hemiparesis, the physician must consider the possibility of hemiplegic migraines along with transient ischemic attacks (TIAs), postictal (Todd's) hemiparesis, and psychogenic disorders. Hemiplegic migraine deficits occasionally become permanent. This condition, a *complicated migraine*, is virtually the same as a stroke. For this reason, women with migraines who are over 35 years of age should usually not take oral contraceptives because of their association with a slightly increased incidence of stroke.

Migraine-Like Conditions

Many people who eat certain foods, take particular medications, or "insult" their body in other ways, develop headaches that mimic migraines. Similarly, these substances can precipitate a typical migraine in susceptible persons. The best-known examples of foods precipitating a headache are the *Chinese restaurant syndrome*, which is caused by monosodium glutamate (MSG), and the *hot dog headache*, which is caused by the nitrites found in processed meats. Another is the *ice cream headache*, caused by any very cold food thatoverstimulates receptors in the pharynx. Despite many claims, few people actually develop headaches after eating foods that contain tyramine, such as ripened cheese, or those that contain phenylethylamine, particularly chocolate.

An interesting headache condition that occurs frequently is the *caffeine-withdrawal headache*. It develops in people who have a steady coffee intake but fail to drink their morning cup(s). This headache, which is often accompanied by anxiety, can be relieved with medications containing caffeine, as well as with black coffee. These headaches pose a dilemma for heavy coffee drinkers, for whom excessive caffeine leads to irritability, palpitations, and gastric burning but forgoing or missing coffee leads to rebound headaches and anxiety.

Antianginal medicines, such as nitroglycerin or isosorbide (Isordil), which contain nitrites or act directly on cerebrovascular tone, may cause headaches. Elderly patients in whom atherosclerosis leads to cerebrovascular insufficiency and poor arteriole muscle tone are particularly vulnerable. Curiously, whereas some calcium channel blockers, such as nifedipine (Procardia), precipitate headaches, others, such as verapamil (Calan), may be useful in prophylaxis.

Migraine-like headaches often occur after strenuous physical activity. Even during sexual intercourse or masturbation, a migraine-like headache, *coital cephalgia*, may develop. Nevertheless, physicians should be cautious in concluding that a severe headache occurring during athletic or sexual activity results from a benign, migrainous vascular change. Such a headache may have resulted from an intracerebral or subarachnoid hemorrhage caused by rupture of a cerebral aneurysm.

Therapy of Migraines

In migraine treatment, several specific steps are usually followed by neurologists:

- **Step 1**. Using a "headache diary," in which patients note the days of headaches and physically and emotionally significant events, physicians and patients might identify the precipitating factors of a migraine. If these factors cannot be avoided, at least they can be anticipated.

- **Step 2**. Abortive medicines, which must be taken immediately, usually consist of vasoactive agents, sometimes in combination with analgesics or sedatives. Medicines beneficial in tension headaches, such as Fiorinal, are often effective in common migraines. If analgesics are ineffective, medicines that consist predominantly of powerful vasoconstrictors, such as Cafergot or Wigraine, may be given to interrupt the vascular changes that lead to the headache. Patients who develop migraines at night may try taking medicine at bedtime. If oral medications are unsatisfactory, suppositories should be tried because they are usually better absorbed, more rapidly effective, and less likely to cause nausea. Sublingual tablets, another alternative, are more socially acceptable but less effective. After taking medicines, patients should remain at rest in a darkened room and, if possible, sleep. If nausea and vomiting are prominent, antiemetic suppositories, which generally contain phenothiazines, should also be used.

- **Step 3**. Prophylactic therapy is usually suggested if headaches occur more than four times a month or if abortive medicines are taken excessively. Prophylactic therapy not only reduces headache frequency and intensity but it also reduces patients' need for all medicines and allays their fear. Propranolol (Inderal), a beta adrenergic blocker, is widely used for migraine prophylaxis, as well as for treatment of angina and essential tremor (Chapter 18). It changes sympathetic tone and counters anxiety. Methysergide (Sansert), which is a congener of LSD that blocks serotonin receptors, is another highly effective prophylactic medicine; however, it may induce mood changes and, if taken for more than 6 months, retroperitoneal fibrosis. Antidepressants, such as amitriptyline, are also effective in migraine prophylaxis. They may be useful not only because they reduce or alter REM sleep, during which many migraine headaches develop, but also because they frequently act as analgesics (Chapter 14). When these commonly used medications fail to suppress migraines, physicians tend to try various medications with unproven or at least inconsistent benefit, including clonidine, antihistamines, and calcium channel blockers.

- **Step 4**. Neither insight-oriented psychotherapy nor classic psychoanalysis has been shown in adequately controlled studies to be an effective migraine treatment. Biofeedback and relaxation therapy have helped small numbers of patients but only for a limited time. All such therapies are less effective in migraines than in tension headaches.

TENSION-MIGRAINE COMBINATION

Descriptions of tension headaches and migraines imply that these conditions are entirely different and readily diagnosed (Table 9-5). However, this distinction may be artificial, and these two headaches may represent only the ends of a spectrum of a single headache disorder. In practice, many patients have a combination of tension headaches and migraines that seems to blend, vary, and recur. This combination is so common that it is virtually a migraine variety.

Whether these headaches are actually separate illnesses or not, physicians should determine what portion of their patients' headaches are migraines. If headaches are at some time unilateral, throbbing, present in the morning, accompanied by nausea, precipitated by menses, or evoked by the other known migraine precipitants, the diagnosis of migraine is appropriate. Physicians should not expect patients to have an aura or even a severe, incapacitating headache before diagnosing migraine. Appropriate therapy remains the prescription of medications, such as propranolol, that are more effective for migraines than for tension headaches. Overall, therapy for combination headaches will be more successful if physicians concentrate on the diagnosis and treatment of the migraine component.

CLUSTER HEADACHES

Cluster headaches are probably caused by a form of cerebrovascular dysfunction different from that suggested for migraines. Since cluster and migraine headaches, however, do result from cerebrovascular imbalance and they share several clinical features, both are referred to as "vascular headaches." Unlike

TABLE 9-5. COMPARISON OF MUSCLE CONTRACTION (TENSION) AND COMMON MIGRAINE HEADACHES

	Tension	Migraine
Age at onset	Middle age	Childhood, adolescence
Location of headache	Symmetric	Hemicranial*
Nature of headache	Dull	Throbbing*
Associated symptoms	None	Nausea, hyperacusis, photophobia
Time of onset	Afternoon	Early or late morning†
Effect of alcohol	Reduces headache	Worsens headache

* In approximately one half of patients.
† May develop during REM sleep and be present on awakening.

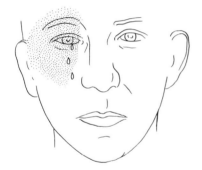

FIGURE 9–4. Patients with cluster headaches usually have unilateral periorbital pain accompanied by ipsilateral tearing and nasal discharge, along with ptosis and miosis (a artial Horner's syndrome).

migraines, cluster headaches have no familial tendency, usually begin between age 20 and 40 years, and affect many more men than women. In fact, they are the only form of chronic headache that develops more frequently in men than in women.

These headaches are called "cluster" because they occur in groups of one to three daily and last from several weeks to a few months. Clusters occur most often in the spring, and cluster-free intervals range from a few months to several years.

The headache itself, which usually lasts only one-half to 3 hours, is located periorbitally. It is nonthrobbing and extraordinarily painful, with pain seeming to bore from the eye straight backward into the head. Characteristic accompaniments are ipsilateral eye tearing, conjunctival congestion, nasal stuffiness, and a partial Horner's syndrome (Fig. 9-4). Headaches can occur randomly throughout the day, but they can also be precipitated by alcoholic drinks, and they have an especially strong tendency to develop during REM sleep. Unlike migraines, cluster headaches are not preceded by an aura or accompanied by nausea. They are not associated with mental changes, but the pain is often so severe that patients speak of wanting to kill themselves.

Treatment with abortive medicines is usually ineffective for a cluster headache because of its abrupt onset and relatively short duration. However, oxygen inhalation at 10 to 12 L/min may provide relief. Even prophylactic treatment with methysergide, propranolol, and amitriptyline may be unsatisfactory. One prophylactic medication is lithium. It was initially tried experimentally because cluster headaches, like manic-depressive illness, were known to be cyclic and to develop in middle-aged persons. Alternatively, steroids, such as prednisone and dexamethasone, are helpful for several weeks. Psychotherapy and biofeedback, however, provide no benefit.

POSTCONCUSSIVE (POSTTRAUMATIC) SYNDROME

After *minor* head trauma, usually as a result of motor vehicle accidents, people are said to have the postconcussive syndrome when they complain of a continual dull headache and neck pain, easy fatigability, insomnia, or personality changes. The most consistent symptoms are irritability, memory loss, and "depression." Compared to the estimated force of impact, the symptoms are unexpectedly severe and prolonged, lasting more than a year in 20 percent of cases.

The neurologic basis is not established. Theories have included microscopic lacerations of meningeal, cerebrovascular, or cerebral structures; shearing of cerebral matter; and, as almost an invariable component, wrenching of cervical muscles, ligaments, and nerve roots ("whiplash" injury). With substantial head trauma, contusion of the tips of the frontal and temporal lobes would explain personality changes and memory impairments.

In this poorly defined entity, the physical examination, CT or MRI scans, EEGs, and most neuropsychologic tests are normal. In some series, brainstem auditory evoked responses (Chapter 15) have been reported to be abnormal. That finding would indicate that the postconcussive syndrome may have an anatomic basis in some patients in brainstem dysfunction.

Important prognostic factors are the patient's premorbid intellectual and personality state, and pending litigation. Highly intelligent and strongly motivated people often do not have any postconcussive disabilities. In particular, soldiers, football players, and children who sustain comparable or more severe head injuries rarely develop the postconcussive syndrome. On the other hand, young adults who have a history of learning disabilities or attention deficit disorders are likely to develop serious incapacity when they sustain physical injury and psychologic shock from a motor vehicle accident.

Mild analgesics, sedatives, and amitriptyline may ameliorate some symptoms. Another aspect of treatment should be directed toward alleviating scalp and neck muscle contraction with muscle relaxants and physical therapy. Psychotherapy would be indicated for posttraumatic anxiety or depression. To eliminate at least one incentive for prolonged disability, litigation should be settled as quickly as possible. In some cases, however, incapacity has continued after settlements were reached.

TRIGEMINAL NEURALGIA (TIC DOULOUREUX)

Trigeminal neuralgia consists of brief, 20- to 30-second jabs of excruciatingly sharp pain extending along one of the three divisions of the trigeminal nerve. The division most often affected is V_2 (Fig. 4-11). Unlike other headaches, this pain can be provoked either by touching certain areas called *trigger zones* or with certain facial movements, such as those made while eating or brushing teeth. Episodes of pain may occur a dozen times daily; however, the neuralgia may recede for many months.

Trigeminal neuralgia affects women twice as often as men and develops relatively late in life, typically between the ages of 50 and 60 years. A lifelong, recurring condition, it is one of the most important causes of headache in the elderly (Table 9-6).

TABLE 9–6. HEADACHES IN THE
ELDERLY*

Brain tumors: glioblastoma, metastasis
Cerebrovascular insufficiency
Cervical spondylosis
Migraines, especially medication-induced
Subdural hematomas
Temporal arteritis
Trigeminal neuralgia (tic douloureux)

* Commonly cited chronic neurologic conditions.

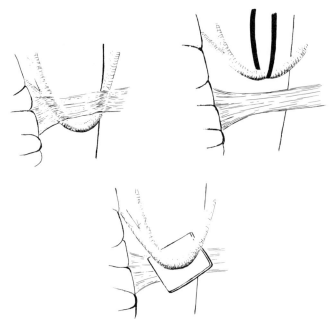

FIGURE 9–5. *Top left,* As pictured through an operating microscope, a patient's right trigeminal nerve is being compressed from below by an aberrant large artery. The brainstem is on the left side of the field and the nerve exists horizontally to the right. *Top right,* In Microvascular decompressive surgery for trigeminal neuralgia, a surgical loop plucks the artery out from under the nerve. *Bottom,* The artery is then fixed to a barrier that protects the trigeminal nerve.

The condition has been shown to originate, in most cases, from an aberrant superior cerebellar artery or other cerebral blood vessel compressing the trigeminal nerve root as it emerges from the brainstem. Another but less frequent cause, accounting for most cases in young adults, is multiple sclerosis. Whatever the cause, treatment is usually begun with carbamazepine (Tegretol). In the majority of patients, in whom an aberrant vessel is responsible for the neuralgia, the most effective procedure is a craniotomy to place a barrier between any vessel compressing the trigeminal nerve and the nerve itself. The technique, which requires use of a microscope, is a major neurosurgical advance (Fig. 9-5). Less risky procedures are injecting percutaneous glycerol and creating radiofrequency lesions in the root of the trigeminal nerve.

ACUTELY OCCURRING OR PROGRESSIVELY SEVERE HEADACHES

Temporal Arteritis

Temporal arteritis is a disease of unknown etiology in which the temporal and other cranial arteries become inflamed. Since histologic examination of affected arteries reveals giant cells, the condition is properly called *giant cell arteritis*.

Patients are almost always older than 55 years. They usually have a dull, continual headache in one or both temples that may radiate toward the jaw ("jaw claudication"). In advanced cases, patients' temporal arteries are reddened and tender. Temporal arteritis is also characterized by signs of systemic illness, such as malaise, low grade fever, and weight loss.

Since untreated arterial inflammation will lead to arterial occlusion, serious complications develop in cases when diagnosis is delayed. Most important, ophthalmic artery occlusion will cause blindness, and cerebral artery occlusion will cause cerebral infarctions. A temporal artery biopsy is the definitive test, but it is often unnecessary, hazardous, or impractical. In over 90 percent of cases, an erythrocyte sedimentation rate (ESR) elevated above 40 mm provides an easily obtainable adequate confirmation. Timely treatment with steroids will quickly relieve the headaches and prevent complications.

Intracranial Mass Lesions

Patients with brain tumors and subdural hematomas often have headaches as their first or most bothersome symptom (Chapter 19). These headaches also are usually dull and either unilateral or generalized. They worsen when intracranial pressure is raised, as when people cough, or early in the morning, when REM sleep occurs. Although brain tumor headaches may awaken patients, most frequently migraines and cluster headaches (which also develop in REM sleep) are the ones that begin during sleep.

When mass lesions cause headache, they also usually produce other signs either of increased intracranial pressure, such as papilledema, or of cerebral impairment, such as seizures or personality changes. But no matter how unlikely is a brain tumor, neurologists order CT or MRI scans in almost all patients with unexplained progressive headaches and an elevated ESR in those over 55 years of age.

Chronic Meningitis

Chronic meningitis, most often from *Cryptococcus*, may cause continual, dull headaches and be accompanied by signs of systemic illness and dementia. These effects can be corrected if the illness is diagnosed early (Chapter 7). Patients who have impaired immune systems, including the elderly, those taking steroids, and those with AIDS, are susceptible. A CT or MRI scan, which must be performed before a lumbar puncture, may show communicating hydrocephalus. The lumbar puncture will yield cerebrospinal fluid (CSF) that has a lymphocytic pleocytosis, low glucose concentration, and possibly positive test results for antigens, such as *Cryptococcus*. Since fungi and tubercle bacilli may take weeks to culture (Chapter 20), the diagnosis must be based on the preliminary CSF results.

Pseudotumor Cerebri

Pseudotumor cerebri (benign intracranial hypertension) is virtually restricted to young obese women who have menstrual irregularities. It gives rise to papilledema and a dull, generalized headache. Pseudotumor appears to be caused by fluid accumulation within the brain interstitium that raises CSF pressure, often to levels over 400 mm H_2O. If untreated, pseudotumor leads to blindness from optic atrophy (Chapter 12). Treatment usually consists of diuretics, weight loss through dieting, repeated lumbar punctures, and sometimes steroids. In refractory cases, CSF shunting procedures are required.

Bacterial Meningitis and Subarachnoid Hemorrhage

In young adults, two life-threatening, headache-producing illnesses are bacterial meningitis and subarachnoid hemorrhage. Bacterial meningitis is usually caused by meningococcus or pneumococcus and often spreads in epidemic fashion among young adults in confined areas, such as dormitories or military training camps. It causes a rapidly developing, severe headache that is accompanied by photophobia, malaise, fever, and nuchal rigidity. At the slightest indication of these symptoms, the CSF must be examined and treatment started with penicillin or another antibiotic.

Viral infections that cause headaches may involve the brain, causing *encephalitis*, or the meninges, causing *viral meningitis*. These conditions, which are usually more benign than bacterial infections, are diagnosed with CSF analysis, CT, and EEG. However, one virus, Herpes simplex, is noteworthy as the most frequent cause of nonepidemic, serious encephalitis. Herpes virus has a predilection for the inferior surface of the frontal and temporal lobes. Thus, in addition to fever, somnolence, and delirium, patients with Herpes encephalitis have partial complex seizures and memory impairment. Some patients who have sustained bilateral temporal lobe damage have developed a human variety of the Klüver-Bucy syndrome (Chapter 16), which was first described in monkeys subjected to surgical removal of both temporal lobes.

The other important acutely occurring headache is caused by *subarachnoid hemorrhage* from a ruptured *berry aneurysm*. In this condition, patients usually suddenly develop an extraordinarily severe headache, prostration, and nuchal rigidity—symptoms similar to those in bacterial meningitis. Subarachnoid hemorrhage often occurs during exertion, including exercise, delivery, straining at stool, and sexual intercourse. However, mild or otherwise atypical subarachnoid hemorrhages ("leaks") are not as dramatic and are often disregarded or confused with common migraines, tension headaches, or a "head cold." The correct diagnosis of subarachnoid hemorrhage may be made from evidence of blood on CT or MRI scans or from CSF that is bloody or xanthochromic (yellow from blood breakdown).

A striking, iatrogenic cause of intracerebral or subarachnoid hemorrhage peculiar to psychiatric practice is the hypertensive reaction to monamine oxidase (MAO) inhibitors. Patients treated with MAO inhibitors can develop severe hypertension with excruciating headaches that culminate in these hemorrhages when patients eat aged cheese, other foods with a high tyramine content, or take dibenzazepine-related medications, meperidine (Demerol), L-dopa (as in Sinemet), or sympathomimetic medications. Commonly used MAO inhibitors—isocarboxid (Marplan), pargyline (Eutron), phenylzine (Nardil), and tranylcypromine (Parnate)—normally cause an accumulation of epinephrine, norepinephrine, and serotonin, which presumably reverses biochemical deficiencies in depression; however, this same process increases the risk of developing hypertensive reactions. Different MAO inhibitors, which are used on an experimental basis in Parkinson's disease to preserve dopamine, are not likely to cause a hypertensive hemorrhage (Chapter 18). If a hypertensive reaction with or without a hemorrhage were to occur, the specific treatment would be 5 mg intravenous phentolamine (Regitine), which is an alpha adrenergic blocking agent. If it is unavailable, chlorpromazine and propranolol are substitutes that will rapidly lower blood pressure.

SUMMARY

In evaluating patients with tension headaches, migraines, and other chronic, recurrent headaches, the diagnosis rests on the history and, to a certain extent, on the patient's response to medicines. Psychologic factors play a limited role in these headaches.

Patients with either acutely occurring or progressively severe headaches are apt to have life-threatening illnesses. A careful neurologic examination and usually also a CT or MRI scan are in order to diagnose a brain tumor, intracranial hematoma, or other mass lesion. Those who might have pseudo-tumor cerebri, meningitis, or subarachnoid hemorrhage usually should have a lumbar puncture. Patients older than 55 years with an unexplained, chronic headache should have an erythrocyte sedimentation rate done as an emergency procedure.

REFERENCES

Abramowicz M (ed): Drugs for migraine. Med Letter 29:27, 1983
Amery WK, Wauquier A (eds): The Prelude to the Migraine Attack. London, Bailliere Tindall, 1987
Barlow CF: Headaches and Migraine in Childhood. London, Spastics International Medical Publications, 1984
Bell NW, Abramowitz SI, Folkins CH: Biofeedback, brief psychotherapy and tension headaches. Headache 23:162, 1983
Bergtsson BA, Malmuall BE: Giant cell arteritis. Acta Med Scand 658(suppl):1, 1982
Blanchard EB, Andrasik F, Arena JG, et al: Nonpharmacologic treatment of chronic headache: Prediction of outcome. Neurology 33:1596, 1983
Bogousslavsky J, Regli F, Van Melle G, et al: Migraine stroke. Neurology 38:223, 1988
Cohen MJ, McArthur DL, Rickles WH: Comparison of four biofeedback treatments for migraine headache: Physiologic and headache variables. Psychosomatics 42:463, 1980
Dalessio DJ (ed): Wolff's Headache and Other Head Pain, 5th ed. New York, Oxford University Press, 1987
Dikmen S, Reitan RM, Temkin NR: Neuropsychological recovery in head injury. Arch Neurol 40:333, 1983
Edelson RN: Menstrual migraine and other hormonal aspects of migraine. Headache 25:376, 1985
Khurana RK: Headache. In Goldstein PJ (ed): Neurological Disorders of Pregnancy. New York, Futura Publishing Company, 1986, pp 247-263
Lance JW: Headaches related to sexual activity. J Neurol Neurosurg Psychiatry 39:1226, 1976
Lauritzen M, Olsen TS, Lassen NA: Regulation of regional cerebral blood flow during and between migraine attacks. Ann Neurol 14:569, 1983
Littlewood JT, Glover V, Davies PTG, et al: Red wine as a cause of migraine. Lancet 1:558, 1988
Martin MJ: Muscle-contraction (tension) headache. Psychosomatics 24:319, 1983
Martin PR, Marie GV, Nathan PR: Behavioral research on headaches: A coded bibliography. Headache 27:555, 1987
Merskey H: Psychiatry and the cervical sprain syndrome. Can Med Assoc J 130:1119, 1984
Noseworthy JH, Miller J, Murry T, et al: Auditory brainstem responses in postconcussion syndrome. Arch Neurol 38:275, 1981
Olesen J: The ischemic hypotheses of migraine. Arch Neurol 44:321, 1987
Raskin NH: Migraine. Psychosomatics 23:897, 1982
Richards W: The fortification illusions of migraines. Sci Am 224:89, 1971
Round R, Keane JR: The minor symptoms of increased intracranial pressure: 101 patients with benign intracranial hypertension. Neurology 38:1461, 1988
Rowe MJ, Carlson C: Brainstem auditory evoked potentials in postconcussion dizziness. Arch Neurol 37:679, 1980
Sacks OW: Migraine: Understanding a Common Disorder. Berkeley, University of California Press, 1985
Schoenhuber R, Gentilini M, Orlando M: Prognostic value of auditory brainstem responses for late postconcussion symptoms following minor head injury. J Neurosurg 68:742, 1988

Solomon S, Guglielmo KM: Treatment of headache by transcutaneous electrical stimulation. Headache 25:12, 1985

Sternbach RA, Dalessio DJ, Kunzel M, et al: MMPI patterns in common headache disorders. Headache 20:311, 1980

Sweet WH: The treatment of trigeminal neuralgia (tic douloureux). N Engl J Med 315:174, 1986

Ziegler DK, Hurwitz A, Hassanein RS, et al: Migraine prophylaxis: A comparison of propranolol and amitriptyline. Arch Neurol 44:486, 1987

QUESTIONS: CHAPTER 9

1–4. A 17-year-old Marine recruit has developed a moderately severe generalized headache, lethargy, and nuchal rigidity.
  1. What disease must be considered first?
  2. What diagnostic procedure must be performed first?
  3. What would the typical result be?
  4. What is the therapy?

5–9. A 45-year-old man has had moderate bitemporal headaches and then the gradual onset of stupor over a 5-day period. He has episodes of unusual repetitive behavior, complaints of unusual smells, and photophobia. On examination he has fever, delerium, mild nuchal rigidity, and bilateral long tract findings.

  5. What might the episodic behavioral disturbances indicate?

  6. What do the delerium and long tract findings suggest?

  7. What is the most common cause of sporadic (nonepidemic) encephalitis?

  8. What areas of the brain are particularly susceptible?

  9. What are the major sequelae of this infection?

  10. A young hypertensive housewife suddenly develops severe right retro-orbital pain, prostration, and a right third cranial nerve palsy. What is the most likely cause?

  11. A middle-aged hypertensive man has the sudden onset of the worst headache of his life while watching television. Although he has nausea and vomiting, he is able to speak coherently. What are the likely possible causes?

  12. An elderly, depressed man has a moderately severe generalized headache and decreased attention span but no "hard" findings. What entities should be given special consideration?

  13. What medicines are known to cause headaches?

14–25. Match the disease with the characteristic symptoms.

14. Tic douloureux	a. Severe ocular pain, "red eye," decreased vision
15. Bell's palsy	b. Papilledema, generalized headache, and menstrual irregularity
16. Pseudotumor cerebri	c. Mastoid pain followed by facial palsy
17. Basilar migraine	d. Lancinating pain in the jaw
18. Subarachnoid hemorrhage	e. Moderate headache, focal seizures, fever
19. Temporal arteritis	f. Mild headache and hemiparesis
20. Angle-closure glaucoma	g. Chronic pain, depressed sensorium
21. Subdural hematoma	h. Temporal pain, blindness, high sedimentation rate
22. Postconcussive headache	
23. Childhood cerebral tumor	

24. Viral meningitis

25. Hemiplegic migraine

i. Prolonged dull headaches inattention, and insomnia
j. Generalized headache, nuchal rigidity
k. Horner's syndrome
l. Headache, nausea, vomiting, and ataxia

26. What features of a headache suggest that it is a migraine?

27. What are common precipitants of migraine headaches?

28. How do migraine headaches in children differ from those in adults?

29. In what neurologic disorders are visual hallucinations experienced?

30–33. At what ages do the following headaches usually occur (more than one age period may be appropriate)?

30. Migraine, classic

31. Migraine, common

32. Cluster

33. Temporal arteritis

a. Childhood
b. Adolescence
c. Middle age
d. Older age

34–37. Which of these headaches are relieved by sleep?

34. Classic migraine

35. Common migraine

36. Cluster

37. Temporal arteritis

38–44. Which of these headaches typically awaken the patient from sleep?

38. Classic migraine

39. Common migraine

40. Brain tumor

41. Subdural hematoma

42. Tension

43. Cluster headaches

44. Conversion reaction

45. In what stage of sleep do migraine and cluster headaches begin?

46. What laboratory tests are associated with migraine headaches?

47. A group of many severe periorbital headaches occurs every winter when the patient goes to Miami. Of which kind of headache is this pattern typical?

48. What are the diseases or conditions that cost industry the largest number of man-hours?

49–51. Which of the following headaches follow family patterns?

49. Migraine headaches

50. Cluster headaches

51. Tension headaches

52–56. Which medicines are useful for the following headaches?

52. Tension headachesa.

53. Infrequently occurring classic migraine

54. Frequent, severe common migraine

55. Cluster headaches

56. Occasionally occurring mild migraine

a. Methysergide (Sansert)
b. Propranolol (Inderal)
c. Cafergot
d. Aspirin compounds
e. Aspirin, phenacetin, caffeine, and barbiturate compounds
f. Lithium

57–60. What are the prominent adverse effects of the following medications?

57. Methysergide (Sansert)

58. Propranolol (Inderal)

59. Cafergot

60. Aspirin

61. Which headache variety is cyclic or periodic, develops in middle-aged persons, and responds to lithium treatment?

62. Which tests are likely to be abnormal in patients with postconcussive syndrome?
   a. CT scan
   b. Lumbar puncture
   c. EEG
   d. Brainstem auditory evoked responses
   e. MRI scan

63. Which procedures may alleviate postconcussive headache?
   a. Neck muscle massage
   b. Use of antidepressant medications
   c. Concluding all litigation
   d. Use of major tranquilizers

64. Which headache variety occurs more often in men than women?
   a. Classic migraine
   b. Common migraine
   c. Pseudotumor cerebri
   d. Trigeminal neuralgia
   e. Tension headaches
   f. Cluster headaches

65. Which therapies are appropriate for pseudotumor cerebri headaches?
   a. Repeated lumbar punctures
   b. Antidepressants
   c. Diuretics
   d. Steroids
   e. Muscle massage
   f. Biofeedback

66–73. Match the headache with its most likely cause:

66. Tic douloureuxa.

67. Hot-dog headache

68. Coital cephalgia

69. Pseudotumor cerebri

70. Temporal arteritis

71. Chinese restaurant syndrome

a. Giant cell inflammation of extra- and intracranial arteries
b. Autonomic nervous system dysfunction
c. Vascular compression of the trigeminal nerve
d. Nitrites
e. Monosodium glutamate
f. Intracerebral fluid retention

72. Nocturnal migraine

73. Antianginal medication-induced headaches

g. Nightmares
h. REM sleep
i. NREM sleep
j. Night terrors
k. Cerebral as well as coronary artery dilation

74. Why might tricyclic antidepressant (TCA) medications be helpful in migraine headaches in people without overt depression?
a. TCAs may improve sleep patterns.
b. TCAs may increase the concentration of serotonin, which is analgesic.
c. TCAs are analgesic themselves.
d. TCAs are endorphins.
e. Such patients may have occult depression.

75. Why is rectal or parenteral administration preferable to oral administration of vasoconstrictors, such as ergotamine, for migraines?

76. Which of the following are reasonable criteria for changing from abortive to prophylactic migraine therapy?
a. More than four migraines monthly
b. Tinnitus from aspirin-containing medications
c. Ergotism
d. Habitual narcotic use
e. Once monthly classic migraines

77. Which conditions are apt to occur in several family members, although not necessarily on a genetic basis?
a. Temporal arteritis
b. Tuberous sclerosis
c. Multiple sclerosis
d. Migraines
e. Absence (petit mal) seizures
f. Cluster headaches
g. Pick's disease
h. Tension headaches

78. During which periods are women's migraines exacerbated?
a. Premenstrually
b. When depressed
c. In the first trimester of pregnancy
d. When nursing
e. Menopause
f. When taking oral contraceptives
g. At menarche
h. During middle age

79. Which observations suggest that serotonin metabolism abnormalities are causally related to the development of migraines?
a. Propranolol (Inderal) is a good prophylactic medication.
b. Dexamethasone suppression tests are abnormal in migraine patients.
c. Platelet serotonin concentrations fall before migraines occur.
d. Reserpine, which depletes serotonin, precipitates migraines.
e. Methysergide (Sansert), which blocks serotonin receptors, prevents migraines.

80. A 35-year-old man, who suffers several migraine attacks a year, developed a uniquely severe headache during sexual intercourse. Two evenings later, such a headache recurred during masturbation. What advice should be given to the patient?

ANSWERS

1. Acute bacterial meningitis, particularly meningococcal, is a common, often fatal disease in military recruits, schoolchildren, and other young people brought to confined areas.

2. The possibility of bacterial meningitis merits immediate investigation with a lumbar puncture for cerebrospinal fluid (CSF) analysis.

3. With bacterial meningitis, the CSF reveals a low glucose concentration (0–40 mg/ 100 mL), high protein concentration (greater than 100 mg/100 mL), and a polymorphonuclear pleocytosis (over 100/mL).

4. Although alternatives have been suggested, penicillin, 20,000,000 U/day intravenously, remains the standard treatment.

5. He may be having partial complex seizures originating in the uncus of the temporal lobe, i.e., "uncinate fits."

6. He probably has cerebral as well as meningeal involvement.

7. Herpes simplex encephalitis is the most common, nonepidemic encephalitis.

8. Herpes simplex encephalitis has a predilection for the temporal lobes, which include the uncus and portions of the limbic system.

9. Temporal lobe inflammation may cause partial complex seizures and, because of the limbic system involvement, profound memory impairment and in rare cases a form of the Klüver-Bucy syndrome (Chapter 16).

10. Although there are many causes of severe retro-orbital pain, a third nerve palsy indicates that a posterior communicating artery aneurysm has ruptured and caused a subarachnoid hemorrhage.

11. Any newly occurring or unique headache is potentially serious. In view of the hypertension, such a headache suggests a cerebral or subarachnoid hemorrhage. Migraine or cluster headaches, which may appear in middleage, might be the correct diagnosis; however, they should be considered only when headaches have become a chronic illness (often requiring months of observation) and when potentially fatal conditions have been excluded.

12. Although elderly people are subject to most forms of headaches, they are prone to develop a variety of conditions (Table 9-6) that probably reflect a depressed immune system, atherosclerotic and fragile cerebral vessels, or iatrogenic disturbances. Also, they may have headache as a symptom of depression.

13. Nitroglycerin, long-acting vasodilators (e.g., Isordil), and some other antianginal medications cause headaches. Reserpine causes a dull frontal pain and nasal stuffiness. The monamine oxidase (MAO) inhibitors cause hypertensive headaches when foods containing tyramine are eaten. Birth control pills can precipitate or exacerbate migrainous headaches.

14. d.

15. c.

16. b.

17. l.

18. j.

19. h.

20. a.

21. f, g, i, or l.

22. i.

23. l.

24. j.

25. f.

26. Typically, a migraine is unilateral (in 50 percent of cases), pulsating, and accompanied by autonomic nervous system dysfunction, e.g., nausea, vomiting, fatigue, and diaphoresis. Classic migraines, which are relatively infrequent (20 percent of migraine sufferers have the classic variety), will be preceded by auras, which are most often visual scotoma.

27. Menses, glare, alcohol, too much sleep, missing meals (hypoglycemia), and relief of stress may precipitate migraines.

28. Although patients of all ages may have visual auras and autonomic dysfunction, these symptoms may be the primary or exclusive manifestation of migraines in children. Children are also more prone than adults to develop the basilar artery migraine variant. Behavioral disturbances, such as agitation or withdrawal, are often more pronounced in children.

29. Migraines, seizures originating in the temporal or occipital lobes, drugs, narcolepsy, and alcohol withdrawal (DTs) all may precipitate visual hallucinations.

30.	a, b, c.	**45.**	REM
31.	a, b, c.	**46.**	Low plasma serotonin
32.	c.	**47.**	A cluster headache
33.	d.	**48.**	Low back pain and headache
34.	Yes	**49.**	Yes
35.	Yes	**50.**	No
36.	No	**51.**	Yes
37.	No	**52.**	d or e.
38.	Yes	**53.**	c.
39.	Yes	**54.**	a or b.
40.	Yes	**55.**	f, sometimes a or b.
41.	Yes	**56.**	d or e.
42.	No	**57.**	Retroperitoneal fibrosis
43.	Yes	**58.**	Bradycardia, asthma, cardiac failure
44.	No		

59. Nausea and vomiting in acute stage; vascular spasm, claudication, and muscle cramps with prolonged use, i.e., ergotism

60. Painful gastric distress, gastroduodenal bleeding, and easy bruisability

61. Cluster headaches were initially treated with lithium because of their similarity to manic-depressive illness.

62. c and d, but neither positive nor negative results have definite diagnostic value.

63.	a, b, c.	**69.**	f.
64.	f.	**70.**	a.
65.	a, c, d.	**71.**	e.
66.	c.	**72.**	h.
67.	d.	**73.**	k.
68.	b.	**74.**	a, b, c, e.

75. Parental or rectal vasoconstrictor medication administration produces effective blood levels much faster than oral administration. Early treatment is essential because, once vasodilation is established, migraines are relatively refractory to vasoconstriction treatments. In addition, when a patient has a migraine, gastric atony prevents absorption of orally administered medications.

76. a, b, c, d.

77. b, c, d, e, g, h. Tension headaches can occur in families, but this tendency presumably does not have a genetic basis.

78. a, c, e, f, g.

79. c, d, e.

80. The patient probably has developed a coital migraine; however, the development of a uniquely severe headache in any patient, especially when it occurs during vigorous activity, might require further evaluation. In particular, a subarachnoid or intracerebral hemorrhage must be considered. A CT scan or lumbar puncture, depending upon the circumstances, is usually performed because the possibility of a potentially fatal subarachnoid hemorrhage should always be borne in mind when confronted with a patient who describes having the "worse headache" of his or her life.

10

Seizures

Seizures, including partial complex seizures, are characterized by specific clinical features and electroencephalographic (EEG) patterns. Also, they are associated with distinctive etiologies, age at onset, and appropriate therapies. The tendency to have recurrent seizures, *epilepsy,** affects about 6 of every 1,000 people.

Seizures can mimic psychiatric disturbances, have prominent cognitive and affective components, and be precipitated by psychotropic medicines. The most specific laboratory test for seizures, the EEG, is also helpful in the diagnosis of metabolic encephalopathy and certain dementias, but it is virtually useless for almost all other conditions.

This chapter reviews the clinical features of the major seizure varieties, their EEG diagnosis, and appropriate anticonvulsants. It emphasizes mental changes brought about by seizures, epilepsy, and anticonvulsants and concludes with a discussion of disorders that can mimic seizures.

EEG

Normal and Abnormal

The routine EEG records cerebral electrical activity detected by "surface" or "scalp" electrodes (Fig. 10-1). (The cost of a routine EEG in 1989 is approximately $175.) Four frequency bands of cerebral activity, called by Greek letters, tend to occur over certain parts of the cerebrum and under particular conditions (Table 10-1).

The normal dominant, or *background*, EEG activity is in the *alpha* range of 8 to 13 cycles-per-second, or Hertz (Hz), and occurs over the occipital region (Fig. 10-2). Alpha activity is prominent when individuals are relaxed with their eyes closed, but it disappears if they open their eyes, concentrate, or become anxious. Thus, it accurately monitors freedom from anxiety and is useful in biofeedback, "alpha training," and other behavior modification techniques. Alpha activity is also lost when people fall asleep or take any medicine that affects mental function, and it slows in the elderly and in almost every neurologic illness that affects the cerebrum.

Beta activity, frequencies faster than 13-Hz, usually has lower voltage and overlies the frontal lobes. Although present in normal persons, its relative proportion is increased when people are concentrating, anxious, or taking minor tranquilizers.

---

* Patients with epilepsy may receive assistance from the Epilepsy Foundation of America, 4351 Garden City Drive, Landover, Maryland 20785, (301) 459-3700.

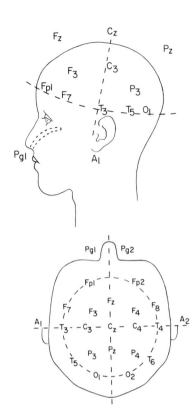

FIGURE 10–1. In the standard array of scalp electrodes, most are named for the underlying brain; odd-numbered ones are on the left and even-numbered on the right. The P_g electrodes are from the nasopharyngeal leads; the C electrodes, the center of the skull; and the A electrodes, the ears.

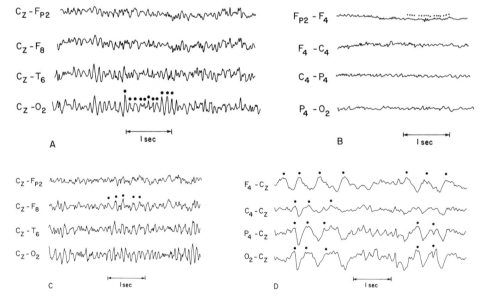

FIGURE 10–2. *A, Alpha* activity is the regular 11-Hz activity overlying the occipital lobe. *B, Beta* activity is the low voltage, irregular 17-Hz activity overlying the frontal lobe. *C, Theta* activity is the 5-Hz activity overlying the right frontal lobe. *D, Delta* activity is the high voltage 2- to 3-Hz activity present over the entire hemisphere.

TABLE 10–1. COMMON EEG RHYTHMS

Activity	Hz (cycles/sec)	Usual Location
Alpha	8–13	Posterior
Beta	>13	Anterior
Theta	4–7	Generalized*
Delta	1–3	Generalized*

* May be focal.

Theta (4- to 7-Hz) and *delta* (1- to 3-Hz) frequencies are usually absent in healthy, alert adults, but are normally seen in children, in all people as they enter deep sleep, and in many people with trivial disturbances. When present diffusely over the entire brain, slow activity may indicate a degenerative condition or metabolic derangement. When found over a particular area or in *phase reversal* (Fig. 10-3), it may indicate a cerebral lesion, but its absence does not exclude one. Overall, since minimal provocation creates EEG slowing, it is nonspecific.

Whatever their frequency, unusually pointed waves, "sharp waves" or "spikes" can indicate a cerebral lesion or a predisposition to epilepsy. When in phase

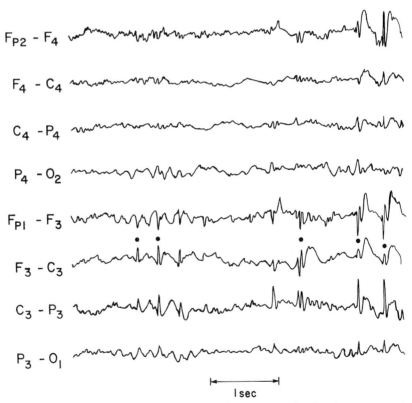

FIGURE 10–3. On at least six occasions (marked by dots), sharp waves and spikes, in *phase reversal*, appear to point toward each other. They originate from the F_3 electrode, which is over the left frontal lobe. A finding of such isolated, phase-reversed sharp waves is associated with seizures; however, without further clinical or EEG evidence, it is insufficient for diagnostic purposes.

reversal, they indicate an irritative focus that is likely to produce a seizure. However, the finding of sharp waves or spikes does not prove that a patient suffers from a seizure disorder, but that he or she has the likelihood of having one.

Uses

Seizures

The EEG is most useful in diagnosing and categorizing seizures. During a seizure (*ictus*), *paroxysmal* EEG activity may arise from either normal or abnormal background activity. Paroxysms usually consist of bursts of spikes, slow waves, or complexes of both.

An EEG should ideally be recorded during the ictus, but seizures rarely occur during routine recordings. When they do, EEGs may be obscured by muscle movement artifacts. The EEGs obtained immediately after the seizure, in the *postictal period*, generally show only slow, low voltage activity, called *postictal depression*. Fortunately, EEGs obtained between seizures, in the *interictal period*, contain specific abnormalities that suffice for definitive diagnosis in up to 80 percent of cases. On the other hand, since about 20 percent of epilepsy patients have essentially normal routine EEGs, normal interictal EEGs do not exclude a diagnosis of seizures.

Several maneuvers are used to evoke diagnostic EEG abnormalities in suspected cases. Patients are usually asked to hyperventilate for about 3 minutes or to look directly into a stroboscopic light during the EEG. If these maneuvers do not yield diagnostic information and if a strong suspicion of seizures persists, an EEG is performed after sleep deprivation. In about one third of epileptic patients, this EEG reveals abnormalities not apparent from routine studies.

In some cases, specially placed electrodes will reveal abnormalities undetectable by scalp electrodes. For example, nasopharyngeal or sphenoidal electrodes can detect discharges from the inferior-medial (mesial or medial) surface of the temporal lobe (Fig. 10-4). Also, electrodes experimentally placed in the subdural space or within the cerebral cortex have revealed an epileptic focus.

Recently introduced techniques, telemetry and cassette recordings, consist of monitoring the EEG, often with simultaneous videotape recording to correlate behavior, for several hours, overnight, or, in difficult cases, several days. The cost of video-telemetry for several hours in 1989 is approximately $500. This long-term continual monitoring is especially valuable in diagnosing partial complex seizures and disorders that mimic seizures, such as pseudoseizures (see below).

Toxic-Metabolic Encephalopathy

A major use of the EEG is in detecting cerebral dysfunction from barbiturates, other drugs, hepatic or renal failure, encephalitis, or other chemical aberration, i.e., toxic-metabolic encephalopathy or "delirium" (Chapter 7). During the initial phases of a toxic-metabolic encephalopathy, when patients may be merely withdrawn or agitated and do not yet display cognitive impairment, the EEG may lose its alpha activity and develop generalized theta and delta activity.

EEG changes are not specific, except that in hepatic or uremic encephalopathy there are characteristic repetitive *triphasic waves* (Fig. 10-5). In hepatic failure, they may appear before the bilirubin levels increase. Most important, although

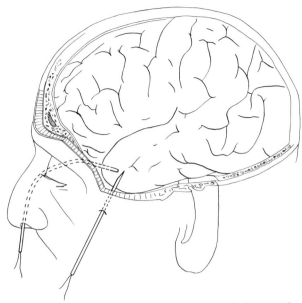

FIGURE 10–4. *Nasopharyngeal electrodes,* which are inserted through the nostrils, reach the posterior pharynx. There, separated by the thin sphenoid bone, they are adjacent to the medial surface of the temporal lobe, which is the focus or origin of about 80 percent of partial complex seizures. (Refer to Figures 20-1 and 20-13 to see the distance between the medial surface of the temporal lobe and the scalp, and also the relationship of the temporal lobe to the sphenoid bone). *Sphenoidal electrodes* are inserted through the skin to reach the lateral, external surface of the sphenoid wing. In this location the electrodes are near the inferior surface of the temporal lobe. (However, specially placed scalp electrodes, new arrays, and critical reading of the EEG, may be just as accurate [Sperling].)

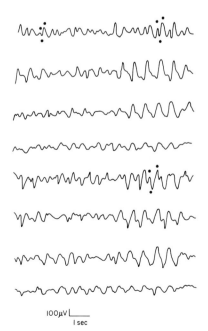

FIGURE 10–5. This EEG obtained from a patient with hepatic encephalopathy reveals typical *triphasic waves,* which can be seen in the first and fifth channel. There is also lack of organized background activity, which would ordinarily be seen clearest in the lowest channel.

100μV

1 sec

most EEG changes found in encephalopathy can be confused with those induced by medications, sleepiness, or congenital injuries, a normal EEG virtually rules out a toxic-metabolic encephalopathy.

Dementia

In early Alzheimer's disease, the alpha background characteristically slows from about 10- to 12-Hz to 8-Hz. Although the background slowing is considered normal in the elderly, virtually all patients with moderately advanced Alzheimer's disease have that or even greater slowing and eventually disorganization. Unfortunately, patients with multi-infarct dementia have similar abnormalities, preventing EEG differentiation between these two conditions (Chapters 7 and 11).

In contrast, the EEG is much more helpful in diagnosing subacute sclerosing panencephalitis (SSPE) and Creutzfeldt-Jakob disease (Chapter 7). In these conditions, where dementia is accompanied by myoclonic jerks, the EEG shows *periodic complexes* (Fig. 10-6).

The EEG is also useful in diagnosing the *locked-in syndrome*, in which people who have sustained pontine or medullary infarctions are alert but cannot speak or move their trunk or limbs (Chapters 2 and 11). Since the cerebrum and upper brainstem are normal, these otherwise devastated people have normal cerebral activity, including cognitive function, and therefore a normal EEG.

Patients with the locked-in syndrome must be differentiated from ones in a *persistent vegetative state*, a condition that typically follows cerebral anoxia from cardiac arrest, drug overdose, or carbon monoxide poisoning. These patients have marked cerebral cortex injury and thus profound dementia accompanied by an inability to speak or move. As would be expected from their extensive

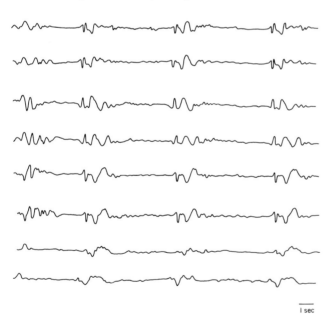

I sec

FIGURE 10–6. *Periodic complexes* are seen in all channels as four fairly regular bursts of electrical activity followed by minimal activity, so-called burst-supression. Periodic complexes are associated with myoclonic jerks, and together they are cardinal features of two dementing illnesses, subacute sclerosing panencephalitis (SSPE), which occurs in children, and Creutzfeldt-Jakob disease, which occurs in the elderly (Chapter 7).

cerebral damage and mental as well as physical incapacity, they have a markedly abnormal EEG.

The EEG is also useful in distinguishing pseudodementia from dementia (Chapter 7). Whereas in pseudodementia the EEG is normal or shows only slightly slowed background activity, in advanced dementia from almost any cause it shows theta and delta activity. Nevertheless, in the many patients who have mixed depression and mild dementia, the EEG is of little help.

Structural Lesions

The EEG does not reliably detect or exclude structural lesions, such as brain tumors, abscesses, cerebrovascular accidents (CVAs), or subdural hematomas. It can be normal in many of these conditions. When abnormal, it cannot distinguish among them. Computed tomography (CT) and especially magnetic resonance imaging (MRI) are more reliable and, despite their expense, are more cost-effective.

Psychiatric Disturbances

Although useful for diagnosing toxic-metabolic encephalopathy, some of the dementias, and the locked-in syndrome, the EEG is inadequate for diagnosing other illnesses that a psychiatrist routinely encounters. Approximately 15 percent of "normal" people have nonspecific EEG changes, such as an occasional spike or slow wave. There is no consensus on the frequency of various EEG abnormalities in different psychiatric illnesses. Further, adults and children with either mental retardation or minimal brain dysfunction have mild, non-specific abnormalities similar to those attributable to age or state of alertness.

In addition, psychotropic medications can induce prominent EEG alterations that can persist for up to 2 months after their withdrawal. Phenothiazines, butyrophenones, tricyclic antidepressants, and lithium may cause background slowing, theta and delta activity, and occasional nonfocal sharp waves. Pheno-thiazines tend to produce these abnormalities in the frontal and temporal lobes. Diazepam (Valium), barbiturates, and some other minor tranquilizer-sedatives typically induce beta activity.

Moreover, these medications do more than merely cause EEG artifacts. Many increase patients' tendency to have seizures (see below). When those with anticonvulsant properties, such as diazepam and barbiturates, are withdrawn abruptly, seizures and sleep disorders are provoked.

Changes in the EEG also follow electroconvulsive therapy (ECT). During and immediately after ECT, EEG changes resemble those of a generalized tonic-clonic seizure and its aftermath. With increasing numbers of treatments, ECT induces more persistent slow-wave activity, lasting up to 3 months over the frontal lobes or the entire cerebrum. ECT-induced slowing of the EEG is generally associated with memory impairment, but also with a more effective treatment of endogenous depression. When ECT is unilateral, EEG slowing is less pronounced and is usually seen much more over the treated side.

VARIETIES OF SEIZURES

Most seizures and varieties of epilepsy are classified either as *partial*, with either elementary (simple) or complex symptoms, or as *generalized*, usually *absences* or *tonic-clonic* (Table 10-2). Partial seizures originate from paroxysmal electrical discharges in a "focus," a discrete region of the cerebral cortex usually injured by a structural lesion. In general, partial seizures with motor symptoms have their focus in the contralateral frontal lobe; those with sensory symptoms, in the parietal lobe; those with visual symptoms, in the occipital or temporal lobe; and those with auditory symptoms, in the temporal lobe.

During and between partial seizures, the EEG typically shows abnormalities in channels overlying the particular focus. Since neither the entire cortex nor deep structures are involved when seizures begin, or often throughout their entire course, consciousness is preserved.

Although partial seizures usually last between several seconds and several minutes, occasionally they continue for hours or days while the discharge remains confined to its original focus. In such cases, called *epilepsy partialis continua* or *focal status epilepticus*, symptoms persist and interfere with normal activity, but routine activity can also continue *despite* the seizure. More often, discharges become more extensive and, enlarging in a slow, brushfire-like manner, involve adjacent areas of the cortex and create additional symptoms. Discharges can also spread over the entire cortex or travel through the corpus callosum to the other cerebral hemisphere. If the entire cerebral cortex is engulfed, *secondary generalization*, patients lose consciousness, develop bilateral motor activity, and have generalized EEG abnormalities.

In contrast to partial seizures, discharges in generalized seizures arise from the thalamus or other subcortical structures and immediately spread upward to the entire cerebral cortex. Also, generalized seizures are usually caused by a genetic disorder or metabolic aberration. Most important, they are characterized by unconsciousness and generalized EEG abnormalities, although not necessarily by gross motor activity. Like partial seizures, generalized seizures can persist, in which cases they are a life-threatening condition called *generalized status epilepticus*.

Partial Seizures

Partial Elementary Seizures

Partial seizures are said to have *elementary* symptoms when their clinical manifestation is only a particular movement, a single sensation, or a simple phenomenon. However, an impaired consciousness, with or without psychologic abnormalities or coordinated motor activity, denotes *complex* symptoms.

Seizures with elementary *motor* symptoms, formerly called "focal motor seizures," usually consist of rhythmic jerking (clonic movement) of a body part

---

TABLE 10–2.   A MODIFIED VERSION OF THE INTERNATIONAL CLASSIFICATION OF EPILEPSIES

Partial (or focal) epilepsies
  Partial seizures with elementary symptomatology
  Partial seizures with complex symptomatology
Generalized epilepsies
  Primary generalized epilepsies
    Absences (petit mal)
    Tonic-clonic (grand mal)

that may be as limited as one finger or as extensive as an entire side (Fig. 10-7). These seizures can develop into focal status epilepticus or undergo secondary generalization. Sometimes, in a "jacksonian march," a seizure discharge spreads along the motor cortex, and movements that began in a finger extend to the entire arm and, then, to the face. After any partial motor seizure, affected muscles may be weakened. A postictal monoparesis or (Todd's) hemiparesis may remain for up to 24 hours. Thus, the differential diagnosis of transient hemiparesis includes transient ischemic attacks (TIAs), hemiplegic migraines, psychologic aberrations, and Todd's hemiparesis.

Seizures with elementary *sensory* symptoms usually consist of tingling or burning paresthesias in regions of the body that have extensive cortical representation, such as the face. Sometimes a sensory loss, a "negative symptom," might be the seizure's only manifestation. Partial elementary seizures with "special sensory" symptoms, consisting of specific but simple auditory, visual, or olfactory sensations, can also occur. Most important, sensory seizures can create vivid and realistic sensations best described as "hallucinations"; however, they are almost always recognized by patients as being the result of cerebral dysfunction, rather than real events.

Auditory symptoms are usually repetitive noises, musical notes, or single words that have no meaning. Visual symptoms usually are "seen" as bright lines, spots, or splotches of color that move slowly across the visual field or, like a view through a kaleidoscope, as stars rotating around the center of vision. Elaborate visual phenomena alone or combined with auditory or emotional symptoms, in contrast, are "complex" symptoms that must be differentiated from these and other visual hallucinations (Table 9-3 and Chapter 12). Olfactory

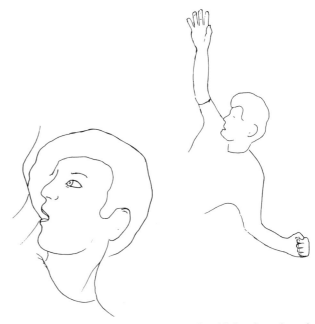

FIGURE 10–7. A patient having a partial seizure with motor symptoms has his head, neck, and eyes deviated toward the right, his right arm extended, and his left flexed. This "adversive posture" suggests that a seizure originated in the left frontal lobe, i.e., in the cerebrum contralateral to the body's direction.

symptoms usually consist of vaguely recognizable smells, such as the most frequent one, burning rubber. Since olfactory hallucinations usually result from discharges in the anterior inferior tip of the temporal lobe, the *uncus*, partial seizures with olfactory symptoms are often called *uncinate seizures* or *fits.* Typically, as discharges spread from the incus to involve larger areas of the temporal lobe, partial complex seizures ensue.

EEG, ETIOLOGY, AND TREATMENT. During partial elementary seizures, EEGs may show spikes, slow waves, or spike-wave complexes overlying the seizure focus. For example, during a seizure with motor symptoms, EEG abnormalities may be prominent in channels over the frontal lobe (Fig. 10-8). During the interictal period, the EEG may continue to reveal occasional spikes in the same channels.

Partial seizures usually begin in late childhood or adolescence but can develop at any age. They can be caused by various cerebral lesions, but depending upon the patient's health and age at the onset of the seizure, particular lesions may be suspected. When young children develop partial seizures, common causes are congenital cerebral injuries, neonatal meningitis, and neurocutaneous disorders, such as tuberous sclerosis (Chapter 13). Thus, children with epilepsy often have mental retardation and "cerebral palsy."

Another cause of partial seizures in childhood is rolandic (centrotemporal) epilepsy, in which seizures consist of facial movements and speech arrest. Unlike most other forms of partial epilepsy, centrotemporal epilepsy is not associated with an underlying structural lesion, but is inherited (in an autosomal dominant pattern) and remits by puberty.

In young adults, common causes of partial elementary seizures are head trauma, arteriovenous malformations (AVMs), and previously asymptomatic congenital injuries. The posttraumatic seizures are not associated with trivial head injuries, but with those that have caused loss of consciousness for more

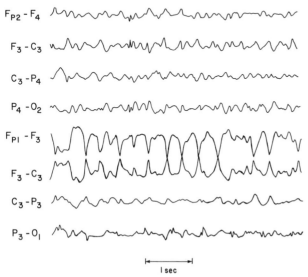

FIGURE 10–8. This EEG obtained during a partial seizure with motor symptoms contains a paroxysm of 4-Hz sharp wave activity with phase reversals referable to the F_3 electrode. Since this electrode overlies the left frontal region, the seizure probably consists of right face or arm motor activity and, in 50 percent of cases, a deviation of the head and eyes to the right.

than 30 minutes, a skull fracture that is depressed (not just linear), or a penetrating wound.

In addition, young adults with serious psychiatric disturbances, particularly autism, are prone to have seizures. In people 40 to 60 years old, primary or metastatic brain tumors are a common cause. Older people are more likely to develop seizures from CVAs than from tumors.

In previous decades, epilepsy was typically treated with combinations of anticonvulsants, but now the preference is to treat with a single anticonvulsant, i.e., *monotherapy*. This approach minimizes side effects, noncompliance, and, in many cases, cost. Standard anticonvulsants for partial seizures are carbamazepine (Tegretol) and phenytoin (Dilantin). These anticonvulsants have replaced phenobarbital and a closely related anticonvulsant, primidone (Mysoline), which both tend to cause sedation and cognitive impairments. Also, barbiturates, particularly when used in children, can cause a "paradoxical reaction" consisting of excitement and hyperactivity, rather than sedation. When seizures tend to occur premenstrually, acetazolamide (Diamox) is useful.

Anticonvulsants may occasionally cause cerebellar atrophy; allergic skin reactions, including the Stevens-Johnson syndrome; hepatitis; or hematologic abnormalities. Much more important, any anticonvulsant, even at therapeutic blood concentration, can induce cognitive impairments and altered affect. Iatrogenic mental impairments can be quite debilitating, and many neurologists choose to permit one or two seizures every several months in certain patients, rather than attempt to suppress all seizures. Inhibition of all seizures is those patients is considered unrealistic and would require such large doses of anticonvulsants that they would become intoxicated. Some patients with mental impairments and frequent seizures actually have had improvement in both problems with reduction in the dose of anticonvulsants or with a switch to monotherapy. The first step in treatment of an epilepsy patient with mental impairments is obviously to minimize the anticonvulsants. Indeed, some patients are unnecessarily maintained on anticonvulsants.

The adverse effects of anticonvulsants are especially important now that carbamazepine and valproate (Depakote) are used to treat mania; excitement resulting from major affective, schizoaffective, or schizophreniform psychosis; and behavioral dyscontrol (Gardner, Placidi). Carbamazepine, the most fully studied anticonvulsant in the treatment of psychiatric conditions, causes less impairment of cognitive function or mood than phenytoin, valproate, phenobarbital, or primidione (Abramowicz, Pedersen, Trimble). In addition, carbamazepine has an antidepressant effect that probably results from its structural similarity to the tricyclic antidepressants (Post). However, some of the success of carbamazepine and valproate may be attributable to the sedation that they induce, and the enthusiasm that they evoke recalls a similar but brief acceptance of phenytoin in treatment of manic-depressive illness and other psychiatric conditions (Turner).

Partial Complex Seizures

Partial complex seizures begin between late childhood and the early thirties and are the single most frequent seizure variety, affecting about 65 percent of epilepsy patients. Many old studies of psychiatric disorders are misleading because they did not acknowledge the preponderance of patients who had partial complex seizures, and they also relied upon patients' descriptions of nonspecific sensations and without EEG correlation. Current studies, which use telemetry, have defined ictal and postictal seizure manifestations and separated them from nonseizure disturbances. Nevertheless, several issues about partial complex seizures remain unsettled. A major one is the genuineness of the broad range of purported ictal symptoms, including violence. Another is the relationship between partial complex epilepsy and interictal mental abnormalities, such as personality disorders, psychosis, and cognitive impairment.

Before describing partial complex seizures, a preliminary note on nomenclature must be inserted. In the past, less cumbersome but less accurate titles, *psychomotor seizures* and *temporal lobe seizures* or *epilepsy* (*TLE*), have been used. The term "psychomotor seizures" is properly applied only to the rare variety of partial complex seizures with exclusively behavioral abnormalities. Likewise, TLE is inappropriate because the seizures originate in the frontal and other lobes rather than in the temporal lobe in about 10 percent of cases, leaving this term at risk of contradicting the location of the focus of the seizure. TLE is also inconsistent with the current classification of seizures based on symptoms, rather than anatomic origin.

As for symptoms of partial complex seizures, about 10 percent of patients have a premonitory sensation, an *aura*, which is not only a warning: it is actually the first part of the seizure. During most of the seizure, patients usually have only a blank stare and are inattentive and uncommunicative. They always (by definition) have impaired consciousness. In most cases, they have memory impairment or total loss, *amnesia*, presumably because the limbic system in the temporal lobe is beset with seizure discharges. Since the amnesia is so striking, it may appear to be a patient's only symptom. (Therefore, partial complex seizures must be strongly considered among the neurologic causes of the acute amnestic syndrome [Chapter 7].)

Usually the only physical sign of partial complex seizures is *automatisms*, which are simple, repetitive, and purposeless face or hand movements, such as swallowing, kissing, and lip smacking, or fumbling, scratching, and rubbing the abdomen (Fig. 10-9). Automatisms are present in more than 80 percent of complex seizures and occur more frequently than psychologic aberrations.

Patients may sometimes assume adversive postures (Fig. 10-7), or perform simple activities, such as standing, walking, pacing, or even driving. It is often unclear, however, whether these usually rote activities are manifestations of a seizure or are naturally occurring actions that have persisted despite the seizure. Likewise, in about 25 percent of cases, patients utter brief phrases or mutter unintelligibly. Many times the actions and words are cued by the environment.

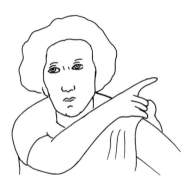

FIGURE 10–9. During partial complex seizures, patients are typically dazed. They perform rudimentary, purposeless actions, such as pulling on clothing. Repetitive, simple body movements, *automatisms*, such as lip smacking, are present in 80 percent of cases.

For example, a child with a partial complex seizure may clutch and continually stroke a nearby stuffed animal while repeating some endearing word. What would distinguish this activity from normal would be the child's impaired consciousness, apparent self-absorption, and subsequent failure to recall the event.

Symptoms might occasionally be complex visual or auditory hallucinations accompanied by an appropriate emotion. Special sensory phenomena that are more elaborate than in partial elementary seizures, however, are notorious but rarely occurring.

Although a wide variety of symptoms could be considered manifestations of seizures, certain ones cannot be accepted in isolation. In particular, the various "experiential phenomena," such as *déjà vu*, *jamais vu*, dream-like states, mind-body dissociations, and floating feelings, are rarely associated with clinical or EEG evidence of seizures. These experiential phenomena are too nonspecific and have been so romanticized that they have virtually no diagnostic value when described by a well-read or flighty patient.

Another frequent disturbance that has a dubious association with partial complex seizures is the *rising epigastric sensation*. This is a perception of a swelling in the abdomen that, as if progressing upward within the body, turns into tightness in the throat and then a feeling of suffocation. Although this symptom could be an aura, it has a striking similarity to a common psychogenic disturbance, *globus hystericus*, in which people also feel tightening of the throat and inability to breathe.

Following a partial complex seizure, which usually has a duration of 2 to 3 minutes, patients typically have confusion, clouding of their sensorium, and a tendency to sleep. If the seizure involved the brain's language centers, patients may have postictal aphasia. Also, for 15 to 30 minutes after the seizure, at least 40 percent of patients have a markedly elevated serum prolactin concentration.

Whatever their ictal manifestions, most partial complex seizures sooner or later undergo secondary generalization. Thus, a guideline for differentiating them from a recurring psychogenic event is that at least every 1 to 2 years partial complex seizures explode into generalized seizures.

Another important but a decidedly uncommon complication of partial complex seizures is *partial complex status epilepticus*. Despite its prevalence in popular literature, only about two dozen cases have been described in neurologic journals, and many were not documented with telemetry. When this condition does occur, patients have 1½ to 24 hours of confusion that is sometimes accompanied by aphasia, automatisms, and other purposeless motor activity (Ballenger). Confusion is so pronounced that patients are incapable of clear thought or complicated activity, much less the homicidal rampages portrayed in novels. However, the attack may be disruptive enough to merit its description, *ictal psychosis*.

ICTAL SEX AND VIOLENCE.   In many people, seizure-symptoms that occur during sexual activity are simply the result of anxiety or hyperventilation. Also, although epileptic patients commonly fumble with buttons or tug at their clothing, and thus may seem to partially undress, true exhibitionism is extraordinarily rare.

Nevertheless, rudimentary sexual activities, such as masturbation, scratching of the perineum, and pelvic thrusting, do occur. For example, in one study, 4 of 61 patients with refractory partial complex seizures had such activity, but it was not accompanied by more complex sexual behavior (Spencer). Only several times has sexual intercourse or orgasm as a seizure symptom been reported in the neurologic literature.

The extent of *ictal violence*, violence as a manifestation of seizures, has been a major controversy. However, by excluding experiential phenomena as being equivalent to a partial complex seizure and relying on telemetry, several reliable observations have been made (Delgado-Escueta, Treiman). Ictal violence occurs in less than 0.1 percent of seizures. In most cases of apparent violence, patients are only combating restraints that are placed during or after the seizure, i.e., "resistive violence." When overt violence occurs, it is not accompanied by a major affective state, such as rage, and it is fragmented, unsustained, and neither directed nor destructive, i.e., ictal violence is not "aggressive." It usually consists only of random shoving, pushing, or kicking, or of verbal abuse, such as screaming. It does not consist of sequential activities or interactions with people or mechanical devices, such as cars or guns. Like other seizures, those with violent manifestations are accompanied by impaired consciousness and usually automatisms, and they are not provoked by social factors, such as threats.

Although almost all neurologists do not accept episodic violence as the sole manifestation of partial complex seizures, a minority have attributed aggressive violence to seizures (Pincus). Likewise, possibly under medical or social pressures, the legal system has occasionally accepted such an explanation. For example, in 15 cases described between 1889 and 1981, seizures have been used in appeal as a defense for murder, homicide, manslaughter, or disorderly conduct.

INTERICTAL MENTAL ABNORMALITIES.

PERSONALITY CHANGES.   The frequently quoted, classic Bear-Fedio studies found that patients with so-called temporal lobe epilepsy had distinctive personality trait abnormalities (Bear). They described patients as being hyposexual, humorless, circumstantial, and overly concerned with general philosophic questions, such as the order of the universe. In addition, those patients characteristically had *hypergraphia*, a tendency to write excessively and compulsively.

Related older studies also suggested that different emotional abnormalities depended upon whether the seizure focus was in the right or left temporal lobe. Right-sided foci supposedly predisposed a patient to anger, sadness, and elation, and left-sided ones to ruminative and intellectual tendencies.

Recent studies, often based on telemetry and strict methodology, have refuted many of these contentions. They find no distinctive personality traits in patients with partial complex epilepsy (Guerrant, Mungas, Stevens). Epileptic patients were found to have the same incidence of behavioral problems as patients with other neurologic disorders, and with few exceptions, patients with partial complex seizures were not beset with more behavioral problems than patients with other varieties of seizures (Dodrill). Likewise, recent evidence indicates there is no difference in personality traits when foci are in different temporal lobes, or even other brain areas (Rodin), and there is no difference in personality traits among patients with different varieties of epilepsy. As a general rule, mental disturbances are associated with a history of onset of seizures in childhood, episodes of status epilepticus, and multiple seizure types; use of two or more anticonvulsants in treatment; and signs of brain damage on neurologic examination or CT or MRI scan.

The studies that purported to show a relationship between specific personality or behavioral characteristics and the side of the lesion usually made several implicit but tenuous assumptions: the patient's left hemisphere was always dominant; the brain, except for the seizure focus, was normal; there was only a single seizure focus; and there were no reciprocal connections between temporal lobes. In retrospect, those numerous studies have remained descriptive. Their data are mostly suggestive (Spiers) and not suitable for diagnostic inferences. They fail to answer practical questions, such as, "Are left-handed, humorless people with hypergraphia statistically likely to have partial complex seizures and, if so, what should be done about it?"

"PSYCHOSIS." In another group of old but frequently cited studies, 10 percent of temporal lobe epilepsy patients were found to have "schizophrenic-like" or "schizophreniform" psychosis; conversely, psychotic epilepsy patients were described as having temporal lobe epilepsy more frequently than either generalized epilepsy or non-neurologic illness (Flor-Henry, Slater). This inter-ictal psychosis, likened to acute but less disruptive idiopathic schizophrenia, was characterized by hallucinations, thought disorders, and paranoid ideation. It usually responded to conventional, orally administered neuroleptics.

The psychosis began on the average at age 30 years and was most often present when epilepsy had begun between ages 5 and 10 years. Therefore, it became symptomatic more than 10 years after the onset of epilepsy. Male epilepsy patients who were left-handed and had a left-sided seizure focus seemed to be more susceptible. Although most studies have reported that the psychosis was more likely to occur when seizures were poorly controlled, some report that it was precipitated by vigorous anticonvulsant suppression of seizures ("forced normalization," see below).

These studies, as the previous ones, must be considered cautiously. Many patients who were diagnosed as having temporal lobe epilepsy had only experiential symptoms or occasional EEG temporal lobe spikes—criteria that by themselves would not now be diagnostic. Also, the high incidence of temporal lobe epilepsy among psychotic patients may be only an appropriate representation of the large proportion (65 percent) of all epilepsy patients who have partial complex seizures. In addition to the usual uncertainty about whether the left hemisphere of epileptic patients is actually dominant, recent studies have questioned the alleged preponderance of left-sided foci in these patients.

In treating this schizophreniform psychosis or more flagrant psychoses in epileptics, high doses of oral neuroleptics and parenterally administered neuroleptics should be used cautiously because they may exacerbate a seizure disorder or precipitate a seizure in someone who has never had one. The neuroleptic with the highest seizure risk is chlorpromazine, haloperidol has a moderate risk, and thioridazine and fluphenazine have the lowest risk (Cummings).

COGNITIVE DETERIORATION. In contrast to the controversy regarding many interictal mental abnormalities, there is general agreement that patients with all varieties of seizures, except for absences, are liable to have mental retardation or develop progressive intellectual (cognitive) deterioration. When epilepsy begins in early childhood, 10 to 25 percent of the children are found to have mental retardation. Thereafter, even without mental retardation, cognitive function decreases. One representative study found that about 50 percent of partial complex seizure patients and 25 percent of generalized tonic-clonic seizure patients developed inattentiveness, impaired memory, and slowed speech (Guerrant). Several factors may contribute cumulatively to progressive cognitive impairments. The most important ones are the frequency and severity of the seizures. In addition to the biochemical and physiologic disruption that the seizures induce, they cause head trauma, cerebral anoxia, and massive electrical discharges. Another factor, as discussed previously, is that anticonvulsants can lead to impairment of memory and concentration. Also, temporal sclerosis may interfere to a progressively greater extent with limbic system function.

CRIME.   Another established interictal trait of epilepsy patients is a high incidence of crime. For example, among incarcerated men, the incidence of epilepsy is at least four times as great as in the general population. However, taking the association of crime and epilepsy at face value is liable to be misleading. Crimes of adult epileptic prisoners are no more violent than those of nonepileptic ones (Whitman). Also, violence is no more prevalent among patients with partial complex seizures than among those with other seizures (Treiman). The consensus is that crime does not originate in epilepsy, but that seizures, head trauma, and other brain injuries lead to conditions, such as poor impulse control and lower socioeconomic status, that predispose persons to crime.

DEPRESSION.   Depression is more prevalent in epileptic patients than in comparably handicapped persons, and it is especially common in individuals who have developed epilepsy in middle age or later. The incidence of suicide is four to five times greater in epilepsy patients than in the general population. Male patients and all those who have partial complex seizures are at greatest risk. In one series, for example, 55 percent of outpatient epileptic patients reported depression, and inpatient epileptic patients were found to have depression with psychotic traits and paranoia (Mendez). This and other studies, however, fail to discern the relative contribution of brain damage, seizures independent of brain damage, and cognitive impairments. The adverse effects of anticonvulsants must be again stressed: in addition to reducing concentration and impairing cognitive function, they often dull the patient's mood and interfere with sleep. Also, when epilepsy patients commit suicide, they frequently take an overdose of anticonvulsants, especially phenobarbital.

Depression may contribute to the clinical problem of recurrent seizures that are inexplicably refractory to routine management. Noncompliance with anticonvulsant regimens or the coexistence of seizures and pseudoseizures may be responsible for that phenomenon. Valuable diagnostic tests in these cases are telemetry with videotape monitoring and frequent determinations of serum anticonvulsant levels.

Tricyclic and heterocyclic antidepressant therapy for epileptic patients must be given cautiously because therapeutic antidepressant doses and serum concentrations can still precipitate seizures. The antidepressants with the greatest risk are moprotiline (Ludiomil), amitriptyline (Elavil, Triavil, and others), and nortriptyline (Pamelor), and those with the least are desipramine (Norpramin), doxepin (Sinequan), alprazolam (Xanax), and monamine oxidase inhibitors (Cummings). Individual psychotherapy, group therapy, and self-help groups can help seizure patients with or without depression.

ACUTE CONFUSION.   An entirely different clinical problem is the acute onset of confusion in an epileptic patient. It is most likely to develop in patients with pre-existing cognitive and physical impairments. The cause is usually anticonvulsant intoxication that is inadvertently induced by changing the medication regimen; however, occasionally the anticonvulsant intoxication is deliberate or the patient has mixed alcohol and anticonvulsants. Other causes of confusion include prolonged seizures, e.g., partial complex or absence status epilepticus, or prolonged postictal confusion. Head trauma occurring during a seizure can be further complicated by intracranial bleeding. A rare and controversial cause is forced normalization, a condition in which epileptic patients reportedly develop psychosis suddenly after (and possibly because) anticonvulsants have controlled the patient's seizures and forced the EEG to be normal (Pakalnis). Overall, the psychiatrist must distinguish between acute confusion and both cognitive decline and the development of depression: acute confusion has several potential causes that are all neurologic and sometimes life-threatening.

EEG AND OTHER TESTS.   During a partial complex seizure, the EEG will typically show paroxysms of spikes, slow waves, or other abnormalities in channels overlying the temporal or frontotemporal region. Even though the seizure focus may be unilateral, EEG abnormalities are found bilaterally in almost all cases because of the presence of additional foci or interhemispheric projections from a single focus.

In the interictal period, the routine EEG reveals spikes or spike and slow-wave complexes over the temporal lobes in about 40 percent of cases. Accompanied by an appropriate history, such EEG abnormalities are specific enough to corroborate the diagnosis. Looking at the situation in reverse, about 90 percent of persons with anterior temporal spikes on the EEG will have had partial complex seizures. Nevertheless, the presence of spikes without an appropriate history should not by itself be considered diagnostic for seizures.

If nasopharyngeal leads, or specially placed scalp leads, and sleep recordings are used, EEG abnormalities will be found in as many as 80 percent of cases (Fig. 10-10). After that test, if cases remain a diagnostic problem, especially where episodic behavioral abnormalities are believed to result from seizures, telemetry must be used. In short, the EEG diagnosis of partial complex seizures should be approached with a routine EEG, which has a 40 percent yield; an EEG with nasopharyngeal leads during sleep, for an 80 percent yield; and then telemetry, with virtually a 100 percent yield.

Since partial elementary and partial complex seizures usually originate from structural lesions, CT or MRI scans are routinely performed (Chapter 20).

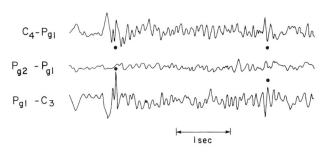

FIGURE 10–10. An interictal EEG with nasopharyngeal electrodes (Pg_1 and Pg_2) shows phase-reversed spikes that routine scalp electrodes may not detect.

They are also performed in most cases of tonic-clonic seizures because clinical and EEG data may not be able to distinguish between primary generalized seizures and partial seizures that have undergone secondary generalization. Cases in which scans might be avoided are those of drug- or alcohol-withdrawal seizures and absences (see below).

In partial seizures, a scan may reveal a structural lesion or temporal lobe atrophy, even when the neurologic examination is normal. It will also reveal most tumors, tuberous sclerosis nodules, large infarctions, and AVMs. However, it may not show medial temporal sclerosis, neonatal injuries, or cryptic temporal lobe vascular malformations.

Positron emission tomography (PET) has been used to study cerebral metabolism during seizures and interictal periods. In partial complex seizures, the affected temporal lobe typically is hypermetabolic during the ictus but hypometabolic interictally. The PET metabolic alterations are not, however, related to the clinical and EEG manifestations of these seizures.

ETIOLOGY.   Lesions that cause partial complex seizures include not only those that cause partial elementary seizures but also temporal lobe hamartomas, astrocytomas, and medial temporal sclerosis. This last condition, which is probably the most common cause of partial complex seizures, is thought to lead to sclerosis of Sommer's sector of the hippocampus and to temporal lobe atrophy. Except for about 10 percent of cases, as noted previously, the lesion is within the temporal lobe. Like other seizures, partial complex seizures may be precipitated by menses, intercurrent illness, and malabsorption of anticonvulsants, but most often the inciting factor cannot be identified.

TREATMENT.   Treatment of partial complex seizures usually begins with the same anticonvulsants used to treat partial elementary seizures. Although monotherapy is preferable, as in elementary seizures, a combination of two or three anticonvulsants is often required. When multiple anticonvulsants are used, it is critical to check the mental status and to follow blood anticonvulsant concentrations.

Patients are sometimes advised to undergo a temporal lobectomy for intractable partial complex seizures. Suitable candidates must have a unilateral, single temporal lobe seizure lesion that is identifiable on clinical, EEG, and radiographic testing. Wada tests (Chapter 8) are performed to avoid postoperative aphasia and the Klüver-Bucy syndrome (Chapters 12 and 16). In properly selected cases, temporal lobectomy reportedly results in a more than 75 percent reduction in seizure frequency. In addition, about 50 percent of patients have a postoperative reduction in rage attacks, aggressive behavior, and psychotic disturbances (Falconer).

Patients with multiple foci causing seizures that undergo secondary generalization may benefit from a *commissurotomy*, a sectioning of the corpus callosum (Chapter 8) that interrupts the spread of discharges between cerebral hemispheres. Despite the extent of the surgery, postoperative deficits are so subtle that special neuropsychologic tests are required to demonstrate its major consequence, the *split-brain syndrome* (Fig. 8-8).

Generalized Seizures

Generalized seizures are characterized by an immediate loss of consciousness accompanied by symmetric, synchronous, paroxysmal EEG discharges. These seizures are usually the result of either an autosomal dominant genetic disorder, a physiologic disturbance, or a metabolic aberration, including drug and alcohol withdrawal. Unlike partial seizures, generalized seizures lack an aura, lateralized motor or sensory disturbances, and focal EEG abnormalities. Also, they practically never result from brain tumors, cerebral infarctions, or other cerebral cortex injuries. Most generalized seizures are of either the absence (*petit mal*) or tonic-clonic (*grand mal*) variety.

Absences

Absence seizures usually begin between ages 4 and 10 years and, unlike other major seizure varieties, usually disappear in early adulthood. However, in about 40 percent of patients, tonic-clonic seizures replace the absences.

Absences, which can occur many times daily, are l-second to 10-second lapses in attention accompanied in almost all cases by automatisms, subtle clonic limb movements, and blinking (Fig. 10-11). Notably, the blinking occurs rhythmically at 3-Hz, which is the frequency of the associated EEG abnormality. Although children do not have retrograde amnesia and they maintain muscle tone and bladder control, their mental and physical activity is interrupted. After the ictus, as though it had never occurred, there is no confusion, agitation, or sleepiness.

Children with unrecognized absences may be misdiagnosed as being inattentive or mentally retarded. More important, they may be misdiagnosed as having partial complex seizures, even though the two conditions can be differentiated (Table 10-3). The distinction is especially important when, on rare occasions, *absence status epilepticus* or "nonconvulsive generalized status epilepticus" leads to a several-hour episode of apathy, psychomotor retardation, and confusion. The attack can be diagnosed only with an EEG, and it can usually be terminated by intravenous administration of diazepam (Valium). This condition usually develops only in children and young adults with a history of absences or other seizures who have suddenly stopped taking their anticonvulsants. As discussed previously, it is a cause of acute confusion in an epileptic patient.

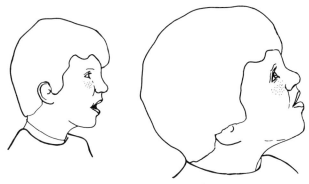

FIGURE 10–11. During a typical absence, this 8-year-old boy has brief, 1- to 3-second staring spells during which he becomes glassy-eyed and mute. Typically he rolls his eyes upward and blinks at 3-Hz. Although he loses consciousness, he maintains bodily tone and does not become incontinent. Absence seizures and the accompanying EEG abnormality (Fig. 10-12) may be demonstrated by having the child count numbers slowly while hyperventilating. Seizures occur when the counting slows or pauses. At the end of the seizure, the child will resume counting at the appropriate number, which indicates that there is no retrograde amnesia.

TABLE 10–3.   COMPARISON OF PARTIAL COMPLEX AND ABSENCE SEIZURES

Feature	Partial Complex	Absence
Aura	Often	Never
Consciousness	Impaired	Lost at onset
Movements	Usually simple, repetitive but may involve some activity	Blinking, and facial and finger automatisms
Postictal behavior	Amnesia, confusion, and tendency to sleep	No abnormality, but amnesia for ictus
Frequency without treatment	1 to 2 per week	Several daily
Duration	2 to 3 minutes	1 to 10 seconds
EEG	Spikes and polyspike and waves, usually over both temporal regions	Generalized 3-Hz spike-and-wave complexes
Anticonvulsants	Carbamazepine, phenytoin	Ethosuximide, valproic acid, clonazepam

EEG, ETIOLOGY, AND TREATMENT.   During an absence, the EEG shows synchronous 3-Hz spike and slow-wave complexes in all channels (Fig. 10-12). Even in the interictal period, occasional asymptomatic bursts of 3-Hz spike and slow-wave complexes lasting 1 to 1.5 seconds may be observed. In patients with absences, either hyperventilation or photic stimulation can precipitate the characteristic clinical and EEG abnormalities. Just as the EEG abnormality is generalized, PET scans performed during absences show increased metabolism in the thalamus and entire cerebral cortex.

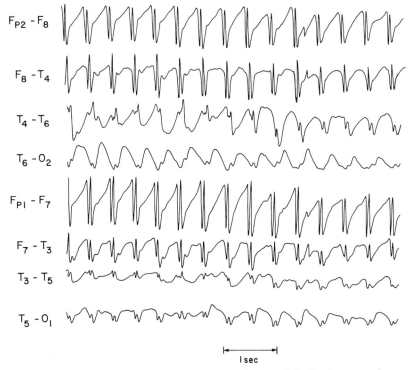

FIGURE 10–12.   During an absence, the EEG characteristically shows regular, symmetric, and synchronous 3-Hz spike-and-wave complexes. The discharge arises from and returns to a normal EEG background.

A patient's relatives also often have absences or 3-Hz spike and slow-wave complexes that can be precipitated by hyperventilation. This finding supports the hypothesis that absences are inherited in an autosomal dominant pattern. In contrast to tonic-clonic seizures, absences are not associated with drug withdrawal, metabolic aberrations, or structural lesions. Therefore, CT and MRI scans are usually not performed.

Absences are treated with ethosuximide (Zarontin), valproic acid, or occasionally clonazepam (Klonopin). Most children readily respond to one or another of these anticonvulsants. After adolescence, anticonvulsants generally can be withdrawn without precipitating recurrence of absences.

Tonic-Clonic Seizures

Tonic-clonic seizures, unlike absences, begin at any age after infancy, persist into adult life, and cause massive motor activity and profound postictal residua. Although patients may have a prodrome of malaise or mood change, tonic-clonic seizures are usually unheralded, explosive events. In the initial tonic phase, patients lose consciousness, roll their eyes upward, and extend their neck, trunk, and limbs as if to form an arch. Subsequently, they undergo a dramatic clonic phase in which their limbs, neck, and trunk are wracked by violent jerks (Fig. 10-13).

A potential diagnostic problem is that, during this terrible episode of tonic-

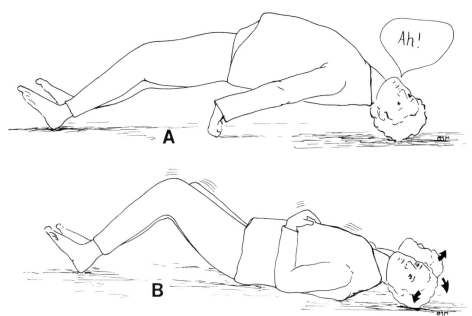

FIGURE 10–13. *A*, This patient in the tonic phase of a tonic-clonic seizure arches his torso and extends his arms and legs. He assumes this position because of the relatively greater strength of the extensor muscles over the flexor muscles. Simultaneous diaphragm, chest wall, and laryngeal muscle contractions force air through a tightened larynx and cause the shrill, epileptic cry. During this phase, patients often bite their tongue and involuntarily force urine out of their bladder. *B*, In the clonic phase, the patient's head, neck, and legs have symmetric and forceful contractions for about 10 to 20 seconds. Saliva, which becomes aerated and often blood-tinged from tongue lacerations, appears as a froth at the mouth. The pupils dilate and the patient sweats profusely. Finally, muscular contractions become progressively less frequent and weaker. The seizure usually ends with a sigh, followed by stertorous breathing. In the immediate postictal period, patients are unresponsive. Before regaining consciousness, they may pass through a state of confusion and agitation, loosely called "postictal psychosis."

clonic activity, the seizure appears similar to a partial seizure that has undergone secondary generalization. Often only a detailed history, a trained observer, or an EEG can resolve the problem.

In the postictal period, which has great diagnostic importance, patients are usually confused, disoriented, and amnesic, both for the ictus and, in a retrograde pattern, the events preceding it. They may be irrational, agitated, and combative. Postictal behavioral disturbances, which can last for several hours, can be so striking as to be misdiagnosed as a functional "postictal psychosis." Such postictal disturbances must also be distinguished from partial complex status epilepticus, anticonvulsant intoxication, and traumatic brain injury.

During the tonic phase, if the superimposed muscle artifact can be eliminated by administering muscle relaxants, the EEG shows repetitive, increasingly greater spikes occurring at about 10-Hz in all channels. In the clonic phase, the spikes, which become less frequent but greater in amplitude, are interrupted by slow waves (Fig. 10-14).

Afterward, the EEG shows postictal depression. The postictal EEG is often the only one available, but it can confirm the diagnosis. Similarly, the EEG is also slow after ECT. Following either a tonic-clonic seizure or ECT-induced seizure, the serum prolactin level rises for 15 to 30 minutes in more than 80 percent of cases. Following a pseudoseizure, in contrast, the EEG is relatively normal, and the prolactin level remains at baseline.

Interictally, 20 to 30 percent of patients with tonic-clonic seizures have asymptomatic, brief bursts of spikes, polyspikes, or slow waves. Seizures and accompanying EEG abnormalities may be precipitated by photic stimulation or hyperventilation.

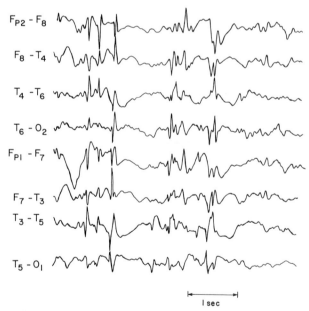

$F_{P2} - F_8$

$F_8 - T_4$

$T_4 - T_6$

$T_6 - O_2$

$F_{PI} - F_7$

$F_7 - T_3$

$T_3 - T_5$

$T_5 - O_1$

I sec

FIGURE 10–14. During a tonic-clonic seizure, the EEG would ideally show paroxysms of spikes, polyspikes, and occasional slow waves in all channels; however, unless a muscle relaxant is administered, muscle artifact obscures this pattern. The interictal background EEG activity usually contains multiple bursts of generalized spikes. In contrast to occasional temporal lobe spikes, this is a pattern that confirms a diagnosis of epilepsy.

ETIOLOGY. Many tonic-clonic seizures are the result of an autosomal dominant trait expressed between the ages of 5 and 30 years. In many of these cases, patients have a history of childhood absences.

Sleep deprivation is one of the most common physiologic disturbances that can precipitate these seizures. In particular, medical house officers who have worked all night are susceptible to tonic-clonic seizures early the following morning. Also, stage I and stage II NREM sleep precipitate tonic-clonic seizures in epileptic patients (Chapter 17). Many epileptic patients have these seizures predominantly or exclusively while asleep, and some patients have seizures almost only on awakening. Occasionally, seizures are precipitated exclusively by stroboscopic light (photoconvulsive epilepsy).

Alcohol in itself does not precipitate seizures. However, binge drinkers often develop hypoglycemia or sleep deprivation that, in turn, triggers seizures. More important, abrupt withdrawal from chronic, excessive alcohol consumption produces "alcohol-withdrawal seizures," which usually occur the day after alcohol abstinence. Although the clinical and EEG manifestations of these seizures are similar to those in genetically determined seizures, the interictal EEG is normal.

Likewise, seizures can be precipitated by abrupt withdrawal from medicines with sedative effects, most notably diazepam (Valium), long- or especially short-acting barbiturates, and anticonvulsants. In contrast to alcohol-withdrawal seizures, drug-withdrawal seizures do not develop until several days after abstinence, and once they begin, they often evolve into status epilepticus.

A small but noteworthy group of children and some adults have absences or tonic-clonic seizures in response to particular sensory stimulation. In this condition, called *reflex epilepsy*, seizures are triggered exclusively by specific stimuli, such as flickering lights, television pictures that have lost their vertical stability, or video games; certain patterns of letters, words, or figures; or even certain sounds, such as musical passages.

TREATMENT. Anticonvulsants commonly used for tonic-clonic seizures are valproic acid, phenytoin, and carbamazepine. As in treatment of partial seizures, neurologists usually attempt to control these seizures with monotherapy. Anticonvulsants are usually given for at least 6 months, except in cases of a single seizure or ones for which a precipitating factor, such as sleep deprivation or alcohol withdrawal, can be identified and avoided.

Any coexisting psychiatric illness must be treated with medications, psychotherapy, or other methods. Improvement in psychiatric illness, especially depression, is often associated with better control of epilepsy. For epileptic patients requiring neuroleptics or antidepressants, the anticonvulsant dosage should be raised only if a seizure occurs. On the other hand, if a nonepileptic patient who is being treated with a neuroleptic or antidepressant develops a seizure, a cerebral lesion must be excluded before attributing the seizure to the medication.

DISORDERS THAT MIMIC SEIZURES

Pseudoseizures

Psychogenic episodes mimicking seizures, *pseudoseizures*, are more prevalent in women, children, and adolescents. Like other psychogenic deficits, pseudoseizures are associated with character disorders, affective illness, and other major psychopathology (Chapter 3). In some epileptic patients, pseudoseizures occur together with seizures and can be responsible for apparently intractable epilepsy. Therefore, although patients may appear to have only pseudoseizures, they should undergo an investigation for seizures, as well as a psychiatric evaluation.

Unlike tonic-clonic seizures, pseudoseizures begin slowly with gradually developing flailing, struggling, alternating limb movements (out-of-phase clonic movements), and similar side-to-side head movements that are often accompanied by sexually suggestive pelvic thrusting (Gates). As fatigue ensues, the movements decline in intensity and regularity, but their duration is often greater than 2 minutes, which is much longer than a tonic-clonic seizure. Also, the movements usually have no tonic phase, and there is usually no tongue-biting, other bodily injury, or incontinence. Despite the apparent generalized nature of the pseudoseizure, consciousness is preserved, and subsequent confusion and retrograde amnesia are absent.

If an EEG were obtained during a pseudoseizure and muscle artifact were eliminated, it would be normal. One performed afterward, which is more feasible, would not show postictal depression. In addition, the serum prolactin concentration, which is usually elevated after a generalized or partial complex seizure, would not rise.

Pseudoseizures with a tonic-clonic appearance are usually a burlesque, but ones mimicking partial seizures are often subtle. Patients who mimic partial elementary seizures usually have apparent memory lapses, episodes of inattention, visual aberrations, other subjective phenomena, or nonspecific sensations, such as dizziness or epigastric sensations. Although these symptoms could be manifestations of seizures, when they result from pseudoseizures, they are variable, last longer than the usual limit of several minutes, and are not accompanied by dulling of the sensorium. Also, pseudoseizures rarely appear to include automatisms or undergo progression to a generalized seizure. Nevertheless, since partial complex seizures may induce bizarre thoughts and behavior, the clinical distinction in most studies is no more reliable than 85 to 90 percent. In difficult cases, long-term (several day) continuous EEG cassette recording, video-monitoring, or other telemetry is usually required to make a reliable diagnosis.

Episodic Dyscontrol Syndrome

The episodic dyscontrol syndrome, which is roughly equivalent to recurrent "rage attacks," consists almost exclusively of violent outbursts, for which the patient typically later claims total amnesia, and dysphoria. In contrast to violent partial complex seizures, episodic dyscontrol outbursts are at least momentarily purposeful, aggressive, and accompanied by a highly charged affect. The violence, which may be preceded by dysphoria, is barbarically destructive and consists of screaming, punching, wrestling, and throwing glasses or bottles. Also unlike seizures, these attacks can be provoked by threats, various other external circumstances, and especially by alcohol consumption. When triggered by alcohol, they can be called *pathologic* or *alcohol idiosyncratic intoxication* (DSM-III-R 291.40).

Episodic dyscontrol attacks are commonplace in young men with diffuse but subtle cerebral damage, especially as a result of either congenital cerebral injury or head trauma. Thus, these attacks are apt to occur among teen boys and young men with minor neurologic impediments and borderline intelligence, who may also have seizures. The coexistence of episodic dyscontrol syndrome and seizures is undoubtedly responsible for some reports of aggression in epileptic patients. Suggested medical treatments for episodic dyscontrol syndrome, in addition to prohibiting alcoholic beverages, have included stimulants, beta blockers, and anticonvulsants, most recently carbamazepine. However, no particular treatment has been proved effective.

Cerebrovascular Disturbances

TIAs resemble partial seizures in that both may involve momentarily impaired consciousness and physical deficits (Chapter 11). In general, however, TIAs have a slower onset, rarely cause loss of consciousness, and tend to begin only when the patient is standing upright. Most closely resembling a partial complex seizure is *transient global amnesia (TGA)*, a variety of TIA in which patients suffer several hours of disorientation, memory impairment, and EEG abnormalities (Chapter 11). It is probably caused by vascular insufficiency of the temporal lobes and may be diagnosed, although with some difficulty, by close attention to clinical and EEG abnormalities. TGA is a well-established cause of the *amnestic syndrome* (DSM-III-R).

Patients with migraine headaches may have episodes of confusion and personality change followed by a tendency to sleep (Chapter 9). They also may have hemiparesis for several hours and abnormal EEGs. In fact, the incidence of seizures in migraine patients is greater than in the general population. Correct diagnosis, which is frequently difficult, relies on the patient's history and response to medications.

Sleep Disorders

Instead of having seizures, some patients with unresponsiveness are actually having sleep attacks associated with hallucinations or momentary loss of body tone, i.e., the *narcolepsy-cataplexy syndrome* (Chapter 17). Unlike seizures, this disturbance has no aura, motor activity, incontinence, or postictal symptoms. Moreover, an EEG during narcolepsy displays rapid eye movement (REM) activity.

Metabolic Aberrations

Of all the possible metabolic aberrations that may cause seizure-like symptoms, medications are probably most often responsible. Many medicines, including some eye drops, produce a wide variety of transient mental alterations. However, they practically never induce movements or stereotyped thoughts. The first diagnostic step, of course, should be to eliminate unnecessary medications for patients with episodic mental aberrations.

Hyperventilation, another common metabolic alteration, induces giddiness, confusion, and other psychologic symptoms that can be confused with seizures (Chapter 3). Severe hyperventilation can precipitate seizures, although this probably occurs only in epileptic individuals.

Hypoglycemia can induce symptoms of a panic attack, as well as of seizures. These complications result from injected insulin, excessive alcohol consumption, and prediabetic states. Similar symptoms also occur when people drink excessive amounts of coffee and skip meals. Although the severity and frequency of symptomatic hypoglycemia are probably overestimated, small frequent meals along with reduction of caffeine intake should remedy most cases.

REFERENCES

Abramowicz M (ed): Drugs for epilepsy. Med Letter *31*:1, 1989

Ballenger CE, King DW, Gallagher BB: Partial complex status epilepticus. Neurology *33*:1545, 1983

Bear DM, Fedio P: Quantitative analysis of interictal behavior in temporal lobe epilepsy. Arch Neurol *34*:454, 1977

Camfield PR, Gates R, Ronen G, et al: Comparison of cognitive ability, personality profile, and school success in epileptic children with pure right versus left temporal lobe EEG foci. Ann Neurol *15*:122, 1984

Cummings JL: Clinical Neuropsychiatry. Orlando, Grune & Stratton, 1985

Delgado-Escueta AV, Bacsal FE, Treiman DM: Complex partial seizures on closed-circuit television and EEG: A study of 691 attacks in 79 patients. Ann Neurol *11*:292, 1982

Delgado-Escueta AV, Mattson RH, King L, et al: The nature of aggression during epileptic seizures. N Engl J Med *305*:711, 1981

Dodrill CB, Batzel LW: Interictal behavioral features of patients with epilepsy. Epilepsia *27*(suppl 2):S64, 1986

Elliot FA: The episodic dyscontrol syndrome and aggression. Neurol Clin *2*:113, 1984

Falconer MA: Reversibility by temporal lobe resection of the behavioral abnormalities of temporal lobe epilepsy. N Engl J Med *289*:451, 1973

Finlayson RE, Lucas AR: Pseudoepileptic seizures in children and adolescents. Mayo Clin Proc *54*:83, 1979

Flor-Henry P: Psychosis and temporal lobe epilepsy. Epilepsia *10*:363, 1969

Gardner DL, Cowdry RW: Positive effects of carbamazepine on behavioral dyscontrol in borderline personality disorder. Am J Psychiatry *143*:519, 1986

Gates JR, Ramani V, Whalen S, et al: Ictal characteristics of pseudoseizures. Arch Neurol *42*:1183, 1985

Geoffroy G, Lassonde M, Delisle F, et al: Corpus callosotomy for control of intractable epilepsy in children. Neurology *33*:891, 1983

Glista GG, Frank HG, Tracy FW: Video games and seizures. Arch Neurol *40*:588, 1983

Guerrant J, Anderson WW, Fischer A, et al: Personality in Epilepsy. Springfield, IL, Charles C Thomas, 1962

Hawton K, Fagg J, Marsack P: Association between epilepsy and attempted suicide. J Neurol Neurosurg Psychiatry *43*:168, 1980

Jabbari B, Bryan GE, Marsh EE, et al: Incidence of seizures with tricyclic and tetracyclic antidepressants. Arch Neurol *42*:480, 1985

Krumholz A: Epilepsy and pregnancy. In Goldstein PJ (ed): Neurological Disorders of Pregnancy. Mount Kisco, NY, Futura Publishing Company, 1986, pp 65-88

Kerson TS, Kerson LA: Understanding Chronic Illness. New York, The Free Press, 1985

Lesser RP, Luders H, Wyllie E, et al: Mental deterioration in epilepsy. Epilepsia *27*(suppl 2):S105, 1986

Lewis DO, Pincus JH, Shanok SS, et al: Psychomotor epilepsy and violence in a group of incarcerated adolescent boys. Am J Psychiatry *139*:882, 1982

Matthews WS, Barabas G: Suicide and epilepsy. Psychosomatics *22*:515, 1981

McElroy SL, Pope HG: Use of Anticonvulsants in Psychiatry: Recent Advances. Clifton, NJ, Oxford Health Care, Inc., 1988

McElroy SL, Keck PE, Pope HG: Sodium valproate: Its use in primary psychiatric disorders. J Clin Psychopharmacol *7*:16, 1987

Mendez MF, Cummings JL, Benson DF: Depression in epilepsy: Significance and phenomenology. Arch Neurol *43*:766, 1986

Mungas D: Interictal behavior abnormality in temporal lobe epilepsy: A specific syndrome or nonspecific psychopathology? Arch Gen Psychiatry *39*:108, 1982

Pakalnis A, Drake, ME, Kuruvilla J, et al: Forced normalization: Acute psychosis after seizure control in seven patients. Arch Neurol *44*:289, 1987

Pedersen B, Dam M: Memory disturbances in epileptic patients. Acta Neurol Scand *74*(suppl 109):11, 1986

Pincus JH: Can violence be a manifestation of epilepsy? Neurology *30*:304, 1980

Placidi GF, Lenzi A, Lazzerni F, et al: The comparative efficacy and safety of carbamazepine versus lithium: A randomized, double-blind 3-year trial in 83 patients. J Clin Psychiatry *47*:490, 1986

Post RM, Uhde TW, Roy-Byrne PP, et al: Antidepressant effects of carbamazepine. Am J Psychiatry *143*:29, 1986

Pritchard PB, Wannamaker BB, Sagel J, et al: Serum prolactin and cortisol levels in evaluation of pseudoepileptic seizures. Ann Neurol *18*:87, 1985

Quesney LF: Clinical and EEG features of complex partial seizures of temporal lobe origin. Epilepsia *27*(suppl 2):S27, 1986

Robertson MM, Trimble MR, Townsend HR: Phenomenology of depression in epilepsy. Epilepsia *28*:364, 1987

Rodin E, Schmaltz S: The Bear-Fedio personality inventory and temporal lobe epilepsy. Neurology *34*:591, 1984

Sherwin I, Peron-Magnan P, Bancaud J, et al: Prevalence of psychosis in epilepsy as a function of the laterality of the epileptogenic lesion. Arch Neurol *39*:621, 1982

Simon RP: Alcohol and seizures. N Engl J Med *319*:715, 1988

Slater E, Beard AW: The schizophrenic-like psychosis of epilepsy. Br J Psychiatry *95*:109, 1963

Solomon GE, Kutt H, Plum F: Clinical Management of Seizures, 2nd ed. Philadelphia, W.B. Saunders, 1983

Spencer SS, Spencer DD, Williamson PD, et al: Sexual automatisms in complex partial seizures. Neurology *33*:527, 1983

Spencer SS, Spencer DD, Williamson PD, et al: Corpus callosotomy for epilepsy. Neurology *38*:19, 1988

Sperling MR, Engle J: Electroencephalographic recording from the temporal lobes: A comparison of ear, anterior temporal, and nasopharyngeal electrodes. Ann Neurol *17*:510, 1985

Spiers PA, Schomer DL, Blume HW, et al: Temporolimbic epilepsy and behavior. In Mesulam M (ed): Principles of Behavioral Neurology. Philadelphia, F. A. Davis, 1985

Staudemire A, Nelson A, Haupt JL: Interictal schizophrenia- like psychoses in temporal lobe epilepsy. Psychosomatics *24*:331, 1983

Stevens JR, Hermann BP: Temporal lobe epilepsy, psychopathology, and violence: The state of the evidence. Neurology *31*:1127, 1981

Stromgren LS, Juul-Jensen P: EEG in unilateral and bilateral electroconvulsive therapy. Acta Psychiatr Scand *51*:340, 1975

Treiman DM: Epilepsy and violence: Medical and legal issues. Epilepsia *27*(suppl 2):S77, 1986

Trimble MR: The psychoses of epilepsy and their treatment. Clin Neuropharmacol *8*:211, 1985

Turner WJ: The usefulness of diphenylhydantoin in treatment of non-epileptic emotional disorders. Int J Neuropsychiatry *3*:8, 1967

Vanderzant CW, Giordani B, Berent S, et al: Personality of patients with pseudoseizures. Neurology *36*:664, 1986

Whitman S, Coleman TE, Patmon C, et al: Epilepsy in prison: Elevated prevalence and no relationship to violence. Neurology *34*:775, 1984

Wyllie E, Luders H, MacMillan JP, et al: Serum prolactin levels after epileptic seizures. Neurology *34*:1601, 1984

QUESTIONS: CHAPTER 10

1–4. Match the EEG with the interpretation (see pages xxx–xxx).

1. Figure 10-EEG-A
2. Figure 10-EEG-B
3. Figure 10-EEG-C
4. Figure 10-EEG-D

a. Spike and polyspike and wave
b. 3-Hz spike and wave
c. Normal
d. Temporal spike focus

5–8. Match the EEG with the associated seizures.

5. Interictal temporal lobe spikes
6. Generalized 3-Hz spike and wave
7. Generalized spike and polyspike and wave
8. Occipital spike and wave

a. Tonic-clonic (grand mal)
b. Partial elementary
c. Partial complex
d. Absence (petit mal)

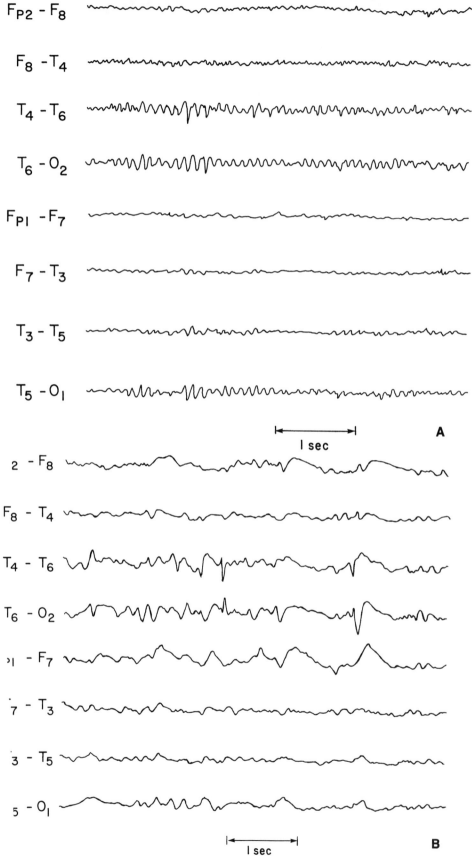

F_P2 - F_8

F_8 - T_4

T_4 - T_6

T_6 - O_2

F_PI - F_7

F_7 - T_3

T_3 - T_5

T_5 - O_1

|← 1 sec →|

A

2 - F_8

F_8 - T_4

T_4 - T_6

T_6 - O_2

_1 - F_7

_7 - T_3

_3 - T_5

_5 - O_1

|← 1 sec →|

B

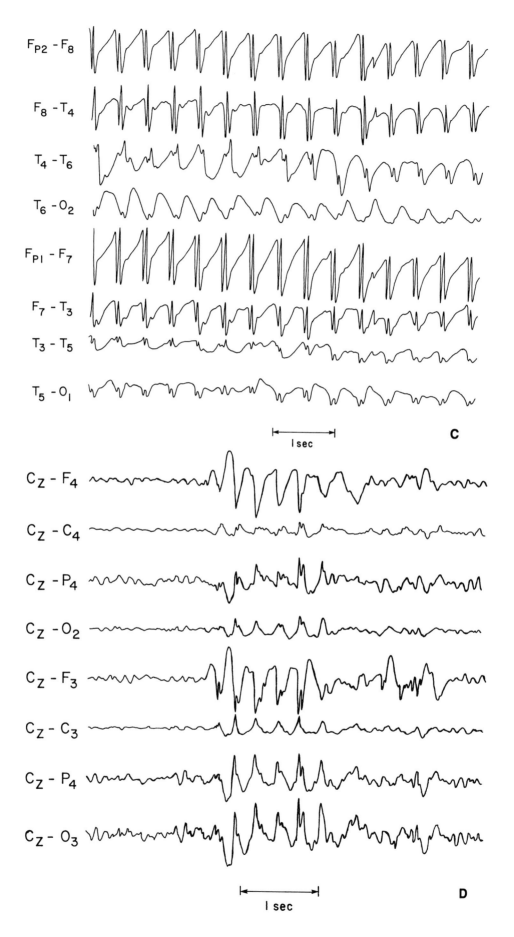

$F_{P2} - F_8$

$F_8 - T_4$

$T_4 - T_6$

$T_6 - O_2$

$F_{P1} - F_7$

$F_7 - T_3$

$T_3 - T_5$

$T_5 - O_1$

I sec

C

$C_Z - F_4$

$C_Z - C_4$

$C_Z - P_4$

$C_Z - O_2$

$C_Z - F_3$

$C_Z - C_3$

$C_Z - P_4$

$C_Z - O_3$

I sec

D

9–16. Match the EEG pattern with its most likely cause.

9. Delta activity, phase reversal
over left occiput

10. Bifrontal beta activity

11. Alpha activity

12. Triphasic waves

13. Rapid extraocular movement artifact

14. Periodic complexes

15. Generalized delta activity

16. Electrocerebral silence

a.   Normal relaxation
b.   Hepatic encephalopathy
c.   Use of sedatives or hypnotics
d.   Brain tumor
e.   Cerebral death
f.   REM sleep; dreaming
g.   Major tranquilizers
h.   Psychoses
i.   Creutzfeldt-Jakob disease

17. In which conditions will an EEG be useful in making a specific diagnosis?
    a. Cerebral tumor
    b. Hepatic encephalopathy
    c. Neurosis
    d. Herpes simplex encephalitis
    e. Cerebral abscess
    f. Creutzfeldt-Jakob disease
    g. Hysteric seizures
    h. Manic-depressive illness
    i. Cerebellar tumor
    j. SSPE
    k. Psychoses
    l. Status epilepticus

18. Match the rare but serious complication of anticonvulsant treatment with its definition.

18. Stevens-Johnson syndrome

19. Forced normalization

20. Paradoxical hyperactivity

    a. Conversion to a normal EEG and suppression of seizure activity that may lead to psychosis
    b. Frequently fatal allergic reaction that primarily involves the gastrointestinal mucosa
    c. Psychosis as an allergic reaction
    d. Excitement instead of sedation, especially with phenobarbital in children and brain-damaged adults

21–24. Identify the following statements as true or false.

21. Use of the EEG in the diagnosis of psychologic disturbance is complicated by drug-induced EEG changes.

22. Diazepam (Valium), meprobamate (Miltown), and barbiturates induce rapid (beta) EEG activity.

23. Tricyclic antidepressants and phenothiazines may induce nonfocal sharp wave EEG activity.

24. The major transquilizers, antidepressants, and lithium may cause slowing of EEG background activity.

25. Carbamazepine (Tegretol) is often used in the treatment of epilepsy patients who are depressed. Which of the following medications has the chemical structure that is the closest to carbamazepine?

a. Lithium
b. Phenytoin
c. Imipramine
d. Haloperidol
e. Phenelzine
f. Tranylcypromine

26–33. Match the visual disturbance with the probable cause.

26. A red blotch of color in the left homonymous field followed by clonic movements of the left arm and leg, then the entire body

27. Loss of central vision in both eyes followed by a throbbing, unilateral headache

28. Fortification scotomata

29. Visualization of the American flag, accompanied by hearing drum beats

30. Seeing and smelling garbage

31. A kaleidoscopic movement of bright lights in the right visual field

32. A "shade of gray" covering one eye for 3 minutes

33. Tremor, sweating, tachycardia, and seeing rodents

a. Amaurosis fugax
b. Partial complex seizure of temporal lobe origin
c. Partial elementary seizure of occipital lobe origin
d. Petit mal seizure
e. Hysteria
f. Tension headache
g. Classic migraine headache
h. Delirium tremens
i. Partial elementary seizures of occipital origin with secondary generalization

34–43. The patient's age when partial (elementary or complex) seizures begin often suggests the cause. Match the cause with the age when it is likely to induce such a seizure.

34. Head injury

35. Congenital cerebral malformation

36. Arteriovenous malformation

37. Glioblastoma

38. Metastatic brain tumor

39. Sinusitis-induced cerebral abscess

40. Cerebrovascular accident

41. Conversion reaction

42. Medial temporal sclerosis

43. Perinatal cerebral hypoxia

a. Childhood, e.g., 3 to 8 years
b. Adolescence, e.g., 13 to 21 years
c. Middle age, e.g., 45 to 65 years

44–46. A 60-year-old man, who has been previously healthy, is brought to the Emergency Room in a state of apparent confusion and excitement. Careful evaluation reveals that he has poor memory for recent and past events, but he can recall his own and his wife's name, and his judgement, language, and other cognitive processes are intact. There are no physical abnormalities. He gradually improves during 2 hours.

44. What is the name of this condition?
a. Delirium
b. Fugue state

    c. Acute amnestic syndrome
    d. Acute confusional state

45. Which one of the following is *not* a frequent cause?
    a. Partial complex seizures
    b. Wernicke-Korsakoff syndrome
    c. Psychogenic disturbances
    d. Medications
    e. Transient global amnesia
    f. Anticonvulsant intoxication

46. When a neurologic cause is responsible, which area of the brain is most often affected?
    a. Temporal lobe
    b. Entire cerebrum
    c. Thalamus
    d. Frontal lobe

47. Is it true, in general, that partial elementary, partial complex, and tonic-clonic seizures are all treated with the same anticonvulsants, but absences are treated with different ones?

48. Which of the following anticonvulsants are most often used for absences?
    a. Phenytoin (Dilantin)
    b. Carbamazepine (Tegretol)
    c. Phenobarbital
    d. Primidone (Mysoline)
    e. Valproic acid (Depakote)
    f. Ethosuximide (Zarontin)

49. A 30-year-old woman, who developed partial complex seizures with psychomotor symptomatology 3 years ago, has developed lethargy and confusion. Which causes of the current difficulties should be considered?
    a. Expansion of a temporal lobe tumor
    b. Development of a subdural hematoma from head trauma
    c. Partial complex status epilepticus
    d. Anticonvulsant intoxication
    e. Development of a systemic disorder, such as renal failure

50. Which of the following physical signs may indicate anticonvulsant intoxication?
    a. Hemiparesis
    b. Ataxia of gait
    c. Nystagmus
    d. Aphasia
    e. Dysarthria
    f. Lethargy or stupor
    g. Dysmetria on heel-shin testing
    h. Tremor on finger-nose
    i. Papilledema

51. In which part of the skull is the temporal lobe located?
    a. Sella
    b. Anterior fossa
    c. Posterior fossa
    d. Middle fossa

52. A rise in the serum prolactin level is detectable after generalized tonic-clonic and partial complex seizures. For what period of time is such a rise detectable?
    a. 24 hours
    b. 12 hours
    c. 2 hours
    d. less than 1 hour

53. Is it true that epileptic people are more likely than nonepileptic people to be convicted of a crime and sent to prison, but that epileptic criminals are no more likely than other criminals to have committed a violent crime?

54. With which of the following disorders is narcolepsy associated?
    a. Genereralized seizures
    b. Manic-depressive illness
    c. Cataplexy
    d. Fugue states

55. A patient's head and eyes deviate to the left and the left arm extends immediately before a generalized tonic-clonic seizure develops. Where did the seizure probably originate?
    a. Cerebellum
    b. Right cerebral hemisphere
    c. Diencephalon
    d. Left cerebral hemisphere

56. What is the frequency with which a child's eyelids blink during an absence?
    a. 8–12/sec
    b. 3/sec
    c. Highly variable
    d. None of the above

57. The EEG:
    a. May have abnormalities in 15 percent of clinically asymptomatic people.
    b. May be abnormal in psychologically disturbed people because of use of psychotropic medications.
    c. Usually has a background activity in the alpha (8–13-Hz) range.
    d. Will be specifically diagnostic in minimum brain dysfunction.
    e. Will be specifically diagnostic in Gilles de la Tourette's syndrome.

58. Partial complex seizures (e.g., psychomotor seizures), compared with absences (petit mal seizures), are:
    a. Longer in duration.
    b. More apt to begin in childhood.
    c. Likely to have an aura and postictal confusion.
    d. Accompanied by automatisms.
    e. Likely to disappear in young adult life.

ANSWERS

1. c.		**13.** f.	
2. d.		**14.** i.	
3. b.		**15.** g.	
4. a.		**16.** e.	
5. c.		**17.** b, d, f, g, j, l.	
6. d.		**18.** b.	
7. a.		**19.** a.	
8. b.		**20.** d.	
9. d.		**21.** True	
10. c.		**22.** True	
11. a.		**23.** True	
12. b.		**24.** True	

25. c.

26. i.

27. g.

28. g.

29. b.

30. b.

31. c.

32. a.

33. h.

34. a, b, c.

35. a.

36. a, b.

37. c.

38. c.

39. b.

40. c.

41. b.

42. a, b.

43. a.

44. c.

45. f.

46. a.

47. Yes

48. e, f.

49. All such causes must be considered; however, in the vast majority of such cases, the cause is anticonvulsant intoxication (d).

50. b, c, e, f, g, h.

51. d.

52. d.

53. Yes

54. c.

55. b.

56. b.

57. a, b, c.

58. a, c.

11

Cerebrovascular Diseases

Cerebrovascular disease is so common that physicians might consider it in the differential diagnosis of most neurologic illnesses in adults. Unfortunately, many physicians have an unjustified pessimism toward patients with cerebrovascular disease and see them as stereotypes, epitomized by the aphorism, "A stroke is a stroke is a stroke." Moreover, many physicians overlook the cognitive changes that accompany cerebrovascular disease. Many of these changes can be predicted by knowing the physical deficits and the course of the illness.

This chapter reviews the salient features of the diagnosis, prevention, and treatment of *transient ischemic attacks* (*TIAs*) and *cerebrovascular accidents* (*CVAs*), conditions that are responsible for well over 95 percent of all cases of cerebrovascular disease.* It stresses the cognitive, language, and affective changes that are frequent manifestations of TIAs or CVAs.

TRANSIENT ISCHEMIC ATTACKS (TIAs)

Transient ischemic attacks are brief interruptions in the blood supply to parts of the brain during which some neurologic function is temporarily lost. Full capacity is usually restored within 3 to 30 minutes, although occasionally not until 12 hours. Most TIAs probably result from platelet emboli that form on the surface of atherosclerotic plaques in the extracranial arteries and break off to travel (embolize) through the cerebral circulation. TIAs are important not only because they cause episodes of neurologic dysfunction but also because they indicate underlying atherosclerotic cerebrovascular disease. Indeed, without treatment, about 5 percent of individuals with TIAs will develop a CVA within 1 year.

Carotid Artery TIAs

The origin of most carotid artery TIAs is thought to be platelet emboli that form on ulcerated atherosclerotic plaques at the bifurcation of the common carotid artery (Fig. 11-1). These arterial plaques are not only a nidus for emboli but they lead also to progressive narrowing (stenosis) of the artery, which eventually can occlude it.

Symptoms of carotid artery TIAs are typically periods of (contralateral) hemiparesis, hemisensory loss, paresthesias, and hemianopsia. Of course, dominant hemisphere TIAs typically cause aphasia.

Since the carotid artery also supplies the ipsilateral eye through its first

---

* Patients with CVAs may receive assistance from the American Heart Association, 7320 Greenville Avenue, Dallas, Texas 75231, (214) 373-6300.

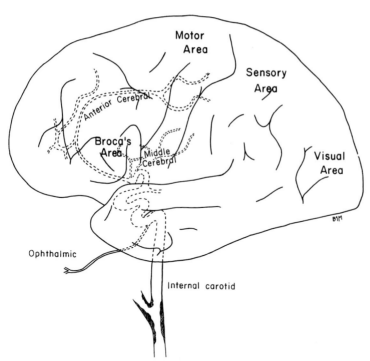

FIGURE 11–1. The common carotid artery bifurcation, which is in the neck, forms the external and internal carotid arteries. Within the skull the internal carotid artery gives rise to the ophthalmic and then branches into the anterior and middle cerebral arteries. Thus, each internal carotid artery perfuses the ipsilateral eye, most of the ipsilateral cerebral hemisphere, and, by collateral circulation, portions of the contralateral hemisphere. Atheromatous plaques at the common carotid artery bifurcation are the source of most platelet emboli and also cause carotid narrowing (stenosis).

The internal carotid arteries trifurcate at the base of the brain into an anterior, middle, and posterior segment. Each *middle cerebral artery* supplies the interior, lateral portion, and midsection of the hemisphere, which contain most of the motor cortex, sensory cortex, and, in the dominant hemisphere, the language arc (Fig. 8-1). Each *anterior cerebral artery* supplies the frontal lobe, including the medial surface of the motor cortex, which contains the motor neurons for the leg. Each *posterior communicating artery* joins with a terminal branch of the basilar artery to form the posterior cerebral artery, which supplies the occipital and most of the temporal lobes.

branch, the ophthalmic artery, TIAs may obscure vision in one eye for several minutes. Individuals with this variety of TIA, *amaurosis fugax*, typically describe a "blanket of gray" coming down slowly in front of one eye (Table 11-1).

Under certain circumstances, confusion and personality changes develop. Most often, transient aphasia, hemi-inattention, or other neuropsychologic problems result from unilateral cerebral ischemia. When a patient with Alzheimer's disease or multi-infarct dementia has a carotid artery TIA, ischemia of one cerebral hemisphere may convert a mild, compensated intellectual impairment into a marked confusional state. A similar situation develops when one carotid artery is markedly stenotic or occluded and the blood supply to both cerebral hemispheres is derived from the other. This single patent carotid artery supplies the contralateral hemisphere through the circle of Willis. In this case, emboli from the patent artery will lead to generalized cerebral ischemia and mental impairment.

Several non-neurologic findings can indicate carotid artery atherosclerosis and, by extension, cerebrovascular and coronary artery disease. A murmur, or

TABLE 11–1. CAROTID ARTERY TIAs

Symptoms
    Ipsilateral amaurosis fugax
    Contralateral hemiparesis, hemianopsia, and/or hemisensory loss
    Aphasia
Associated findings
    Carotid bruit
    Retinal artery emboli
Noninvasive tests
    Ultrasonography
    Digital intravenous arteriography (DIVA)
Invasive tests
    Arteriography
Therapy
    Medical: platelet inhibitors, e.g., aspirin
    Surgical: carotid endarterectomy

bruit, over the carotid artery bifurcation may suggest an arterial stenosis or at least roughening. Although the implication of a bruit in asymptomatic individuals is controversial, the consensus is that a carotid endarterectomy (see below) is not necessarily warranted. Another indication of carotid stenosis is a retinal artery embolus (Hollenhorst plaque), which can be seen by examination of the fundus. These emboli are comprised of atheromatous material from the ipsilateral carotid artery.

In the elderly, particularly those with diabetes or hypertension, carotid artery TIAs are probably the most common cause of several minutes of motor or sensory impairments, monocular visual loss, or confusion. Other causes of *transient motor or sensory loss,* which is an important clinical situation, include the following: impaired cerebral blood flow from cardiac arrhythmias; a sensory seizure; postictal (Todd's) hemiparesis (Chapter 10); migraine attacks (Chapter 9); metabolic derangements, such as hypoglycemia; and psychogenic disturbances (Chapter 3).

Laboratory Tests

Since TIAs are precursors of strokes and might be confused with other conditions, many neurologists recommend a series of tests to confirm that diagnosis and to search for the atherosclerotic plaques. A routine evaluation includes an electrocardiogram (ECG) and sometimes a 24-hour study of the cardiac rhythm (a Holter monitor). An EEG might be performed if there is a possibility that the patient is having seizures. A CT or MRI scan is almost always performed to exclude CVAs and cerebral mass lesions. On the other hand, lumbar punctures and skull x-ray films are not indicated. Several noninvasive techniques provide reasonable visualization of carotid artery stenosis. For example, ultrasound imaging (Doppler studies) and digital intravenous arteriography (DIVA) are accurate, carry little risk, and do not require hospitalization.

Therapy

Nonsurgical (medical) therapy is effective and preferred in most patients. Neurologists generally prescribe aspirin (one tablet daily) because it is the most readily available and safe platelet inhibitor. Some medicines, such as, sulfinpyrazone (Anturane) and dipyridamole (Persantine), which also interfere with platelet function, might be indicated in people who cannot tolerate the side effects of aspirin.

For carefully selected patients with carotid artery stenosis, *carotid endarterectomy* is indicated. In this procedure, the artery is briefly opened for the removal of an atheromatous plaque. Even in experienced hands, however, it entails at least a 2 percent risk of cerebrovascular accident, myocardial infarction, or death. The formerly popular *extracranial-intracranial arterial bypass* procedure, in which a surgeon anastomosed a scalp artery to a superficial branch of the middle cerebral artery through a small hole in the skull, has been shown to be ineffective relative to its risks.

Basilar Artery TIAs

The two vertebral arteries join to form the basilar artery. This group of vessels, which is usually called the *vertebrobasilar system* or simply the *basilar artery*, supplies the brainstem, cerebellum, and the inferomedial portion of the temporal lobes (Fig. 11-2).

The mechanism of basilar artery TIAs is probably similar to that of carotid artery TIAs except that atherosclerotic plaques are found at the origin of the vertebral arteries (in the chest) and at their junction (at the undersurface of the brain). Since these locations are inaccessible to surgeons, a basilar endarterectomy cannot be performed.

Symptoms and signs of basilar artery TIAs are distinctly different from those of carotid artery TIAs (Table 11-2). Instead of having lateralized physical or mental deficits, which are manifestations of ischemia of one cerebral hemisphere, patients with basilar artery TIAs have deficits that result from patchy ischemia of the brainstem cranial nerve nuclei and cerebellar tracts. Typical symptoms are tingling around the mouth (circumoral paresthesias), dysarthria,

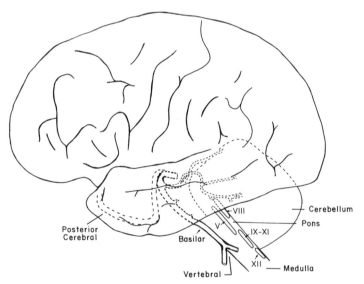

FIGURE 11-2. The two vertebral arteries join to form the basilar artery. This vertebrobasilar complex supplies the brainstem, cerebellum, and the inferomedial portions of the temporal lobes. Atheromatous plaques form at the junction of the vertebral arteries. (The Roman numerals refer to cranial nerves.)

TABLE 11–2. VERTEBROBASILAR ARTERY TIAs

Symptoms
  Vertigo, vomiting, tinnitus
  Circumoral paresthesias
  Dysarthria, dysphagia
  Transient global amnesia
  Drop attacks
Associated findings
  Nystagmus
  Ataxia
Noninvasive tests
  Digital intravenous arteriography (DIVA)
Therapy
  Medical: aspirin
  Surgical: none

nystagmus, ataxia, and vertigo. On rare occasions, when all blood flow through the basilar artery is momentarily interrupted and the entire brainstem becomes ischemic, a patient will have a *drop attack*, which is a brief loss of consciousness and body tone.

During a basilar artery TIA, patients are usually incapacitated by vertigo and nausea. Vertigo, an important symptom that should not be confused with other conditions, is the sensation of either revolving in space or feeling one's surroundings revolve. No substitutes should be accepted by the thoughtful physician. In particular, the common complaint of "dizziness" is without value because it can also mean lightheadedness, giddiness, anxiety, confusion, or imbalance.

Ultrasonography and DIVA are not useful in assessing the vertebrobasilar system. Although arteriography would demonstrate stenotic areas, this procedure is usually not performed because it is risky, and moreover, vertebrobasilar stenosis is ultimately not surgically accessible. Medical therapy for basilar artery TIAs follows the same guidelines as for carotid artery disease. Intracranial-extracranial arterial bypass procedures are not beneficial.

Transient Global Amnesia

A noteworthy but rare phenomenon associated with basilar artery TIAs is *transient global amnesia*. This condition, which is often precipitated by exertion in older people, probably results from ischemia of the posterior cerebral arteries. These vessels are terminal branches of the basilar artery and supply the temporal lobes (Fig. 11-2). Since the temporal lobes contain portions of the limbic system structures (Fig. 16-5), ischemic attacks that affect both posterior cerebral arteries result in 3 to 24 hours of memory impairment and personality change. A recurrence rate of about 10 percent can be expected.

While in a state of transient global amnesia, patients are apathetic and disoriented, and characteristically they have profound anterograde and spotty retrograde amnesia. Nevertheless, their general knowledge remains intact, and under the circumstances, their affect is appropriate. Transient global amnesia is a frequently cited cause of the *acute amnestic syndrome* (Chapter 7) and a transiently altered mental status (Table 9-3). Although transient global amnesia most closely mimics partial complex seizures, it would probably be distinguished

TABLE 11–3. CEREBROVASCULAR ACCIDENTS (CVAs)

Carotid artery
  Anterior cerebral
    Contralateral lower extremity paresis
    Muteness, apathy, pseudobulbar palsy*
  Middle cerebral
    Contralateral hemiparesis, homonymous hemianopsia, and hemisensory loss
    Aphasia and related syndromes
    Hemi-inattention
  Posterior cerebral
    Contralateral homonymous hemianopsia
    Alexia without agraphia
Vertebrobasilar system
  Basilar artery
    Total occlusion: coma or locked-in syndrome
    Occlusion of branch: cranial nerve palsy with contralateral hemiparesis, internuclear ophthal-
      moplegia
  Vertebral artery
    Lateral medullary (Wallenberg's) syndrome

* When both anterior cerebral arteries are infarcted.

from a seizure by lack of motor activity, epileptiform EEG changes, and subsequent rise in the serum prolactin level (Chapter 10).

CEREBROVASCULAR ACCIDENTS (CVAs)

In contrast to the brief neurologic deficits in TIAs, CVAs cause permanent physical and mental deficits. Although numerous causes have been identified, most CVAs result from arterial thromboses, emboli, or hemorrhages. *Risk factors* for CVAs have been elucidated. The incidence of CVAs rises in almost exponential fashion after the age of 65 years, but still about 20 percent of CVA victims are under the age of 65 years. An even more important risk factor than age, because it is prevalent and its effects can be attenuated, is hypertension. It leads to CVAs in middle-aged as well as older adults, and it is probably the cause of *multi-infarct dementia* (see below). Moreover, hypertension induces atherosclerosis, which is another major risk factor. Antihypertensive medications have reduced the incidence of CVAs and other complications of hypertension; however, these medications themselves may cause some problems (see below).

Cardiac valvular disease, myocardial infarctions, atrial fibrillation, and possibly mitral valve prolapse are also risk factors because, in each of these conditions, thromboses tend to form on the endocardial surface and embolize to the brain. Other important risk factors are cigarette smoking and heavy alcohol consumption. Oral contraceptives in some studies have been implicated as a risk factor; however, their adverse influence may be confined to women who smoke or have migraine headaches. Curiously, some risk factors for coronary artery disease, such as lack of exercise and cholesterol-rich diets, carry relatively little risk for CVAs.

Thromboses and Emboli

In thrombotic or embolic CVAs, the area of the brain that the artery supplies becomes infarcted and the surrounding region becomes edematous. Some clinical recovery seems to occur because the edema resolves; however, the infarcted tissue is functionless and a permanent scar with epileptogenic potential (Chapter 10).

The majority of CVAs are caused by either a thrombosis that propagates within an atherosclerotic cerebral artery or an embolus that originates within a carotid artery, i.e., an "arterial-arterial embolus." Related causes of CVAs are cardiac emboli (especially from atrial fibrillation), sickle cell disease, drug abuse, vasculitis, and blood dyscrasias. In short, the causes of CVAs are abnormalities of the cerebral vessels, heart, or blood.

A disproportionate number of CVAs occur during sleep, although many develop in a stuttering fashion over 1 or 2 days. The most pronounced deficit in cerebral infarction occurs between the third to tenth days when edema is most severe. A mild unilateral or bilateral headache sometimes accompanies a cerebral thrombosis.

Since each of the major cerebral arteries supplies a particular area of the brain, a characteristic neurologic deficit is associated with each artery (Fig. 11-1 and Table 11-3). The *middle* cerebral artery infarction (Fig. 20-8), which is the most common, is associated with contralateral hemiparesis, hemisensory loss, homonymous hemianopsia and, with dominant hemisphere lesions, aphasia. Hemi-inattention and related neuropsychologic deficits may be present when the lesion is in the nondominant hemisphere. With an *anterior* cerebral artery infarction, the contralateral leg will be paretic, but if both anterior cerebral arteries have infarctions, bilateral frontal lobe damage may cause pseudobulbar palsy, dementia, apathy, muteness, abulia, and the other signs of the "frontal lobe syndrome" (Chapter 7). With a *posterior* cerebral artery infarction, a contralateral homonymous hemianopsia will result.

Several discrete intellectual impairments, such as aphasia, are associated with cerebral hemisphere infarctions. However, patients could also have dementia if they sustained one massive cerebral infarction, if both frontal lobes were injured, or if many small infarctions accumulated to cause multi-infarct dementia.

Infarctions in the distribution of the basilar artery cause brainstem or cerebellar injuries. In contrast to cerebral hemisphere infarctions, *small* brainstem infarctions are accompanied by no impairment of language or intellectual function. *Large* brainstem infarctions usually cause coma if not immediate death. However, patients who survive brainstem infarctions of any size usually have no cognitive impairment, sometimes despite having severe physical incapacity (see below, the Locked-In Syndrome).

Precise localization of brainstem infarctions is often desirable for practical as well as academic reasons. Lesions of the midbrain cause ipsilateral oculomotor nerve and contralateral paresis (Fig. 4-8). Pontine lesions cause ipsilateral abducens nerve and contralateral paresis (Fig. 4-10). Midline pons or midbrain infarctions cause the MLF syndrome (Chapters 12 and 15). Finally, lateral medullary infarctions (Wallenberg's syndrome) cause ipsilateral limb ataxia, palatal paresis, Horner's syndrome, and alternating hypalgesia (Fig. 2-10).

Once the lesion is localized to the brainstem, the physician can usually conclude that the patient's mental function is intact. For example, a patient with a left sixth cranial nerve palsy and right hemiparesis is unlikely to have aphasia.

Hemorrhages

Hemorrhagic cerebrovascular disease, the most ominous condition, occurs when a ruptured cerebral artery sprays a jet of blood directly into the brain. Hematomas often develop in the pons, cerebellum, or putamen (Fig. 18-1). Brain damage is usually extensive and often fatal.

Although thromboses develop slowly or intermittently and are relatively painless, most hemorrhages are abrupt in onset and are accompanied by headaches, nausea, and vomiting. In many cases, patients quickly lapse into stupor with profound neurologic deficits.

Most patients cannot be helped. However, several forms of hemorrhage can be treated. An important condition is the hemorrhage induced by monamine oxidase inhibitors (Chapter 9). Another relatively common condition that any physician might encounter in older, hypertensive patients is *cerebellar hemorrhage*. This hemorrhage characteristically causes occipital headache, gait ataxia, dysarthria, and lethargy. Evacuation of a cerebellar hematoma is feasible and may be life saving. *Subarachnoid hemorrhages* are usually the result of rupture of a berry aneurysm (a balloon-like arterial dilation). Ruptures often occur during exertion and cause an extraordinarily severe headache and nuchal rigidity; however, they may produce no physical deficits. Although the clinical features of a subarachnoid hemorrhage are occasionally confused with those of a migraine headache (Chapter 9), a CT or MRI scan of the head will usually reveal blood at the base of the brain. Also, lumbar puncture will yield bloody CSF in hemorrhages of recent onset and xanthochromic CSF in those more than several days old (Chapter 20).

CEREBROVASCULAR ACCIDENTS AND COGNITIVE CHANGES

Although atherosclerosis leads to TIAs and CVAs, atherosclerosis itself does not cause intellectual, emotional, or other psychologic abnormalities. In other words, "hardening of the arteries" does not cause dementia.

Once a CVA has developed, however, cognitive changes can be a prominent feature. Specific abnormalities caused by CVAs are associated with certain physical deficits. For example, dominant hemisphere CVAs that cause aphasia or Gerstmann's syndrome are associated with right-sided hemiparesis, reflex abnormalities, and homonymous hemianopsia. Likewise, nondominant parietal lobe CVAs that cause hemi-inattention, anosognosia, and constructional apraxia are associated with left-sided sensory and visual abnormalities (Chapter 8).

Deficits can, in a sense, be additive. Dementia has been found when many small CVAs have damaged a total quantity of brain, estimated to be 50 to 150 cc, irrespective of the location of the injuries. *Multi-infarct dementia* accounts for 8 to 40 percent of all cases of dementia. It is similar to *état lacunaire* in which hypertensive cerebrovascular disease causes multiple small cerebral scars (lacunes) measuring 0.5 to 1.5 cm in diameter. With successive infarctions, patients have a stepwise decrease in intellectual function and emotional stability associated with progressive physical impairments, such as paresis, clumsiness, rigidity, and reflex abnormalities. Signs of frontal lobe injury often predominate. Patients usually have partial recovery after each "mini-infarction."

Multi-infarct dementia differs from Alzheimer's disease in that it has a stepwise worsening with some partial remissions and relatively prominent physical signs. Otherwise, the distinction is difficult. The cognitive and other psychologic changes in multi-infarct dementia are similar to those found in Alzheimer's disease. The *Hachinski test* might be helpful (see References) in identifying multi-infarct dementia, but most other neuropsychologic tests cannot reliably distinguish between the two. Early in both conditions, the EEG is either normal or contains only some nonspecific slowing. Although CT and MRI scans show small areas of infarction in multi-infarct dementia, in both conditions the scans usually show atrophy.

Cerebrovascular accidents of the cerebral hemisphere may cause partial complex and other seizures because about 5 percent of cerebral infarctions become irritative scars. Therefore, in patients with cerebrovascular disease, brief generalized confusion may result from TIAs, transient global amnesia, or partial complex seizures.

Another important and probably often overlooked psychologic manifestation of a CVA is depression. Above and beyond despair attributable to physical disabilities, 30 percent to 60 percent of patients with CVAs have been found to have depression. Moreover, depressed CVA patients have a greater functional impairment than nondepressed patients with similar physical deficits. This discrepancy has been attributed to the interference of depression with rehabilitation programs. Although CVAs affecting the left frontal pole have been closely associated with depression, the correlations are inconsistent. Also, clinicians may confuse depression with pseudobulbar palsy, nonfluent aphasia, anosognosia, or aprosody (Chapter 8). Antidepressant medications have been found to be helpful and have minimal side effects in many but not all patients with depression after a stroke.

In addition to CVA-induced depression, some mood changes may be iatrogenic. Many antihypertensive medications, such as methyldopa (Aldomet) and propranolol (Inderal), impair mental function by reducing cerebral blood flow, acting as false neurotransmitters, or otherwise interfering with neuronal function. Diuretics can also cause confusion and seizures when they lower the serum sodium concentration below 120 to 125 mEq/mL. Also, when patients taking these medications suddenly stand up, they may develop orthostatic hypotension. Cerebral blood flow is reduced, and it causes lightheadedness, vertigo, and confusion. Patients can even lose consciousness.

Locked-In Syndrome

Numerous patients who have sustained multiple CVAs are rendered completely demented, mute, and quadriplegic. Among CVA patients who have been devastated, especially when assessing their cognitive capacity for legal purposes, physicians should search for the rare patient who has the *locked-in syndrome*. In this important condition, patients, even though mute and quadriplegic, have intact cognitive capacity. Moreover, these patients, who can only voluntarily move their eyes and eyelids, are able to communicate.

The locked-in syndrome usually results from infarction of the inferior portion (base or ventral surface) of the pons or medulla (bulb) when a branch of the basilar artery is occluded (Fig. 11-3). Patients are mute because of severe bulbar palsy and quadriplegic because of interruption of the corticospinal tract. Similar clinical situations have been found in some patients who have unusually severe cases of myasthenia gravis or the Guillain-Barré syndrome (Chapters 5 and 6),

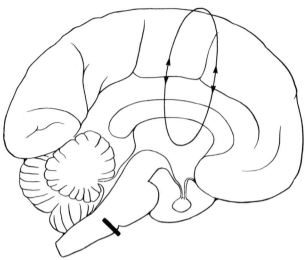

FIGURE 11–3. The locked-in syndrome usually results from an infarction of the ventral surface of the lower brainstem. A lesion in this area (*indicated by the bar*) would sever the corticospinal tracts and directly injure cranial nerves nine through twelve, but the lesion would not damage the reticular activating system, which governs attention.

More important, the cerebral cortex and upper brainstem are still intact and able to maintain normal interactions. There is no damage to the cognitive, language, or visual areas of the brain, which are all in the cerebral cortex. Also, the cerebral centers governing eye movement and their connections to the upper brainstem, which contains the ocular motility cranial nerves, remain intact (Fig. 12-12).

The reverberating circuits between the thalamus and the cerebral cortex (indicated by the loop), which generate the organized relatively regular background EEG activity, are also intact. Thus, the EEG of patients with the locked-in syndrome is relatively normal.

If all peripheral and cranial nerves are impaired in severe cases of Guillain-Barré syndrome or myasthenia gravis, these patients too could have the locked-in syndrome. In these cases, however, patients' eyes and eyelids would be immobile, and they could not communicate with blinks or eye movement.

although in these cases the neurologic damage is to the peripheral nervous system.

In the locked-in syndrome, whatever the cause, the cerebral cortex, upper brainstem, dorsal surface of the bulb, and their interconnections are all intact. Thus, patients are alert, have normal cognitive and affective capacity, and can purposefully move their eyes and eyelids. Given sufficient clues, they will maintain a normal sleep-wake schedule. Their EEGs are usually normal.

The medical and social management of patients who have the locked-in syndrome should be altered to reflect their normal cognitive and affective capacity. They can understand people talking and reading to them. They can be expected to participate in decisions regarding their care. Some patients who have suffered a brainstem infarction can partially recover. Patients debilitated from myasthenia gravis or the Guillain-Barré syndrome often totally recover.

Physicians should carefully examine patients who are unable to speak or move their limbs but can voluntarily look from side to side. An examination for the locked-in syndrome should begin by asking patients to blink a certain number of times. If patients respond, a system of communication can be developed. At least one patient has been able to communicate freely using eyelid blinks in Morse code. If the patients can blink their eyelids meaningfully, the physician should test their ability to see and calculate. Afterward, more detailed mental status testing might be undertaken to determine their capacity to make decisions. Evaluation of mute but attentive patients can uncover occasional cases where an intact mind had been unrecognized.

Persistent Vegetative State

Patients who have sustained extensive cerebral damage resulting in permanent and total incapacity, both mental and physical, are said to be in the *persistent vegetative state*. In this condition, which has also been known as "akinetic mutism" or "coma vigil," patients are awake or arousable, but they are entirely unaware of their surroundings and devoid of cognitive capacity. They have only spontaneous, random eye movements and reflex eyelid blinks. As with patients in the locked-in syndrome, they are mute and quadriplegic.

Most of them will have been in coma, a state of being unarousable, for periods of days or weeks preceding their evolution to the vegetative state. The underlying illnesses have usually been cerebral anoxia from cardiac arrest or drug overdose, profound hypoglycemia, major head trauma, or advanced Alzheimer's disease. In any case, the cerebral cortex and often the underlying cerebral tissue are typically destroyed (Fig. 11-4). The brainstem, being relatively unaffected by these conditions, becomes independent of cerebral control. It then operates by reflex to regulate the body's vegetative functions, such as breathing and swallowing. Once patients have been in this state for 1 month, there is little chance of recovery, although they often survive for years.

Unlike patients in the locked-in syndrome, those in the persistent vegetative state have no cognitive or affective capacity. They cannot understand speech, read, or appreciate visitors' emotions. They do not respond to questions or

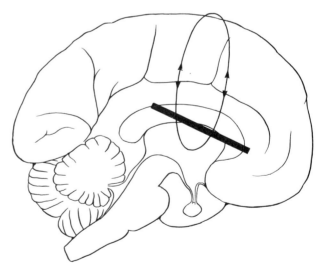

FIGURE 11–4. The persistent vegetative state, which can be caused by cerebral anoxia or numerous other conditions, results from extensive damage to the cerebral cortex or the cerebral tissue immediately underlying it (*indicated by the bar*). Such injury impairs all cerebral function, including cognitive ability, purposeful motor activity, vision, and speech. Also, since the cerebral hemispheres are damaged, their interactions (*indicated by the loop*) with the brainstem produce an abnormal EEG.

Patients in the vegetative state may have roving eye movements because the brainstem is intact (Fig. 12-12). However, aside from some reflex quality, the movements are random and incapable of being meaningful.

requests, and they do not communicate with their eyes or eyelids. Their EEG is abnormal. Positron emission tomography (PET) scans show marked reduction in cerebral cortex metabolism.

The persistent vegetative state is much more common than the locked-in syndrome. Although patients in the persistent vegetative state do not require endotracheal intubation, respirators, or mechanical supports, their medical and nursing requirements are enormous. Living in nursing homes and acute care hospitals, they are maintained by nasogastric tubes, urinary catheters, and continuous nursing care (Fig. 11-5). The cost for each patient and the number of patients affected make this condition a financial burden to the public.

The problem is not only its economic impact. Many patients, while in better health, had expressed desires that they "not live like a vegetable." Several ethical and legal contests, starting with the case of Karen Ann Quinlan, have explored the limits of maintaining patients, who have no mental function and no reasonable expectation of recovery, when medical care is administered against their explicit or implicit wishes. The issue of maintaining anyone in this state, given society's limited resources, has also been raised. Without necessarily entering into a debate or making any moral judgment, the role of the physician, at this time, would be at least to demonstrate a patient's loss of cognitive and affective function, to ascertain that the patient did not have the locked-in syndrome or a correctable cause of dementia, to demonstrate an abnormal EEG, and to discuss the prognosis with colleagues and family members.

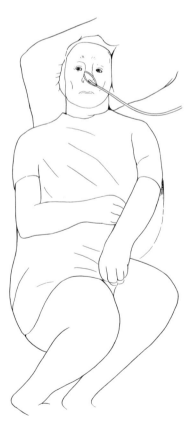

FIGURE 11–5.   Patients in the persistent vegetative state assume a decorticate (flexed or fetal) posture because of extensive cerebral damage. Although they are awake, have roving eye movements, and do not require a respirator, they are mute, virtually motionless, and unable to respond to visitors or examiners. Patients are dependent on nasogastric tubes or intravenous solutions for nourishment, and on urinary catheters. They are vulnerable to aspiration pneumonia, urinary tract infections, and pressure sores.

Laboratory Tests in CVAs

In most cases the diagnosis of a CVA is made on the basis of the clinical evaluation and confirmed with a CT or MRI scan (Chapter 20). Alternative diagnoses are brain tumor, abscess, subdural hematoma, and systemic illness with neurologic complications, such as vasculitis (Chapter 19).

Either type of scan will indicate the existence and location of almost all CVAs, except those that are fresh or small. They can exclude subdural hematomas and the other structural lesions. In contrast, skull x-rays are superfluous. An EEG is also not helpful because it cannot reliably indicate the location or cause of most structural lesions. Angiography is done in selected cases to diagnose carotid stenosis, cerebral aneurysms, and vascular malformations.

Examination of the CSF via a lumbar puncture is used to diagnose a subarachnoid hemorrhage when scans are unavailable or equivocal. It is also indicated when meningitis or encephalitis is suspected. However, it is not usually performed when a CVA or an intracranial mass lesion is present (see Transtentorial Herniation, Chapter 19).

Therapy of CVAs

During the initial phase of a CVA, careful attention is paid to maintaining a patent airway and supporting vital bodily functions. Fluids are given in liberal amounts, and salts must be repleted in order to ensure adequate cerebral perfusion. There is no proven benefit to use of steroids, anticoagulants, oxygen, or vasoactive medicines. If the patient is not alert or the gag reflex is diminished, all nutrition is provided intravenously, medications are given parenterally, and nasopharyngeal secretions must be cleared by frequent suctioning.

Decubitus ulcers (bedsores) must be prevented because they are unsightly and malodorous and can lead to infection and potentially fatal sepsis. Physicians usually order air mattresses, sweat-absorbent bed surfaces (e.g., artificial sheepskins), and elbow and heel cushions for paretic limbs. Nurses should reposition the patient every 2 hours. Since urinary incontinence adds to the likelihood of developing a bed sore, makes patients cold and wet, and creates odors repugnant to family and staff, indwelling or condom catheters are often used.

The patient's bed should be placed against the wall so that all visitors and staff must approach the patient from the side without perceptual impairment. For example, after suffering a left hemiparesis and a left homonymous hemianopsia, the patient should be placed with his or her left side against the wall so that people approach from the right, and important objects (e.g., call-buttons, television, clock, and pictures) can be seen and grasped.

The family should help by orienting the patient and bringing a luminous dial clock, a calendar, and a family picture. They should help reposition the patient and passively move paretic limbs to avoid contractures. The family might locate appropriate rehabilitation facilities.

Traditional physical therapy will often maintain muscle tone, forestall bedsores, and prevent contractures. Therapy will usually help patients with simple hemiparesis to regain their ability to walk, circumvent some impediments, and avoid maladaptive but expeditious physical compensations.

Most physical and psychologic recovery occurs spontaneously. Hemi-inattention and anosognosia resolve over a period of 1 to 3 weeks. However, aphasias usually improve to almost their fullest extent in 4 to 6 weeks, and then deficits are usually permanent. Speech therapy may help with dysarthria and offer patients encouragement. "Cognitive and perceptual skill training" for impaired mentation, sensory impairment, and visual loss has also not been shown to be effective.

Various psychologic aberrations may require medication. In particular, depression and pathologic crying, which is often a manifestation of pseudo-bulbar palsy, can be treated with antidepressants. Likewise, agitation, over-whelming anxiety, and hallucinations can be treated with neuroleptics. Control of these aberrations permits some patients to accept deficits, restraints, and therapies. When a patient's sleeping schedule is disrupted, mild hypnotics are necessary; however, phenobarbital and other barbiturates should be avoided because they tend to create agitation in brain injured patients, i.e., a paradoxical reaction.

SUMMARY

Signs of cerebrovascular disease are usually attributed to TIAs or CVAs of either the carotid or vertebrobasilar (basilar) artery circulation. Carotid artery TIAs, which cause amaurosis fugax and cerebral dysfunction, are believed to result from platelet emboli that originate on atherosclerotic plaques at the carotid artery bifurcation. Standard treatment, which depends upon the clinical situation, is either carotid endarterectomy or an antiplatelet agent, usually aspirin. Basilar TIAs, which usually cause vertigo, occasionally cause transient global amnesia, which is an important form of acute amnesia. These TIAs are not amenable to surgery but are also treated with aspirin.

Cerebrovascular accidents in the carotid circulation produce contralateral physical deficits and a tendency to have seizures. Depending upon which hemisphere is injured, patients have specific psychologic disturbances, such as aphasia with left middle cerebral artery infarctions and hemi-inattention with right middle cerebral artery infarctions. However, despite having specific deficits, patients with these or similar single infarctions usually do not have dementia. They often have depression, which tends to interfere with their rehabilitation, but it may respond to antidepressant medications.

Multiple small cerebral infarctions lead to multi-infarct dementia. This form of dementia is clinically similar to Alzheimer's dementia except that its course is intermittently progressive and the examination reveals prominent motor and reflex abnormalities.

Cerebrovascular accidents of the brainstem produce certain combinations of cranial nerve palsies and hemiparesis. In contrast to cerebral CVAs, brainstem CVAs usually do not cause depression or dementia. The most important although rare example of brainstem infarction is the locked-in syndrome, which is the result of a ventral pons or medulla infarction. Patients with this condition have devastating paresis and mutism; however, they have normal cognitive capacity, which they can express only by eye movement, and relatively normal EEGs.

Another important condition is the persistent vegetative state. In contrast to the locked-in syndrome, it is a common condition that is usually caused by extensive cerebral hypoxia that has rendered patients physically and mentally permanently disabled. Patients in the persistent vegetative state may be awake, but they are mute and unresponsive, and have markedly abnormal EEGs.

REFERENCES

Abbott RD, Yin Y, Reed DM, et al: Risk of stroke in male cigarette smokers. N Engl J Med *315*:717, 1986

Carter LT, Howard BE, O'Neil WA: Effectiveness of cognitive skill remediation in stroke patients. Am J Occup Ther *37*:320, 1983

Dupont RM, Cullum CM, Jeste DV: Poststroke depression and psychosis. Psychiatr Clin North Am *11*:133, 1988

Finklestein SP, Weintraub RJ, Karmouz N, et al: Antidepressant drug treatment for poststroke depression: Retrospective study. Arch Phys Med Rehabil *68*:772, 1987

Gill JS, Zezulka AV, Shipley MJ, et al: Stroke and alcohol consumption. N Engl J Med *315*:1041, 1986

Goodstein RK: Overview: Cerebrovascular accident and the hospitalized elderly—A multidimensional clinical problem. Am J Psychiatry *140*:141, 1983

Grotta JC: Current medical and surgical therapy for cerebrovascular disease. N Engl J Med *317*:1505, 1987

Hachinski V: Multi-infarct dementia. Neurol Clin *1*:27, 1983

Hale G: The Source Book for the Disabled. Philadelphia, The Saunders Press, 1979

Ishii N, Nishihara Y, Imamura T: Why do frontal lobe symptoms predominate in vascular dementia with lacunes? Neurology *36*:340, 1986

Keith L: A synthesis of studies on stroke rehabilitation. J Chron Dis *35*:133, 1982

Kerson TS: Understanding Chronic Illness. New York, The Free Press, 1985

Kritchevsky M, Squire LR, Zouzounis JA: Transient global amnesia: Characterization of anterograde and retrograde amnesia. Neurology *38*:213, 1988

Levy DE, Sidtis JJ, Rottenberg DA, et al: Differences in cerebral blood flow and glucose utilization in vegetative versus locked-in patients. Ann Neurol *22*:673, 1987

Miller JW, Petersen RC, Metter EJ, et al: Transient global amnesia: Clinical characteristics and prognosis. Neurology *37*:733, 1987

Perry J: Rehabilitation of the neurologically disabled patient: Principles, practice, and scientific basis. J Neurosurg *58*:799, 1983

Reding MJ, Orto LA, Winter SW, et al: Antidepressant therapy after stroke. Arch Neurol *43*:763, 1986

Robinson RG, Kubos KL, Starr LB, et al: Mood disorders in stroke patients. Brain *107*:81, 1984

Robinson RG, Lipsey JR, Rao K, et al: Two-year longitudinal study of poststroke mood disorders: Comparison of acute-onset with delayed-onset depression. Am J Psychiatry *143*:1238, 1986

Ross ED, Rush AJ: Diagnosis and neuroanatomical correlates of depression in brain-damaged patients. Arch Gen Psychiatry *38*:1344, 1981

Sinyor D, Amato P, Kaloupek DG, et al: Post-stroke depression: Relationships to functional impairment, coping strategies, and rehabilitation outcome. Stroke *16*:1102, 1986

Starkstein SE, Robinson RG, Price TR: Comparison of patients with and without poststroke major depression matched for size and location of lesion. Arch Gen Psychiatry *45*:247, 1988

QUESTIONS: CHAPTER 11

1–10. Match the neurologic deficit with the most likely artery of infarction.

[Deficit]	[Artery]
1. Hemiparesis with relative sparing of leg	a. Right posterior cerebral
	b. Left posterior cerebral
2. Lower extremity monoparesis	c. Anterior cerebral
	d. Middle cerebral
3. Monocular blindness from optic nerve ischemia	e. Right middle cerebral
	f. Left middle cerebral
	g. Ophthalmic
4. Left homonymous hemianopsia	h. Vertebral or posterior inferior cerebellar
5. Left palate paresis, limb ataxia	i. Perforating branch of basilar
6. Right third cranial nerve palsy with left hemiparesis	j. Anterior spinal
	k. Basilar

7. Right hemiparesis with aphasia

8. Quadriplegia and mutism with intact mentation

9. Left sixth and seventh cranial nerve palsy with right hemiparesis

10. Coma, quadriparesis

11–20. Match the type of transient neurologic deficit with the artery involved (a, b, both, or neither).

[Deficit]	[Artery]
11. Transient global amnesia	a. Carotid
12. Amaurosis fugax	b. Basilar
13. Paresthesias of right arm and aphasia	
14. Vertigo, nausea, nystagmus, and ataxia	
15. Drop attacks	
16. Dizziness, malaise, headache	
17. Diplopia	
18. Dysarthria	
19. Transient hemiparesis	
20. Transient right hemiparesis without aphasia	

21–30. A 74-year-old man has had a left-sided headache for 5 days, a nonfluent aphasia, right hemiparesis with hyperreflexia, a Babinski sign, and right homonymous hemianopsia. Which of the following should be considered as likely possibilities?

21. Cerebral hemorrhage

22. Subarachnoid hemorrhage

23. Brain tumor

24. Subdural hematoma

25. Basilar artery occlusion

26. Carotid artery occlusion

27. Brain abscess

28. Conversion reaction

29. Cerebral embolus

30. Multiple sclerosis

31–36. A 65-year-old man sustains a cerebrovascular accident, after which he is alert but mute and unable to move his arms or legs. He has paresis of the palate, bilateral hyperreflexia, and Babinski signs. He responds to verbal and written questions by blinking his eyelids.

31. Does this man have a fluent, nonfluent, or global aphasia?

32. Is his vision impaired?

33. Is there evidence of cerebral damage?

34.   How would the EEG appear?

35.   What is this syndrome called?

36.   Where is the lesion?

37–41.   A 64-year-old man, who had sustained a right cerebral infarction the previous year, is admitted after the sudden, painless onset of right hemiparesis and mutism. He now has bilateral paresis and no verbal output. Although his eyes are frequently open, he fails to respond to either voice or gesture.

37.   Where is the probable site of the recent injury?

38.   What is the probable cause?

39.   Would the EEG be normal?

40.   If he were not paralyzed, would he be able to write?

41.   Would he have bulbar or pseudobulbar palsy?

42–52.   A 20-year-old woman awakens from sleep and finds that she has a mild left hemiparesis. Which are the possible causes of her deficit?

42.   Cerebral thrombosis associated with oral contraceptives

43.   Cerebral vasculitis from lupus, drug abuse, etc.

44.   Cerebral embolus from mitral stenosis

45.   Cerebral embolus from drug abuse

46.   Rupture of a cerebral arteriovenous malformation

47.   Cerebral embolus from an atrial myxoma

48.   Compression of the right carotid artery during a stuporous sleep

49.   Infarction from sickle cell disease

50.   A prolonged postictal (Todd's) paresis

51.   A transient paresis of hemiplegic migraine

52.   Multiple sclerosis

53–56.   A 20-year-old woman is brought to the Emergency Room by her family because she is suddenly unable to speak or move her right side. She looks directly forward but does not follow commands. On inspection of her fundi, her eyes constantly evert. She seems to respond to visual images in all fields. The right arm and leg are flaccid and immobile, although her face is symmetric. Deep tendon reflexes are symmetric, and no pathologic reflexes are elicited. She does not react to noxious stimuli on the right side of her face or body.

53.   Where is the apparent lesion?

54.   (a) What pathologic features usually found with such a lesion are not present in the patient? (b) What nonpathologic features are present?

55.   What is the most likely origin?

56.   What readily available laboratory tests would lend great support to the diagnosis?

57–61.   A 70-year-old man has the sudden onset of an occipital headache, nausea, vomiting, and an inability to walk. He has no paresis, but a downward drift of the right arm, and symmetrically active deep tendon reflexes with normal plantar response. He has dysmetria on right finger-nose and heel-shin movements and ataxia of gait.

57.   Where is the lesion?

58.   Which side?

59. What is its origin?

60. Why is there a "drift" of the right arm?

61. What is the consequence of increased size of the lesion?

62–65. A 75-year-old man has moderate, unremitting left-sided headaches and development of right-sided hemiparesis with hyperreflexia and a Babinski sign. On admission, he has neither aphasia nor visual field loss. During the initial 3 days in the hospital, however, he develops stupor with a dilated, unreactive left pupil and bilateral Babinski signs.

62. Where is the lesion?

63. What are the possible causes?

64. Which would be the most appropriate diagnostic test?

65. What is the origin of the pupillary abnormality?

66–67. Found wandering about in a confused manner, a 45-year-old woman is brought to the Emergency Room. She is lethargic, inattentive, and confused but not aphasic. Her pupils are equal and reactive, and her fundi are normal. Extraocular movements are full. All her extremities move well. She has hyperactive deep tendon reflexes and bilateral Babinski signs.

66. Where is the lesion?

67. What is the most likely cause?

68. Which of the following varieties of CVAs most often appears as patients awaken in the morning?
    a.   Cerebral hemorrhage
    b.   Cerebral thrombosis
    c.   Cerebral embolus
    d.   Subarachnoid hemorrhage

69. Which of the varieties of CVAs described in question 68 most often develop during sexual intercourse?

70. Which of the following CVA risk factors is the most important and correctable?
    a.   Advanced age
    b.   High cholesterol diet
    c.   Obesity
    d.   Cigarette smoking
    e.   Hypertension
    f.   Lack of exercise

71. Which of the following is the standard therapy for vertebrobasilar artery TIAs?
    a.   Endarterectomy
    b.   Surgical anastomosis
    c.   Coumadin
    d.   Aspirin

72. Which of the following is thought to be the most important cause of multi-infarct dementia?
    a.   Carotid bifurcation atherosclerosis
    b.   Cerebral emboli
    c.   Generalized atherosclerosis
    d.   Hypertension

73. Which of the following is the greatest difference between Alzheimer's disease and multi-infarct dementia?
    a.   Quality of dementia
    b.   CT findings
    c.   EEG findings
    d.   Clinical course

74. A 28-year-old man has had a 3-day history of increasing left arm weakness and clumsiness, and also a mild generalized headache. Examination reveals only hyperactive deep tendon reflexes in the mildly paretic left arm. Routine medical evaluation reveals no abnormalities. Both CT and MRI scans show a large right cerebral lesion with a sharply defined border. Of the following, which is the most likely cause of the patient's neurologic difficulties?

    a. Cerebral infarction
    b. Cerebral hemorrhage
    c. Toxoplasmosis
    d. Glioblastoma
    e. Meningioma

75–86. Match the condition(s) with the sign.

[Sign]

75. Mutism

76. Quadriparesis

77. Voluntary eye movement

78. Results from cerebral hypoxia

79. Results from lower brainstem infarction or embolus

80. Relatively normal EEG

81. Cognitive capacity intact

82. Cognitive capacity lost

83. Due to lesion in base of pons that spares reticular activating system

84. Due to lesion that damages virtually all of cerebral cortex or underlying cerebrum

85. Can be caused by Guillain-Barré syndrome or myasthenia gravis

86. Can be caused by insulin injections, as in attempted murder

[Condition]
    a. Locked-in syndrome
    b. Persistent vegetative state

ANSWERS

1. d.		**11.**	b (posterior cerebral arteries).
2. c.		**12.**	a (ophthalmic arteries).
3. g.		**13.**	a.
4. a or e.		**14.**	b.
5. h.		**15.**	b.
6. i.		**16.**	Neither
7. f.		**17.**	b.
8. i.		**18.**	a or b.
9. i.		**19.**	a or b.
10. k.		**20.**	b.

21.   No. Cerebral hemorrhages usually are suddenly occurring catastrophic processes.

22.   No. The headaches would be sudden and incapacitating. Nuchal rigidity would be present.

23.   Possibly, but the course is somewhat too rapid.

24.   Unlikely. Although the headache and hemiparesis are consistent, the aphasia and hemianopsia are rare with masses outside of the brain substance, i.e., extra-axial lesions.

25.   No. He would be comatose.

26.   Good choice. This is a typical story of progressive carotid stenosis.

27.   Possibly, but brain abscesses are rare.

28.   No. There are objective neurologic findings: asymmetric deep tendon reflexes and a Babinski sign.

29.   No. These occur suddenly, but the deficit itself is compatible.

30.   No. The headache, limited extent of the lesion, and age at onset, are incompatible.

31.   No. There is no evidence of aphasia. He can understand spoken language and respond appropriately.

32.   No. He can read written questions.

33.   No. The palatal and other motor pareses may be the result of brainstem damage. Cortical processes seem to be intact.

34.   The EEG might appear normal because cortical functions are intact.

35.   Locked-in syndrome

36.   The lesion is in the ventral surface of the lower brainstem, i.e., the base of the pons.

37.   The new lesion is in the left (dominant) hemisphere.

38.   The sudden, painless onset suggests a thrombotic or embolic CVA.

39.   The EEG will be abnormal because of extensive cerebral damage.

40.   No. Aphasic patients generally have difficulty in all modes of communication.

41.   He would probably have pseudobulbar palsy because of bilateral cerebral infarctions. Moreover, since he has evidence of no cognitive function and the EEG is abnormal, if he makes no improvement in 1 month, he can then be said to be in a persistent vegetative state.

42–49.   All yes. CVAs in young people are the result of diseases of the heart, blood, or blood vessels.

50–52.   All yes. These other processes, not strictly cerebrovascular, may mimic strokes.

53.   A patient who seems to have global aphasia and a right hemiparesis would usually have a left hemisphere lesion.

54.   a. She does not have the usual paresis of the lower (right) face, asymmetric deep tendon reflexes, Babinski signs, or a right homonymous hemianopsia. b. Eversion of the eyes during inspection is always a voluntary act. Inability to perceive noxious stimuli is rare in cerebral lesions, and a sharply demarcated sensory loss (splitting the midline) is not neurologic.

55.   Hysteria, malingering, or other psychogenic disturbance

56.   A normal EEG and CT scan

57.   The lesion is located in the cerebellum.

58. The abnormal findings are referable to the ipsilateral cerebellar hemisphere, which in this case is the right.

59. In view of the patient's age and the sudden onset, a CVA is most likely. Since it is painful, a cerebellar hemorrhage must be considered primarily.

60. The right arm drifts downward probably not on the basis of a mild paresis (because strength is normal and no corticospinal tract findings were elicited), but because damage to the cerebellar system disturbs coordination.

61. If the hemorrhage were to expand, the brainstem would become compressed, resulting in coma and death.

62. In view of the left-sided headaches and contralateral hemiparesis, the lesion would be on the "left side" of the CNS. Since there is no language or visual disturbance, the physician cannot initially be certain that the deficit is referable to the cerebral hemisphere, rather than the brainstem. The development of transtentorial herniation makes it clear, however, that in retrospect the lesion was in the left supratentorial (cerebral) compartment.

63. The rapid demise with transtentorial herniation suggests that a mass lesion continued to expand. An occlusion of the internal carotid artery with subsequent cerebral swelling and herniation is possible, but a subdural hematoma is more likely. Tumors, arteriovenous malformations, and abscesses are less common causes (Chapter 19).

64. The most appropriate diagnostic test would be a CT or MRI scan. Presumably, routine history, physical examination, and initial hematologic and chemistry tests would have been done on admission. By the time he "herniates," however, emergency measures must be instituted and those preliminary studies postponed.

65. The dilation and unreactivity of the left pupil are caused by compression of the third cranial nerve as the subdural hematoma squeezes the temporal lobe through the tentorial notch.

66. The woman has delirium. Since she has no lateralizing signs or indications of increased intracranial pressure, one cannot say that she has a "lesion."

67. Causes of diffuse neurologic dysfunction are metabolic alterations (uremia, hypoglycemia), postictal confusion, infectious processes (encephalitis), and intoxications (alcohol, barbiturates).

68. b.		**71.** d.	
69. d.		**72.** d.	
70. e.		**73.** d.	

74. c. Further inquiry revealed that the patient was a homosexual, and laboratory testing revealed that he had acquired immune deficiency syndrome (AIDS). This condition is typically complicated by the development of cerebral toxoplasmosis. The scans are consistent with this condition.

Cerebral infarction in a 28-year-old man is unlikely. Also, the scans in cerebral infarctions usually have a "pie-shaped" pattern. Cerebral hemorrhage is typically a suddenly occurring event, associated with blood-density on CT and MRI scans. A glioblastoma would be rare in a 28-year-old individual, and the scans would have indicated an infiltrating tumor. A meningioma is likewise rare in young adults, and when it does occur, it is extra-axial and slowly growing.

75. Both		**81.** a.	
76. Both		**82.** b.	
77. a.		**83.** a.	
78. b.		**84.** b.	
79. a.		**85.** a.	
80. a.		**86.** b.	

12

Visual Disturbances

Because visual disturbances are so frequent, psychiatrists should be aware of the rudiments of ophthalmology, including those major ocular, neurologic, and systemic illnesses that can cause visual impairment.* This chapter discusses several common clinical problems likely to occur in psychiatric patients, including decreased visual acuity, visual field loss, glaucoma, and certain psychologic aberrations affecting vision.

APPROACH TO THE PATIENT

The physician should determine the specific nature of visual symptoms (Table 12-1). The initial examination (Table 12-2) includes inspecting the globe, or "eyeball" (Fig. 12-1); assessing visual acuity, visual fields, and optic fundi; and testing pupil reflexes and ocular movement. Examinations for special cases, such as psychogenic blindness and visual agnosia, are discussed later in the chapter.

DECREASE IN VISUAL ACUITY

Visual acuity is routinely determined by having the patient read from either a Snellen wall chart or a hand-held card (Fig. 12-2). A person with "normal" visual acuity is someone who can read ⅜-inch letters at a distance of 20 feet. This acuity, which is the reference point of the system, is designated 20/20. People with 20/40 acuity must be at 20 feet to see what a normal person can see as far as 40 feet.

Optical Disturbances

In *myopia*, because of either too "thick" a lens or too "long" a globe, people have increasingly blurred vision at increasingly greater distances (Fig. 12-3). Myopia first becomes troublesome during adolescence when it causes difficulty with seeing blackboards, watching movies, and driving. Since reading and other close activities are unimpaired, people with myopia are said to be "nearsighted."

In its counterpart, *hyperopia* or hypermetropia (farsightedness), the lens is too "thin" or the globe too "short." People with hyperopia have increasing visual difficulty at increasingly shorter distances. In *presbyopia*, a related optical

---

* Patients with visual impairment may receive assistance from many organizations, including the American Foundation for the Blind, 15 West 16th Street, New York, New York 10011, (212) 620-2000.

TABLE 12–1. SALIENT FEATURES OF A PATIENT'S HISTORY

Is the symptom in one or both eyes?
What is the primary symptom?
  Decreased visual acuity
  Visual field loss (one or both eyes)
  Diplopia: direction(s)
  Visual distortions or hallucinations, including halos around lights
What associated symptoms are present?
  Ocular: pain, scintillations
  Neurologic: headache, paresis, ataxia, impotence
  Systemic: fever, malaise, nausea, excessive thirst
Is there a history of any of the following conditions?
  Diabetes, hypertension, syphilis
  Use of psychotropic, anticholinergic, antituberculous, other medications
  Abuse of tobacco, alcohol, or methanol
  Exposure to hallucinogens or industrial toxins
Is there a family history of visual disturbances, especially glaucoma?

condition that begins in middle age, the lenses are not able to focus on closely held objects. Both patients with hyperopia and those with presbyopia have difficulty reading and sewing, and they tend to hold newspapers and needles away from themselves. "Reading glasses" correct the problem.

In addition to these ocular conditions, use of certain medications can lead to important optical disturbances. The foremost is *drug-induced accommodation paresis*, in which patients also have visual acuity impairment for closely held objects (Fig. 12-4). Normally, when a person looks at a closely held object, a parasympathetically mediated *accommodation reflex* contracts the ciliary body muscles, which thickens the lens to focus the image on the retina. However, medications with anticholinergic properties, particularly the tricyclic antidepressants, block this reflex and thus cause blurred vision. (They also occasionally

TABLE 12–2. SALIENT FEATURES OF A PATIENT'S EXAMINATION

Gross evaluation of the globe (eyeball)
  Injection of conjunctival vessels*
  Clarity of cornea and lens
  Inspection for Kayser-Fleischer rings (Chapter 18)*
  Corneal reflex
Determination of visual acuity
  Naked eye
  Corrected with eyeglasses or lens
Determination of visual fields
  Confrontation (Fig. 4–2)
Inspection of fundi
  Optic disk: color, clarity of margins
  Retina: color, hemorrhages,* exudates,* pigment deposit*
  Vessels: arterial pulsations,* venous pulsations
Testing of pupils
  Size, shape, and equality
  Light reflex
  Accomodation
Measurement of extraocular movement
  Position at rest
  Position when looking horizontally or vertically (diplopia,* nystagmus*)
  Strength of orbicularis oculi (eyelids)
  Paresis with fatigue

* Abnormalities.

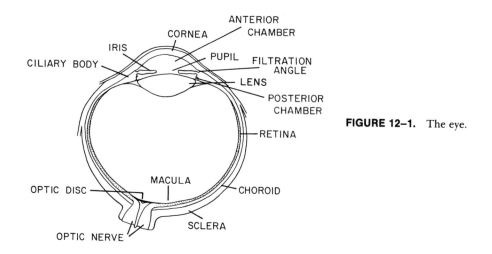

FIGURE 12–1. The eye.

precipitate glaucoma by causing pupillary dilation.) Amitriptyline and doxepin and, to a lesser extent, the other tricyclics and the tetracyclic antidepressants can cause accommodation paresis without causing other anticholinergic side effects, such as dry mouth, constipation, and urinary hesitancy. Even trazodone, which has a different chemical structure, produces the same effects. In contrast, phenothiazines, butyrophenones, and the minor tranquilizers have little or no anticholinergic activity or associated blurred vision.

Abnormalities of the Lens, Retina, and Optic Nerve

Cataracts (loss of lens transparency) result from complications of old age (senile cataract), trauma, diabetes, myotonic dystrophy (Chapter 6), and, par-

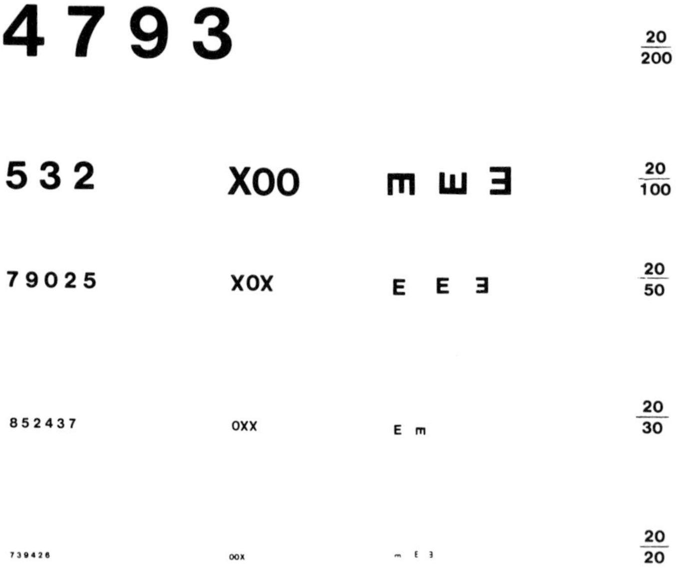

4 7 9 3 $\frac{20}{200}$

5 3 2   XOO   ⌶ ⫲ Ǝ $\frac{20}{100}$

7 9 0 2 5   XOX   E E Ǝ $\frac{20}{50}$

8 5 2 4 3 7   OXX   E m $\frac{20}{30}$

7 3 9 4 2 8   OOX   E Ǝ $\frac{20}{20}$

FIGURE 12–2. This hand-held visual acuity chart should be held 14 inches from the patient. The acuity is that line which can be read without a mistake. Each eye should be tested individually, and for neurologic evaluations, glasses or contact lenses should be worn.

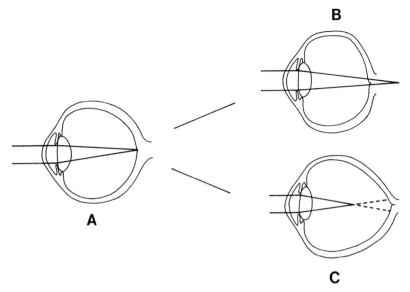

FIGURE 12–3. Image focusing in myopic and hyperopic eyes. *A,* In normal eyes, the lens focuses the image onto the retina. *B,* In hyperopic eyes, the shorter globe or improperly focusing lens causes the image to fall behind the retina. *C,* In myopic eyes, the longer globe or improperly focusing lens causes the image to fall in front of the retina.

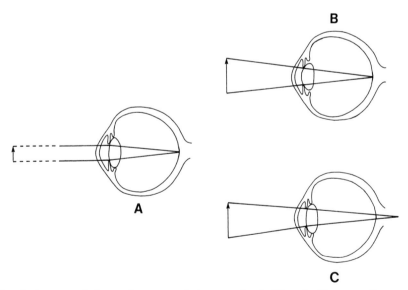

FIGURE 12–4. *A,* Accommodation and accommodation paresis: *A,* When looking at a distant object, parallel light rays are refracted slightly by a relatively flat lens onto the retina. *B,* Accommodation: When looking at a closely held object, ciliary muscle contraction increases the curvature of the lens, greatly refracting the light rays. *C,* Accommodation paresis: If the ciliary muscles are paretic, the lens cannot form a rounded shape. Its weakened refractive power can only focus the light rays from closely held objects behind the retina; however, parallel light rays from distant objects are still focused on the retina. Therefore, with accommodation paralysis, closely held objects will be blurred, but distant ones will be distinct.

ticularly, phenothiazines. For example, chlorpromazine (Thorazine) given in large doses, such as 300 mg daily for 2 years, induces minute opacities in the sclera, cornea, and lens. Fortunately, phenothiazine-induced cataracts rarely impair vision.

Pigmentary changes in the retina that can interfere with vision can be manifestations of congenital injuries, degenerative diseases, diabetes, or use of phenothiazines. Patients who have received thioridazine (Mellaril) in massive doses, such as 2,000 mg daily for 1 month, sometimes develop retinal pigment accumulations similar to those observed in retinitis pigmentosa (Fig. 12-5). However, phenothiazine-induced retinal pigmentary deposits usually cause no visual loss.

In contrast, optic nerve injuries almost always produce marked visual loss, and sometimes also psychiatric symptoms. One example is olfactory groove or sphenoid wing *meningiomas* (Chapter 19 and Fig. 20-5), which compress the adjacent optic nerve. When they grow into the frontal or temporal lobe, these tumors can trigger partial complex seizures and induce intellectual and personality changes. Another example is pituitary tumors, such as *adenomas* or *craniopharyngiomas*, which can grow upward to compress the optic chiasm and hypothalamus and downward to damage the pituitary gland (Fig. 19-4). Compression of the optic chiasm causes optic atrophy and bitemporal hemianopsia, and compression of the hypothalamus and pituitary causes headache, decreased libido, diabetes insipidus, and loss of secondary sexual characteristics.

Inflammation of the optic nerve, *optic* or *retrobulbar neuritis*, causes sudden, painful visual loss in one eye (Fig. 12-6). The pupil will usually have a preserved but diminished reaction to light (reactivity) during the initial attack. Since patients are usually otherwise in good health, the optic disk appears normal, and the pupil is still reactive, patients might be misdiagnosed as suffering from a psychogenic disturbance (Chapter 3). In fact, at least one third of optic

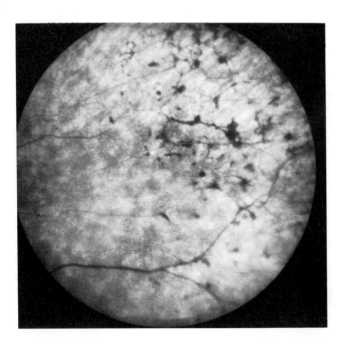

FIGURE 12–5. Hyperpigmentation that appears similar to black bone spicules is seen in retinal changes induced by thioridazine (Mellaril).

FIGURE 12–6. The long segment of the optic nerve behind the eye, the retrobulbar portion, is subject to multiple sclerosis and other inflammatory conditions. The resulting condition, called *optic* or *retrobulbar neuritis*, causes pain and loss of vision (Fig. 15-2). However, in the early stages, optic neuritis does not cause any observable change in the optic disk, which is the bulbar portion of the nerve.

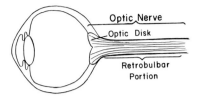

neuritis patients ultimately develop multiple sclerosis (Chapter 15). With recurrent optic neuritis attacks, whether or not part of multiple sclerosis, the optic nerve can become atrophic, the pupil unreactive, and the eye blind.

Another inflammatory condition of the optic nerve is *temporal*, or *giant cell*, *arteritis*. Typically affecting old people, it causes headaches, malaise, weight loss, and sometimes the appearance of depression. If temporal arteritis is not promptly treated with steroids, optic nerve and cerebral infarctions could ensue (Chapter 9). Finally, methanol intoxication, which occasionally occurs in alcoholics, and chronic papilledema, often from brain tumors or pseudotumor cerebri, are associated with optic atrophy, blindness, and sometiems mental aberrations.

GLAUCOMA

Glaucoma is characterized by elevated intraocular pressure because of decreased outflow of aqueous humor through the *filtration angle* of the anterior chamber of the eye (Fig. 12-7). Two common varieties, based on the configuration of the angle, are recognized, and one of them occasionally results from psychotropic medications. If either condition remained untreated, glaucoma would damage the optic nerve and cause irreparable visual loss.

Open-angle or *wide-angle glaucoma* occurs far more frequently than closed-angle glaucoma. It usually begins after the age of 40 years and often occurs in

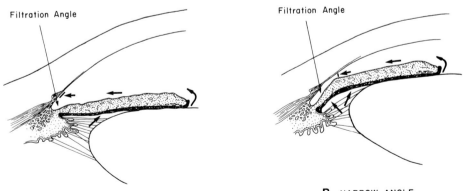

A OPEN ANGLE   **B** NARROW ANGLE

FIGURE 12–7. *A*, Open-angle glaucoma: The aqueous humor is not drained despite access to the absorptive surface of the angle. Impaired flow from the eye leads to gradually increased intraocular pressure (glaucoma). *B*, Narrow-angle glaucoma: When the iris is pushed forward, as may occur during pupil dilation, the angle is narrowed or even closed. Blockage of flow of aqueous humor, which usually occurs suddenly, leads to acute angle-closure glaucoma.

individuals who have family members with this variety of glaucoma. Since symptoms are usually absent at the onset, it might be diagnosed only by an ophthalmologist detecting elevated intraocular pressure. Later, when some vision is lost, the optic cup is abnormally deep and permanently damaged. The lack of symptoms in the initial phase of open-angle glaucoma is the primary reason why yearly ophthalmologic examinations that include measurements of intraocular pressure are recommended for all people older than 40 years. Open-angle glaucoma is usually responsive to topical medications (eye drops), such as pilocarpine, that constrict the pupil and improve aqueous outflow from the filtration angle. Other suitable topical medications, such as timolol (Timoptic), reduce the production of aqueous humor; however, this medication and others may be absorbed systemically and cause cardiovascular changes and psychologic aberrations. Marijuana reportedly lowers intraocular pressure, but standard topical medications are more effective. Because of the effectiveness of medications, open-angle glaucoma seldom requires surgical treatment.

Psychotropic medications do not precipitate open-angle glaucoma. Patients known to have it may be given heterocyclic antidepressants and other psychotropic medications as long as their glaucoma treatment is continued under the care of an ophthalmologist.

The other variety of glaucoma, *angle-closure, closed-angle,* or *narrow-angle glaucoma,* is characterized by elevation of intraocular pressure caused when the iris blocks the outflow of aqueous humor at the angle. Patients with narrow-angle glaucoma, like those with open-angle glaucoma, usually are older than 40 years and often have a family history, but they also have congenitally narrow angles. Only a few have had preceding symptoms, such as seeing halos around lights. In contrast to the relatively normal appearance of the eye in open-angle glaucoma, in acute angle-closure glaucoma, the vessels are engorged, the eye red, the pupil dilated, and the cornea hazy. Even more striking, the eye and forehead are painful, and vision is markedly impaired.

Prompt treatment is mandatory. Topical and systemic medications open the angle (by constricting the pupil) and also reduce the production of aqueous humor. In addition, surgery or laser iridectomy is usually necessary to create a passage for the aqueous humor directly through the iris to the angle.

In addition to developing spontaneously, angle-closure glaucoma is sometimes iatrogenic. For example, when the pupils are dilated for ocular examinations, the "bunched-up" iris can block the angle. Similarly, it can be precipitated by medications with anticholinergic properties, such as the heterocyclic antidepressants, because they also dilate the pupil. However, the incidence of glaucoma complicating antidepressant use is very low—far lower than the amount of discussion in the literature might lead one to expect.

Since measuring the intraocular pressure before medications are prescribed does not predict who will develop angle-closure glaucoma, few rules are practical. In general, everyone over the age of 40 years should have their intraocular pressure measured annually. As previously stated, patients who are already treated for either form of glaucoma may continue to receive psychotropic medications under ophthalmologic care. Individuals known to have narrow angles should be given antidepressants with caution.

From a different perspective, just as psychotropic medications can cause ocular problems, ophthalmologic medicines, when systemically absorbed, can cause psychiatric problems. In particular, medications with anticholinergic effects can induce frightening physical or psychologic symptoms, such as confusion or anxiety. Another example is the beta blocker timolol (Timoptic), which can cause lightheadedness, depression, or fatigue. Children are particularly susceptible. When they receive scopolamine and other atropine-like eye drops for ocular examination, they can develop agitation.

CORTICAL BLINDNESS AND RELATED PHENOMENA

Patients with cortical blindness do not perceive visual stimulation because of bilateral occipital lobe (visual cortex) damage. Cortical blindness usually results from devastating cerebral injuries, such as bilateral occlusion of the posterior cerebral arteries, occipital head trauma, cerebral anoxia, multiple cerebral infarctions, or multiple sclerosis. Notably, since the optic nerves and brainstem remain intact, the pupils of patients with cortical blindness are normal in size and reactivity to light.

Anton's Syndrome

An important psychologic ramification of cortical blindness is the dramatic phenomenon known as *Anton's syndrome.* In this condition, patients with cortical blindness not only insist that, or act as if, their vision is intact, but with prompting they also go on to "describe" their room, clothing, and various other objects. Its hallmarks are an implicit denial of blindness (similar to that in anosognosia) and the resultant confabulation. Anton's syndrome occurs most frequently in patients with preceding cognitive impairment and predominantly nondominant hemisphere damage. For example, an elderly gentleman, who has just sustained a posterior right cerebral infarction and had had a left posterior cerebral infarction the previous year, ascribed his inability to see the examiner's blouse first to poor lighting and then his disinterest in it. When pressed, still denying his blindness, he confabulated by calmly describing the garment as "lovely" or "attractive," and at times elaborating that it was a "dark, fine silk."

Agnosia

Another associated phenomenon, *visual agnosia*, is a perceptual inability to identify an object by sight despite an intact visual system and absence of aphasia and dementia. For example, patients with visual agnosia are unable to write or say the word "key" when a key is shown to them although they are able to make a drawing of it, describe its use, and say "key" when one is placed in their hand. Visual agnosia, which also results from cerebral cortical damage, differs from aphasia in that when vision is bypassed (when patients touch objects), language function is normal. Also, the site of the damage in visual agnosia is not as well established as in aphasia (Fig. 8-1).

Visual agnosia is a major aspect of the infamous, experimentally produced *Klüver-Bucy syndrome*, which is produced in monkeys by resection of both temporal lobes (Chapter 16). The loss of a good portion of their limbic system results in visual agnosia so severe that the monkeys not only touch all objects but they also put any object they wish to identify into their mouth ("psychic blindness"). Their behavior is repetitive, compulsive, and indiscriminate. Likewise, the human Klüver-Bucy syndrome induces a rough equivalent of psychic blindness, *oral exploration*, in which patients place inedible objects in or near their mouth. Compared to the monkeys, this tendency is muted. People only kiss, lick, or put common hospital or household objects into their mouth briefly, absentmindedly, and intermittently.

Color agnosia, a variety of visual agnosia that also results from damage to the cerebral cortex, is an inability to identify (by speaking or writing) an object's color despite a normal ability to match colored cards, read Ishihara plates (pseudoisochromatic numbered cards), and say the colors of well-known objects, such as the sky. It differs from common color blindness, which is a sex-linked inherited retinal abnormality. In another variety, *prosopagnosia*, patients with bilateral occipitotemporal lesions cannot recognize *familiar* faces, although they can identify people by voice, dress, mannerisms, and other nonfacial characteristics (Chapter 8). Patients with right cerebral lesions are said to have impaired ability to match pairs of pictures of *unfamiliar* faces, and these patients do worse than those with left hemisphere lesions in attempting to identify pictures of people that are taken from different angles (the Facial Recognition Test). This deficit is probably a manifestation of visuospatial impairments that result from nondominant parietal lobe lesions (Chapter 8). Overall, visual agnosia, its varieties, alexia, and anomias are apt, in clinical practice, to be found almost only in combination with other neurologic deficits.

Psychogenic Blindness

A completely different situation is *psychogenic blindness*. Neurologists go to great lengths to diagnose this disorder even though it is usually self-limited, rare, and not indicative of major psychopathology. An uninhibited examiner simply might make child-like facial contortions or ask the patient to read some four-letter words. The patient's reaction to these provocations would reveal an ability to see. When only one eye is affected by psychogenic blindness, colored or polarized lenses will often confuse (or fatigue) a patient into revealing that vision is present. A vertically striped cylinder (drum) spun in front of any patient with a normal visual system will produce involuntary (*opticokinetic*) nystagmus. Likewise, looking at a large, moving mirror forces anyone with normal vision to follow visually the movement of their own image. Visual evoked response (VER) testing can show diagnostically helpful electrical potentials (Chapter 15). Alternatively, having patients wear lenses with negligible optical value may also reveal their normal vision. Also, this maneuver may permit patients to extract themselves from psychogenic blindness without embarrassment.

A special disturbance is *tubular or tunnel vision* (Fig. 12-8), a pattern inconsistent with the laws of optics, which dictate that the visual area expands with increasing distance. An important exception to this law, however, is the classic migraine (Chapter 9), which can cause peripheral vision constriction and make it appear to patients that they are looking through tubes.

Nonpsychogenic Visual Hallucinations

Visual hallucinations can sometimes result from a seizure or other abnormal stimulation of the visual cortex (see Table 9-3). The visions tend to be repetitive

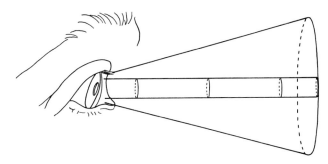

FIGURE 12–8. The area seen by a person normally increases conically in proportion to the distance from the object. In *tubular* or *tunnel vision*, which defies the laws of optics, the visual area is constant despite increasing distance.

and stereotyped for the individual. Partial *elementary* seizures, which originate in the occipital lobe (Chapter 10), induce hallucinations that are "seen" in both eyes and usually consist of displays of brightly colored, slowly moving simple geometric forms lasting from a few seconds to several minutes. The displays can develop during sleep and appear within an area of hemianopsia. In contrast, partial *complex* seizures, which usually result from temporal lobe discharges, are apt to cause detailed but often fragmented visions in which objects appear distorted. In addition, these hallucinations are often accompanied by related sounds, thoughts, and emotions and, characteristically, impairment of consciousness. A typical visual hallucination from a partial complex seizure might be a glimpse of the stripes of the American flag and a few notes of *God Bless America*. The experience would be similar from seizure to seizure and might reoccur several times in a day.

Hallucinations can also be associated with narcolepsy. In this case, they are essentially dreams that have intruded into a patient's consciousness. They occur upon falling asleep (hypnagogic) or awakening (hypnopompic) and are associated with the flaccid, areflexic paresis characteristic of dream-filled (REM) sleep (Chapter 17). Characteristically, the hallucinations, like dreams, are composed of varied sounds, rich thoughts, and strong emotions, as well as intricate visions.

Classic migraine headaches, in which the visual cortex may be irritated by ischemia, are usually preceded by crescentic scotomata with scintillating borders that enlarge and move slowly across the visual field (Fig. 9-2). Most scotomata last from 1 to 20 minutes before yielding to the actual headache, but sometimes they are the sole manifestation of a migraine. In some cases, patients have visual aberrations associated with nonmigrainous conditions, such as an homonymous hemianopsia, which is associated with middle cerebral artery infarctions.

Visual hallucinations are caused by many illicit drugs, such as mescaline and lysergic acid diethylamide (LSD), alcohol, and numerous medicines, including scopolamine, atropine, cimetidine, propranolol, and L-dopa (Sinemet). Likewise, *delirium tremens*, or DTs, caused by alcohol withdrawal, consists of visual hallucinations accompanied by agitated confusion (delirium), sweating, and tachycardia. Typically, these substance-induced hallucinations are accompanied by psychologic and physical excitement.

Finally, visual hallucinations can be produced by any sudden visual loss. Those from cortical blindness, namely Anton's syndrome, are one example. Another is that of soldiers who, following eye wounds, have periods of "seeing" brightly colored forms and even entire scenes. Similarly, eye surgery in the elderly is occasionally followed by visual hallucinations, disorientation, and agitation. Some physicians suggest that this complication results from spontaneously discharging unstimulated cortical neurons, whereas others believe that it results from sensory deprivation superimposed on dementia. Whatever the reason, bilateral ophthalmologic surgical procedures in the elderly should be avoided.

VISUAL FIELD LOSS

Visual field loss patterns (Fig. 12-9) are a reliable guide to the location of a lesion. And the location, in turn, suggests the cause. In general, the following rules apply.

Monocular quadrantanopsias, hemianopsias, scotomata, and blindness are usually the result of optic nerve injury.

Homonymous quadrantanopsias and hemianopsias almost always result from visual tract injuries between the optic chiasm and the occipital cortex (Fig. 4-1). The most common situation is a middle cerebral artery infarction that results in a contralateral homonymous hemianopsia accompanied by hemiparesis and hemisensory loss. An homonymous superior quadrantanopsia (Fig. 12-10), although rare, is noteworthy because it may be the only physical manifestation of a contralateral temporal lobe lesion that produces partial complex seizures. Another noteworthy loss is an homonymous hemianopsia that excludes the center of vision (macular sparing) because it is said to be diagnostic of occipital lobe lesions. However, this rule has been challenged, and even if true, it is an impractical guide because such fine visual field determinations are beyond the ability of a nonspecialist.

The visual field loss most commonly associated with mental aberrations is the left homonymous hemianopsia. It is often accompanied by left sensory

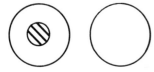

LEFT CENTRAL SCOTOMA

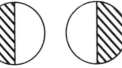

BITEMPORAL HEMIANOPSIA

BITEMPORAL SUPERIOR QUADRANTANOPSIA

LEFT HOMONYMOUS HEMIANOPSIA

FIGURE 12–9. Uniocular *central scotomata* may be caused by migraine attacks, optic neuritis, or other ipsilateral optic nerve injuries. *Bitemporal superior quadrantanopsia* is usually caused by lesions of the optic chiasm, such as pituitary adenomas or craniopharyngiomas. *Bitemporal hemianopsias* are caused by more advanced compression of the optic chiasm by the same lesions. *Homonymous hemianopsias*, with or without macular sparing, are most often caused by contralateral cerebral lesions, such as infarctions.

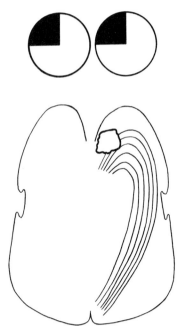

FIGURE 12–10. Large anterior temporal lobe lesions may interfere with forward-sweeping optic tract fibers. Thus, these lesions, which are rare, may cause a contralateral superior quadrantanopsia, as well as partial complex seizures.

inattention, visuospatial impairments, and, when left hemiparesis is present, anosognosia (Chapter 8 and Fig. 2-8).

Bitemporal quadrantanopsias and hemianopsias indicate a lesion at the optic chiasm. The vast majority are pituitary adenomas, which, as discussed previously, compress the optic chiasm, cause optic atrophy, and lead to hypopituitarism.

CONJUGATE OCULAR MOVEMENT

Both eyes move together in a paired, coordinated (*conjugate*) manner so that people can look laterally and can follow moving objects. Abnormalities in the conjugate ocular movement system are often prominent manifestations of neurologic injury. Also, subtle abnormalities have been associated with psychiatric illnesses.

Conjugate ocular movement originates in *cerebral conjugate gaze centers* located in the frontal lobes. When a person is at rest, each cerebral center continuously emits impulses that go through a complicated pathway to move the eyes contralaterally. Since the effect of each center is counterbalanced, the eyes remain midline (Fig. 12-11). When a person wants to look to one side, the contralateral cerebral gaze center becomes increasingly active. For example, when someone wants to look toward an object on the right, the impulses of the left cerebral gaze center increase, and as if it pushes the eyes away, the eyes turn to the right. If this person also wanted to reach for the object, the left cerebral corticospinal center, which is adjacent to the gaze center, would mobilize the right arm.

The activity of the conjugate gaze center is increased during partial seizures. Not only do partial seizures cause the eyes to move contralaterally but since they usually envelop the adjacent corticospinal tract, they can also deviate the head contralaterally and produce tonic-clonic activity of the contralateral limbs.

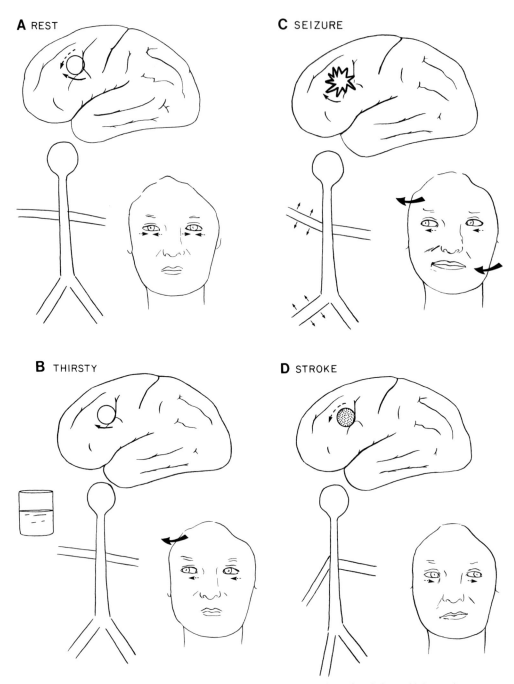

FIGURE 12–11. *A*, At rest, the eyes are midline because the impulses of each frontal lobe conjugate gaze center are balanced, each "pushing" the eyes contralaterally. *B*, Voluntarily increased activity of the left cerebral gaze center drives the eyes to the right (contralaterally). *C*, Involuntarily increased cerebral activity also drives the eyes contralaterally. Also, with left cerebral seizure activity, the right arm and leg develop tonic-clonic activity. *D*, A CVA destroys the left cerebral gaze center, permitting the right center to push the eyes toward the lesion. It also destroys the cerebral motor strip, causing contralateral paresis. This common CVA is characterized by the eyes "looking" away from the hemiparesis.

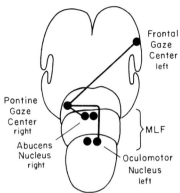

FIGURE 12–12. When looking to the right, the left frontal conjugate gaze center stimulates the right (contralateral) pontine gaze center, which, in turn, stimulates the right (adjacent) abducens nerve nucleus and, through the left medial longitudinal fasciculus, the left (contralateral) oculomotor nerve nucleus.

By contrast, when patients have unilateral destructive cerebral injuries, such as cerebrovascular accidents (CVAs), the activity of the gaze center on that side is reduced, and the activity of the other center, being unopposed, pushes the eyes toward the injured side. For example, with a left cerebral infarction, the eyes deviate toward the left, and since the corticospinal tract is generally involved, the right side of the body is paralyzed. This example illustrates the sayings, "When the eyes look away from the paralysis, the stroke is cerebral" and "The eyes look toward the stroke."

Each cerebral gaze center works by stimulating a contralateral *pontine gaze center*. In contrast to the cerebral center, each pontine center pulls the eyes toward its own side (Fig. 12-12). Thus, a pontine infarction allows the eyes to be pulled toward the opposite side. For example, if the right pontine gaze center were damaged, the eyes would deviate to the left. In addition, because the right pontine corticospinal tract would be damaged, the left limbs would be paralyzed. With a pontine lesion, the eyes "look toward the paralysis."

Each pontine gaze center stimulates the adjacent abducens nucleus and, through the *medial longitudinal fasciculus (MLF)* (Figs. 15-3 and 15-4), the contralateral oculomotor nucleus. Innervation of one abducens nucleus and

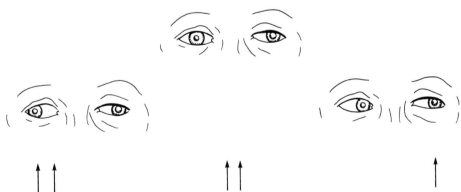

FIGURE 12–13. Left oculomotor (third cranial) nerve palsy. In the *center picture*, a patient looks ahead. The left upper lid is lower, the pupil larger, and the eye deviated slightly laterally. Since the eyes are dysconjugate, the patient sees two arrows (diplopia) when looking ahead. In the *picture on the left*, the patient looks to the right. Since the paretic left eye fails to cross medially beyond the midline (i.e., it fails to adduct), the eyes are more dysconjugate, and there is greater diplopia. In the *picture on the right*, the patient looks to the left. The eyes are almost conjugate, and there is little or no diplopia.

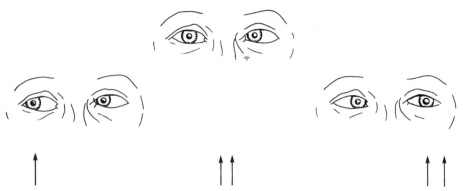

FIGURE 12–14. A left abducens (sixth cranial) nerve palsy. In the *center picture*, a patient looks ahead. The patient's left eye is deviated medially. The eyes are dysconjugate, and the patient sees two arrows when looking ahead. In the *picture on the left*, the patient looks to the right. The eyes are conjugate, and the patient sees only a single arrow. In the *picture on the right*, the patient looks to the left. The paretic left eye fails to cross the midline laterally, i.e., it fails to abduct. The exaggeration of the dysconjugate gaze increases the diplopia.

the other oculomotor nucleus is necessary for conjugate lateral eye movement. If both abducens nuclei were simultaneously stimulated, both eyes would turn outward, and if both oculomotor nuclei were stimulated, both eyes would turn inward. When the MLF is injured, as often occurs in MS and brainstem CVAs, the *MLF syndrome (internuclear ophthalmoplegia)* develops. In this condition, the cranial nuclei and nerves are normal, but the eyes cannot move conjugately (Chapter 15).

Another important ocular movement abnormality is *nystagmus* (rhythmic horizontal or, less often, vertical or rotatory eyeball oscillation). Although nystagmus is often caused by labyrinthitis, in many cases it is caused by various neurologic injuries, including multiple sclerosis, brainstem infarction, Wernicke-Korsakoff syndrome, alcohol intoxication, and drug use. Therefore, the presence of nystagmus can suggest that patients are taking diazepam (Valium), barbiturates, or other hypnotic medications. Also, since nystagmus is routinely found in seizure patients who take therapeutic doses of phenytoin (Dilantin) or phenobarbital, its absence suggests noncompliance with an anticonvulsant regimen.

Ocular movement disturbances have also been described in patients with schizophrenia and, less frequently, affective psychosis. Such patients have been found to have abnormalities in conjugate ocular movements when tracking rapidly moving targets (*smooth pursuit eye movements*). The smooth pursuit abnormality, which does not appear to be caused by either inattention or medication, is postulated to originate in a disorder "above" the pontine gaze center. Similar smooth pursuit eye movement abnormalities have been reported in patients with Huntington's disease (Chapter 18). These ocular movement impairments have been linked to dopamine excess.

DIPLOPIA

Diplopia ("double vision") is rarely the result of ocular abnormalities, such as a dislocated lens. Instead, it is almost always caused by neurologic disorders, including oculomotor or abducens cranial nerve injury, brainstem (but not cerebral) infarction, and extraocular muscle paresis. Sometimes, however, it can be psychogenic.

Oculomotor (third cranial) nerve injury results in ptosis, pupil dilation, lateral deviation of the eye, and diplopia that is greatest when the patient looks away from the resting position of the eyes (Fig. 12-13). Abducens (sixth cranial) nerve injury results in medial deviation of the eye and diplopia when looking laterally, but neither in ptosis nor pupil abnormality (Fig. 12-14).

Although diplopia is frequently the result of cranial nerve injury, several conditions are important variations. When myopic adults read or drive while fatigued, they develop momentary diplopia because of ocular muscle fatigue. Also, myasthenia gravis causes diplopia, which is initially transient and never associated with pupil abnormalities (Chapter 6).

On the other hand, although congenital ocular muscle weakness, *strabismus*, causes dysconjugate gaze, children do not have diplopia because the brain suppresses the image from the weaker eye. However, with continuous suppression of the vision of that eye, the eye will actually become blind (*amblyopic*). Thus, babies and children with a "crossed" or "lazy eye" often have the "good" eye patched several hours each day to force them to use the visual and muscle systems of the weak eye.

Finally, patients can have psychogenic diplopia. Usually, it is intermittent and in all directions of gaze. There is, of course, no observable abnormality. Nonetheless, physicians must be careful not to overlook subtle neurologic conditions, especially myasthenia gravis and internuclear ophthalmoplegia. In another psychogenic disturbance, children or young adults, as if looking at the tip of their nose, fix their eyes in a downward and inward position. This ocular movement is a burlesque that can be overcome by inducing opticokinetic nystagmus.

HORNER'S SYNDROME AND ARGYLL-ROBERTSON PUPILS

Horner's syndrome, which consists of ptosis, miosis, and anhidrosis, should not be confused with an oculomotor nerve injury even though ptosis is the most prominent sign of both conditions (Fig. 12-15). In Horner's syndrome there is neither impairment of ocular motility nor diplopia, and the pupil of the affected eye is small. Moreover, the syndrome results from injury to the sympathetic tract anywhere along its roundabout course. The sympathetic nerves begin in

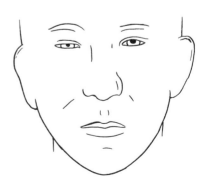

FIGURE 12–15. Horner's syndrome, which may be found in brainstem, spinal cord, carotid artery, or thoracic lesions, consists of miosis (a small pupil), ptosis, and, with special testing, anhidrosis (loss of sweating).

the brainstem, descend in the cervical spinal cord, ascend through the chest, and, wrapped around the carotid artery, finally innervate the pupil, eyelid, and facial sweat glands. Thus, Horner's syndrome can be caused by lateral medullary infarctions (Wallenberg's syndrome); cervical spinal cord injury; apical lung (Pancoast's) tumors; and, because of a carotid artery abnormality, cluster headaches.

Argyll-Robertson pupils, which also must be differentiated from oculomotor nerve injury, are irregular, asymmetric, and small (1–2 mm). In addition, they are characteristically unreactive to light but do constrict normally when patients look at closely held objects, i.e., during accommodation. The impaired light reflex with intact accommodation has given rise to the saying, "Argyll-Robertson pupils are like prostitutes; they accommodate but do not react." Although Argyll-Robertson pupils have historically been a manifestation of syphilis, the majority of cases today result from diabetic autonomic neuropathy.

REFERENCES

Abramowicz M (ed): Amoxapine (Ascendin). Med Letter *23*:39, 1981
Abramowicz M (ed): Maprotiline (Ludiomil). Med Letter *23*:58, 1981
Abramowicz M (ed): Trazodone (Desyrel). Med Letter *24*:47, 1982
Aldrich MS, Alessi AG, Beck RW, et al: Cortical blindness: Etiology, diagnosis, and prognosis. Ann Neurol *21*:149, 1987
Asaad G, Shapiro B: Hallucinations: Theoretical and clinical overview. Am J Psychiatry *143*:1088, 1986
Bauer RM, Rubens AB: Agnosia. In Heilman KM, Valenstein E (eds): Clinical Neuropsychology, 2nd ed. New York, Oxford University Press, 1985
Damasio AR, Damasio H, Hoesen GWV: Prosopagnosia: Anatomic basis and behavioral mechanisms. Neurology *32*:331, 1982
Hamilton JD: Thioridazine retinopathy within upper dosage limit. Psychosomatics *26*:823, 1985
Keane JR: Neuro-ophthalmic signs and symptoms of hysteria. Neurology *32*:757, 1982
Lieberman E, Stoudemire A: Use of tricyclic antidepressants in patients with glaucoma. Psychosomatics *28*:145, 1987
Lipton RB, Levy DL, Holzman PS, et al: Eye movement dysfunctions in psychiatric patients: A review. Schizophr Bull *9*:13, 1983
Reid WH, Rakes S: Intraocular pressure in patients receiving psychotropic medications. Psychosomatic *24*:665, 1983
Remick RA: Anticholinergic side effects of tricyclic antidepressants and their management. Prog Neuro-Psychopharmacol Biol Psychiatry *12*:225, 1988
Rizzo JF, Lessell S: Risk of developing multiple sclerosis after uncomplicated optic neuritis: A long-term prospective study. Neurology *38*:185, 1988
Siever LJ, Haier RJ, Coursey RD, et al: Smooth pursuit eye tracking impairment. Arch Gen Psychiatry *39*:1001, 1982

QUESTIONS: CHAPTER 12

1. Which findings characterize Argyll-Robertson pupils?
   a.   Miosis
   b.   Ptosis
   c.   Irregular shape
   d.   Unreactivity to light
   e.   Unresponsiveness to accommodation

2. Which medications are associated with transient visual impairment because of accommodation paresis?
   a.   Butyrophenones
   b.   Amitriptyline

    c. Imipramine
    d. Phenobarbital
    e. Phenytoin

3. Which of the following cause cataracts that interfere with vision?
    a. Myotonic dystrophy
    b. Diabetes mellitus
    c. Ocular trauma
    d. Chlorpromazine

4. A 20-year-old soldier develops loss of vision in the right eye. The eye is painful, especially when moved voluntarily. No ocular or neurologic abnormalities are found, except for a relative decrease in light reaction in the right eye. After 1 week, vision returns, except for a small central scotoma. What illness is he likely to have had?

5. What is the prognosis in the case presented in question 4?

6. Which laboratory procedure will identify dysfunction of the optic nerve in patients with clinical symptoms and signs indicative of multiple sclerosis and also help distinguish patients with visual impairments from those with psychogenic impairments?

7. What are the characteristics of open- or wide-angle glaucoma?
    a. Chronicity
    b. Acute onset
    c. Hereditary predisposition
    d. Onset after age 40
    e. Raised intraocular pressure
    f. Precipitated by tricyclic antidepressant medications
    g. Absolute contraindication to use of tricyclic antidepressant medications
    h. Usually responsive to ocular or systemic medical therapy

8. What are the characteristics of closed- or narrow-angle glaucoma?
    a. Chronicity
    b. Acute onset
    c. Hereditary predisposition
    d. Onset after age 40
    e. Painful eye
    f. "Steamy" cornea
    g. Headache
    h. Precipitated by antidepressant medications
    i. Surgical treatment

9. Should patients with closed- or narrow-angle glaucoma be given tricyclic antidepressant medications?

10–15. Match the usual field loss (10–15) with the underlying illness (a–f) [answers may be used more than once]:

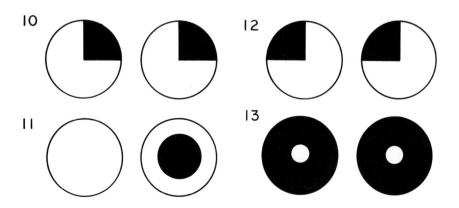

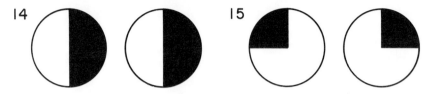

a. A 25-year-old woman has paraparesis and ataxia.
b. A 35-year-old woman has insidious onset of loss of peripheral daytime vision and all nighttime vision. Her mother has a similar illness.
c. A 30-year-old man has episodes of seeing the American flag and hearing the first five bars of "America the Beautiful."
d. A 21-year-old man has loss of bodily hair, gynecomastia, and diabetes insipidus.
e. A 70-year-old man has global aphasia and right hemiplegia and hemisensory loss.
f. A 75-year-old man has fluent (receptive, Wernicke's) aphasia.

16–26. Match the characteristics of the visual hallucination with the source.

16. Associated musical hallucinations

17. Flashes of bright lights in the contralateral visual field

18. Associated olfactory hallucinations

19. Rotating blotches of color

20. Formed hallucinations with impaired consciousness

21. Postictal aphasia

22. Throbbing unilateral headache

23. Nausea and vomiting

24. Simple blocks and stars of color

25. Twisting, complicated multicolored lights

26. Faces with distorted features or coloring
    a. Seizures that originate in the occipital lobe
    b. Seizures that originate in the temporal lobe
    c. Classic migraine headaches

27–28. Match the symptom (27–28) with the possible origins (a–d).

27. Diplopia when looking to the right

28. Diplopia when looking to the left
    a. Left third nerve palsy
    b. Left sixth nerve palsy
    c. Right third nerve palsy
    d. Right sixth nerve palsy

29–30. Match the actions that cause blindness with the etiology.

29. Staring directly into the sun

30. Drinking nonethanol alcohols
    a. Methanol optic nerve injury
    b. Pigmentary retinal degeneration
    c. Retinal burns

31. What are the common causes of ptosis?
    a. Third nerve palsy
    b. Sixth nerve palsy

    c. Pancoast tumor
    d. Multiple sclerosis
    e. Myasthenia gravis
    f. Hysteria

32. What are the common causes of internuclear ophthalmoplegia?
    a. Multiple sclerosis
    b. Polio
    c. Muscular dystrophy
    d. Hysteria
    e. Heroin overdose
    f. Brainstem cerebrovascular infarctions

33. Which abnormality is reported to occur in patients with schizophrenia and, to a lesser extent, affective psychosis?
    a. Internuclear ophthalmoplegia
    b. Nystagmus
    c. Ptosis
    d. Conjugate gaze paresis
    e. Smooth pursuit abnormalities

34. A 70-year-old man awakens with a right hemiparesis, vertigo, and his eyes deviated to the right. Which of the following conditions will also be found?
    a. Aphasia
    b. Right homonymous hemianopsia
    c. Dementia
    d. Nystagmus

35. Which conditions indicate that the dopamine system is involved in conjugate eye movement?
    a. Internuclear ophthalmoplegia
    b. Nystagmus
    c. Pontine gaze center movement
    d. Oculogyric crisis

36. Which conditions have a predilection for people older than 65 years?
    a. Myopia
    b. Presbyopia arteritis
    c. Macular degeneration
    d. Classic migraines
    e. Temporal or giant cell arteritis
    f. Glaucoma
    g. Cataracts
    h. Optic neuritis

37. A 70-year-old man suffers a cerebral infarction. Afterward, he has a right homonymous hemianopsia, right hemisensory loss, and a mild right hemiparesis. Although he can both say and write the names of objects that he feels, he has a peculiar inability to name objects that he only sees, even when they are presented to his left visual field. What is the name of this condition and where is the lesion located?

38. Match the visual disturbance with the etiology.
    1. Psychic blindness   a. Carotid stenosis
    2. Night blindness   b. Occipital infarction
    3. Cortical blindness   c. Conversion reaction
    4. Transient monocular blindness   d. Bilateral temporal lobe injury
                                 e. Vitamin A deficiency

39–46. Match the condition (39–46) with the neuropsychologic condition (a–j).

39. Cannot recognize familiar faces

40. Despite visual loss, willfully but erroneously describes hospital room and physician

41. Following cardiac arrest, blindness with normal pupil light reflex. In addition, although alert, mental impairment is prominent

42. Cannot identify a red card, although able to match it to another red card and read a red-colored number on the Ishihara plates

43. Despite only a right homonymous hemianopsia, inability to read. Writing ability is normal.

44. Congenital inability to read Ishihara plates

45. Inability to name common objects under any circumstances

46. Cannot name objects when seen, but can name objects when described or felt
   a.   Cortical blindness
   b.   Visual agnosia
   c.   Color agnosia
   d.   Color blindness
   e.   Prosopagnosia
   f.   Anton's syndrome
   g.   Wernicke-Korsakoff syndrome
   h.   Alexia without agraphia
   i.   Congenital cerebral injury
   j.   Aphasia

ANSWERS

1.   a, c, d.

2.   b, c.

3.   a, b, c.

.   He probably had an episode of optic neuritis.

5.   Most patients who have optic neuritis have no recurrences. However, about one third of male patients and three quarters of female patients later develop multiple sclerosis.

6.   Visual evoked responses (VER), which are essentially analyses of the EEG when light is shown into the subject's eyes, will indicate the presence and location of impairment of the visual system. It is a sensitive procedure that permits detection of asymptomatic optic nerve lesions.

7.   a, c, d, e, h.

8.   b, c, d, e, f, g, h, i.

9.   Patients with closed- or narrow-angle glaucoma may take tricyclic antidepressants once therapy for glaucoma has been instituted.

10.   c. The patient may have partial complex (e.g., psychomotor) seizures and a right superior quadrantanopsia as the result of a left temporal lobe lesion. *or* f. The patient may have a left temporal lobe lesion giving him aphasia and a contralateral superior quadrantanopsia.

11.   a. The patient has spinal cord, cerebellar, and right optic nerve injury, probably as the result of multiple sclerosis.

12.   c. The patient may have psychomotor seizures and a left superior quadrantanopsia as the result of a right temporal lobe lesion.

13.   b. The patient and her mother have preservation only of the central vision during daytime. If examination of her fundi showed clumping of retinal pigment, the diagnosis of retinitis pigmentosa would be certain. These visual fields might also be obtained from someone having tunnel vision.

14. e. The patient probably has a dominant hemisphere lesion, such as a cerebrovascular accident or tumor, giving a right homonymous hemianopsia.

15. d. The patient has a large pituitary tumor causing panhypopituitarism and bitemporal hemianopsia.

16. b.	**25.** b, c.
17. a, c.	**26.** b, c.
18. b.	**27.** a, d.
19. a.	**28.** b, c.
20. b.	**29.** c.
21. b.	**30.** a.
22. c.	**31.** a, c, e.
23. c.	**32.** a, f.
24. a, c.	

33. e. These patients are reported to have smooth pursuit abnormalities. Also, since they are heavily medicated, they may have oculogyric crises.

34. d. This patient has an infarction in the left brainstem at the pontine level. Thus, he would not have signs of cerebral injury, such as aphasia, hemianopsia, or mental impairment. He would have nystagmus. Also, injury to the left facial and abducens nerve nuclei would result in left upper and lower facial paresis and medial deviation of the left eye.

35. d. Oculogyric crises are precipitated by phenothiazines, including those used for nonpsychotic conditions, such as nausea and vomiting.

36. b, c, e, f, g. The prevalence of these conditions, which are readily found in a large number of people, will increase astronomically as the population ages. Combinations of these conditions may occur together in the same older person. Whatever the cause of a visual impairment, it is a major threat to the mental well-being of older people, especially those with intellectual or emotional impairment or other sensory deprivations.

37. The lesion is probably in the left parietal and occipital region. The patient has visual agnosia, a condition in which patients cannot process visually acquired information. Additional testing might reveal Gerstmann's syndrome or alexia without agraphia (Chapter 7)—conditions also resulting from posterior dominant hemisphere lesions. His problem is not aphasia because language function is normal as evidenced, once vision is circumvented, by his normal writing and speaking ability.

38. 1–d (Klüver-Bucy syndrome); 2-e; 3-b; 4-a (amaurosis fugax).

39. e.

40. f.

41. a.

42. c.

43. h.

44. d.

45. j.

46. b.

13

Congenital Cerebral Injuries

Many common congenital neurologic disorders that cause lifelong physical and mental impairment can be readily diagnosed by routine clinical evaluation. Such disorders include varieties of cerebral palsy and neurocutaneous disturbances. By contrast, the brain injuries said to cause hyperactivity and certain learning disabilities are often so difficult to define that their nature remains controversial.

CEREBRAL PALSY

Cerebral palsy (CP)* is a nonscientific but generally accepted descriptive term for the permanent neurologic *motor system* impairments that result from cerebral injuries sustained in utero, during infancy, or in early childhood. Characteristically, children and adults with CP suffer from spastic paresis of the limbs, a choreoathetotic movement disorder, or both. In addition, depending upon the variety of CP, they frequently, but not necessarily, have mental retardation, seizures, or other concomitants of cerebral injury. After childhood, the particular handicap changes little as the child grows into adult life. In other words, the CP deficits are static or nonprogressive. Although the cause of CP can be any condition that damages the brain from gestation through age 5 years, in most cases CP is associated with prematurity, low birth weight, anoxia during delivery, or neonatal hyperbilirubinemia. Recent medical advances that prevent or treat these conditions have been responsible for the decline in incidence to 1 per 1,000 live births. Nevertheless, thousands of adults as well as children are handicapped by cerebral injuries that occurred perinatally.

During the clinical evaluation, the physician might accept as diagnostic of CP a history of perinatal cerebral injury followed by a permanent, relatively stable motor impairment (Table 13-1). In these cases, it is not always necessary to perform CT, MRI, EEG, or other tests. Rather, the physician should concentrate on the problem at hand and evaluate the patient's mental and physical abilities (Table 13-2). *Since many patients with CP have normal intelligence, despite major motor*

---

* Patients with cerebral palsy or virtually any brain injury before age 5 years may receive assistance from the United Cerebral Palsy Foundation, 66 East 34th Street, New York, New York 10016, (212) 481-6300. Patients with neurocutaneous disorders may receive assistance from the Tuberous Sclerosis Association of America, P.O. Box 44, Rockland, Massachusetts 02370, (617) 947-8893; or the National Tuberous Sclerosis Association, 4351 Garden City Drive, Landover, Maryland 20785, (301) 459-9888; and The National Neurofibromatosis Foundation, 14l Fifth Avenue, Suite 7S, New York, New York 10010, (212) 460-8980.

**TABLE 13–1. HISTORICAL FEATURES OF
CEREBRAL PALSY**

Description of deficit
  Motor impairment
    Paresis: extent, degree
    Movement disorder: nature, age of onset
  Delayed acquisition of motor skills
  Associated conditions
    Mental retardation
    Seizures
Search for cause
  Maternal health
    Personal or familial neurologic illness
    Prenatal illness or abnormalities
      Infections, medications, etc.
      Vaginal bleeding, paucity of fetal movements
  Delivery
    Prematurity
    Low weight for date
    Prolonged labor, fetal distress
    Obstetric complications
  Neonatal period
    Low Apgar score
    Cyanosis, unresponsiveness
    Seizures
    Jaundice

deficits, movement disorders, and hearing impairments, the physician should never conclude that a person has mental impairment or retardation without full, detailed, and specialized mental status evaluations.

Varieties of CP

Of the many clinical varieties of CP, the two that occur most commonly and have the greatest descriptive value are *spastic* and *extrapyramidal* (choreoathetotic) CP. Each has a characteristic motor impairment and a predictable association with seizures and mental retardation.

TABLE 13–2. PHYSICAL FINDINGS OF CEREBRAL PALSY (CP)

Motor Deficits
  Signs of spastic CP
    Gross impairment: paresis/spasticity, growth arrest, pseudobulbar palsy
    Subtle impairment: unequal size of hands or feet, toe walking (from shortened heel cords),
      hand preference, e.g., right-handedness before the age of 18 months
  Signs of extrapyramidal CP
    Choreoathetosis
    Chorea: intermittent, rapid, jerky involuntary movements of the shoulders and hips
    Athetosis: continual, slow, writhing involuntary movements of the hands and feet
Associated conditions
  Intellectual impairment, i.e., mental retardation
  Seizures (generalized, focal motor or psychomotor)
  Impairment of special senses
    Visual: strabismus, myopia, blindness
    Auditory: deafness
    Vocal: dysarthria

Spastic CP, which accounts for approximately 70 percent of cases, is characterized by paralysis with marked muscular hypertonicity (spasticity). Since the paralysis results from cerebral damage, it is invariably accompanied by hyperactive DTRs, clonus, and Babinski signs. Also, since cerebral damage has occurred before childhood growth, the affected extremities are characteristically foreshortened, i.e., have *growth arrest*. The spasticity and growth arrest create as much disability as the paresis.

Subcategories of spastic CP are based on the pattern of deficit: diplegic (paresis of both legs), hemiplegic (arm and leg), and quadriplegic (all limbs). More extensive cerebral damage causes more extensive paresis, a greater incidence of seizures, and more severe mental retardation.

Diplegic CP is symmetric paresis, primarily of the legs (Fig. 13-1). Patients display toe walking and a scissors gait because of the spasticity. Short tendons keep the knees, ankles, and toes straight, drawn together (adducted), and pointed downward (extended). The usual cause of spastic diplegia is prematurity and low birth weight, leading to periventricular injury that damages the corticospinal tract fibers of the legs (Fig. 7-7). Since cerebral damage is relatively mild and limited, both seizures and mental retardation occur in only about 25 percent of cases, which is much less frequent than in the other forms of spastic CP. Recent developments in neonatal intensive care have greatly reduced the incidence of this form of CP.

Hemiplegic CP is spastic hemiparesis that usually affects the face and the arm more than the leg (Fig. 13-2). Hemiplegic cerebral palsy patients resemble adults with middle cerebral artery occlusions, but they have growth arrest of the affected limbs. In particular, their thumb and great-toe nail beds will be smaller on the paretic side. Also, a contracted Achilles tendon forces them to walk on the toes of the affected foot. Another feature of hemiplegic CP is abnormal early development of hand preference, e.g., right-handedness.

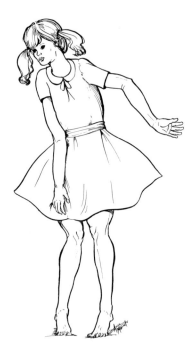

FIGURE 13–1. Spastic diplegia. This 10-year-old girl with low-normal intelligence has straightening and in-turning of the legs, a tiptoe stance, and scissors-like gait. She also has uncoordinated, awkward movements of her arms (posturings).

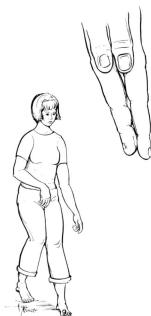

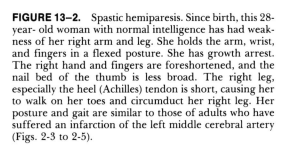

FIGURE 13–2. Spastic hemiparesis. Since birth, this 28-year-old woman with normal intelligence has had weakness of her right arm and leg. She holds the arm, wrist, and fingers in a flexed posture. She has growth arrest. The right hand and fingers are foreshortened, and the nail bed of the thumb is less broad. The right leg, especially the heel (Achilles) tendon is short, causing her to walk on her toes and circumduct her right leg. Her posture and gait are similar to those of adults who have suffered an infarction of the left middle cerebral artery (Figs. 2-3 to 2-5).

Whereas hand preference normally is apparent only after 2 years of age, exclusive use of one hand much before that time suggests palsy of the other.

More important, since the right hemisphere can become dominant when the left is injured in infancy, people who have had congenital left hemisphere damage might become right hemisphere dominant. These individuals would be left-handed with normal language development, and would have right hemiparesis (Chapter 8). In contrast, adults who sustain left cerebral hemisphere injuries almost always have aphasia, as well as right hemiparesis.

The cerebral damage in spastic hemiparesis is generally more severe and extensive than in spastic cerebral diplegia. Thus, seizures, including the partial complex variety, or mental retardation develop in approximately 50 percent of cases.

Quadriplegic CP is paresis of all four limbs that is usually accompanied by pseudobulbar palsy. Since it results from severe, extensive cerebral damage, often caused by anoxia during delivery, 75 percent of these individuals suffer from seizures and mental retardation. In contrast, cervical spinal cord birth injury causes a non-CP form of quadriplegia. In these cases, when there is no cerebral damage, there are no seizures, pseudobulbar palsy, or mental retardation.

Extrapyramidal CP, the other major category, accounts for 15 percent of cases. It is characterized by *choreoathetosis*, an involuntary writhing (athetosis) of the face, tongue, hands, and feet punctuated by jerking movements (chorea) of the trunk, arms, and legs (Fig. 13-3). Choreoathetosis is usually symmetric, but in some cases it is nearly unilateral. Like all involuntary movement disorders, it disappears during sleep and tends to be aggravated by anxiety (Chapter 18). Movements frequently prevent appropriate hand use and interfere with walking. They also affect the vocal mechanics of the larynx, pharynx, and diaphragm so that patients have marked dysarthria. In addition, deafness is a frequent complication.

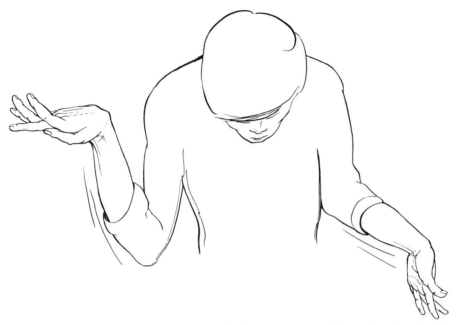

FIGURE 13–3. Choreoathetosis. A 13-year-old girl, since the age of 3 years, has had slow sinuous movements (athetosis) of the wrists, hands, and fingers. The movements force her hands into flexion at the wrist and her fingers into extension and overlapping positions. Quick, jerk-like movements (chorea) are superimposed intermittently.

Choreoathetosis is usually caused by either anoxia at birth or neonatal hyperbilirubinemia and the resultant damage to the basal ganglia called *kernicterus*. Even though the basal ganglia damage occurs perinatally, since involuntary movements might not be apparent until walking and some fine motor movements are present, choreoathetosis is often detected only when children are older than 2 years. More important, since the cerebral cortex can be relatively or entirely spared in kernicterus, this form of extrapyramidal CP is associated with the lowest incidence of cerebral cortical injury. Overall, only about 10 percent of patients have seizures, and many have normal intelligence. Despite considerable impediments, many have completed college or other advanced education. These patients are liable to be underrated by a superficial social, academic, or medical evaluation.

Finally, *mixed forms* of CP—combinations of spastic paraparesis and choreoathetosis—account for about 15 percent of CP cases. The clinical patterns reflect the most severe, extensive cerebral and basal ganglia damage, which is usually the result of a combination of jaundice, anoxia, and prematurity. As would be expected, this degree of damage is associated with the highest incidence of seizures or mental retardation—95 percent.

In summary, seizures or mental retardation are found in increasingly greater incidence in choreoathetosis (10 percent), diplegia (25 percent), hemiplegia (50 percent), quadriplegia (75 percent), and mixed CP (95 percent).

Rehabilitation

Adequate assessment of the intellectual capabilities of patients is necessary, especially in the extrapyramidal forms of CP. Special schooling is required in many, but not all, cases. Hearing aids vastly improve the capabilities of some patients, and newly developed electronic typewriters permit some patients with severe dysarthria to communicate by print or voice output.

Attempts at physical rehabilitation must be made from many approaches. Braces and other mechanical devices may augment strength, and corrective surgery that transposes or lengthens tendons will ameliorate spasticity and contractures. Muscle relaxants, such as baclofen (Lioresal), can also reduce spasticity.

Although choreoathetosis is difficult to treat, neuroleptics and sedatives may suppress some movement. Experimental surgical procedures involving ablation of deep cerebral structures reportedly reduce athetosis, but with considerable risk and uncertain benefit.

Control of seizures is difficult. Often two or more anticonvulsants are required, causing oversedation, hyperactivity, or other side effects. Particularly when there is mental retardation, as is often the case, anticonvulsants can exacerbate behavioral disturbances.

Myelomeningocele, another congenital disorder, is a sac-like protrusion of the lower spinal cord, the cauda equina, and their meningeal coverings through a defect of the lumbosacral spine. Poor development of the lumbosacral nerves yields areflexic paraparesis and incontinence. Moreover, myelomeningoceles are associated with comparable cranial abnormalities that cause hydrocephalus and mental retardation (Arnold-Chiari malformations). Unless defects are surgically corrected within several days after birth, fatal bacterial meningitis develops.

Myelomeningoceles result from neural tube closure defects that have been attributed to genetic abnormalities and exposure to toxins. A woman who has a child with myelomeningocele will have a 10 percent chance of having the same abnormality in future pregnancies. Affected fetuses can be detected by sampling amniotic fluid, testing maternal serum for alpha-fetoprotein, or performing an ultrasound examination. This condition has been the focus of emotional public debates about "fetal screening" and responsibility for severely handicapped infants.

NEUROCUTANEOUS DISORDERS

The neurocutaneous disorders are a group of illnesses, largely inherited in an autosomal dominant pattern, that cause a combination of skin and neurologic abnormalities. The skin and brain, sometimes together with the peripheral nerves, retina, and related organs, are affected together, presumably because they all derive from the ectodermal layer of the embryo.

The clinical manifestations of the neurocutaneous disorders are often not apparent until late childhood. Although these conditions usually remain stable through adult life, in some cases the neurologic abnormality changes from a benign to a malignant condition. Of the many neurocutaneous disorders in the literature, only the three most clinically important ones—tuberous sclerosis, neurofibromatosis, and Sturge-Weber syndrome—are discussed below.

Tuberous Sclerosis

Tuberous sclerosis is characterized by cutaneous *adenoma sebaceum*, epilepsy that is often intractable, and progressive mental impairment. Adenoma sebaceum, which develops by puberty, is an aggregation of smooth, firm nodules of the skin of the chin, nose, and cheeks (Fig. 13-4). The adenomas resemble acne; however, acne "pimples" have a liquid (pus) center and inflammation at the periphery, and they are found on the trunk, as well as the face.

Dementia, the most salient feature, typically begins in childhood and progresses slowly in association with the growth of cerebral *tubers*. These characteristic lesions are potato-like brain nodules, 1 to 3 cm in diameter, that compress brain tissue, irritate the surrounding cortex to cause seizures, and sometimes undergo malignant transformation. In most cases, tubers cannot be removed because they are too numerous and too deep. The combination of progressive mental impairment, epilepsy, and poor prognosis forces many patients into institutions. However, possibly 40 percent of patients have a relatively benign form of the illness with few seizures and little or no mental retardation.

Neurofibromatosis

Neurofibromatosis or von Recklinghausen's disease seems to be inherited in only 50 percent of cases and sporadically occurring in the others. It is characterized by multiple *café au lait* spots and neurofibromas. Although as many as 40 percent of patients may have some intellectual impairment, mental retardation is present in only 2 to 5 percent and there is no tendency toward psychosis.

Café au lait spots are flat and light brown (Fig. 13-5). They are found in at least 10 percent of normal people, but they indicate neurofibromatosis when more than six are present and each is larger than 1.5 cm. Neurofibromas, another cutaneous lesion, are subcutaneous papule-like growths measuring a few millimeters to several centimeters. They generally emerge along peripheral nerves and are visible subcutaneously (Fig. 13-6). Neurofibromas can occur all over the body and reach grotesque proportions: Joseph Merrick, the famous 19th-century "Elephant Man," is an example.

Neurofibromas are usually benign and create no functional impairment; however, occasionally they grow to compress the spinal cord, an important nerve root, or the cauda equina. They can also induce extraordinary growth of a limb. Most important, they sometimes develop on the acoustic or optic cranial nerves, causing acoustic neuromas or optic gliomas. These intracranial neurofibromas can be removed surgically, although sometimes the affected nerve must be sacrificed. Excision of peripheral neurofibromas, however, is not feasible because virtually all peripheral nerves are involved. Café au lait spots can be blanched using lasers.

Recent genetic work indicates that this condition actually includes two main varieties and possibly several minor ones. The von Recklinghausen's variety,

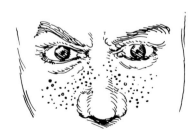

FIGURE 13–4. Tuberous sclerosis. The cutaneous component, adenoma sebaceum, which is prominent on this patient's malar surface, is several millimeters in diameter, firm, and uniformly pale without surrounding inflammation.

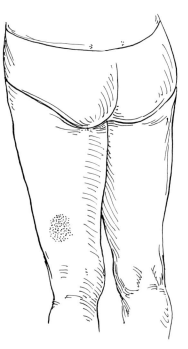

FIGURE 13–5. Café au lait spot. This flat, light brown skin lesion, when found in a group of six or more with each being greater than 1.5 cm, indicates neurofibromatosis.

the more common, causes café au lait spots and neurofibromas that affect the peripheral nerves. It is an autosomal dominant disorder that has been attributed to an abnormal gene localized to chromosome 17. The other major variety is characterized by bilateral acoustic neuromas and other intracranial or intraspinal tumors. This variety is also an autosomal dominant genetic disorder, but has been localized to chromosome 22.

Sturge-Weber Syndrome

Sturge-Weber syndrome, or *encephalo-trigeminal angiomatosis*, which is usually not hereditary, consists of vascular malformations in the face and in the ipsilateral cerebral hemisphere. The vascular malformations of the skin of the face cause a deep red discoloration (port-wine stain) in the region of one or more divisions of the trigeminal nerve (Fig. 13-7). Since the first division is the one most often affected, the most common cutaneous abnormality involves the anterior scalp, forehead, and upper eyelid (Fig. 4-11). By contrast, most people

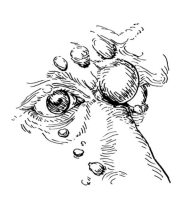

FIGURE 13–6. Neurofibromas. Although typically less than 0.5 cm, neurofibromas often grow to several centimeters on the face, trunk, and limbs.

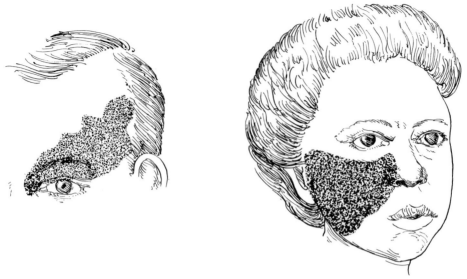

FIGURE 13–7. The cutaneous angiomatosis of Sturge-Weber syndrome involves one or more divisions of the distribution of the trigeminal nerve (see Fig. 4-11).

with small, patchy port-wine stains and infants with small forehead or facial angiomas, such as strawberry nevi, do not have Sturge-Weber syndrome.

The cerebral component of the Sturge-Weber syndrome is a calcified vascular abnormality in the meninges with underlying cerebral atrophy. When cerebral damage is extensive, patients have homonymous hemianopsia, spastic hemiparesis, mental retardation, and epilepsy.

SUBTLE BRAIN INJURY

Attention Deficits and Hyperactivity

In the *Diagnostic and Statistical Manual of Mental Disorders, Third Edition, Revised* (DSM-III-R), a refocused concept of minimal brain dysfunction (MBD) is *attention-deficit hyperactivity disorder (ADHD)*. ADHD is characterized by varying degrees of age-inappropriate inattention, impulsivity, and hyperactivity. Despite the change in designation, most children with ADHD, like those with MBD, are hyperactive. Moreover, as with MBD, their classroom behavior responds to stimulants such as methylphenidate (Ritalin). However, stimulants have less effect on shortened attention spans and learning disabilities, and scattered reports suggest that they may induce or exacerbate tics or Tourette's syndrome (Chapter 18).

Only 5 to 15 percent of ADHD cases are associated with a diagnosable neurologic disease, which is almost always cerebral palsy or mental retardation. Most children with overt brain damage from cerebral anoxia or head trauma have reasonable attention spans and no hyperactivity. Also, any hyperactivity they do have rarely improves with stimulants.

Many ADHD symptoms are undoubtedly manifestations of delayed cerebral maturation, rather than brain injury. Slowed myelination of the frontal lobes and limbic system is said to retard age-appropriate fine and gross motor skills, intellectual ability, and socialization. Since cerebral maturation brings development of very important inhibitory influences, a child with slow neurologic development may have uncontrollable reactions to newly presented stimulation, excessive motor and reflex activity ("disinhibition"), and unrestrained fears and fantasy.

Learning Disabilities

Learning disabilities are also considered a manifestation of congenital brain injury and are often described in children with ADHD or MBD. Although learning disabilities obviously can result from various social, emotional, or neurologic problems, several important neurologic-based (neuropsychologic) disabilities have been described. The DSM-III-R diagnostic criteria for developmental disorders of arithmetic, expressive writing, reading, and language preclude a neurologic origin, but careful neurologic examinations often reveal telltale signs of brain injury. In fact, several disorders seem to be the childhood counterparts of adult-onset syndromes.

Children with reading impairment, often called "developmental dyslexia," or in DSM-III-R, *developmental reading disorder* (315.00), frequently display right-sided hyperactive DTRs and other lateralized signs referable to a dominant hemisphere injury—which would be the congenital counterpart of aphasia and right hemiparesis (Chapter 8). In a disability that mimicks Gerstmann's syndrome, which results from a dominant parietal lobe injury (Chapter 8), children have dyslexia with impairment of arithmetic skills (dyscalculia), impairment of left-right identification, and poor handwriting (dysgraphia). Neuropsychologic learning disabilities have also been associated with nondominant hemisphere injury. In particular, older children and young adults with dyslexia have impaired spatial perception and a paucity of gesture and vocal emotion (prosody, Chapter 8) that are associated with left-sided clumsiness, hyperactive DTRs, and other lateralized signs.

Physical Signs

On the other hand, physical signs held by some to suggest subtle congenital brain injury, the "soft signs," might be merely manifestations of delayed cerebral maturation. Few soft signs have been statistically correlated with learning disabilities because examiners' criteria for identifying these signs and determining the learning disability have been notably subjective and inconsistent. In addition, we are all aware from our own experiences, including observation of our medical colleagues, that many people have excellent learning skills despite poor social graces, handwriting, and athletic abilities.

However, all this is still problematic. Language impairments are found in boys much more often than girls, and left-handedness is disproportionately more frequent. Children with dyslexia reportedly have slowed or irregular rapid alternating movements (dysdiadochokinesia, Chapter 2), incoordination, unsteadiness, and impaired fine motor movements, e.g., in buttoning clothing. In addition, children with delayed CNS maturation or actual injury often have "overflow" movements: excessive, unnecessary, or contralateral actions that usually occur when a skilled, repetitive task is attempted (Fig. 13-8). They also

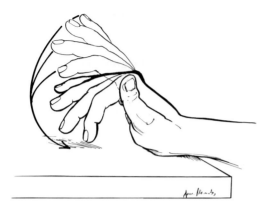

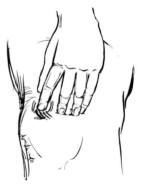

FIGURE 13–8. Synkinetic, mirror, or overflow movements are exemplified by movements of the fingers of either or both hands when the boy is asked to tap only his right index finger on the desk. These movements are seen in normal children younger than 10 years. In children of this age with congenital hemiparesis, the movements are found primarily in the nonhemiparetic ("the good") hand, but in older children with congenital hemiparesis, they are found equally in both hands.

have persistent fidgety finger and body movements, called "adventitious" or "choreiform" movements, that are similar to those seen in Sydenham's chorea, Tourette's syndrome, choreoathetotic CP, or mere restlessness. Curiously, frontal release signs (Chapter 7), which are often found in adults who sustain cerebral injuries, are not described in children with suspected brain injury.

Other commonly cited soft signs are unilateral "posturing" while walking on the sides of feet (Fig. 13-1), asymmetric DTRs, unsustained clonus, and inability to move the eyes without head motion. However, these and many overflow movements may be manifestations of lack of normal motor inhibition ("disinhibition"), rather than combinations of abnormalities of the basal ganglia and corticospinal tract. Disinhibition may result merely from delayed myelination of the frontal lobes and the corpus callosum, which is the pathway for interhemispheric inhibitory tracts. Since cerebral myelination is usually complete only by 10 years of age, clumsiness and unnecessary motor activity are often normal in younger children. In older children and adults, such findings are soft signs of cerebral injury.

Some childhood motor disturbances are especially important. Speech difficulties (dysarthrias), whether or not they are associated with brain injury, possibly indicate a major pathologic condition and almost always interfere with school performance. They may be caused by pseudobulbar palsy, athetosis, cleft palate, and hearing impairment. Childhood gait impairments, which are always important, may be due to spastic diplegia (see above), Duchenne's muscular dystrophy (Chapter 6), and torsion dystonia (Chapter 18). Dysconjugate ocular gaze usually results from simple ocular muscle imbalance (strabismus); however, when it is found in combination with face, head, ear, and hand abnormalities, it is associated with cerebral dysfunction. Moreover, persistent deviation of one eye will lead to loss of vision in that eye, i.e., *amblyopia*.

Laboratory Findings

Although some series report that dyslexic children have occipital lobe abnormalities or reversal of the usual planum temporale (language area) asymmetry, there are no specific CT or MRI abnormalities in ADHD or MBD children. Routine EEG abnormalities, reportedly present in 25 to 75 percent of cases, include dominant frequency slowing, interhemispheric asymmetry, and sharp waves; however, these abnormalities, like soft signs, depend on the examiner, the patients studied, and the criteria applied. Also, the EEG changes are even more likely than the soft signs to be age-related, nonspecific, or even induced by movement, sleep, and medications.

Sophisticated studies, such as spectral analysis and evoked potentials, of children with learning disabilities have found only inconsistent, diffuse, or multifocal abnormalities that do not have a clear relation to cerebral language areas. In short, laboratory evaluation cannot provide confirmation of a diagnosis of ADHD.

Differential Diagnosis

Of the many possible causes of childhood neurologic impairments, the physician must give first consideration to congenital cerebral and sensory injuries: cerebral palsy, mental retardation, and visual or auditory impairments. One condition that particularly affects children and elderly adults is adverse reactions to common medications. For example, phenobarbital, cough medications, and antihistamines may cause hyperactivity. Migraines in children may cause hyperactivity and behavioral disturbances that mimic seizures, gastrointestinal difficulties, and mental alterations. Finally, both absences (petit mal) and partial complex seizures may develop in childhood and cause inattentiveness, learning disabilities, and behavioral changes (Chapter 10).

Outcome

Almost 50 percent of children who have had ADHD grow up to be indistinguishable from other adults. In them, childhood hyperactivity became controlled, if not by nervous system maturation, then by social constraints, and the repercussions of their learning disabilities were avoided by choosing appropriate occupations.

Nevertheless, some ADHD children grow up to become ADHD adults in whom erratic behavior, poor organization, and inattentiveness reflect persistent subtle cerebral dysfunction and possibly further superimposed injury from trauma, alcohol, and drug abuse. So-called rages, episodic dyscontrol, and idiosyncratic (pathologic) alcohol intoxication (Chapter 10) may partly result from congenital brain injury. These ADHD adults, like their childhood counterparts, are clearly liable to have paradoxical reactions to barbiturates, other sedatives, and alcohol. Likewise, some have reportedly benefited from stimulants and others from carbamazepine (Tegretol).

REFERENCES

Abramowicz M (ed): Methylphenidate revisited. Med Letter *30*:51, 1988

Bellak L: ADD psychosis as a separate entity. Schizophr Bull *11*:523, 1985

Chervenak FA, Isaacson G, Mahoney MJ: Advances in the diagnosis of fetal defects. N Engl J Med *315*:305, 1986

Cranberg LD, Filley CM, Hart EJ, et al: Acquired aphasia in childhood: Clinical and CT investigations. Neurology *37*:1165, 1987

Elliott FA: The episodic dyscontrol syndrome and aggression. In Symposium on the Borderland Between Neurology and Psychiatry. Neurol Clin 2:113, 1984

Ferry PC: Infant stimulation programs: A neurologic shell game? Arch Neurol *43*:281, 1986

Golden GS: Neurobiological correlates of learning disabilities. Ann Neurol *12*:409, 1982

Haslam RHA, Dably JT, Johns RD, et al: Cerebral asymmetry in developmental dyslexia. Arch Neurol *38*:679, 1981

Herskowitz J. Rosman PN: Pediatrics, Neurology, and Psychiatry—Common Ground. Behavioral, Cognitive, Affective, and Physical Disorders in Childhood and Adolescence. New York, Macmillan, 1982

Johnston RB, Stark RE, Mellits ED, et al: Neurological status of language-impaired and normal children. Ann Neurol *10*:159, 1981

Mannuzza S, Klein RG, Bonasura N, et al: Hyperactive boys almost grown up. II. Status of subjects without a mental disorder. Arch Gen Psychiatry *45*:13, 1988

Nass R: Mirror movement asymmetries in congenital hemiparesis. Neurology *35*:1059, 1985

National Institutes of Health Consensus Development Conference: Neurofibromatosis. Arch Neurol *45*:575, 1988

Nelson KB, Ellenberg JH: Antecedents of cerebral palsy: Multivariate analysis of risk. N Engl J Med *315*:81, 1986

Orsini DL, Satz P: A syndrome of pathological left-handedness: Correlates of early left hemisphere injury. Arch Neurol *43*:333, 1986

Pebenito R: Developmental Gerstmann syndrome: Case report and review of the literature. J Dev Behav Pediatr *4*:229, 1987

Rodriguez-Gomez M (ed): Neurocutaneous Diseases: A Practical Approach. Stoneham, MA, Butterworths, 1987

Sorensen SA, Mulvihill JJ, Nielsen A: Long-term follow-up of von Recklinghausen neurofibromatosis. N Engl J Med *314*:1010, 1986

Voeller KKS, Hanson JA, Wendt RN: Facial affect recognition in children. Neurology *38*:1744, 1988

Weintraub S, Mesulam MM: Developmental learning disabilities of the right hemisphere: Emotional, interpersonal, and cognitive components. Arch Neurol *40*:463, 1983

Weiss G, Hechtman LT: Hyperactive Children Grown Up: Empirical Findings and Theoretical Considerations. New York, The Guilford Press, 1986

Wender PH, Wood DR, Reimherr FW: Pharmacological treatment of attention deficit disorder, residual type (ADD, RT, "Minimal Brain Dysfunction," "Hyperactivity") in adults. Psychopharmacol Bull *21*:222, 1985

QUESTIONS: CHAPTER 13

1–11.   Match the neurocutaneous disorder with its manifestations:

1. Acoustic neuroma

2. Cutaneous lesions resembling rhinophyma

3. Progressive dementia

4. Neurofibromas

5. Adenoma sebaceum

6. Cauda equina syndrome

7. Intractable epilepsy

8. Café au lait spots

9. Facial angiomatosis

10. Optic glioma

11. Epilepsy

a. Tuberous sclerosis
b. Von Recklinghausen's disease
c. Sturge-Weber syndrome

12–17. Which of the following disorders causes episodic changes in mood or inattentiveness in children?

12. Migraines

13. Partial complex seizures

14. Antihistamines

15. Cerebral palsy

16. Sedative medications

17. Absences

18. In which of the following conditions will CT or MRI provide useful diagnostic information?
  a. Attention deficit disorder
  b. Absences
  c. Migraines
  d. Hydrocephalus
  e. Sturge-Weber syndrome
  f. Learning disabilities
  g. Tuberous sclerosis
  h. Tourette's syndrome

19. Which of the following procedures or developments has helped reduce the incidence of congenital brain injury or abnormality?
  a. Prenatal chromosome analysis
  b. Neonatal exchange transfusion
  c. Fetal cardiac monitoring during labor
  d. Amniocentesis
  e. Ultrasound examinations
  f. Prevention of RH incompatibility

20. Children who sustain any brain injury until the age of 5 years are all eligible for assistance by most programs that serve CP children (True/False).

21. Which of the following is (are) *not* usually found in children with mental retardation?
  a. Dyslexia
  b. Dysarthria
  c. Hyperactivity

22. Which of the following is (are) *not* usually found in children with cerebral palsy?
  a. Dyslexia
  b. Dysarthria
  c. Hyperactivity
  d. Seizures

23. Adults with penetrating head injuries (e.g., gunshot wounds) frequently have:
  a. Aphasia
  b. Paresis
  c. Cerebral palsy
  d. Hyperactivity
  e. Seizures
  f. Mental retardation

24. A 1-year-old boy has a stroke because of sickle cell disease. This results in mild right hemiparesis. Which of the following will probably be additional consequences?
  a. Chorea
  b. Aphasia
  c. Seizures
  d. Spastic cerebral palsy
  e. Stunted growth of right arm
  f. Minimal brain dysfunction

25–30.   Match the disorder with the cause.

25.   Choreoathetosis

26.   Spastic quadriplegia

27.   Spastic hemiparesis

28.   Deafness

29.   Seizure disorder

30.   Cortical blindness

    a.   Cervical cord injury
    b.   Kernicterus
    c.   Cerebral anoxia
    d.   Stroke in utero

31.   List the following types of cerebral palsy in the order of increasing frequency of the likelihood of mental retardation.
    a.   Choreoathetosis
    b.   Spastic diplegia
    c.   Spastic quadriplegia
    d.   Spastic hemiplegia
    e.   Mixed spastic choreoathetosis

32.   Which of the above types of CP has the lowest incidence of seizures?

33.   Which of the above may not be apparent until as late as 2 years of age?

34.   Which is the most commonly encountered form?

35.   In which form are the legs affected more than the arms?

36.   A 10-year-old boy is observed to have "fidgety" movements of the hands and feet and facial grimacing. Which of the following disorders may be present in childhood and may be manifested by such movement disorders?
    a.   Cerebral palsy
    b.   Minimal brain dysfunction
    c.   Sydenham's chorea
    d.   Wilson's disease
    e.   Tourette's syndrome

37–43.   True or False

37.   The predominant EEG frequencies are slower in young children than young adults.

38.   Theta frequencies are slower than alpha frequencies.

39.   Sleeping during an EEG will alter the background activity.

40.   Changes in attention will alter the EEG rhythms.

41.   Eye opening will alter the EEG.

42.   Some medications will alter the EEG.

43.   Children will normally have scattered theta activity on an EEG.

ANSWERS

1. b.   **3.** a.

2. a.   **4.** b.

5.	a.		**25.**	b.
6.	b.		**26.**	a or c.
7.	a.		**27.**	d.
8.	b.		**28.**	b.
9.	c.		**29.**	c or d.
10.	b.		**30.**	c.
11.	a,c.		**31.**	a, b, d, c, e.
12.	Yes		**32.**	a.
13.	Yes		**33.**	a.
14.	Yes		**34.**	d.
15.	No		**35.**	b.
16.	Yes		**36.**	a, b, c, d, e.
17.	Yes		**37.**	True
18.	d, e, g.		**38.**	True
19.	a, b, c, d, e, f.		**39.**	True
20.	True		**40.**	True
21.	c.		**41.**	True
22.	c.		**42.**	True
23.	a, b, e.		**43.**	True
24.	c, d, e.			

14

Neurologic Aspects of Pain

Recent discoveries in anatomy and pharmacology have led physicians to view pain as a clinical entity, rather than simply a symptom. Using this new information combined with empirically derived therapies, physicians can now at least ameliorate pain and its affective component, suffering. Rational treatment can be offered to patients who have pain from cancer and other progressive disorders (malignant pain) or from healed and nonprogressive injuries (nonmalignant pain).*

This chapter first reviews the *endogenous opioids* of the central nervous system (CNS)—the most important discovery. It outlines the pathways that convey pain from injuries to the CNS and those pathways that provide pain relief (analgesia). Emphasizing the treatment of malignant pain, it then describes the ways in which analgesia is produced by the endogenous opioid system, pain relieving medicines (analgesics), and certain surgical procedures. Afterward, clinical aspects and treatment of several common nonmalignant pain syndromes are discussed.

ENDOGENOUS OPIOIDS

Endogenous opioids, often called *endorphins* (endogenous morphine-like substances), are modified amino acid chains (polypeptides) synthesized in the CNS. They are located in the limbic system, dorsal horn of the spinal cord, and other CNS sites. They bind onto the same CNS receptors as the "exogenous" opioids, particularly morphine (Table 14-1), and produce the same effects—analgesia, mood elevation (euphoria), sedation, and respiratory depression. Like morphine, with repeated administration of endogenous opioids, increasingly greater quantities are required to produce their effects (*tolerance*), and physical signs of withdrawal occur upon abstinence (*dependence*). Naloxone (Narcan) reverses the effects of endogenous opioids just as it does the effects of morphine. Indeed, the narcotic antagonist effect of naloxone is so reliable that *naloxone reversibility* is the criterion for determining whether the effect of an analgesic is mediated by the opioid pathways.

The beta endorphins and adrenocorticotropin (ACTH) are derived from a large common precursor (Fig. 14-1). The "runners' high" and the initial painlessness described by wounded soldiers are postulated to result from

---

* Patients may receive help from multidisciplinary groups by contacting the International Pain Foundation, 909 N.E. 43rd Street, Suite 306, Seattle, Washington 98105-6020.

TABLE 14–1.　GLOSSARY

Beta endorphin: An endogenous opioid, concentrated in the pituitary gland and secreted with ACTH. It consists of amino acid numbers 61–91 of beta lipotropin and gives rise to the enkephalins (Fig. 14–1).

Beta lipotropin: A 91-amino-acid polypeptide, which may be an ACTH fragment, gives rise to beta endorphin. However, it has no opioid activity itself, i.e., beta lipotropin is not an endogenous opioid.

Endogenous opioids: Polypeptides (amino acid chains) found within the CNS that create effects similar to those of morphine and other naturally occurring opioids. The effects of endogenous opioid and naturally occurring opioids are characteristically reversed by nalkoxone (Narcan).

Endorphins: Endogenous morphine-like substances; a term virtually synonymous with endogenous opioids.

Enkephalins: Short (5-amino-acid) polypeptide endogenous opioids that include met-enkephalin and leu-enkephalin. They are found primarily in the amygdala, brainstem, and dorsal horn of the spinal cord.

Naloxone (Narcan): A pure opioid antagonist that reverses all effects of endogenous and naturally occurring opiods.

Substance P: An 11-amino-acid polypeptide that is probably the primary pain neurotransmitter at the first synapse of the primary afferent neuron.

endogenous opioids secreted along with ACTH from the pituitary gland in people who are under stress.

PAIN AND ANALGESIA PATHWAYS

Peripheral Systems

Painful tissue inflammation liberates prostaglandins, arachidonic acid, and bradykinin, which all stimulate specific peripheral nerve receptors (nociceptors). Pain may be alleviated at this very first step while the process is still in the "periphery," with aspirin, acetaminophen (Tylenol), steroids, and nonsteroidal anti-inflammatory agents. These medicines are analgesic in large part because they inhibit synthesis of prostaglandins or in other ways reduce tissue inflammation.

Pain, whether it originates from pressure, heat, or inflammation, is carried by two types of peripheral nerve fibers, the primary afferents or first-order neurons. *A delta* fibers are thinly myelinated fibers of small diameter that convey

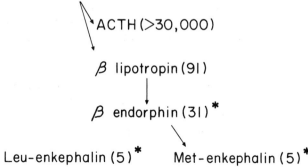

FIGURE 14–1. A large precursor molecule (not pictured) gives rise to ACTH and beta lipotropin, which are often released together. Beta lipotropin gives rise to beta endorphin and met-enkephalin, but another precursor gives rise to leu-enkephalin. (The asterisks denote the important endogenous opioids, and the numbers within parentheses are the amino acid units in the polypeptide chains.)

sharp or pricking sensations from the skin and mucous membranes. *C fibers*, unmyelinated but also small, convey diffuse, prolonged, and burning sensations as well as noxious sensations from the viscera. Pain transmission along these fibers may be dampened by stimulation of other sensory fibers. This analgesic effect may explain why people instinctually massage an injury at a proximal site as, for example, a person with a sprained ankle will rub the lower leg.

The famous "gate theory" of analgesia explains this common observation. It suggests that stimulation of large diameter, heavily myelinated fibers that carry vibration and position sensation, *A beta* fibers, inhibits pain transmission by the small fibers with little or no myelin. The gate theory has given rise to *transcutaneous electrical nerve stimulation (TENS)*, in which electric current stimulation reduces pain.

A more direct way of reducing pain is to interrupt (block) the entire peripheral nerve by an injection of a local anesthetic or a neurolytic substance, such as alcohol. *Nerve blocks* are useful in chest and abdominal pain because the thoracic and lumbar nerve roots can be injected with alcohol as they emerge from the vertebrae. However, this technique is usually not feasible for painful limbs because it usually causes paresis, as well as analgesia. Nor is it practical in treating facial pain within the first division of the trigeminal nerve (Fig. 4-11), since analgesia involving the cornea leads to corneal ulcerations.

Sometimes sympathetic plexus or ganglia blockade is helpful. For example, in pancreatic carcinoma, the celiac plexus might be injected with alcohol, and in the shoulder-hand syndrome, the cervical (stellate) ganglia can be injected.

Central Systems

Pain Transmission to the Brain

The peripheral nerve fibers enter the CNS at the dorsal horn of the spinal cord. They synapse either immediately or after ascending a few segments. At many of these synapses, the fibers release the polypeptide *substance P*, which is believed to be a major neurotransmitter for pain in the spinal cord (Fig. 14-2). After the synapse, a second-order neuron crosses to the other side of the spinal cord and ascends contralaterally to the injury, within the *lateral (neo) spinothalamic tract*, to the brain (Figs. 2-6 and 2-14). There are also other, less well-defined spinal cord tracts, such as the paleospinothalamic tracts, which ascend both ipsilaterally and contralaterally.

Tracts carrying pain synapse primarily in the thalamus. However, because they also synapse in the reticular activating system, other regions of the brainstem, and, most important, the limbic system, pain notoriously affects mood and sleep.

To provide analgesia in selected cases of malignant pain, the spinothalamic tract may be interrupted by severing the lateral portion of the spinal cord contralateral to the pain. This technique, called a *cordotomy*, is particularly useful when patients have intractable pain confined to a single limb or one side of the trunk. However, it is not suitable for more generalized pain because bilateral cordotomy, which would be required, is often complicated by respiratory drive impairment (Ondine's curse) and loss of bladder control.

Although severing a pathway to the thalamus reduces pain, destroying tracts connecting the thalamus to the cortex does not. For example, performing a

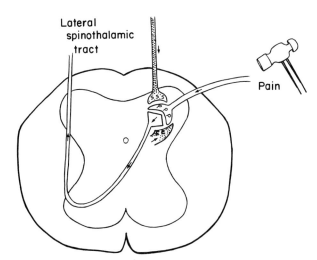

FIGURE 14–2. Painful sensations are conveyed along the *A delta* and *C* fibers of the peripheral nerves. These fibers enter the dorsal horn of the spinal cord where, probably utilizing *substance P* (P), they synapse with neurons giving rise to the lateral spinothalamic and other tracts that ascend to the brain. Two (*stippled*) pain-dampening analgesic systems play upon the dorsal horn synapse. One tract descends from the brain and releases *serotonin* (S). The other system is comprised of spinal interneurons that release *enkephalins* (E).

frontal lobotomy reduces suffering but not the presence of pain. Also, as can commonly be observed, patients with cerebrovascular accidents still feel pain although their affect is blunted.

Analgesic Pathways in the Spinal Cord and Brain

Not all pain-carrying peripheral nerves synapse in the dorsal horn to give rise to the lateral spinothalamic tract. Some form an analgesic pathway by a synapse onto short neurons, *interneurons*, which play back upon the primary afferent neurons. By releasing enkephalins, this pathway inhibits pain transmission. It has a powerful analgesic effect that can be mimicked by intrathecal injections of morphine and reversed by naloxone. In fact, such narcotic injections can provide long-lasting relief of pain in the lower trunk, pelvis, or legs.

Other analgesic pathways, located in a descending spinal cord tract, are in the *dorsolateral funiculus*. These pathways originate in the brainstem and also relieve pain by playing on the primary afferent neurons and the ascending spinal cord pain pathways. Unlike most other analgesic pathways, these fibers release *serotonin*.

The analgesic effect of serotonin has important clinical correlations. The antidepressant medications useful in pain treatment presumably induce analgesia by raising serotonin concentrations in analgesic pathways. The medications' analgesic effects are noted to occur in patients without overt depression and, in depressed patients, before there is an improvement in mood. Also, lower dosages of antidepressants are required to treat pain than depression. Since studies have shown that substances that deplete serotonin intensify pain, lowered serotonin levels in depressed patients are believed to make them more susceptible to pain.

Certain brainstem structures give rise to analgesic tracts. For example, the gray matter that surrounds the brainstem's third ventricle and aqueduct has tracts that can release large amounts of endogenous opioids. When this area is stimulated, patients have profound analgesia (see below).

THERAPIES

A variety of medications can now be given and combined with psychologic therapies for pain control. They can be the basis for reducing pain and suffering, and, at least, can give patients respite and some control over their situation.

Non-narcotic Analgesics

Non-narcotic analgesics are relatively potent and rarely apt to cause serious side effects (Table 14-2). Aspirin remains the standard, and two tablets (600 mg) have about the same potency as two common narcotics: 65 mg of propoxyphene (Darvon) or 50 mg of oral meperidine (Demerol). Since aspirin, steroids, and nonsteroidal anti-inflammatory agents are analgesic in large measure because they inhibit the synthesis of prostaglandins, they are more effective if taken before pain develops rather than after. For example, pain can be partly prevented by prophylactic use of analgesics before dental procedures, menses, and headaches.

Aspirin, steroids, and nonsteroidal agents act at the site of injury, i.e., *peripherally*. When they are given in combination with narcotics, which act *centrally* on CNS opioid pathways, they enhance narcotic analgesia. Thus taking two tablets of aspirin will increase the potency of morphine. For example, aspirin, indomethacin, or other anti-inflammatory medicines are routinely given in combination with narcotics for treatment of metastases to bone. Non-narcotic analgesics alone, however, provide limited analgesia. Once their maximum benefit is achieved, additional quantities will not increase analgesia (the "ceiling effect").

Narcotics

Narcotics, the most potent analgesics (Table 14-3), are particularly useful in cancer patients who have moderate, incessant, or distressing pain. These medicines can be administered orally, intramuscularly, intravenously, or in-

TABLE 14–2. NON-NARCOTIC ANALGESICS

Medication	Dose† (mg)	Interval
Acetaminophen (Tylenol and others)	650	q4h
Aspirin	650	q4h
Nonsteroidal anti-inflammatory agents,		
e.g., diflunisal (Dolobid),	500	q8–12h
ibuprofen (Motrin, Advil, Nuprin),	400	q4–6h
indomethacin (Indocin),	25–50	q8h°
naproxen (Naprosyn),	375	q12h
sulindac (Clinoril)	150	q12h

† All administered orally, typical dose schedules.
° Long-acting preparation available.

TABLE 14–3. NARCOTIC ANALGESICS

Medication	Route	Dose (mg)	Interval
Codeine†	Oral	30–60	q4h
Hydromorphone	Oral	4–8	q3–4h
(Dilaudid)	IM	.75–1.5	q3h
Levorphanol	Oral	2–4	q4h
(Levo-Dromoran)	IM	1–2	q4h
Meperidine	Oral	50–150	q3–4h
(Demoral)	IM	50–150	q3–4h
Methadone	Oral	10–20	q12h
	IM	5–10	
Morphine	Oral	30–60	q3–4h
	IM	10	q3–4h
Morphine long-acting			
(MS Contin)	Oral	30	q12h
(Roxane SR)	Oral	30	q8–12h
Oxycodone†	Oral	5–10	q4h
(Percocet)			
Propoxyphene†	Oral	65–120	q4h
(Darvon)			

† Sufficient for mild to moderate pain.

trathecally. Continual intravenous infusion can provide a particularly satisfactory steady state of analgesia and rest. In the future, narcotics may be administered by transdermal or intranasal absorption.

Narcotics should be given on a regular prophylactic basis, such as every 2 to 4 hours, rather than at the onset of pain. When analgesics must be requested by the patient and then given by nurses only after pain begins, the delay in treatment makes pain difficult to alleviate. Moreover, the patient, worried about the recurrence of pain and about obtaining relief, becomes anxious and preoccupied with obtaining drugs.

As tolerance almost invariably develops or pain increases as the disease progresses, ever more frequent and larger doses are required. Greater doses or more potent preparations of narcotics, which should be administered generously, can increase the analgesia, i.e., they have no ceiling effect. Long-acting, sustained-release oral and intramuscular preparations of morphine are now available (Table 14-3), and high doses can be given to cancer patients without causing respiratory depression. Addiction is not a realistic consideration in seriously or terminally ill patients, and it rarely occurs in patients with normal premorbid mental health who develop a painful limited illness.

Side effects can be anticipated. Constipation can be prevented with a combination of laxatives, such as senna (Senokot), and stool softeners, such as docusate sodium (Colace). Nausea, often a devastating problem, may be caused by the underlying illness, radiotherapy, chemotherapy, or the narcotics themselves. Patients should be given vigorous and preferably prophylactic treatment with antiemetic suppositories, injections, or pills. Some caution is necessary because most antiemetics are composed of phenothiazines. Synthetic marijuana, dronabinol (Marinol), and related preparations, such as Nabilone (Cesamet), have been approved as antiemetics, but their benefit is not established, and they can cause mental aberrations. Metaclopramide (Reglan) is more effective, but like phenothiazines it can cause dystonic reactions and parkinsonism.

One particular difficulty with narcotics is that their effects are highly dependent upon the route of administration. The same dose that is given orally may produce an overdose if given intramuscularly or intravenously. If the situation were reversed, undertreatment may precipitate drug-seeking behavior, symptoms of narcotic withdrawal, and recurrence of pain.

The use of several narcotics is fraught with special difficulties. Meperidine (Demerol), although one of the most frequently prescribed narcotics, is usually unsatisfactory. It is poorly absorbed when taken orally, and changing the routes of administration leads to complications. More important, when meperidine is given for several days, especially in patients with renal insufficiency, accumulation of its toxic metabolite, normeperidine, often causes dysphoria and other mental aberrations, tremulousness, myoclonus (Chapter 18), and seizures.

Another problematic narcotic is heroin. Not only is its effectiveness in relieving pain and improving mood no greater than an appropriate dose of morphine but also the potential for abuse is much greater. In "Brompton's cocktail" and its variations, heroin is combined with cocaine, chloroform water (for flavor), phenothiazines (for nausea), and gin or another alcoholic beverage. These concoctions, which have received wide publicity, are no better than adequate doses of morphine and antiemetics.

Finally, narcotics that possess narcotic antagonist properties, such as pentazocine (Talwin) and butorphanol (Stadol), have limited use. They were developed, quite rationally, to prevent addiction by incorporating narcotic antagonist properties into narcotic analgesics; however, they were found to be quite addictive. Also, they have psychotomimetic properties, and injections of pentazocine lead to skin and muscle necrosis. Moreover, because of their narcotic antagonism, a change from a morphine-like narcotic to one of these mixed agonist-antagonist drugs will, like undertreatment, produce withdrawal symptoms and pain recurrence.

The effectiveness of narcotics has one major disadvantage: once strong analgesics are no longer necessary, patients resist discontinuing narcotics. They may rightfully fear a return of the pain and suffering and the development of withdrawal symptoms. Although the issue is complex, narcotics should be discontinued when unnecessary. Their use leads to confusion between abstinence, tolerance, and symptoms of the illness. They engender drug-seeking behavior and themselves induce side effects. Exceptions may be appropriate, however, for rare individuals who have no alternative treatment for severe chronic pain and do not have abusive, destructive drug-seeking behavior.

There are several ways to discontinue narcotics. If the original narcotic was given in only small or irregular doses, it can be abruptly stopped. For intermittent use of mild to moderately powerful narcotics, such as Percodan, the best method is to reduce the total dose to 25 percent of the usual daily dose and then taper and discontinue the remainder over 7 to 10 days. If the narcotic was more potent and given continuously for a long time or if the patient is very anxious about withdrawal, an equivalent dose of methadone can be substituted for an additional week before it is tapered. Hospitalized patients who agree to certain structured programs are given placebos in the final stages of drug withdrawal. As narcotics are withdrawn, non-narcotic analgesics should be substituted. Also, when patients have physical or mental discomfort, they might be helped by a minor tranquilizer or an ataractic, such as hydroxyzine (Vistaril) or, curiously, clonidine (Catapres).

Psychotropic Medications

Adding tranquilizers to analgesics is often beneficial because together they tend to alleviate anxiety, restore sleep patterns, and reduce painful muscle spasms. Antidepressants can also treat the affective components of the painful illness. However, they do not decrease requirements for narcotics.

Antidepressants have been beneficial in many studies. Their clearest indication is when pain is accompanied by depression, but they are also useful with patients who do not have overt depression. They frequently provide sufficient analgesia for chronic nonmalignant pain. As mentioned before, they may produce analgesia by increasing serotonin concentrations in CNS analgesic pathways.

The most common practice is to use amitriptyline in a low dose, such as 25 mg, taken at bedtime. Doses are increased gradually, usually to a range of 75 mg to 150 mg at bedtime. Other tricyclic antidepressants that have been useful in pain suppression include imipramine and doxepin.

Stimulation-Induced Analgesia

Scientific data suggest that acupuncture is an effective form of analgesia in some people with mildly to moderately painful injuries. For securing analgesia, the "meridians," which are the traditional regions in which needles are placed, have been shown to be less important than dermatomes (Figs. 2-15 and 16-2). Since acupuncture induces a rise in CSF endorphins and the analgesia is naloxone-reversible, acupuncture is presumed to work through the endogenous opioid system (Table 14-4).

A frequently effective treatment for chronic musculoskeletal disorders is TENS, the technique in which an electrical stimulus is applied to the skin just proximal to the painful region. It is believed to be analgesic because stimulation of the underlying large nerve fibers causes "gating." Some types of TENS also probably work through the endogenous opioid system.

In a method that is theoretically similar to TENS, *dorsal column stimulation*, electrodes are inserted directly onto the dorsal columns of the spinal cord. The analgesia provided by the procedure is typically short-lived, and the risks are substantially higher than with TENS, but selected patients may benefit.

Stimulation of the CNS has been taken a step further in recent years. Neurosurgeons have implanted electrodes into the periventricular and peria-

TABLE 14–4. ANALGESICS MEDIATED BY THE ENDOGENOUS OPIOID SYSTEM*

Acupuncture
Narcotics
Placebo
Stimulation
    TENS (transcutaneous electrical nerve stimulation)
    Dorsal column stimulation
    Periaqueductal gray matter and other deep brain stimulation

* Since these analgesics are partially or entirely reversed by naloxone (Narcan), their effects are considered to be mediated by the endogenous opioid system. In contrast, analgesia induced by tricyclic antidepressants and hypnosis is not reversed by naloxone.

queductal gray matter and adjacent brainstem regions. Stimulation of these sites, which may release stores of endogenous opioids, can produce profound analgesia.

Placebos, Hypnosis, and Behavioral Therapies

Placebos, which are commonly given by physicians either deliberately or when they prescribe ineffectual medications, will produce a definite but brief period of analgesia in about 30 percent of patients. They are most effective for acute, severe pain, especially when patients have anxiety, and least effective for continual mild pain. Contrary to popular notion, a beneficial response to placebo does not mean that a patient's pain is psychogenic. Since the analgesic effect of placebos is partially naloxone-reversible, placebos probably stimulate the endogenous opioid system.

Hypnosis is useful for a limited period in a wide variety of chronic painful conditions including cancer. It differs from placebo therapy because patients' ability to be hypnotized does not correlate with their response to placebos, and hypnosis-induced analgesia is not naloxone-reversible, i.e., hypnosis is not a placebo.

Cognitive therapy, behavior modification, operant conditioning, and other psychologic therapies have been recommended when the response to the usual treatments is insufficient, or when the pain is out of proportion to the organic etiology. They have also been used in cases of abnormal behavior, narcotic abuse, or when family members have begun to reinforce the pain. Widely used behavioral therapies are relaxation, desensitization, and distraction. Likewise, biofeedback, which is helpful in muscle contraction and migraine headaches, may have a role for certain individuals.

NONMALIGNANT PAIN SYNDROMES

Although agonizing pain is generally associated with malignancies, several nonmalignant pain syndromes create—for numerous people—comparable pain and suffering. Many of these syndromes occur frequently. Herniated intervertebral disks, diabetic neuropathy, and headaches have already been discussed. The treatment of each of these syndromes can vary widely, but several neurologic guidelines can be suggested. Both patients and physicians should accept that most of these conditions are chronic illnesses that cannot be cured. Their goals should be to achieve living with the pain, reduction of the suffering, and, despite persistent pain, restoration of occupational and social function. All goals should be clearly stated, acceptable to the patient, and attainable within several months.

Medications should usually consist of combinations of non-narcotic analgesics, anti-inflammatory agents, and, for reasons discussed previously, a tricyclic antidepressant. If narcotic analgesics must be given, they are usually appropriate only for a preplanned, limited period. Anticonvulsant medications may be helpful. For example, phenytoin (Dilantin) is sometimes useful in pain that has a lancinating quality. Likewise, carbamazepine (Tegretol), which is structurally similar to the tricyclic antidepressants, is useful in trigeminal neuralgia and certain other painful conditions.

With all these medications available, physicians tend to overmedicate patients. They should consider supplementing or replacing medications with nonpharmacologic modalities including supportive psychotherapy, hypnosis, cognitive-behavior techniques, and physical therapy.

Primary care physicians should be encouraged to refer patients for psychiatric consultation not only for evaluation for depression and other routine indications but also when patients have vegetative symptoms regardless of the apparent connection to the pain. A psychiatric consultation should also be recommended when the pain or disability is refractory to several courses of medical treatment, when excessive medications are required, or when many diagnostic or surgical procedures have been unsuccessful. The consultation should be obtained early and as an integral part of the evaluation. It should not be an afterthought, last resort, or a method that merely passes the patient to another physician.

The psychiatrist might find that the pain is a symptom of several different psychiatric conditions described in the *Diagnostic and Statistical Manual of Mental Disorders, Third Edition, Revised (DSM-III-R)*: *schizophrenia, depressive disorders, somatoform pain disorder, hypochondriasis,* and *malingering.* If pain is the only symptom, *conversion disorder* cannot be diagnosed by using DSM-III-R criteria. Most cases of chronic pain in community and acute-care medical hospital patients are related to depression or a somatoform disorder. The problem in these cases is almost always seemingly excessive pain following one or two bodily injuries. During the evaluation, the psychiatrist should concentrate on the suffering, disability, and family dynamics that result from the pain. Also, possibly unlike the evaluation performed by many psychiatrists, the painful part of the patient's body should be physically examined: the touching would have a therapeutic benefit, albeit primitive, and possibly diagnostic usefulness.

In pain patients, the symptoms of depression may be atypical. Their mood changes may be subtle, and their concern with the pain and its implications may be substituted for typical symptoms of depression. Sometimes the pain is said to be a "depressive equivalent," "masked depression," or "dysthymic pain disorder." In some patients, pain can be assumed to be closely related to depression but not an actual manifestation of it. The prevalence of chronic pain in depressed patients and, likewise, of depression in chronic pain patients is high. Chronic pain patients, like depressed patients, are often found to have vegetative signs with mental changes, such as impaired concentration and irritability. Also, they have the "neurotic triad" (high scores on hysteria, hypochondriasis, and depression) on the Minnesota Multiphasic Personality Inventory (MMPI) and characteristic patterns on a widely used test that measures pain's affective and sensory dimensions, the "McGill Pain Questionnaire" (Fig. 14-3).

Postmastectomy Axillary Pain

During a radical mastectomy, a surgeon routinely explores the axilla and removes pectoral muscles and lymph nodes. This portion of the procedure usually involves cutting the cutaneous branch of the first thoracic nerve root, the intercostobrachial nerve. Several weeks postoperatively, some women develop searing pain in the axilla extending to the inner aspect of the upper arm, well beyond the lateral end of the incision. This pain can be distinguished from common "incisional pain," which is only mildly to moderately intense, has an

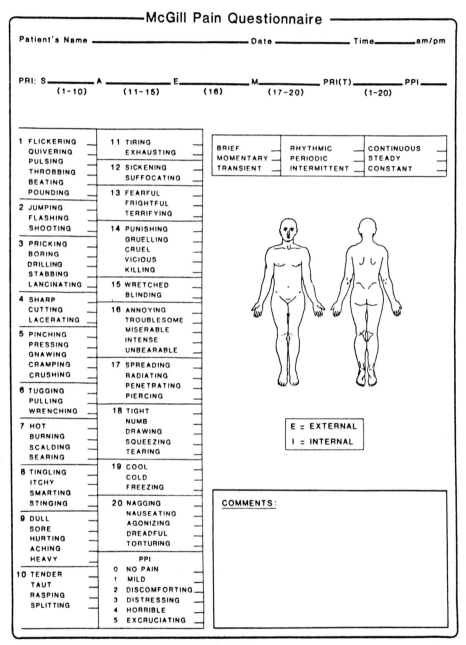

──────── McGill Pain Questionnaire ────────

Patient's Name ──────────────── Date ─────── Time──────am/pm

PRI: S────── A ────── E──────── M────── PRI(T)────── PPI──
     (1-10)   (11-15)   (16)   (17-20)   (1-20)

1 FLICKERING QUIVERING PULSING THROBBING BEATING POUNDING	11 TIRING EXHAUSTING
2 JUMPING FLASHING SHOOTING	12 SICKENING SUFFOCATING
3 PRICKING BORING DRILLING STABBING LANCINATING	13 FEARFUL FRIGHTFUL TERRIFYING
4 SHARP CUTTING LACERATING	14 PUNISHING GRUELLING CRUEL VICIOUS KILLING
5 PINCHING PRESSING GNAWING CRAMPING CRUSHING	15 WRETCHED BLINDING
6 TUGGING PULLING WRENCHING	16 ANNOYING TROUBLESOME MISERABLE INTENSE UNBEARABLE
7 HOT BURNING SCALDING SEARING	17 SPREADING RADIATING PENETRATING PIERCING
8 TINGLING ITCHY SMARTING STINGING	18 TIGHT NUMB DRAWING SQUEEZING TEARING
9 DULL SORE HURTING ACHING HEAVY	19 COOL COLD FREEZING
10 TENDER TAUT RASPING SPLITTING	20 NAGGING NAUSEATING AGONIZING DREADFUL TORTURING

BRIEF	RHYTHMIC	CONTINUOUS
MOMENTARY	PERIODIC	STEADY
TRANSIENT	INTERMITTENT	CONSTANT

E = EXTERNAL
I = INTERNAL

COMMENTS:

PPI
0 NO PAIN
1 MILD
2 DISCOMFORTING
3 DISTRESSING
4 HORRIBLE
5 EXCRUCIATING

FIGURE 14–3. The McGill Pain Questionnaire. The patient is asked to mark the one adjective in each group that best describes the pain. Those objectives numbered 1 to 10 are sensory; 11 to 15, affective; 16, evaluative; and 17 to 20, miscellaneous. Their value is based on their position in the group, and the sum of their values is the "pain rating index (PRI)."

The patient is also asked to sketch the location of the pain on the drawings and indicate if it is deep (internal) or superficial (external). In the "comments" box, the patient is expected to note symptoms that might be accompanying the pain, such as insomnia, anorexia, or lassitude. (Reprinted from Melzack R (ed): Pain Measurement and Assessment. New York, Raven Press, 1983. With permission of Raven Press.)

itching quality, and occurs only along the incision. Postmastectomy pain, like many other forms of pain, worsens at night. It is also provoked when the patient moves her arm. The pain and loss of the pectoral muscles restrict shoulder motion and may lead to a "frozen shoulder."

Assuming that a patient's primary physician is simultaneously excluding other causes of pain in the axilla, such as tumor infiltration of the brachial plexus, infection in the incision, and radiation fibrosis, patients may be treated with non-narcotic analgesics and amitriptyline. Pain may also be reduced by massaging the painful skin with a damp cloth after applying a vapocoolant, such as ethylchloride spray, or by TENS. Patients should exercise to increase shoulder mobility and upper arm strength.

When postmastectomy pain develops, even though it does not carry prognostic significance, it intensifies the mastectomy's psychologic impact. No matter how tempting, pain at or near the site of a mastectomy should not readily be attributed to psychogenic factors.

Postherpetic Neuralgia

Acute Herpes zoster infection causes a red maculopapular and then a vesicular skin eruption, *shingles*, in the distribution of one or two nerve dermatomes. Although any dermatome may be affected, the thoracic dermatomes followed by the first branch of the trigeminal nerve, which includes the cornea, are most commonly affected. The infection is caused by reactivated varicella (Herpes) virus that has lain dormant in dorsal (sensory) nerve root ganglia. It is especially common among elderly people, patients with lymphoproliferative disorders, and individuals with immunosuppression, including acquired immune deficiency syndrome (AIDS).

The acute infection causes moderate pain, described as continual and burning. Sometimes the onset of the pain precedes the appearance of the skin lesions by 2 or 3 days. The skin lesions clear within several weeks, and in most cases, the pain recedes. The infection leaves a band of scarred skin with decreased sensation. If a major motor nerve were involved, muscle weakness and atrophy would be present. During this period, narcotic analgesics are appropriate. An antiviral agent, acyclovir (Zovirax), may speed healing of the vesicles, shorten the duration of the pain, and prevent the spread of the infection into the eye.

After the resolution of the skin lesions, some patients develop severe pain with a lancinating quality, a condition known as *postherpetic neuralgia*. Overall, 10 to 20 percent of Herpes zoster patients are affected with postherpetic neuralgia, but the proportion is much greater in people older than 65 years. The pain can last for months and cause anorexia, insomnia, and mood changes.

The severity of postherpetic neuralgia justifies the routine use of narcotics. Possibly more than in many other conditions, a trial of amitriptyline is indicated. As in other chronic pain syndromes, carbamazepine and phenytoin have often been suggested, but studies have shown that they are helpful only for relieving the lancinating aspect of the pain. Individual reports have advocated using fluphenazine or perphenazine. A novel approach to analgesia has been recently introduced for the treatment of postherpetic neuralgia: a skin cream containing capsaicin (Zostrix) reportedly depletes substance P and thereby interrupts pain transmission. Physical measures, such as TENS, acupuncture, and ethylchloride sprays, have been reported to be helpful in individual cases.

Causalgia

Causalgia is a particularly painful condition that follows an injury of a major peripheral nerve or nerve plexus of the arm or leg (Table 5-1). It is usually produced by a penetrating injury, such as a gunshot wound; however, a seemingly minor compressive or traction injury can be responsible. Some authors note that causalgia-like pain ("thalamic" or "central" pain, see below) can also result from injuries in any area of the CNS.

Within 2 months after a nerve injury, patients may develop a relentless burning sensation superimposed on an irritating numbness. Affected limbs are often rendered useless. A patient may carefully guard a hand by wearing a sling and a glove or protect a foot by using crutches.

The characteristic pain has accompanying skin changes called "trophic" or "sudomotor," in which the skin may become smooth, shiny, pale, and scaly. The nails tend to be long and brittle. Although the affected skin may have excessive sweating, *hyperhidrosis*, it is usually sweatless, cool, and dry.

The best treatment for causalgia is blockade of the regional sympathetic ganglia with an injection of an anesthetic agent. For example, patients with causalgia of the hand benefit from a lidocaine or alcohol injection into the stellate (sympathetic) ganglion that, being adjacent to the upper cervical vertebrae, is readily accessible. Alternatively, an intravenous infusion of an affected limb with guanethidine, which blocks alpha and beta adrenergic sympathetic ganglion receptors, reportedly produces noninvasive and diagnostically important relief. TENS may provide some relief, and a large variety of drugs has been advocated.

Causalgia is a particularly important condition for psychiatrists. On an academic level, it illustrates an unusual relationship between the sympathetic and peripheral nervous systems. On a clinical level, patients are in pain, and they are apt to be misdiagnosed. Patients' inability to use their affected limb may seem disproportionately great. Also, they tend to be preoccupied with the limb and go to extravagant lengths to protect it.

Phantom Limb Pain

Phantom limb pain is pain in the region of an amputated limb. For example, a man may have his leg severed at the thigh in an automobile accident, and weeks later he may still feel pain as though it were centered in his ankle. The pain is often accompanied by nonpainful sensations, such as feelings of purposeful movement. However, phantom limb pain is different from pain at the site of a surgical incision, called *stump pain*, which is usually attributed to scar tissue and nerve damage (neuromas) at the incision site. Phantom and stump pain, of course, may occur together.

Phantom limb pain varies in nature, severity, and accompanying psychologic symptoms. It usually begins soon after a traumatic amputation of a limb and has a self-limited duration of several weeks. It is more likely to develop in patients older than 35 years, if the limb were chronically painful before the amputation (as occurs with osteomyelitis), or if the amputation were traumatic. Since most cases of phantom pain result from war, the patients are usually young or middle-aged men. Many have lost their ability to walk or work. Some have more extensive injuries, including loss of several limbs or their genitalia.

Medical treatment alone is insufficient. Carbamazepine, phenytoin, and conventional analgesics are inconsistently beneficial. TENS and acupuncture have been effective only in isolated cases. Physicians have claimed benefit by stump and forehead muscle relaxation and by inducing the sensation that the phantom limb is shrinking to the point that it disappears.

Thalamic Pain

Thalamic infarctions, which themselves are painless, initially cause contralateral hemianesthesia. Depending on other structures that are damaged, hemianesthesia may be accompanied by hemiparesis or hemiataxia.

The condition, also called the *Déjérine-Roussy syndrome* or *central pain*, is characterized by various painful sensations on the hemianesthetic side of the body, which are felt most strongly in the face and hand. In trying to ward off the pain, patients wear hats, long sleeves, and gloves.

Some authors advocate using carbamazepine or phenytoin; however, in most cases these anticonvulsants as well as conventional analgesics do not provide sustained relief. Even narcotics are not satisfactory. Physical therapy and supportive psychotherapy may be temporizing as the pain typically subsides after 6 to 12 months.

Whiplash

When an automobile is struck from behind, the heads of the driver and passengers are thrown backward, i.e., the neck is suddenly hyperextended because the neck muscles are too weak and too slow to counteract the unexpected force. The hyperextension of the neck suddenly applies severe traction on the neck muscles and anterior spine ligaments, and compresses the cervical intervertebral disks and nerve roots. Immediately following the hyperextension, the head naturally rebounds forward, i.e., the neck is suddenly flexed. Unlike the hyperextension, the flexion is limited—as the chin strikes the chest or forehead hits the dashboard. Although the flexion may be less extreme than the extension and the sequence may be reversed, it places yet another and opposite stress on the soft tissues of the neck. This rapid back-and-forth movement of the head and neck is commonly known as a "whiplash."

Whiplash pain is felt in the neck and shoulder muscles, down the arms, and often along the length of the spine. Patients feel as though they cannot bend or turn their neck and that their neck and back muscles are continuously in spasm. In addition, despite the lack of direct head trauma, patients may also have symptoms associated with the postconcussive syndrome, such as headache, insomnia, poor memory, and inattentiveness (Chapter 9). Whiplash injury typically prevents patients from working for 3 to 6 months. Protracted litigation may be associated with even more protracted disability.

The treatment of chronic whiplash injury is notoriously unsuccessful. If possible, occupational, psychologic, and legal issues must all be identified and settled. Medical treatment consists of non-narcotic analgesics, muscle relaxants, and psychotropic medications. Since soft tissues are usually damaged, physical therapy is important. Some patients respond better to passive treatment, such as immobilization of their neck muscles by wearing a foam rubber cervical collar and having moist heat applied for 20 minutes four times daily. Others do better with cervical traction and exercises. Some physicians advocate injections of steroids and local anesthetics into "trigger points" of muscle spasm.

Chronic Low Back Pain

Acute low back pain may be caused by a herniated intervertebral disk, vertebral body facet displacement, or life-threatening illnesses, such as osteomyelitis or metastatic (especially prostatic) cancer. Patients with all these conditions usually have readily demonstrable abnormalities on clinical examination, electromyograms, or CT or MRI scans.

In contrast, *chronic* low back pain rarely has an identifiable cause. Subtle degenerative or inflammatory changes are postulated to have developed in the lumbar vertebrae, their facets, the spine ligaments, or other soft tissues. Few patients have a herniated disk.

Most patients complain of continual, moderate, dull pain in the low back that may be intensified by straining, bending, or prolonged sitting or standing. The pain is not associated with demonstrable paresis despite patients' complaints that they are "weak" in the low back or both legs and they cannot move freely.

Of all the chronic pain syndromes, low back pain is one of the most closely associated with depression. In addition, medications frequently prescribed as analgesics or muscle relaxants, such as diazepam (Valium), may themselves induce psychologic aberrations, including further depression, and engender drug-seeking behavior. Since low back pain cases frequently involve motor vehicle accident insurance, Workers' Compensation Insurance, and litigation, many individual's neurologic, psychiatric, and legal problems become inextricable.

The usual medications are combinations of non-narcotic analgesics, anti-inflammatory agents, and muscle relaxants. TENS may be helpful. Physical therapy, even if it consists only of warm baths or passive exercises, is usually beneficial. Surgery should be avoided. For a flare-up, bedrest, corsets, warm baths, or massages can reduce the pain. Chiropractic spinal manipulation has been shown, in somewhat flawed studies, to be helpful in reducing pain and mobilizing patients. This improvement has been attributed to the doctor-patient relationship and the literal laying-on of hands.

The length of the bedrest has traditionally been 10 to 14 days, but recent studies suggest that 2 days is equally effective. Often pelvic traction is used, but the weights usually applied (10 pounds to 20 pounds) produce no mechanical benefit other than to enforce bedrest. Hospitalization can give certain patients a thorough evaluation, intensive physical therapy, and possibly a refuge under the aegis of a hospitalization for medical reasons.

REFERENCES

Abramowicz M (ed): Nabilone and other antiemetics for cancer patients. Med Letter *29*:2, 1988
Bonica JJ: Management of Pain, 2nd ed. Philadelphia, Lea & Febiger, 1989
Deyo RA, Diehl AK, Rosenthal M: How many days of bed rest for acute low back pain? N Engl J Med *315*:1064, 1986
Dworkin RH, Richlin DM, Handlin DS, et al: Predicting treatment response in depressed and non-depressed chronic pain patients. Pain *24*:343, 1986
Fields HL: Pain. New York, McGraw-Hill Co., 1987
France RD, Houpt JL, Skott A, et al: Depression as a psychopathological disorder in chronic low back pain patients. J Psychosomat Res *30*:127, 1986

Hadler NM: Medical Management of the Regional Musculoskeletal Diseases. Orlando, Grune & Stratton Inc, 1984

Hadler NM: Regional back pain. N Engl J Med *315*:1090, 1986

Merskey H: Psychiatry and the cervical sprain syndrome. Can Med Assoc J *130*:1119, 1984

Merskey H: Regional pain is rarely hysterical. Arch Neurol *45*:915, 1988

Nuzzo JL, Warfield CA: Thalamic pain syndrome. Hosp Pract *20*:32C, 1985

Payne R, Foley KM (eds): Cancer Pain. Med Clin North Am *71*:1987

Plumb LR: Diagnosis and management of whiplash. Pain Analgesia *2*:3, 1986

Portenoy RK, Duma C, Foley KM: Acute herpetic and postherpetic neuralgia: Clinical review and current management. Ann Neurol *20*:651, 1986

Raj PP: Practical Management of Pain. Chicago, Year Book Medical Publishers, 1986

Schott GD: Mechanisms of causalgia and related clinical conditions. Brain *109*:717, 1986

Reich J, Tupin JP, Abramowitz SI: Psychiatric diagnosis of chronic pain patients. Am J Psychiatry *140*:1495, 1983

Schwartzman RJ, McLellan TL: Reflex sympathetic dystrophy. Arch Neurol *44*:555, 1987

Sherman RA, Sherman CJ: Prevalence and chracteristics of chronic phantom limb pain among American veterans. Am J Physical Med *62*:227, 1983

Sternbach RA: The Psychology of Pain, 2nd ed. New York, Raven Press, 1986

Spiegel K, Kalb R, Pasternak GW: Analgesic activity of tricyclic antidepressants. Ann Neurol *13*:462, 1983

QUESTIONS: CHAPTER 14

1–7. Match the substance with its effect on the pain pathways.

1. Morphine
2. Endogenous opioids
3. Serotonin
4. Substance P
5. Enkephalin
6. Beta endorphin
7. Nonsteroidal anti-inflammatory agents

a. Reduce tissue inflammation and reduced fever
b. Interfere with prostaglandin synthesis
c. Provide analgesia by acting on the CNS
d. Pain neurotransmitter in the spinal cord
e. Liberated in a spinal cord descending analgesic tract

8. Which properties of morphine are *not* shared with endogenous opioids?
   a. Tolerance
   b. Effective in deep brainstem structures and spinal cord
   c. Causes mood changes, as well as analgesia
   d. Reversibility with naloxone
   e. Commercial availability
   f. Causes respiratory depression

9–17. What is the composition of these substances?

9. Leu-enkephalin
10. ACTH
11. Morphine
12. Beta endorphin
13. Heroin acid polypeptide
14. Beta lipotropin
15. Met-enkephalin
16. Serotonin
17. Substance P

a. 11-amino-acid polypeptide
b. 5-amino-acid polypeptide
c. Diacetyl morphine
d. Greater than 30,000 amino
e. An indole
f. An alkaloid of opium
g. 91-amino-acid polypeptide
h. 31-amino-acid polypeptide

18. Which of these fibers do not carry pain sensation?
    a. A delta
    b. C
    c. A beta

19. In which spinal cord tract does most pain sensation ascend?
    a. Fasciculus gracilis
    b. Fasciculus cuneatus
    c. Lateral corticospinal tract
    d. Lateral spinothalamic tract

20. In which tract do pain-dampening fibers that utilize serotonin descend within the spinal cord?
    a. Lateral spinothalamic tract
    b. Dorsolateral funiculus
    c. Fasciculus gracilis
    d. Dentorubral tract

21. Which forms of analgesia are mostly naloxone-reversible?
    a. Acupuncture
    b. Narcotic administration
    c. TENS
    d. Aspirin
    e. Hypnosis
    f. Placebo
    g. Stimulation of periventricular gray matter

22. Why would the addition of aspirin or acetaminophen increase the effectiveness of narcotics?
    a. They are also narcotics.
    b. They actually do not increase analgesia.
    c. They stimulate endogenous opioid release.
    d. They interfere with prostaglandin synthesis.
    e. They increase serotonin reuptake.

23. Why are tricyclic and other antidepressants sometimes helpful in treatment of chronic pain?
    a. They treat depression.
    b. They help restore restful sleep patterns.
    c. They increase serotonin levels, which act to decrease pain.
    d. They alter autonomic system activity.
    e. They themselves are analgesics.

24. What are the potential complications of mixedagonist-antagonist narcotics, such as pentazocine
    a. Normeperidine accumulation
    b. Addiction
    c. Delirium
    d. Respiratory depression
    e. Can precipitate withdrawal in patients previously using meperidine (Demerol)

25. What are the potential complications of meperidine (Demerol) use?
    a. Marked undertreatment when the same dose is given orally as intramuscularly
    b. Normeperidine toxicity
    c. Overdose when the same dose is given parenterally as orally
    d. Stupor
    e. Seizures
    f. Tremulousness

26. Which one of the following features is *not* a characteristic of causalgia?
    a. The sympathetic nervous system is involved.
    b. The skin usually becomes shiny and often scaly.
    c. The pain is usually relieved with blockade of the sympathetic ganglia.

    d.   The trunk and abdomen are often involved.
    e.   It originates from major motor nerve trunk or more proximal portions.

27. Which features are present in the phantom limb but not stump (incisional) pain?
    a.   Patients have pain at the site of the amputated limb.
    b.   Patients have the sensation that the limb is still present.
    c.   Patients have a sensation that the limb is capable of movement.
    d.   There is extensive damage to non-neurologic as well as neurologic tissues.

28. Which of the following is *not* a complication of infarction of the thalamus and its surrounding structures?
    a.   Hemianesthesia
    b.   Hemiataxia
    c.   A tendency to cover the face and involved limb
    d.   Abnormal sweating
    e.   Dysesthesia

29. What are the causes of postherpetic pain?
    a.   A varicella virus
    b.   A Herpes virus
    c.   Chicken pox
    d.   Immunosuppression
    e.   Trauma

ANSWERS

1. c.		**13.** c, f.	
2. c.		**14.** g.	
3. e.		**15.** b.	
4. d.		**16.** e.	
5. c.		**17.** a.	
6. c.		**18.** c.	
7. a, b.		**19.** d.	
8. e.		**20.** b.	
9. b.		**21.** a, b, c, f, g.	
10. d.		**22.** d.	
11. f.		**23.** a, b, c, e.	
12. h.			

24. b, c, d, e. Also, pentazacine (Talwin) can cause skin and subcutaneous scarring (sclerosis).

25. a, b, c, d, e, f.

26. d.

27. b, c.

28. d.

29. a, b, c, d.

15

Multiple Sclerosis Episodes

Multiple sclerosis (MS)* is the most common disabling neurologic illness of North American and European young adults. It is characterized by multiple episodes of multiple neurologic deficits. In its early stages only subtle, evanescent disturbances may be present. Multiple sclerosis may then be confused with other neurologic conditions or a psychogenic disorder. In its later stages, various mental disturbances, induced by combinations of neurologic and psychologic factors, may complicate the illness. Despite new tests, the diagnosis of MS and its complications rests on clinical grounds.

ETIOLOGY

A condition of unknown etiology, MS occurs when 1 mm to 3 cm patches of "white matter," the myelin sheaths of CNS axons, become inflamed, then sclerotic, and eventually stripped of myelin. Demyelinated patches, called *plaques*, are scattered or disseminated throughout the optic nerves, brain, and spinal cord. (MS is consequently called "disseminated sclerosis" in the United Kingdom.) Even though the bodies and axons of the nerves are relatively spared, demyelination impairs impulse transmission and causes neurologic deficits. These deficits seem to resolve as the inflammation subsides, but as more plaques develop with repeated attacks, neurologic deficits accumulate.

Multiple sclerosis occurs 50 percent more frequently in women than in men and about 10 times more frequently in close relatives of MS patients than in the general population. Spouses, however, are not especially vulnerable. The mean age of onset is 33 years, with virtually all cases developing between 15 and 50 years. Some patients suffer their first or subsequent attacks following infection, childbirth, physical trauma, electrical injury, or psychologic stress, but there is no significant evidence that any of these factors is the cause of MS.

Although the cause of MS is not known, immunologic abnormalities have been found. For example, patients have increased frequency of particular HLA and other histocompatibility antigens, as well as decreased suppressor T lymphocytes. Also, as in subacute sclerosing panencephalitis (SSPE) and several other chronic debilitating neurologic illnesses, the CSF of MS patients often has a high measles antibody titer, and they tend to have contracted measles at an older age than other persons.

---

* Patients with MS may receive assistance from the National Multiple Sclerosis Society, 205 East 42nd Street, New York, New York 10017, (212) 986-3240.

Epidemiologic studies have shown that the incidence of MS is greatest in patients who have lived, at least through age 15, in cool northern latitudes (above the 37th parallel) in the United States, Europe, and the Soviet Union. Likewise, in Australia, the incidence is greater in the cool, southernmost region. In particular, the incidence of MS is higher in Boston than New Orleans; extremely low in Central Africa, Latin America, and Japan; and higher in Northern Europeans who emigrated as adults to Israel than in those who emigrated as children. Curiously, a small focus of MS cases has been recently found in Key West, Florida.

Epidemiologic information has suggested that dogs may transmit the infectious agent. One major study found that MS had practically never been diagnosed before World War II in the Faeroe Islands, which are near the coast of Scotland, but after the war the islanders suffered a virtual epidemic. The onset of MS was attributed to British troops and their canine mascots who had occupied the islands. Another study found that a significantly greater number of American MS patients, compared to individuals without MS, had kept dogs and other small indoor pets while children.

CLINICAL MANIFESTIONS

Initial manifestations may range from trivial impairment lasting several days to a group of debilitating disturbances that remain for several weeks and do not fully recede. On the average, 2 to 3 years elapse before a recurrence (exacerbation) develops. Then the initial symptoms, accompanied by additional ones, generally recur. Most patients have a course characterized by exacerbations, then partial remissions, and finally accumulated impairments. However, from the outset, about 10 percent have steady deterioration. Regardless of their initial course, many patients reach a state in which they are partially or fully blind, confined to a wheelchair, unable to speak distinctly, and overwhelmed by seemingly unwarranted bouts of emotion. On the other hand, about one third of patients have no functional disability 10 years after the diagnosis.

Although many symptoms may occur during the illness, the initial and more frequent ones result from demyelination of the heavily myelinated CNS (white matter) tracts in the spinal cord, brainstem, and optic nerves. Only when accumulated extensive demyelination has accumulated in the voluminous cerebral white matter, late in the course, does MS produce significant mental impairment. Since the unmyelinated cerebral cortical "gray matter" is relatively spared, MS patients rarely develop signs of cerebral cortical dysfunction, such as seizures or aphasia. Likewise, since the basal ganglia are unmyelinated, involuntary movement disorders (Chapter 18) are virtually never manifestations of MS.

In classic descriptions, the cardinal manifestations of MS were dysarthria, nystagmus, and tremor—Charcot's *triad*. Today, the constellation of symptoms that is most often described by patients as being troublesome includes incontinence, impotence, and impairment of gait. This change apparently results from today's earlier diagnosis of MS and greater personal openness.

The most frequently encountered symptoms of MS are paresis, sensory disturbances, ataxia, ocular impairments, bladder and sexual dysfunction, and mental disturbances (Fig. 15-1). Almost all MS patients develop paresis, if not

INITIAL AND CUMULATIVE MANIFESTATIONS OF MS

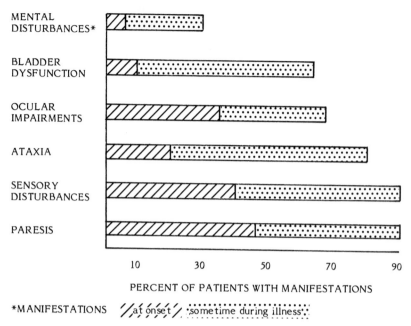

FIGURE 15–1.   Initial and cumulative manifestations of multiple sclerosis.

at the onset of illness, then soon afterward. They usually have paraparesis from spinal cord involvement (Fig. 2-17), but rarely hemiparesis from cerebral involvement. In both cases, since the CNS is damaged, patients have hyperactive DTRs and Babinski signs (Chapter 2). Spinal cord involvement is indicated by a characteristic electrical sensation that extends from the neck down the spine when the neck is flexed (*Lhermitte's sign*). More important, spinal cord demyelination causes muscle spasticity that leads to gait impairment, painful leg spasms, and bladder and sexual disturbances.

Multiple sclerosis patients almost always develop ataxia and other manifestations of cerebellar injury. Typically, they have gait ataxia (Fig. 2-13) that causes them to spread their feet widely apart and lurch forward. When the ataxia is subtle, it can only be elicited by having the patient walk heel-to-toe (*tandem gait*). Other manifestations of cerebellar involvement are intention tremor (Fig. 2-11), dysdiadochokinesia, and arrhythmic, disconcerting head rocking (*titubation*).

In addition, MS patients' speech is impaired by ataxia. The result is a variety of dysarthria called *scanning speech* that is characterized by irregular and prolonged pauses between syllables, and uneven cadence. For example, when asked to repeat a pair of short syllables, such as "ba . . . ga . . . ba . . . ga . . . ," the patient might place unequal emphasis on each syllable, blur them together, or pause excessively.

Sensory disturbances, which are a prominent feature of MS, result from cerebral or spinal cord plaques. Patients have hypalgesia or paresthesias in scattered areas of their limbs or trunk, or below a particular spinal cord level (Fig. 2-15). Notably, since patients' descriptions of their sensory disturbances often overshadow objective findings and do not conform to commonplace neurologic patterns, those patients with only sensory disturbances are liable to be misdiagnosed as suffering from a psychogenic condition.

Ocular impairments, which are often early MS manifestations, include impaired visual acuity and disordered ocular motility. Visual acuity impairment results from attacks of *retrobulbar (optic) neuritis*, which is an inflammatory condition of the retrobulbar portion of the optic nerve (Fig. 12-6). Optic neuritis causes both an irregular area of visual loss in one eye, a *scotoma* (Fig. 15-2), and pain when that eye is moved. Since the optic disk is unaffected, ophthalmoscopic examination reveals no abnormality. This discrepancy between visual loss and normal ophthalmoscopy has given rise to the saying, "The patient sees nothing and the physician sees nothing." As an optic neuritis attack subsides, the pain leaves, and most, if not all, vision returns. However, with repeated attacks, progressive visual loss ensues, and the disk becomes atrophic.

About 25 percent of patients have had overt optic neuritis as their initial symptom, and the majority have had it at some time during their illness. New electrophysiologic studies have shown that almost all MS patients have had asymptomatic, if not symptomatic, optic neuritis. On the other hand, only 20 to 40 percent of young adults who develop optic neuritis as an isolated condition will later develop MS. Therefore, although optic neuritis is a common MS symptom, a single, isolated attack of optic neuritis is not diagnostic of MS.

Multiple sclerosis also causes two ocular movement disturbances: *nystagmus* and the characteristic *internuclear ophthalmoplegia (INO)*, which is also called the *medial longitudinal fasciculus (MLF) syndrome*. Nystagmus results from brainstem or cerebellar MS involvement. Although MS-induced nystagmus is clinically indistinguishable from nystagmus caused by other conditions (Chapter 12), it frequently occurs in combination with dysarthria and tremor (Charcot's triad).

Internuclear ophthalmoplegia, which causes diplopia on lateral gaze, results when demyelination or other MLF damage interrupts nerve impulse transmission to the oculomotor nuclei (Figs. 15-3 and 15-4). Although a unilateral INO may result from lupus in young adults or from basilar artery infarctions in elderly patients, bilateral INO is virtually pathognomonic of MS. Only botulism and myasthenia gravis, because they cause paresis of several cranial nerves, may create a confusingly similar picture of abnormal ocular motility.

Bladder dysfunction, which is a sign of spinal cord MS, not only impairs the functional capabilities of patients and causes psychologic repercussions but it is also associated with sexual impairment (Chapter 16). It results from a combination of spasticity and paresis of the external sphincter of the bladder (Fig. 15-5), paresis of the lower abdominal muscles, and bladder and sphincter incoordination (*dyssynergy*). Affected patients initially have frequent, small, and precipitous urinations, and also incontinence during sleep and sexual intercourse. Later in the illness, patients develop urinary retention and complete incontinence. Many require intermittent or continuous catheterization, which burdens them with the risk of infection, as well as esthetic problems.

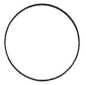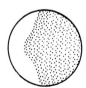

FIGURE 15–2.   Optic (retrobulbar) neuritis causes pain on eye movement and impaired vision in a large, irregular area (a *scotoma*), which typically includes the center of vision (also see Fig. 12-6).

MEDIAL LONGITUDINAL
FASCICULUS (MLF)

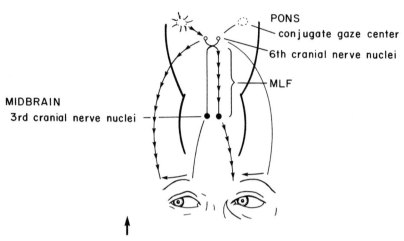

FIGURE 15–3.   When looking laterally, the pontine conjugate gaze center stimulates the adjacent abducens (sixth) nerve nucleus and, though the *medial longitudinal fasciculus (MLF)*, the contralateral oculomotor (third) nerve nucleus. Thus, when looking to the right, the right abducens and the left oculomotor nuclei are both stimulated (also see Fig. 12-12).

INTERNUCLEAR
OPHTHALMOPLEGIA

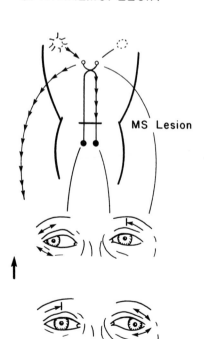

FIGURE 15–4.   In *internuclear ophthalmoplegia (INO)*, interruption of the MLF prevents impulses from reaching the oculomotor nuclei. Since the oculomotor nuclei themselves are intact, the pupils and eyelids are normal in both eyes. When looking to the right, because the oculomotor nuclei are not stimulated, the left eye fails to adduct. The right eye abducts, but nystagmus develops. With bilateral INO, which is characteristic of MS, neither eye adducts, and the abducting eye has nystagmus.

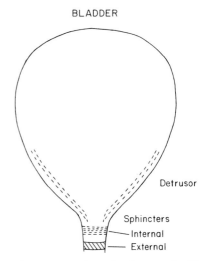

FIGURE 15–5. Normal urinary bladder emptying (urination) occurs when the detrusor (wall) muscle contracts and *both* sphincter muscles relax. Urination requires reflex parasympathetic stimulation (to contract the detrusor and relax the internal sphincter), as well as voluntary action (to relax the external sphincter).

Urinary retention occurs with either anticholinergic medications or excessive sympathetic activity. Both inhibit detrusor contraction and internal sphincter muscle relaxation. Retention occurs with spinal cord injury because the external sphincter is then spastic and paretic, and also because, when the detrusor contracts, the sphincters fail to relax (dyssynergy).

Sexual impairment, (Chapter 16), with or without bladder dysfunction, plagues about 85 percent of MS patients. Men may have premature or retrograde ejaculation and impotence. They also have reduced fertility, partly because of sexual impairment and partly because spinal cord MS leads to lowered and abnormal sperm production. An interesting new technique that induces erections in MS men with erectile dysfunction is injections of papaverine and other substances directly into the penis (Chapter 16).

Women with MS tend to become unarousable and anorgasmic. They remain fertile, and during pregnancy MS is stable or improved; however, the postpartum period is associated with exacerbations. The delivery itself, when the spinal cord is affected, can be complicated by spastic abdominal and pelvic muscle contractions, unstable blood pressure, and other signs of autonomic dysfunction.

MENTAL ABERRATIONS

As would be expected, depression at the onset of MS is the most common disturbance; however, patients in remission may be troubled less by depression than by overt physical disabilities, social impairments, and anxiety. Studies have indicated that when depression occurs in MS patients, it may not always be simply a psychologic response to the illness but possibly a manifestation of cerebral involvement. Depression is found more frequently in MS patients than in those with other chronic neurologic and non-neurologic conditions that yield comparable physical impairments. Also, depression is especially frequent in MS during exacerbations, late in the course of the illness, or when intellectual function is compromised.

In view of the consequences of MS, the apparent elevation of mood in some patients, the so-called euphoria, has been a striking paradox. Certainly, some euphoric patients have been protecting themselves psychologically by denial or have been masking depression. Others simply have been feeling relief as an MS attack subsides. Also, following hospitalization there is often a remission of symptoms and reduced anxiety, and patients become overjoyed.

In addition to these psychodynamic mechanisms for euphoria, it may also be induced by MS treatments that are based on high-dose ACTH, prednisone, or other steroid medications (see below, Steroid Psychosis). Also, laughing and other superficial aspects of euphoria may be manifestations of pseudobulbar palsy (Chapter 4). Moreover, since euphoria is associated with physical deterioration and subtle, if not overt, intellectual impairment, it probably results partly from advanced cerebral involvement.

Intellectual impairments clearly result from extensive cerebral demyelination. Although the cerebral cortical gray matter is usually spared in MS, it may be extensively undercut, irritated by numerous plaques, or damaged in other ways with advanced disease. Thus overt intellectual impairment does not appear until late in the course of the disease, when physical incapacity is pronounced. Until then, only subtle, nonspecific intellectual changes can be detected. Demonstrating them requires complex neuropsychologic tests, such as the Wechsler Adult Intelligence Scale (WAIS) and the Halstead Category Test.

The late development of intellectual changes in MS distinguishes it from Alzheimer's disease and CVAs. In Alzheimer's disease, which affects the gray matter virtually exclusively, intellectual impairment occurs first and becomes pronounced before physical impairment develops. CVAs typically damage both gray and white matter and cause combined intellectual and physical impairment. Particularly with multi-infarct dementia, intellectual and physical deficits progress together (Chapter 11).

Sometimes the mental disturbances of MS mimic psychosis. However, the incidence of psychosis in MS patients is remarkably lower than that found in other neurologic illnesses, including Alzheimer's disease, head trauma, and partial complex epilepsy. In MS, psychotic disturbances probably originate from intellectual impairment and sensory deprivation. Other causes may be steroid therapy, which can lead to steroid psychosis (see below), or delirium from systemic infection. In general, psychiatrists should initially assume that psychotic behavior and even less pronounced mental aberrations in MS patients are organic in nature, and perhaps manifestations of cerebral demyelination, drug therapy, or a concomitant physical condition.

LABORATORY TESTS

The diagnosis of MS, like that of such common illnesses as migraine headaches and herniated intervertebral disks, can be based on the patient's history and neurologic examination. Laboratory tests, although potentially useful in certain cases, are often superfluous, as well as expensive. They are indicated, however, when symptoms are vague, few objective signs are present, or, more important, when only a single overt attack has occurred or a single CNS area is involved. Some tests indicate exacerbations of MS, quiescent as well as active disease, or prior asymptomatic attacks. Unfortunately, no single test is diagnostic, and many false-negative and false-positive results occur.

The "hot-bath test," which still has historic interest, has fortunately fallen into disuse. In this test people who were suspected of having MS were immersed in a very warm bath for about 30 minutes. If the warmth precipitated neurologic deficits that resolved as the patient's temperature returned to normal, a diagnosis of MS was strongly supported. However, the test occasionally produced disabilities, such as paraparesis, which did not remit.

Routine CSF protein analysis during an MS attack will often reveal that, although protein concentration is normal (40 mg/100 ml) or only slightly elevated, the gamma globulin portion will be elevated (9 percent or greater). In contrast, in other chronic inflammatory CNS illnesses, including fungal meningitis, neurosyphilis, and SSPE, the CSF is characterized by marked elevations in total protein concentration and percent of gamma globulin.

A more specific diagnostic indicator is the presence of CSF *oligoclonal bands*. The substance constituting these bands is actually a discrete IgG protein, similar to an antibody, that is found in more than 90 percent of patients with either quiescent or active MS. It may, however, also be found in chronic inflammatory CNS illnesses, including neurosyphilis and acquired immunodeficiency syndrome (AIDS). Another diagnostically important CSF substance is *myelin basic protein*. It is found, presumably because of myelin breakdown, in MS exacerbations and several rare neurologic illnesses, such as leukodystrophies and central pontine myelinolysis. It is usually not found in normal CSF or in chronic MS. The cost of such CSF analyses, which require a lumbar puncture, is about $250 (in 1989).

Although routine EEGs are not diagnostically helpful, electrophysiologic *evoked response tests* can reveal visual, auditory, or sensory pathway impairment. The tests are based on repetitive stimulation of these heavily myelinated pathways, which evokes a characteristic electrical response that may be detected with scalp electrodes similar to those used for EEGs. With any injury, the delay (*latency*) between the stimulus and response is prolonged and often abnormal in form. Evoked response tests are particularly useful in demonstrating asymptomatic demyelinating lesions, the presence of which would indicate that a neurologic illness has affected multiple CNS areas. For example, if a patient has deficits referable only to the spinal cord, but evoked response tests reveal an optic nerve injury, the physician would know that at least two CNS areas were injured, and therefore MS would be a likely diagnosis. The cost of evoked response testing is about $300 to $800.

Visual evoked responses (*VERs*), which are the most reliable of these tests, reveal any optic nerve abnormality. Visual evoked responses are performed by recording the latency as a patient stares at a rapidly flashing checkerboard pattern on a television screen. The cerebral responses are computer-averaged and made into a composite pattern that minimizes background or random electrical activity ("noise"), and displays a characteristic wave pattern, a response that would otherwise be undetectable.

Prolonged latencies and otherwise abnormal patterns are found in virtually all cases of MS with optic neuritis. Abnormal results are also found with other optic nerve lesions, such as optic nerve gliomas or astrocytomas (Chapter 19), congenital injury (Chapter 13), and optic neuritis when it occurs apart from

MS. Visual evoked responses are also helpful in distinguishing ocular from cortical blindness and in identifying psychogenic visual loss (Chapter 12).

Brainstem auditory evoked responses (BAERs) measure responses to a series of clicks in each ear. They are helpful not only in indicating MS brainstem involvement but also in characterizing hearing impairments, diagnosing acoustic neuromas, and evaluating hearing in people unable to cooperate, such as infants and those with autism or psychogenic disturbances.

Somatosensory evoked responses involve application of various stimuli to a patient's arms or legs. Multiple sclerosis or other spinal cord injury will cause abnormal latencies.

Computed tomography (CT) can occasionally demonstrate areas of demyelination that are indicative of MS plaques in either the cerebral or cerebellar white matter. In addition, since asymptomatic as well as symptomatic plaques can be demonstrated, CT can show that a neurologic disease is disseminated. However, CT does not demonstrate abnormalities that are small, in the spinal cord, or in the location or quantity that would be predicted by the clinical examination.

Magnetic resonance imaging (MRI) is the better test to identify demyelination of optic nerve, spinal cord, or brain. Some MS plaques are indistinguishable from lesions due to other illnesses, but MS lesions are typically more numerous and widely distributed (Fig. 20-17).

Although MS patients have immunologic impairments, the appropriate tests are technically difficult and the results imprecise. For example, although CSF measles antibody titers can be measured, elevated levels are a nonspecific reaction that are found in other neurologic conditions. Likewise, histocompatibility antigens and suppressor T lymphocytes are not specific enough markers to be diagnostic.

THERAPY

Systemically administered high-dose ACTH, prednisone, or other steroid medications are widely used because they are believed to foreshorten MS attacks and even reduce the residual deficits. Although steroid treatment may lead to mental aberrations, it is rarely complicated by opportunistic infections, such as TB or cryptococcal meningitis, as happens in lupus or renal transplantation treatment. More potent immunosuppressants are sometimes used, but their slight additional benefit, compared to their risks, has made their acceptance limited.

Physical therapy helps to preserve muscle tone, prevent decubitus ulcers, and provide maximum mobility. Depending upon the nature of a patient's bladder dysfunction, medication alone, such as imipramine (Tofranil) might be sufficient; however, self-catheterization or external sphincter removal may be necessary. Spasticity, another common problem, usually requires baclofen (Lioresal), diazepam (Valium), or other muscle relaxants.

Since depression is so common, physicians are justified in using antidepressant medications. In addition to elevating mood, they may improve sleep and reduce some of the pain associated with the patient's immobility and spasticity; however, antidepressants with anticholinergic effects must be used cautiously because they may precipitate urinary retention. Almost all patients with established MS can benefit from MS clinics or self-help groups that provide psychologic support and practical information.

STEROID PSYCHOSIS

A wide variety and degree of intellectual, emotional, and behavioral aberrations—loosely termed "steroid psychosis"—can result from treatment of MS with ACTH, prednisone, or other steroid medications. These mental aberrations also occur during steroid treatment of various systemic inflammatory conditions, such as rheumatologic disorders and lupus, organ transplant rejection, and acute asthma; in patients with conditions that overproduce steroids, such as Cushing's syndrome; and in athletes who surreptitiously use steroids for energy and body building.

When steroid medications are given in high dosage they cause euphoria, ravenous appetite, and insomnia. They also often produce a fine, rapid tremor that mimics anxiety-induced and essential tremors (Chapter 18). In some cases, which supposedly cannot be predicted by the presence or absence of a premorbid psychiatric disturbance, steroids produce agitation, hallucinations, and delusions. Although rare patients have been described as being depressed, the typical clinical picture is increased physical and mental activity.

The problem usually begins 1 to 4 days after high-dose steroid treatment is started, and the onset is related to the biologic activity of the medication. Expressed in biologic equivalents of prednisone, the incidence increases from 4 percent of patients receiving less than 40 mg prednisone daily to 20 percent of patients receiving more than 80 mg daily. If steroid treatment is discontinued, the symptoms recede, leaving no permanent damage.

Steroid psychosis in a patient with a systemic inflammatory disease on high-dose steroids poses a clinical dilemma. In illnesses where the brain may be directly involved, such as lupus, abruptly decreasing the steroids might worsen the underlying disease's cerebral involvement. In addition, at a time when the body is under stress and consequently requires increased steroids, stopping them may cause shock from adrenal insufficiency. As a general rule, when confronted with this dilemma, until a thorough evaluation is completed, steroids should be maintained or increased, and psychotic disturbances should be treated with major tranquilizers. Alternatively, according to a few reports, lithium has also been effective. However, tricyclic antidepressants may exacerbate the condition.

CONDITIONS THAT MIMIC MS

Several physically incapacitating conditions that frequently develop in young people may resemble MS. Even with CSF analyses and electrophysiologic tests, they may be difficult to diagnose.

The Guillain-Barré syndrome, for example, is a demyelinating disorder of the peripheral nervous system (PNS), which generally strikes young and middle-aged adults (Chapter 5). Patients may have paraparesis or quadriparesis, mild sensory loss, and in severe cases respiratory insufficiency. Since Guillain-Barré syndrome affects PNS myelin, its paresis, unlike that of MS, is symmetric, accompanied by flaccidity and areflexia, and likely to resolve completely. In addition, since the Guillain-Barré syndrome is a PNS illness, it does not cause optic neuritis, INO, or mental disturbances.

Brainstem astrocytomas, which occur in children as well as young adults, mimic MS because they invade the corticospinal, cerebellar, and sensory tracts and also the MLF. Cerebral astrocytomas, which occur in young adults and older individuals, cause hemiparesis but also, unlike MS, produce headaches and seizures. Most important, neoplasms produce steadily worsening symptoms and signs referable to a single CNS area, and can be diagnosed with CT or MRI scan.

Although acquired immune deficiency syndrome (AIDS) usually begins with signs of systemic illness, such as fever, malaise, lymphadenopathy, and opportunistic infections, it also frequently produces seizures, hemiparesis, and dementia. The neurologic abnormalities are often caused by brain or spinal cord lymphomas or infections with toxoplasmosis (Chapter 7). Neurologic illness from AIDS should not be confused with MS because it has a typically unremitting course and is associated with signs of systemic illness.

Like MS, systemic lupus erythematosus (lupus or SLE) and other vascular inflammatory diseases may produce multiple CNS abnormalities in individuals 15 to 40 years old. Although some series include common symptoms, such as headache or neurosis, as being its first manifestation, lupus rarely causes serious neurologic or psychiatric problems at its onset. Patients usually develop these symptoms during exacerbations of the illness, and particularly in its terminal phase. Approximately 75 percent of lupus patients eventually develop neurologic or psychiatric complications. The neurologic complications have been attributed to an arteritis produced by immune complexes. In addition, patients can have neurologic problems from the hypertension, uremia, opportunistic infections, and treatment with steroids and other immunosuppressant medications.

The multisystem nature of lupus causes several notable clinical patterns. Mental aberrations can be associated with systemic symptoms, certain PNS injuries (Table 5-2), and movement disorders (Table 18-4). Mental aberrations, which can take the form of either dementia or delirium (Chapter 7), can occur in young adults (Table 7-2). Also, as in Lyme disease, CNS and PNS symptoms can be associated with joint pains (Chapter 5). Lupus causes neuropathy, mononeuropathy multiplex, and other PNS abnormalities. It usually causes a delirium that mimics psychosis, and supposedly it also causes affective disorders, phobias, and autistic behavior. Other common manifestations are seizures and cerebral and brainstem stroke syndromes, of which a characteristic consequence is chorea. Overall, among the numerous potential neurologic complications of lupus, the most common are the "three S's": seizures, strokes, and psychosis.

In patients with paraparesis only, alternative diagnoses are spinal cord disorders, which include combined-system disease (B_{12} deficiency), cervical spine degeneration, and spinal meningiomas. Thus, a spine CT or MRI, myelogram, and a serum B_{12} level determination are typically obtained.

Despite the many neurologic conditions that mimic MS, it is probably most commonly confused with psychogenic disorders (Chapter 3). An individual with either MS or a psychogenic disorder may have common symptoms, such as blurred vision, clumsiness, sexual impairments, and nonspecific sensory losses. If the neurologic examination fails to reveal definitive, abnormal neurologic signs, further investigations with MRI scans, VERs, and possibly CSF analysis are indicated.

REFERENCES

Adelman DC, Saltiel E, Klinenberg JR: The neuropsychiatric manifestations of systemic lupus erythematosus: An overview. Semin Arthritis Rheum *15*:185, 1986

Baretz RM, Stephenson GR: Emotional responses to multiple sclerosis. Psychosomatics *22*:117, 1981

Birk K, Rudick R: Pregnancy and multiple sclerosis. Arch Neurol *43*:719, 1986

Bluestein HG, Pischel KD, Woods VL: Immunopathogenesis of the neuropsychiatric manifestations of systemic lupus erythematosus. Springer Semin Immunopathol *9*:237, 1986

Dalos NP, Rabins PV, Brooks BR, et al: Disease activity and emotional state in multiple sclerosis. Ann Neurol *13*:573, 1983

Hall RCW, Popkin MK, Stickney SK, et al: Presentation of the steroid psychoses. J Nerv Ment Dis *167*:229, 1979

Hallpike JF, Addams CWM, Tourtelloutte WW (eds): Multiple Sclerosis: Pathology, Diagnosis and Management. Baltimore, Williams & Wilkins, 1983

Honer WG, Hurwitz T, Li DKB, et al: Temporal lobe involvement in multiple sclerosis patients with psychiatric disorders. Arch Neurol *44*:187, 1987

Huber SJ, Paulson GW, Shuttleworth EC, et al: Magnetic resonance imaging correlates of dementia in multiple sclerosis. Arch Neurol *44*:732, 1987

Joffe RT, Lippert GP, Gray TA, et al: Mood disorder and multiple sclerosis. Arch Neurol *44*:376, 1987

Kirkeby HJ, Poulsen EU, Petersen T, et al: Erectile dysfunction in multiple sclerosis. Neurology *38*:1366, 1988

Korn-Lubetzki I, Kahana K, Cooper G, et al: Activity of multiple sclerosis during pregnancy and puerperium. Ann Neurol *16*:229, 1984

Kurtzke JF, Hyllested K: Multiple sclerosis in the Faroe Islands. Neurology *36*:307, 1986

Kurtzke JF, Beebe GW, Norman JE: Epidemiology of multiple sclerosis in US veterans: III Migration and the risk of MS. Neurology *35*:672, 1985

Lyon-Caen O, Jouvent R, Hauser S, et al: Cognitive function in recent-onset demyelinating diseases. Arch Neurol *43*:1138, 1986

McArthur JC, Young F: Multiple sclerosis in pregnancy. In Goldstein PJ (ed): Neurological Disorders of Pregnancy. Mt. Kisco, NY, Futura Publishing Company, 1986

Minderoud JM, Leemhuis JG, Kremer J, et al: Sexual disturbances arising from multiple sclerosis. Acta Neurol Scand *70*:299, 1984

Omdal R, Mellgren SI, Husby G: Clinical neuropsychiatric and neuromuscular manifestations in systemic lupus erythematosus. Scand J Rheumatol *17*:113, 1988

Patterson MB, Foliart R: Multiple sclerosis: Understanding the psychologic implications. Gen Hosp Psychiatry *7*:234, 1985

Scheinberg LC, Holland NJ (eds): Multiple Sclerosis: A Guide for Patients and Their Families, 2nd ed. New York, Raven Press, 1987

Schiffer RB: The spectrum of depression in multiple sclerosis. Arch Neurol *44*:596, 1987

Valleroy ML, Kraft GH: Sexual dysfunction in multiple sclerosis. Arch Phys Med Rehabil *65*:125, 1984

van den Burg W, van Zomeren AH, Minderhoud JM, et al: Cognitive impairment in patients with multiple sclerosis and mild physical disability. Arch Neurol *44*:494, 1987

QUESTIONS: CHAPTER 15

1–5. A 25-year-old policeman develops paraparesis and markedly impaired visual acuity in his left eye over 4 days. Aside from a delayed light reaction in the left eye and lower extremity hyperactive deep tendon reflexes with Babinski signs accompanying the paraparesis, his neurologic examination is normal.

1. Which of the following disorders are possible causes of his disturbances?
   a. Spinal cord tumor
   b. Hysteria
   c. Multiple sclerosis

    d. Postvaccination encephalomyelitis
    e. Wilson's disease

  2. Which areas of the nervous system are most likely to be involved?
    a. Right occipital lobe and thoracic spinal cord
    b. Thoracic spinal cord and left optic nerve
    c. Sacral spinal cord and left optic nerve

  3. After 3 weeks, he becomes ambulatory and finds that his vision is almost normal. One year later, however, he develops dysarthria, ataxia, and tremor of the arms. Where is the new lesion?
    a. Cerebrum
    b. Cerebellum
    c. Brainstem
    d. Spinal cord

  4. Although a diagnosis cannot be made with complete assurance, this patient's illness is typical of a certain disorder. What is it?

  5. A year after the episode of cerebellar dysfunction, he develops paraparesis, urinary and fecal incontinence, and complete loss of sensation below the umbilicus. What diagnostic procedure is indicated?
    a. Cranial computed tomography
    b. Visual evoked responses
    c. Myelography
    d. None of the above

  6. Use of which of the following substances is associated with optic neuritis?
    a. Tobacco
    b. Oral contraceptives
    c. Ethyl alcohol
    d. Methyl alcohol
    e. Penicillin
    f. Heroin

  7. With which of the following conditions is optic neuritis associated?
    a. Rubella
    b. Gonorrhea
    c. Multiple sclerosis
    d. Combined-system disease
    e. Sarcoidosis
    f. Vasculitis

  8. Which of the following conditions may lead to internuclear ophthalmoplegia?
    a. Multiple sclerosis
    b. Subdural hematoma
    c. Hysteria
    d. Lupus erythematosus
    e. Pontine gliomas
    f. Brainstem infarctions

  9–12. A 60-year-old man has difficulty walking, lower back pains that radiate to the trunk and legs, loss of position sense (but intact pain and touch sense) in the feet, and pupils that are small and unreactive to light. Strength in the lower extremities is normal, but deep tendon reflexes are absent. He walks with a broad-based gait.

  9. What is the origin of the gait disturbance?
    a. Cerebellar disturbance
    b. Spinal cord compression
    c. Multiple sclerosis
    d. Hysteria
    e. Dysfunction of tracts of the spinal cord

  10. Although the pupils were small and unreactive to light, they were found to accommodate, i.e., become smaller when the patient looks at a closely held object. What is the pupillary disturbance called?

11. Although the patient had dysfunction of two parts of the nervous sytem, he did not have multiple sclerosis. What disease is he most likely to have?

12. What laboratory test would be most helpful in confirming the clinical impression?

13–17. A 32-year-old man develops blindness and weakness and sensory loss of the right arm and leg. Deep tendon and plantar reflexes are normal. Pupils are equal and reactive to light. He recovers spontaneously after 2 days and is asymptomatic for 1 month. Then he develops paraparesis. Although he cannot perceive pain below the umbilicus, he can distinguish warm from cold and perceive vibration and position sense. Deep tendon, plantar, anal, and cremasteric reflexes are normal.

13. If the patient's right-sided weakness has been the result of cerebral multiple sclerosis or other lesions, with which of the following would his condition be associated?
    a. Weakness of the lower face on the right
    b. Weakness of the lower face on the left
    c. Alterations in the deep tendon reflexes on the right
    d. A flexor plantar response
    e. An extensor plantar response

14. In the second episode, the preservation of temperature sensation despite loss of pain sensation indicates which of the following?
    a. Lateral spinothalamic tract impairment
    b. Posterior column impairment
    c. A peripheral neuropathy
    d. None of the above

15. In multiple sclerosis, blindness is usually the result of retrobulbar or optic neuritis that often leads to optic atrophy. Under these circumstances, what are the pupillary reactions?
    a. The pupils are normally reactive to light.
    b. The light reflex is impaired.

16. With spinal cord injuries, how are the cremasteric and anal reflexes altered?

17. What is the origin of the patient's multiple symptoms that have occurred multiple times?

18–24. Match the ocular movement disorder with the cause(s).

18. Pupillary dilation, ptosis, and paresis of adduction

19. Bilateral ptosis

20. Bilateral horizontal nystagmus

21. Bilateral horizontal nystagmus, unilateral paresis of abduction, and areflexic DTRs

22. Nystagmus in abducting eye and paresis of adduction of other eye

23. Ptosis bilaterally, paresis of adduction of one eye, and normal pupils

24. Nystagmus in adducting eye and paresis of abduction of other eye
    a. Wernicke's encephalopathy
    b. Labyrinthitis
    c. Psychogenic disorders
    d. Myasthenia gravis
    e. Multiple sclerosis
    f. Midbrain infarction
    g. None of the above

25–28. With which conditions are the following laboratory results associated?

25. Anti-ACh receptor antibodies

26. CSF oligoclonal bands

27. CSF myelin basic protein

28. Antistriational antibodies

a. MS in its chronic phase
b. MS in its acute phase
c. Psychogenic disorders
d. Generalized myasthenia gravis
e. Fungal meningitis
f. Myasthenia with underlying thymoma

29. Of the natives of the following cities, who would have the highest and the lowest MS incidence?
   a. New Orleans
   b. Boston
   c. Tokyo

30. Which of the following people have the highest and lowest incidence of MS?
   a. Native Israelis (Sabras)
   b. European immigrants to Israel
   c. Black Africans

31. In which situations do visual evoked responses (VERs) show prolonged or otherwise abnormal latencies?
   a. Asymptomatic optic neuritis
   b. Retrobulbar neuritis
   c. Almost all patients with longstanding MS
   d. Patients with psychogenic blindness
   e. Optic nerve gliomas

32. In MS patients, with which finding(s) is urinary incontinence associated?
   a. Leg spasticity
   b. Ataxia
   c. Spasticity of the external sphincter of the bladder
   d. Sexual impairment
   e. Internuclear ophthalmoplegia (MLF syndrome)

33. Which symptoms typically develop only late, if at all, in the course of MS?
   a. Pseudobulbar palsy
   b. Internuclear ophthalmoplegia
   c. Optic neuritis
   d. Bladder dysfunction
   e. Neurologic-induced mental changes
   f. Depression
   g. Sexual dysfunction
   h. Dementia

34. Which of the following conditions often leads to multiple CNS lesions in young adults?
   a. Lupus
   b. Acquired immune deficiency syndrome (AIDS)
   c. Myasthenia gravis
   d. Bacterial endocarditis
   e. Postvaccination demyelination (encephalomyelitis)

35. Which of the following conditions may lead to "euphoria" in MS patients?
   a. Pseudobulbar palsy
   b. Medications
   c. Cerebral cortex demyelination
   d. Extensive cerebral demyelination
   e. Depression
   f. Remission of an acute attack
   g. Partial complex seizures

36. Although the geographic studies suggest that an environmental factor causes MS, they may also reflect that certain genetic pools (races) are more susceptible to MS. Which of the following factors can suggest a genetic predilection?

    a. VER studies
    b. HLA studies
    c. Israeli immigrant studies
    d. Failure of spouses to contract MS

37. Which of the following conditions are said to precipitate MS exacerbations?
    a. Pregnancy
    b. Depression
    c. Hot baths
    d. Lack of exercise
    e. Hyperthyroidism
    f. Anxiety
    g. Cold weather
    h. Electrical injury

38. In a patient who suddenly developed paraparesis, urinary incontinence, and a T-10 sensory level, which test is the best in indicating a lesion in the CNS in addition to the obvious one in the spinal cord?
    a. CSF oligoclonal bands
    b. CSF myelin basic protein
    c. EEG
    d. CT of the head
    e. VERs
    f. Hot bath test

ANSWERS

1. a. No. Spinal cord tumors would create spastic paraparesis, but they would be unable to cause visual impairment.
    b. No. Hysteria might lead to visual and motor complaints; however, people with hysteria cannot mimic abnormal light, DTR, or plantar reflexes.
    c. Yes. The policeman might have multiple sclerosis affecting the optic nerve and spinal cord.
    d. Yes. Inflammatory reactions to vaccinations, especially for smallpox and rabies, leads to CNS demyelination syndromes that mimic multiple sclerosis.
    e. No. Wilson's disease produces movement disorders and changes in mental status.

2. b. The patient has retrobulbar neuritis and impairments of the thoracic spinal cord.

3. b.

4. Multiple sclerosis

5. d. With another episode of neurologic deficit, the diagnosis of multiple sclerosis can be made with even greater assurance. Although the current event is also compatible with spinal cord compression by a tumor, as well as another episode of multiple sclerosis, the possibility of such a young man developing a second neurologic illness is so remote that a myelogram is unjustified. The other diagnostic procedures are clinically irrelevant.

6. a, c, d.

7. c, d, e, f.

8. a, d, e.

9. e. The gait disturbance is entirely explainable by loss of proprioception in the lower extremities. Loss of reflexes and pupillary abnormalities suggest that the disease is not psychogenic.

10. Argyll-Robertson pupils

11. Tabes dorsalis from syphilis

12. Positive serology, e.g., VDRL, on the spinal fluid

13. a, c, e.

14. d. Pain and temperature sensation both travel in the spinothalamic tract. Their dissociation defies the usual laws of neurology.

15. b. With optic nerve injuries that cause blindness, the pupils are unreactive to direct light. Moreover, in acute optic neuritis, attacks are accompanied by pain.

16. Cremasteric and anal reflexes, both superficial reflexes, are suppressed by both central and peripheral nervous system injuries. Their presence is evidence that the nervous system is physiologically intact.

17. Few illnesses cause recurring symptoms and signs. This patient does not, however, suffer from multiple sclerosis because he has no objective evidence of neurologic dysfunction. On the contrary, he has evidence of a psychogenic disorder.

18. f.

19. d.

20. a, b, e.

21. a.

22. e.

23. d.

24. g.

25. d.

26. a, b, and e.

27. b and e.

28. f.

29. Highest-Boston; lowest-Tokyo.

30. Highest-European immigrants; lowest-Black Africans.

31. a, b, c, e.

32. a, c, d.

33. a, e, h.

34. a, b, d, e.

35. a, b, d, e, f.

36. b, c, d.

37. a, b, c, f, h.

38. e.

16

Neurologic Aspects of
Sexual Function

Whatever its psychology, sexual function requires complex neurologic pathways. This chapter describes how many patients with neurologic illness have predictable sexual impairments, but that patients with certain neurologic illnesses, even when incapacitated in many ways, have no sexual impairment. Patients' sexual potential and limitations should be known by both the patients and their physicians.* This chapter reviews current psychiatric terminology and the neurologic basis of sexual function and dysfunction. Diagnostic techniques and recently introduced mechanical and physiologic treatments are discussed.

The *Diagnostic and Statistical Manual of Mental Disorders, Third Edition, Revised* (*DSM-III-R*) describes a *female sexual arousal disorder (302.72)* and its counterpart in the male, *male erectile disorder (302.72)*, which is a new and useful term. Within each of those disorders, lack of a physiologic response in the genitals is given diagnostic weight equal to a lack of psychologic response, "lack of a subjective sense of sexual excitement." The DSM-III-R also describes several orgasmic disorders: *inhibited female orgasm (302.73)*, *inhibited male orgasm (302.74)*, and *premature ejaculation (302.75)*. Neurologists, on the other hand, do not use codified definitions of sexual dysfunction, but broadly recognize *arousal disorders*, *erectile dysfunction*, *anorgasmy*, and changes in the *libido*. Also, neurologists continue to diagnose *impotence*, which is a nonspecific and pejorative term, when they really mean erectile dysfunction, anorgasmy, or diminished libido.

NEUROLOGIC FUNCTION

Two main neurologic pathways, one originating in the brain and the other in the genitals, convey neurologic impulses that lead to erection or clitoral engorgement (genital arousal). Both pathways involve the central nervous system (CNS), the peripheral nervous system (PNS), and the autonomic nervous system (ANS).

In one pathway, various cerebral stimuli, such as erotic pictures, sleep-related events, and emotional responses, are converted to excitatory neurologic impulses. Most of them travel down the spinal cord (part of the CNS) and exit at its sacral region to be carried by the *pudendal nerve* (part of the PNS). Branches of the pudendal nerve supply the genital muscles and skin (Fig. 16-1).

---

* NPT studies are newly developed, sophisticated polysomnographic recordings performed in sleep disorder centers (Chapter 17) and cost about $1,000 in 1989.

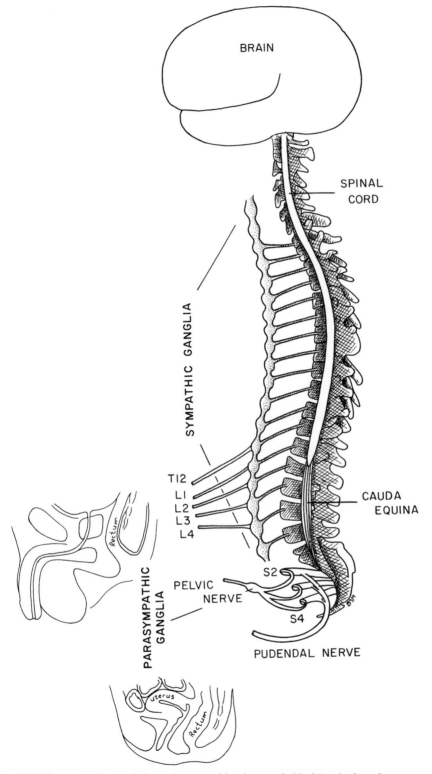

FIGURE 16–1.   The genitals are innervated by the sacral (S2–S4) spinal cord segments and also, in a virtually parallel and complementary manner, by the sympathetic and parasympathetic components of the autonomic nervous system.

Some impulses of this pathway, as if diverted to a subsidiary pathway, exit the lower spinal cord to join *sympathetic* or *parasympathetic* ANS ganglia. The ANS innervates the genitals, reproductive organs, bladder, sweat glands, and artery wall muscles. Stimulation of the ANS first induces vascular distention, which results in genital arousal, and then a complex series of ANS-mediated events produce orgasm. The sympathetic and parasympathetic components of the ANS depend on different neurotransmitters: acetylcholine in the parasympathetic and monoamines in the sympathetic. These components also have different actions in arousal, orgasm, and ejaculation; however, their roles are complementary, and they share vulnerabilities to the same injuries, medications, and psychologic inhibition.

The other pathway, which is shorter and less complicated, originates in sensory receptors in the genitals and loops back through the spinal cord. Although some impulses from genital stimulation pass through the pudendal nerve and continue up the spinal cord to the brain, those in the *genital-spinal cord reflex* synapse in the sacral region of the spinal cord and return, via the ANS, to the genitals. Erotic stimulation of the genitals, which requires this pathway, produces arousal and orgasm.

NEUROLOGIC IMPAIRMENT

A neurologic cause of sexual impairment is indicated when no arousal or orgasm occurs during either cerebral or genital stimulation, when men have no erections on awakening, or when individuals have certain neurologic illnesses (Table 16-1). Physical signs of a neurologic cause should be sought not only on the routine neurologic examination (Table 1-1) but also on examinations of sexually related (extrasexual) functions (Table 16-2).

Since ANS function is crucial, signs of its impairment, which can be subtle, are particularly important. For example, *orthostatic hypotension*, usually defined as a fall of 10 mm Hg in blood pressure on standing, is strong evidence of diabetic, medication-induced, or spontaneous ANS impairment. *Anhidrosis*, lack of sweating, in the groin and legs, which is usually accompanied by hairless and sallow skin, is another sign. Urinary incontinence is usually a manifestation of severe ANS impairment; however, more common causes, such as prostatism or stress incontinence, are often responsible. Finally, *retrograde ejaculation*, another sign, can be detected by examining a urine sample obtained after

TABLE 16–1. INDICATIONS OF NEUROLOGIC SEXUAL IMPAIRMENT

Continual erectile dysfunction
   Absence of morning erections
   No erection or orgasm during masturbation or sex with different partners
Related somatic complaints
   Sensory loss in genitals, pelvis, or legs
   Urinary incontinence
Certain neurologic conditions
   Spinal cord injury
   Diabetic neuropathy
   Multiple sclerosis
   Herniated intervertebral disk
   Use of medications

TABLE 16–2.   SIGNS OF NEUROLOGIC SEXUAL IMPAIRMENT

Signs of spinal cord injury
 Paraparesis or quadriparesis
 Leg spasticity
 Sensory level
 Urinary incontinence
Signs of autonomic nervous system injury
 Orthostatic hypotension or lightheadedness
 Anhidrosis in groin and legs
 Urinary incontinence
 Retrograde ejaculation
Signs of peripheral nervous system injury
 Loss of sensation in the genitals, "saddle area," and legs
 Paresis and areflexia in legs
 Scrotal, cremasteric, and anal reflex loss*

* Also found with spinal cord injury.

orgasm. Microscopic examination of this urine, which appears cloudy to the naked eye, reveals sperm.

With either spinal cord or peripheral nerve injury, weakness and a sensory loss below the waist or one confined to the genitals, anus, and buttocks—the "saddle area" (Fig. 16-2)—might be present. Plantar and deep tendon reflex testing will indicate which system is responsible. With either CNS or PNS impairment, the scrotal, cremasteric, and anal ("superficial") reflexes (Fig. 16-3) will be absent.

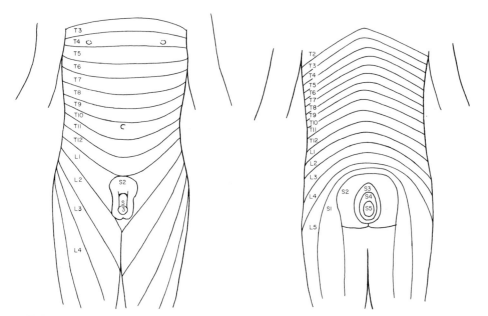

FIGURE 16–2.   The sacral dermatomes (S2–S5) innervate the skin overlying the genitals and anus, but lumbar dermatomes innervate the legs.

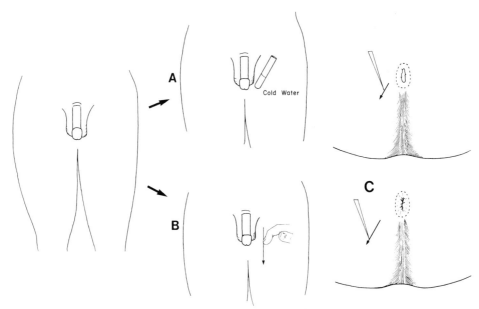

FIGURE 16–3. *A*, The *scrotal reflex*: Normally when a cold surface is applied to the scrotum, the testicle retracts and the skin surface contracts. *B*, The *cremasteric reflex*: Likewise, when the inner thigh is stroked, the testicle retracts and the skin surface contracts. *C*, The *anal reflex*: When the perianal skin is scratched, the anus tightens.

Laboratory Tests

In the most important test, the *nocturnal penile tumescence (NPT) study*, erections are monitored during 1 to 3 nights and correlated with rapid eye movement (REM) sleep.* Normal males, from infancy to old age, have erections and other manifestations of ANS activity, such as tachycardia, during 90 percent or more of REM sleep, regardless of its overt dream content. Since NPT studies directly measure sexual function, they are more accurate than the traditional evaluation that was based on the man's history. During NPT studies, some men with sexual impairment, when freed from social and psychologic influences, are found to have erections. Results of NPT and other physiologic studies have shown that, contrary to the traditional assumption that erectile dysfunction results from psychogenic impairment, at least 50 percent of men with erectile dysfunction have underlying neurologic or other physical abnormalities.

The determination of blood flow in the penis, another new diagnostic technique, is valuable in men with peripheral vascular disease, atherosclerosis, diabetes, or pelvic injuries. This testing, using noninvasive Doppler-based instruments, measures the blood pressure in the dorsal artery of the penis and its microcirculation. Electrophysiologic studies, similar to nerve conduction velocities (Chapter 6), can detect nerve damage. Also, radioimmunoassay of

* Men with sexual dysfunction and their partners may receive assistance from Impotents Anonymous (IA), 119 South Ruth Street, Maryville, TN, (615) 983-6094. Patients with spinal cord injury may receive assistance from veterans associations, The National Multiple Sclerosis Society (see Chapter 15), or the March of Dimes, 1275 Mamaroneck Avenue, White Plains, New York 10605, (914) 428-7100.

serum prolactin and gonadotropic hormone concentrations can reveal abnormalities in the hypothalamic-pituitary-gonadal axis.

Mechanical and Physiologic Treatment of Erectile Dysfunction

Several techniques can produce credible erections in a man with erectile dysfunction resulting from neurologic injury, vascular insufficiency, or certain other physiologic abnormalities. A mechanical penile prosthesis surgically implanted in the penis can mimic an erection. The device can be either a rigid or semirigid rod or an inflatable, balloon-like apparatus. Unfortunately, they are all prone to mechanical failures, infections, or aesthetic difficulties. Also they are costly. In 1989, the insertion of a rod cost about $3,000 and, of an inflatable device, about $12,000. Most insurance companies do not cover the expense. Nevertheless, the majority of men and their partners are satisfied with the prosthesis.

A novel and promising technique, but one not yet approved for general use, is injection of vasoactive medications directly into the penis, at the base of the corpus cavernosum (the erectile tissue), several minutes before intercourse. The smooth muscle relaxant, papaverine, and the alpha adrenergic blocker, phentolamine (Regitine), injected alone or together induce erections that permit enjoyable intercourse and orgasms. These erections usually subside spontaneously, but they can be aborted with epinephrine. Although this procedure has been complicated by priapism and rarely by ischemia, it is gaining popularity and even has been suggested to treat selected cases of psychogenic erectile dysfunction.

NEUROLOGIC ILLNESSES ASSOCIATED WITH SEXUAL IMPAIRMENT

Since sexual function is dependent on the CNS, PNS, and ANS, it is vulnerable to various neurologic illnesses. Some textbooks, although technically correct, list dozens of such illnesses, but only a few are responsible for the majority of cases. As a general rule, if a neurologic illness associated with sexual impairment is present, the physician should assume that the sexual impairment has a neurologic rather than a psychologic basis. On the other hand, treatment of psychologic or behavioral disturbances may enable a partially impaired person with neurologic disease to function.

Spinal Cord Injury

Each year hundreds of people sustain spinal cord injuries, usually from automobile, horseback riding, diving, and trampoline accidents; knife or bullet wounds; or multiple sclerosis (MS) (Chapter 15). In these people, arousal and orgasmic disorders, sexual impairment, as well as other manifestations of spinal cord injury—spastic paraparesis or quadriparesis, urinary incontinence, and sensory loss (Chapter 2)—depend on the site and completion of the injury. Although libido should remain intact, spinal cord injury often leads to a diminished libido and other psychologic problems.

Upper Spinal Cord Injury

When the cervical or thoracic spinal cord is completely transected, ascending sensory and descending neurologic impulses are totally interrupted. When the cervical portion is severed, quadriparesis develops, and when the thoracic portion is severed, paraparesis develops. Although in either case, the injury prevents the patient from sensing genital tactile stimulation, in lower thoracic spinal cord injuries, breast sensation and its erotic capacity are preserved.

With upper spinal cord lesions, the genital-spinal cord reflex remains intact. These patients retain the capacity for having genital arousal and orgasm, but they are unable to feel either, and their erections are usually too weak for intercourse. Moreover, orgasms may produce an excessive, almost violent ANS response, *autonomic hyperreflexia*, which causes hypertension, bradycardia, nausea, and lightheadedness.

Accompanying the loss of genital sensation, spinal cord injury patients lose sensation for bladder fullness, and they generally require catheters. Urinary tract and genital infections are common. Men become infertile because of inadequate and abnormal sperm production, but women continue to ovulate, menstruate, and retain their capacity to conceive and bear children.

With incomplete spinal cord injuries, as in MS and many nonpenetrating injuries, sexual and extrasexual deficits and autonomic hyperreflexia are less pronounced. However, erectile dysfunction and varying degrees of anorgasmy affect most patients.

Lower Spinal Cord Injury

When the lumbar or sacral spinal cord is transected, the critical genital-spinal cord reflex is interrupted, and stimulation cannot produce pleasurable sensation, arousal, or orgasm. As in upper spinal cord transection, patients have paraparesis and urinary incontinence, but since the ANS continues to innervate the genitals, fertility in both men and women is preserved.

Poliomyelitis and Other Exceptions

Before the Salk and Sabin vaccines were introduced, many people suffered from poliomyelitis (polio), a motor neuron disease that causes trunk and limb paresis. Since intellect, sensation, involuntary muscle strength, and ANS functions were characteristically spared (Chapter 5), polio victims had full libido, genital sensation, bladder control, sexual function, and fertility. Another devastating motor neuron disease that does not affect sexual or bladder function is amyotrophic lateral sclerosis (ALS). Extrapyramidal illnesses (Chapter 18), such as choreoathetosis, dystonia, Wilson's disease, Huntington's disease, and parkinsonism, despite causing difficulties with mobility, also do not impair sexual desire, sexual function, or fertility.

Diabetes Mellitus

Sexual impairment, especially retrograde ejaculation and erectile dysfunction, eventually affects almost 50 percent of diabetic men. It is the first sign of diabetes in about 5 percent of patients. Diabetic sexual impairment results from ANS and PNS injury, and also from atherosclerosis of the arteries of the genitals (see below). Since the bladder and genitals have common ANS inner-vation, erectile dysfunction and urinary incontinence coincide in diabetics. The bladder of affected patients is typically large, flaccid, and poorly controlled (Fig. 16-4). Patients also have anhidrosis and orthostatic hypotension, but curiously they do not necessarily have other complications of diabetes, such as retinopathy, nephropathy, or peripheral vascular disease. Although diabetic sexual impairment should not directly lessen the libido, psychologic repercus-sions, as in spinal cord injury, can be debilitating. Some diabetic men with erectile dysfunction have low testosterone concentrations, and some have hyperprolactinemia. In general, however, testosterone therapy has only a placebo effect.

Descriptions of sexual impairment in diabetic women conflict. For example, Kolodny found that 35 percent of diabetic women had anorgasmy and that sexual impairment was related to neuropathy; however, Ellenberg found that diabetic women were no more prone than nondiabetic ones to sexual impairment

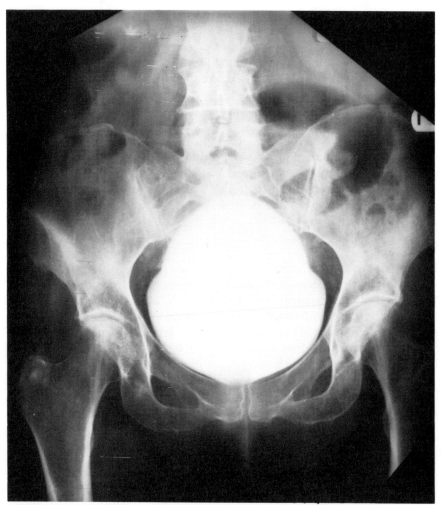

FIGURE 16–4.   A patient had diabetes mellitus complicated by impotence and urinary incontinence, which are typically associated with a large, flaccid bladder. His intravenous pyelogram (IVP) reveals a distended bladder, which is the large white circular area.

and that diabetic women, even those with profound neuropathy, had full sexual function. All agree that vaginal infections are more common in diabetic women, and although these women remain fertile, pregnancies are more often complicated by miscarriages and fetal malformations.

Multiple Sclerosis

Intermittent or permanent sexual impairment in MS patients results from patches of spinal cord demyelination (Chapter 15). Sexual impairment can be the sole symptom, and when it is found with vague sensory disturbances, the patient may be misdiagnosed as hysteric. MS often eventually brings about devastating deficits, of which sexual impairment is only one aspect.

Multiple sclerosis causes premature ejaculation, erectile dysfunction, retrograde ejaculation, and anorgasmy. In its early stages, patients might have few extrasexual deficits, but when episodes develop repeatedly, the incidence of sexual impairment, urinary incontinence, and extrasexual deficits all rise dramatically. Although fertility is preserved in women, pregnancies are associated with exacerbations. The fertility of men is impaired because of decreased sperm production, as well as sexual dysfunction.

Medication-Induced Impairment

Although hundreds of medications are implicated, only a few categories consistently impair sexual function. In most cases, in view of their pharmacology, this effect could be predicted. The tricyclic and, possibly to a lesser extent, other antidepressants cause sexual impairment, probably because they interfere with parasympathetic activity (Table 16-3). Likewise, anticholinergic medications, which are often given to counteract the parkinsonian side effects of phenothiazines, cause sexual impairment. All these medicines tend to cause dry mouth, orthostatic hypotension, accommodation paresis (Fig. 12-4), and urinary

---

TABLE 16-3. PSYCHIATRIC MEDICATIONS ASSOCIATED WITH SEXUAL DYSFUNCTION*

Tricyclic and heterocyclic antidepressants
    Amitriptyline (Elavil†)
    Imipramine (Tofranil†)
    Nortriptyline (Aventyl†)
    Trazodone (Desyrl°)
Monamine oxidase inhibitors
    Isocarboxazid (Marplan)
    Phenelzine (Nardil)
Other antidepressants
    Amoxapine (Asendin)
    Lithium (Eskalith†)
Antipsychotics
    Chlorpromazine (Thorazine†)
    Haloperidol (Haldol†)

---

* Decreased libido, erectile dysfunctions, or anorgasmy. For fuller listing of medications, see Abramowicz M (ed): Drugs that cause sexual dysfunction. Med Letter *29:*67–70, 1987.
† And other brands.
° Can cause priapism.

hesitancy (Fig. 15-5). Phenothiazines and butyrophenones cause sexual impairment possibly also because of their anticholinergic properties and because they increase prolactin levels.

The libido can be diminished by numerous medications, particularly those that are narcotic, anticholinergic, hypnotic, or tranquilizing. Antihypertensive medications that affect the CNS as well as the ANS are apt to reduce the libido. In this group, reserpine, propranolol (Inderal), and methyldopa (Aldomet) are the most commonly cited medications, but package inserts or the *Medical Letter* should be consulted.

Miscellaneous

Atherosclerosis of the dorsal artery and smaller vessels of the penis commonly causes erectile dysfunction. The atherosclerosis can be associated with aging, diabetes, hypertension, or surgery of aortic aneurysms or the coronary arteries. When penile vessel evaluations indicate vascular disease, various arterial reconstructive procedures, including grafting, can be attempted. However, in cases where vascular disease or surgery has caused nerve damage or spinal cord infarction, the prognosis is poor.

Extensive prostate surgery damaging the pudendal nerves is another common cause of erectile dysfunction. With the current procedures, transurethral

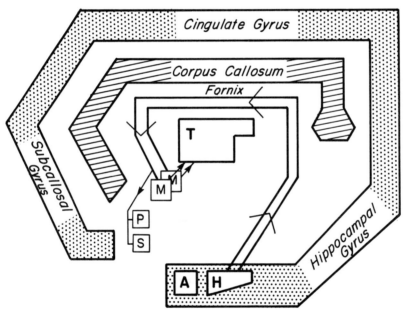

FIGURE 16–5. This schematic portrayal of the *limbic system* shows its essential components. The *limbic lobe or cortex*, which virtually encircles the corpus callosum, consists of the *cingulate gyrus* (*stippled*); its anterior extension into the frontal lobe, the *subcallosal gyrus*; and its posterior extension into the temporal lobe, the *hippocampal formation* (H). The *amygdala* (A) receives connections from the cerebral cortex, cingulate gyrus, and the hypothalamus. In turn, the amygdala and other subcortical structures are connected, in a bidirectional pathway in the *fornix*, to the *mammillary bodies*, which are a segment of the hypothalamus, and the adjacent *preoptic* (P) and *septal* (S) regions. The *mammillothalamic tract* connects the mammillary bodies with the *anterior nucleus of the thalamus* (T). Connections between the thalamus and the cingulate gyrus (not pictured) complete circuits within the limbic system and between the limbic system's amygdala and hypothalamus and the cerebral cortex and brainstem.

prostatectomy (TURP) and suprapubic prostatectomy, these nerves are usually spared.

Herniated lumbar intervertebral disks occasionally compress the sacral nerve roots (Chapter 5). When disks herniate, patients develop distressing, radiating low back pain. Examination usually reveals signs of nerve root compression that include foot paresis, urinary retention, and Lasègue's sign (Fig. 5-7). In cases of herniated disk, sexual impairment would be a minor part of the patient's problem.

Patients are difficult to evaluate when they have sexual impairment that they attribute to chronic low back pain. Their pain must be considered carefully, but neurologists are reluctant to accept it as the primary cause of sexual impairment. On the other hand, patients who have undergone myelography, laminectomy, and related operations on the lower spine might have developed nerve root injury from surgical trauma or postoperative *arachnoiditis* (inflammation of the covering of the nerve roots). These patients often have unarousability, severe low back pain, and signs of nerve root compression from extensive nerve root damage.

LIBIDO

From a neurologic viewpoint, the *limbic system* is the source of the libido (Fig. 16-5). Illnesses that damage the limbic system, usually through injury of the frontal or temporal lobe, hypothalamus, or the entire brain, alter the libido. With few exceptions, those injuries reduce the libido.

Isolated limbic system injury is rarely encountered. The closest example is the experimentally produced *Klüver-Bucy syndrome*, in which rhesus monkeys display increased heterosexual, homosexual, or autosexual activity and other behavioral changes following bilateral anterior temporal lobectomies with removal of both amygdalae. Their increased sexuality is accompanied by placidity, continual tactile activity, and placing inedible objects in their mouth, which is called "psychic blindness" or *oral exploration* (similar to visual agnosia, Chapter 12).

In humans, a modified form of this syndrome, the *human Klüver-Bucy syndrome*, has been observed following bilateral temporal lobe injury from trauma, Herpes simplex encephalitis, infarctions, or, rarely, Alzheimer's disease or Pick's disease. These patients, like the experimental monkeys, are placid, have a tendency to eat excessively, and have oral exploration. In contrast to the monkeys, heterosexual and masturbatory activity is increased in only about one half of the patients, and most patients only make suggestive gestures. Also, despite their oral tendencies, these patients usually do not become obese. Overall, they are usually more impaired by aphasia, memory impairment (amnesia), or dementia than by their sexual proclivities.

Increased sexual activity can also result from cerebral excitatory substances, including Sinemet, hallucinogens, and amyl nitrate. Similarly, several neurologic illnesses, in which cerebral "inhibitory centers" are damaged, are associated with unrestrained urges. For example, people with mild mental retardation, Alzheimer's disease, parkinsonism, cerebral palsy, or merely old age all might have uninhibited sexual actions.

Otherwise, neurologic damage usually results in decreased libido. Pituitary, hypothalamic, and diencephalic lesions have occasionally been associated with hypersexuality, but usually such injuries are characterized by hyposexuality and appetite changes. For example, the Wernicke-Korsakoff syndrome and transient global amnesia, conditions in which limbic system structures are injured, are characterized by temporary memory impairment but not by libido changes (see Acute Amnestic Syndromes, Chapter 7).

Partial complex epilepsy, which characteristically originates in temporal lobe dysfunction, is sometimes associated with limited sexual activity. During seizures, patients may initiate rudimentary masturbation or even partially undress. However, during seizures, they do not engage in heterosexual activity, and during interictal periods, patients are prone to hyposexuality (Chapter 10).

The libido is vulnerable to neurologic sexual impairments because lack of sexual satisfaction decreases demand, as through a "negative feedback loop." For example, men with MS or diabetes who have chronic erectile dysfunction often abandon their sexual desires. Thus, the classic question posed to people with sexual dysfunction, "Is the problem decreased libido or impotence?" is sometimes like asking them about the chicken and the egg.

Patients with chronic pain characteristically have a decreased libido. They may be suffering from depression and may also be consuming potent analgesics. Most important, pain interferes with pleasure from any source. Although libido persists despite mild fatigue, hunger, and fear, the dampening effect of pain is popularly acknowledged in the classic refusal, "Not tonight, honey, I have a headache."

REFERENCES

Abramowicz M (ed): Drugs that cause sexual dysfunction. Med Letter *29*:67, 1987

Abramowicz M (ed): Intracavernous injections for impotence. Med Letter *29*:95, 1987

Boller F, Frank E: Sexual Dysfunction in Neurologic Disorders: Diagnosis, Management, and Rehabilitation. New York, Raven Press, 1982

Bradley WE: Etiology of impotence in diabetes mellitus. Neurology *33*:101, 1983

Comfort A (ed): Sexual Consequences of Disability. Philadelphia, George F. Strickley Co, 1978

Dechesne BH, Schellen AM: Sexuality and Handicap: Problems of Motor Handicapped People. Springfield, IL, Charles C. Thomas, 1986

DeLeo D, Magni G: Sexual side effects of antidepressant drugs. Psychosomatics *12*:1076, 1983

Ellenberg M: Diabetic neuropathy. In Ellenberg M, Rifkin H. Diabetes Mellitus: Theory and Practice, 3rd ed. New York, Medical Examination Publishing Co, 1983, pp 777–802

Ford JR, Duckworth B: Physical Management of the Quadriplegic Patient. Philadelphia, F. A. Davis, 1987

Hale G (ed): Sex Instruction for the Physically Handicapped. Philadelphia, W.B. Saunders, 1979

Karacan I: Nocturnal penile tumescence as a biologic marker in assessing erectile dysfunction. Psychosomatics *23*:349, 1982

Kirkeby HJ, Poulsen EU, Petersen T, et al: Erectile dysfunction in multiple sclerosis. Neurology *38*:1366, 1988

Kolodny RC, Masters WH, Johnson VE: Textbook of Sexual Medicine. Boston, Little, Brown, and Co, 1979

Lilly R, Cummings JL, Benson DF, et al: The human Klüver-Bucy syndrome. Neurology *33*:1141, 1983

McCulloch DK, Young RJ, Prescott RJ, et al: The natural history of impotence in diabetic men. Diabetologia *26*:437, 1984

Monat RK: Sexuality and the Mentally Retarded: A Clinical and Therapeutic Guidebook. San Diego, College-Hill Press, 1982

Mooney TO, Cole TM, Chilgren RA: Sexual Options for Paraplegics and Quadriplegics. Boston, Little Brown, and Co, 1975

Pedersen B, Tiefer L, Ruiz M, et al: Evaluation of patients and partners 1 to 4 years after penile prosthesis surgery. J Urol *139*:956, 1988

Sidi AA, Reddy PK, Chen KK: Patient acceptance of and satisfaction with vasoactive intracavernous
  pharmacotherapy for impotence. J Urol *140*:293, 1988
Spark RF: Neuroendocrinology and impotence. Ann Intern Med *98*:103, 1983

QUESTIONS: CHAPTER 16

1. A 40-year-old man complains of longstanding erectile dysfunction. He has severe low back pain, mild hypertension, and borderline diabetes. Which conditions should be considered as possible causes of his sexual dysfunction?
   a.   Herniated lumbar intervertebral disk
   b.   Antihypertensive medications
   c.   Diabetic neuropathy
   d.   Psychogenic factors
   e.   All of the above

2. A 24-year-old man who complains of premature ejaculation also had episodes of unsteady gait, diplopia, and paraparesis. Which of the following might a neurologic examination reveal?
   a.   Internuclear ophthalmoplegia
   b.   Absent abdominal reflexes
   c.   Ataxia of gait
   d.   Babinski signs
   e.   Hyperactive deep tendon reflexes

3. Which of the following conditions might cause retrograde ejaculation?
   a.   Ovarian dysfunction
   b.   Diabetic autonomic neuropathy
   c.   Psychogenic influence
   d.   Use of guanethidine (Ismelin)
   e.   Sexual inexperience

4. The physician might assume that patients with neurologic illness will have sexual dysfunction. With which illnesses is the assumption valid?
   a.   Dominant hemisphere infarctions
   b.   Nondominant hemisphere infarctions
   c.   Parkinsonism
   d.   Poliomyelitis
   e.   Amyotrophic lateral sclerosis

5. Medications as well as particular illnesses cause erectile dysfunction and other forms of sexual impairment. In which illness is iatrogenic sexual dysfunction likely to be encountered?
   a.   Psychosis
   b.   Migraine headache
   c.   Hypertension
   d.   Low back pain
   e.   Duodenal ulcer

6. During sleep, when do erections and emissions occur?

7. With which situations is fertility lost?
   a.   Women with cervical spinal cord transection
   b.   Men with cervical spinal cord transection
   c.   Men with diabetes mellitus and neuropathy
   d.   Women with diabetes mellitus and neuropathy

8. With which conditions are erections still possible?
   a.   Severe diabetic autonomic neuropathy
   b.   Use of clonidine (Catapres) or enalapril (Vasotec)
   c.   Sacral spinal cord transection
   d.   Cervical spinal cord transection

    e. Upper thoracic spinal cord transection
    f. Multiple sclerosis

9. With which conditions are cremasteric reflexes lost?
    a. Severe diabetic autonomic neuropathy
    b. Psychogenic difficulties
    c. Sacral spinal cord injury
    d. Frontal meningiomas

10. A 35-year-old man suffers low back pain after falling down a flight of stairs. Among his complaints a month later is impotence. Examination reveals loss of pinprick sensation from the waist down to the toes but intact position, vibratory, and warm-cold sensation. Deep tendon and cremasteric reflexes are intact, and plantar reflexes are flexion. To what could the impotence be attributed?
    a. Spinal cord injury
    b. Autonomic nervous system dysfunction
    c. Peripheral neuropathy
    d. Multiple sclerosis
    e. None of the above

11. In monkeys, with which of the following is the Klüver-Bucy syndrome associated?
    a. Psychic blindness
    b. Apathy
    c. Frontal lobectomy
    d. Loss of amygdalae
    e. Increased homosexual, heterosexual, and autosexual activity

12. In humans who have had bilateral temporal lobe damage, which of the following conditions are almost always found?
    a. Memory impairment, aphasia, or both
    b. Placing food and inedible objects in their mouths
    c. Hypersexuality
    d. Rage attacks

13. Which of the following conditions is likely to lead to transient or permanent temporal lobe or limbic system damage?
    a. Herpes simplex encephalitis
    b. Alcoholism
    c. TIAs of the posterior cerebral arteries
    d. Herpes zoster

14. With which of the following are pituitary tumors associated?
    a. Headaches
    b. Hyperprolactinemia
    c. Optic atrophy
    d. Homonymous superior quadrantanopsia

15. In normal males, which of the following are associated with REM-induced erections?
    a. Dreams with no overt sexual content
    b. Most dreams with even frightful or anxiety-producing content
    c. Increased pulse and blood pressure
    d. Increased cerebral blood flow
    e. An EEG that appears, aside from eye movement artifact, as though the patient were awake

16. In treatment of men with erectile dysfunction, injections into the corpus cavernosum of which substances will produce erection?
    a. Epinephrine
    b. Phentolamine
    c. Papaverine
    d. Morphine

ANSWERS

1. e. This man might have sexual impairment because of the various medical or psychogenic disorders.

2. a, b, c, d, e. The patient is likely to have MS with cerebellar, brainstem, and spinal cord involvement. Between episodes, when the patient is likely to have residual neurologic signs (a–e), he may also have sexual dysfunction. Premature ejaculation and impotence are often a manifestation of quiescent MS that has affected the spinal cord.

3. b, d. In retrograde ejaculation, semen is propelled by involuntary mechanisms into the bladder instead of the urethra. It is always the result of neurologic or local muscular dysfunction.

4. None of these answers is correct. Each condition may cause bodily weakness; however, sexual drive, genital sensation, and orgasmic reactions are all preserved.

5. a, c, e. Medications that cause sexual impairments are usually those with anticholinergic properties, such as neuroleptics and ulcer therapy medications, and antihypertensive medications.

6. During REM sleep, when dreams usually occur, erections and orgasm occur. Erections are also characteristically present on awakening.

7. b. Men with upper spinal cord injury have low sperm counts and produce abnormal sperm. Women are able to conceive and bear children despite spinal cord injury. Both men and women with diabetes remain fertile.

8. b, d, e, f. Erections are possible provided that the lumbosacral spinal cord and the sacral autonomic nervous system are intact. Thus, men with either severe diabetic autonomic neuropathy or sacral spinal cord damage will be unable to have erections. When the spinal cord damage is incomplete, as in patients with MS, or is located in the cervical region, erectile function may be preserved. Sexual dysfunction with use of medications is inconsistent. Newly introduced antihypertensives (b) usually do not cause sexual dysfunction.

9. a, c. Cremasteric reflexes require that the pudendal nerves, autonomic nervous system, and lower spinal cord be intact. When impotence is accompanied by a loss of these reflexes, neurologic impairment must be considered.

10. e. Since the patient has no objective neurologic deficit, none of the neurologic illnesses is indicated. In fact, the dissociation of pinprick and warm-cold sensation cannot be caused by a structural lesion because both sensations travel in the same nerve pathways.

11. a, b, d, e. The monkeys, subjected to temporal lobectomy with removal of the amygdalae, have oral exploratory behavior. Although their vision is intact, they do not identify objects by their appearance. They are said to have visual agnosia. Also, the monkeys characteristically lose extreme emotion. Sometimes appearing fearless, they are actually apathetic. Most striking, they have increased and indiscriminate sexual activity.

12. a, b. The human variety of the Klüver-Bucy syndrome is characterized by impaired language function and memory, the tendency to eat excessively, and, as with monkeys, placing inedible objects in their mouths. Contrary to expectations, patients with this syndrome have little increased sexual appetite or violent outbursts. Also, they are usually not obese.

13. a, b, c. Herpes simplex virus has a predilection for the frontal and temporal lobes. It is a frequent cause of encephalitis that often leads to memory impairment and partial complex seizures. Although Herpes zoster usually does not infect the CNS, it often causes painful postherpetic neuralgia. Posterior cerebral TIAs cause ischemia of the temporal lobes. They are associated with confusion and memory impairment and are called "transient global amnesia." Chronic alcohol abuse can cause the Wernicke-Korsakoff syndrome, which is associated with hemorrhage into the mammillary bodies and other parts of the limbic system.

14. a, b, c, d.

15. a, b, c, d, e.

16. b, c. Men who have erectile dysfunction because of multiple sclerosis, diabetes, and other conditions can obtain an erection by injections of phentolamine (Regitine) or papaverine into the dorsum of the penis. The erection can be reversed by an epinephrine injection. The procedure can be complicated by priapism or ischemia.

17

Sleep Disorders

The incidence of sleep disorders is so high that they qualify as a public health problem. For example, about 10 percent of Americans are unhappy about the quality or quantity of their sleep, and 3 to 10 percent use sleeping pills (sedatives or hypnotics). Moreover, people who habitually sleep too little (less than 2 hours) or too much (greater than 10 hours) have increased morbidity and mortality.

In the last two decades, the study of sleep and its disorders has given rise to an entirely new branch of medical practice.* Using the *polysomnogram* (*PSG*), which is a recording of the electroencephalogram (EEG), electromyogram (EMG), ocular movements, and vital signs of sleeping people, investigators have studied normal patterns, variations, and disorders. In addition, they have examined biologic correlates of dreaming, nighttime behavior, and psychologic status. This chapter reviews the patterns, as measured by clinical studies and PSG, of normal sleep and of sleep disorders characterized by too little or fragmented sleep (insomnia), excessive sleepiness, and sleep disruptions.

NORMAL SLEEP

Two distinct phases of sleep recur throughout a normal night. Their most salient difference is that dreaming and rapid, conjugate, horizontal movement of the eyes take place together in one phase, called *rapid eye movement* (*REM*) *sleep*. The other phase, *nonrapid eye movement* (*NREM*) *sleep*, is longer and has other qualities (Table 17-1). A proposed explanation for the pattern is that the locus ceruleus and the median raphe, two deep brainstem structures, have reciprocal functions and that their cyclic activity alternately triggers REM and NREM sleep. Also, studies indicate that during REM sleep, dopamine, norepinephrine, and epinephrine activity decreases, and acetylcholine activity increases. During NREM sleep, serotonin activity increases.

REM Sleep

Since most people who are awakened during a REM period report that they were having a dream, REM sleep has become synonymous with dreaming. The dreams that occur during REM sleep are intellectually complex, on a superficial level at least, and rich in visual imagery. The vigorous eye movements are attributed to people watching or feeling themselves participating in a dream.

Aside from the eye movements and uninterrupted breathing, there is a

---

* Patients with sleep disorders may receive assistance from the Association of Sleep Disorders Centers, 701 Welch Road, Suite 2226, Toronto, CA 94304.

TABLE 17–1. STAGES OF NORMAL SLEEP

| Stage | Graduation | Movement | | EMG | EEG |
		SOMATIC	OCULAR		
NREM 1	Light sleep	Persistent facial tone and repositioning movements of body every 15–20 minutes	Slow, rolling eye movements	Continual activity	Loss of alpha activity
2	Intermediate sleep	Same	Absent	Slight reduction	Sleep spindles and K complexes
3	Deep or slow-wave sleep	Same	Absent	Further reduction	Increased proportion of slow-wave (1 to 3-Hz) activity
4	Deepest or slow-wave sleep	Same	Absent	Further reduction	Greatest proportion of 1 to 3-Hz activity
REM	Activated or paradoxical sleep	Absence of all muscular movement and tone, except for brief episodes of facial and limb movement	Rapid, conjugate eye movements	Silent	Low voltage activity, ocular movement artifacts

virtual absence of muscle movement and muscle tone in the head, trunk, and limbs during REM sleep. The muscles are paretic and flaccid, and their deep tendon reflexes (DTRs) cannot be elicited (areflexia). EMGs show no electrical activity in the chin and limb muscles (Fig. 17-1). The lack of muscle activity acts as though benign paralysis prevented people from acting on their dreams.

Despite the sleeping person's motionlessness, so much autonomic nervous system activity takes place in REM sleep that it has been called "activated" or "paradoxical" sleep. For example, there are increases in pulse, blood pressure, intracranial pressure, cerebral blood flow, and muscle metabolism. Also, regardless of the content of dreams, penile erections occur (Chapter 16).

The EEG is also surprisingly active. Aside from eye-movement artifact, it is similar to EEGs in wakefulness. Overall, in REM sleep, the bodily activities and EEG, but not the EMG, are more similar to those in wakefulness than to those in NREM sleep.

NREM Sleep

NREM sleep is divided into four stages that are distinguished by progressively greater depths of unconsciousness and by slower and higher voltage EEG patterns. In all stages of NREM sleep, the eyes have slow, rolling motions, and only brief, rudimentary thoughts are formed. Also in contrast to REM sleep, muscle tone is present, DTRs can be elicited, and EMG activity is present in the chin and limb muscles (Fig. 17-2).

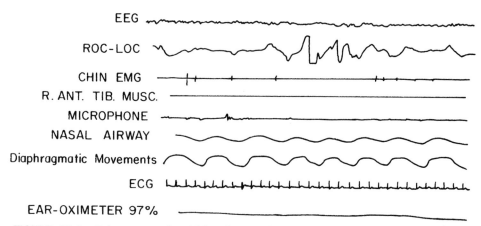

FIGURE 17–1. Polysomnography (PSG) of REM sleep characteristically shows that the EEG channel has low voltage, fast activity and the channel referable to ocular movement (ROC-LOC) indicates rapid eye movement (REM) by the large-scale, quick movements. Electromyography (EMG) of the chin and right anterior tibialis muscles shows virtually no activity, which indicates absence of muscle movement and tone. The microphone channel indicates a little noise, which may be a snore. The airway and diaphragm channels indicate normal breathing and air movement.

Although there is a generalized decrease in autonomic nervous system function, important hypothalamic-pituitary (neuroendocrine) activity occurs. For example, the daily secretion of growth hormone occurs almost entirely during NREM, about 30 to 60 minutes after sleep begins. Likewise, serum prolactin concentrations are highest soon after sleep begins. In contrast, cortisol is secreted in five to seven discrete late nighttime episodes, which accumulate to yield the day's highest cortisol concentration at about 8:00 AM. Overall, the third and fourth stages of NREM sleep, which are called *slow-wave* or *deep NREM* sleep, provide most of the physical recuperation derived from a night's sleep. As if the immediate role of sleep were to revitalize the body, these stages occur predominantly in the early night. As the sleep continues, it becomes lighter and more filled with dreaming.

Patterns

People usually fall asleep 5 to 10 minutes after retiring; however, this interval, *sleep latency*, is highly variable because it is influenced by numerous psychologic and physical factors. Once asleep, people enter NREM sleep and pass in

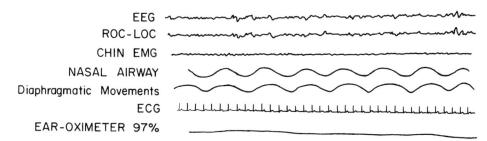

FIGURE 17–2. A PSG of stage 1 of NREM sleep shows some slow EEG activity but not the higher voltage, very slow EEG activity of deep or slow-wave NREM sleep. The PSG also shows, in the ROC-LOC channel, no substantial ocular movement, i.e., no REM activity. The chin muscles have tone as indicated by continual, low voltage EMG activity. Breathing and cardiac activity are normal.

succession through its four stages. After about 70 to 110 minutes of NREM sleep, they enter the initial REM period, which lasts for about 10 minutes. The interval from falling asleep to the first REM period, *REM latency*, which normally averages 90 minutes, is critical in affective and sleep disorders.

The NREM-REM cycle repeats itself throughout the night with a periodicity of about 90 minutes. REM periods, occur four or five times nightly and are progressively longer and more frequent (Fig. 17-3). In later sleep, body temperature falls to the day's lowest point (the nadir). The final REM period merges with awakening. Thus, a person's final dream may be influenced by surrounding morning household activities, and when men awake they usually have erections.

Variations

Effects of Age

As people grow older, they spend less time sleeping and dreaming. Neonates sleep 16 to 20 hours a day, with about 50 percent of that time in REM sleep. Young children spend 10 to 12 hours sleeping at night and during afternoon naps, with about 30 percent in REM sleep.

Adults average 6 to 8 hours, with 20 to 28 percent in REM sleep. In those adults who are accustomed to relatively little sleep, the proportion of deep NREM sleep is greatly increased whereas that of REM remains constant. Therefore, in these cases, the *quantity* of deep NREM sleep tends to be preserved at the expense of REM sleep.

The elderly sleep somewhat less than young adults and have sleep that is fragmented by multiple brief awakenings especially in its later half. These individuals obtain part of their sleep during daytime naps not only after meals and in the late afternoon, which are times of normal sleepiness, but irresistibly at any time, including during social activities. Their REM periods, instead of being longer and more frequent in the later night, change neither in duration nor frequency. The total REM time is decreased.

Sleep onset and awakening times in the elderly are usually earlier, (i.e., are *phase advanced*), so that elderly people typically both go to sleep and awaken

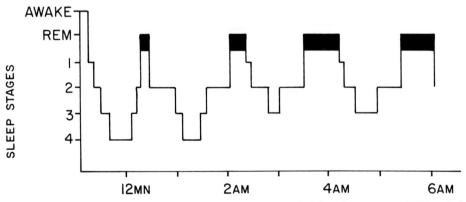

FIGURE 17–3. In the conventional representation of a normal night's sleep pattern, REM periods start about 90 minutes after sleep begins, i.e., the REM latency is 90 minutes. REM periods then recur somewhat more frequently and in longer duration throughout the night. NREM sleep progresses through regular although progressively lighter stages.

early. In the elderly, unlike younger adults, reductions in sleep are taken at the expense of stages 3 and 4 NREM sleep. In addition to these variations, the elderly have an increased incidence of inadequate sleep because of medication-induced insomnia, medical illnesses, and various sleep disorders, including leg movements, REM behavior disturbances, and sleep apnea syndrome (see below).

Sleep Schedules

For most adults, social and occupational demands determine a morning awakening time and, indirectly, an evening bedtime. These external considerations usually override emotional makeup, early conditioning, physical activities, and possibly an intrinsic sleep mechanism.

However, some people, "night owls" or "owls," prefer to remain awake late into the night and to sleep until early afternoon. They gravitate toward the entertainment industries and other nighttime work, and they form friendships with other owls. These people are well-adjusted to their sleep rhythm and must be distinguished from those who, handicapped by their daytime sleep schedule, are said to have "delayed sleep phase syndrome" (see below). In contrast, "larks" arise early in the morning. Their work, which is more conventional, is more productive in the morning than in the afternoon.

PSG recordings have confirmed common observations of groups of normal people. College students and the elderly often seem to be perpetually tired or sleepy. Some children and adolescents never seem to need sleep. On the other hand, when adolescents are always sleepy, abnormal physical or emotional factors are probably responsible.

Sleep Deprivation

Important changes occur during the night following sleep deprivation. Adults who have worked all night or children skipping their customary afternoon nap, for example, have a short sleep latency and a lengthened sleep time. Also, they have a characteristic *REM rebound*: the first REM period occurs early (short REM latency) or even immediately (*sleep-onset REM*); subsequent REM periods, compared with normal ones, are generally longer; and REM sleep occupies a greater proportion of sleep time. In short, as is commonly known, after missing sleep, a normal person immediately falls deeply asleep, immediately starts to dream a great deal, and sleeps late the next morning.

REM rebound also occurs following withdrawal from sedatives, hypnotics, and alcohol—substances that selectively suppress REM sleep. REM-onset sleep, a characteristic feature of REM rebound, is also found consistently in narcolepsy and, intermittently, in other sleep disorders (see below).

CLASSIFICATION OF SLEEP DISORDERS

The classification in the *Diagnostic and Statistical Manual of Mental Disorders, Third Edition, Revised, (DSM-III-R)* reflects the long-established classification of the *Association of Sleep Disorders Centers (ASDC)* Table 17-2). Although the DSM-III-R classification may be better known in the psychiatric community, the ASDC classification is preferable. It is more comprehensive and scientific. Unlike the DSM-III-R, the ASDC classification considers laboratory data, particularly the results of PSG studies, as diagnostic criteria. Moreover, since

TABLE 17–2. CLASSIFICATIONS AND EXAMPLES OF SLEEP DISORDERS

DSM-III-R*	ASDC°
Dyssomnias	Disorders of Initiating and Maintaining Sleep
Insomnia	(Insomnia)
Primary (307.42)	Psychophysiologic, transient or permanent
Related to	Associated with personality, affective, or psy-
another mental disorder	chotic disorders
(nonorganic) (307.42)	Related to drug and alcohol use
a known organic factor (780.50)	As result of medical illness
Hypersomnia	Disorders of Excessive Somnolence
Primary (780.54)	Narcolepsy
Related to	Sleep apnea
another mental disorder	Myoclonus or restless legs
(nonorganic) (307.44)	
a known organic factor (780.50)	
Sleep-Wake Schedule Disorder (307.45)	Disorders of the Sleep-Wake Schedule
	Jet lag, work shift change
	Delayed sleep phase syndrome
Parasomnias	
Sleep terror disorder (307.46)	Dysfunctions Associated with Sleep, Sleep
Sleepwalking disorder (307.46)	Stages, or Partial Arousals (Parasomnias)
Dream anxiety (nightmare) disorder	Night terrors
(307.47)	Enuresis
Other parasomnias (307.40)	Sleepwalking

* *Diagnostic and Statistical Manual of Mental Disorders*, Third Edition, Revised.
° Association of Sleep Disorder Centers.

its terminology is used by most neurologists, other clinicians, and researchers in sleep disorders, the ASDC classification will be followed in this chapter.

In the near future the ASDC classification will be revised to reclassify sleep and arousal disorders into dyssomnias, parasomnias, and sleep disorders associated with medical or psychiatric conditions. Although similar to the current DSM-III-R criteria, the descriptions of the dyssomnias will recognize that individuals have sleep abnormalities that may cause combinations of insomnia and somnolence, and that insomnia is often the cause of somnolence.

Disorders of Initiating and Maintaining Sleep (Insomnias)

The inability to fall or remain asleep, *insomnia*, is characterized by shorter sleep time, lighter sleep, or frequent arousals. People usually have insomnia because of psychiatric disturbances, including substance abuse, and medical illnesses. It may also be a consequence of a disorder° of excessive somnolence or a parasomnia. However, insomnia is usually not the result of an esoteric sleep disorder. In fact, most people who claim that they have too little or fragmented sleep will have normal sleep when studied by PSG.

Although PSG is a major technical advance, it is a costly study (in the vicinity of $2,000) that is not appropriate for most patients with insomnia. Its greatest usefulness is in the diagnosis of disorders of excessive somnolence and in certain behavioral, neurologic, or medical disorders that are present only during sleep. As for patients with insomnia, the first step would be to define the characteristics of their sleep disturbance (Table 17-3) within the context of a complete clinical evaluation. If specific treatments for medical and psychiatric conditions do not relieve the insomnia, then PSG and other sleep center studies should be considered.

TABLE 17–3. SALIENT HISTORICAL FEATURES OF PATIENTS WITH INSOMNIA OR EXCESSIVE DAYTIME SLEEPINESS*

A. Nighttime sleep
    1. What is the usual bedtime and time of falling asleep and awakening?
    2. What is the time spent sleeping compared with that spent in bed?
    3. What activities precede bedtime: (e.g., sex, food, medications, exercise)
    4. When asleep, is the patient apt to have any of the following interruptions?
        Nightmares or night terrors, sleepwalking, bedwetting
        Seizure-like activity
        Excessive snoring or apnea pauses
        Restless legs or generalized myoclonus
        Headaches, chest pain, or other medical symptoms
B. Daytime sleep
    1. Are there afternoon or evening naps?
        Are they restful?
        Are they irresistible or not preceded by a feeling of fatigue?
        Do they occur at inappropriate times?
    2. Are there episodes of loss of bodily tone?
        Does the patient slump suddenly and unexpectedly, especially following laughter or excitement?
        Does the patient have loss of tone in a single muscle group, such as those in the jaw or knees?
C. If left to his or her own schedule, would the patient be more alert and productive in the morning or night? And would such a self-determined schedule provide 6 to 8 hours of continual, restful sleep?
D. General health
    1. Does the patient suffer from medical illness?
    2. Does the patient take any medications with a stimulating or sedating effect?
    3. Does the patient use alcohol habitually?
    4. Does the patient use coffee or other caffeine-containing beverage or food regularly or in the evening?

* Proper history may only be obtained from a bed partner.

Drug and Alcohol Related Insomnia

Many people have insomnia because they take medicines, such as steroids, aminophylline, or pseudoephedrine (Actifed), which have stimulant effects. Some individuals consume excessive caffeine, the most common stimulant, in coffee (which has 60 to 140 mg of caffeine per cup), cola drinks (25 to 55 mg per cup), and many headache medicines, e.g., 130 mg in two Excedrin tablets. Many Americans easily and often inadvertently ingest such a large amount of caffeine (250 to 500 mg per day) that it causes "caffeinism": insomnia, agitation, tremulousness, palpitations, gastric distress, diuresis, and "caffeine-withdrawal headaches" (Chapter 9).

Other common causes of insomnia are sedatives, hypnotics, or alcohol. Although these substances generally induce sleep, they cause insomnia when used chronically or excessively because they disrupt sleep cycle periodicity, reduce deep NREM sleep, delay the onset of REM sleep, and shorten REM periods. Their interference with REM sleep can be so great that they can completely suppress it.

A similar problem affects people who suddenly abstain from chronic use of alcohol, sedatives, neuroleptics, or hypnotics, especially short-acting barbiturates. They may develop *drug withdrawal insomnia*, in which insomnia is associated with excessive daytime sleepiness and physical and psychologic agitation. When they are finally able to fall asleep, the abstainers have REM rebound, as though their previously suppressed REM sleep were trying to catch up. Abrupt withdrawal from alcohol or barbiturates may also lead to generalized, tonic-clonic seizures.

The elderly, who are prone to insomnia, inadvisedly take inordinate quantities of both prescription and over-the-counter sleeping pills. They often become psychologically dependent on these medicines. Not only are hypnotics rarely effective if taken for longer than 1 month but they can also aggravate insomnia (*medication-induced insomnia*). Also, when individuals who have Alzheimer's disease or other brain damage take hypnotics, instead of being sedated they may, in a "paradoxical reaction," develop agitation, psychologic aberrations, and hallucinations.

Insomnia in Psychiatric Illness

In patients with major depression, especially the elderly, PSGs show a short REM latency. Not only does the first REM period occur before 60 minutes but it is also abnormally long and intense. Although the total amount of REM sleep is about the same in normal and depressed individuals, in those who are depressed, REM periods occur in relatively rapid succession in the early night, leaving the later night almost devoid of REM. This preponderance of REM sleep in the depressed person's early night is similar to that in the normal person's later night.

Depressed individuals, as well as many others, have increased sleep latency and then intermittent awakenings throughout the night. In other words, they have difficulty falling asleep and then staying asleep. Their sleep is restless and shorter because they tend to arise early in the morning, i.e., they have "early terminal awakening." Unlike the normal situation, when depressed individuals have a reduction in total sleep, deep NREM sleep is reduced. The implication of this PSG data is that lack of restorative sleep contributes to the feeling of lethargy in depression.

Although the short REM latency is characteristic of depression, it is not diagnostic. About 15 percent of patients with depression have normal or even prolonged REM latency. Moreover, short REM latency is found in some patients with nonaffective psychiatric disorders; people with sleep deprivation, such as those who withdraw from alcohol, neuroleptics, and other medicines; those with narcolepsy; and those with medical illness. In mania and acute agitation, REM sleep can be abolished, and total sleep time can be markedly reduced. When sleep does occur in mania, REM latency is shortened.

In addition to their abnormal sleep patterns, depressed individuals have related neuroendocrine abnormalities. Their body temperature nadir occurs several hours earlier than is normal. Likewise, they have earlier excretion of cortisol and the norepinephrine metabolite MHPG. Overall, the earlier onset of so many features of sleep—the first REM period, the bulk of REM sleep, the temperature nadir, and nocturnal hormone excretion—is a result of the forward movement of the normal circadian rhythm, called a *phase shift advance*. It is as though, when depressed people fall asleep, they speed ahead into the middle of the sleep stage pattern and neuroendocrine cycle of normal people.

Schizophrenic patients vary in their sleep patterns according to the activity of the disorder. In acute schizophrenia, the total sleep time is decreased, and sleep occurs in small segments throughout the day. Patients with chronic schizophrenia, in contrast, have essentially normal sleep patterns and, interestingly, can distinguish their dreams from hallucinations.

A frequently occurring but underrecognized disorder is *pseudoinsomnia*, or "subjective insomnia without objective findings." In this condition, people complain of not sleeping long or deeply enough, but PSGs show a normal pattern and duration of sleep. This discrepancy, usually along with other complaints, suggests that the symptom originates from psychologic disturbances. Sometimes the misperception of sleeplessness approaches the level of a delusion.

Disorders of Excessive Somnolence

Excessive somnolence or *daytime sleepiness* is manifested by a feeling of fatigue and a tendency to nap one or more times throughout the day. Many cases can be attributed to psychiatric and medical illnesses, or are part of other sleep disorders, such as insomnia. The majority of individuals without these underlying conditions have *narcolepsy*, *sleep apnea*, or myoclonus or *restless legs*—very important, relatively recently defined conditions.

Narcolepsy

Narcolepsy is a condition in which multiple, brief, irresistible episodes (attacks) of sleep intrude into the waking hours of patients, whose days are dominated by sleepiness. Narcolepsy is the keystone of three other associated disorders, each of which is an aspect of REM sleep: *cataplexy*, *sleep paralysis*, and *sleep hallucinations*. Together they form the *narcoleptic tetrad*, but the much more common condition is restricted to the *narcolepsy-cataplexy syndrome*. Nevertheless, the primary feature of narcolepsy is excessive sleepiness, and the other factors are of secondary importance.

Although its cause is not yet established, recent studies indicate that narcolepsy has a genetic basis. Virtually 100 percent of white and Japanese narcolepsy patients, compared to 22 percent of controls, have a certain major histocompatibility complex designated human leukocyte antigen (HLA) DR2. This antigen has been found to be coded by a locus on the short arm of chromosome 6. It is not found uniformly in blacks with narcolepsy.

Narcolepsy almost always starts between adolescence and age 25 years. The first symptom of the adolescents and young adults who are developing narcolepsy is excessive daytime sleepiness. Subsequently, sleepiness may be complicated by cataplexy and occasionally the other problems. Unlike sleep apnea, men and women are affected equally.

Most narcolepsy attacks are preceded by a feeling of overwhelming fatigue and occur when the patient is comfortable and safe. Unlike boredom-induced naps, narcolepsy attacks can start when patients are standing, engaged in activities that require constant attention, or having a lively interchange. Narcolepsy patients have a compelling need to sleep. Their sleep attacks typically occur about 12 times weekly at the onset and 24 times weekly later in the illness. Each attack usually lasts 10 to 15 minutes, but it can be interrupted by noise or movement. Although the sleep is brief, it is refreshing for at least 1 to 2 hours.

Attacks characteristically start with a REM period, sleep-onset REM, rather than with the normal preliminary NREM phases (Fig. 17-4). Sometimes REM latency in narcolepsy is so short, it is virtually absent, and these episodes appear to have sleep-onset REM. A standard test for narcolepsy, the *multiple sleep latency test (MSLT)*, is based on the short or nonexistent REM and sleep latencies in

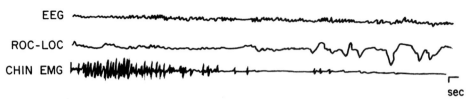

FIGURE 17–4. A PSG during the start of a narcoleptic attack shows the characteristic, almost immediate onset of rapid eye movement (REM) accompanied by loss of (chin) muscle EMG activity. Although such REM-onset sleep is characteristic of narcolepsy, it is also found following sleep deprivation and withdrawal of a tricyclic antidepressant or sedative. The multiple sleep latency test (MSLT), which is a standard laboratory test for narcolepsy, measures sleep latency and REM latency during five daytime naps. Results indicate narcolepsy when the sleep latency averages 5 minutes or less and if, in two or more episodes, the naps have REM-onset sleep.

daytime naps. Likewise, nighttime sleep, which is restless, has a sleep-onset REM and also multiple, brief, spontaneous awakenings.

Cataplexy, which usually begins about 4 years after the onset of narcolepsy, consists of episodes of sudden weakness that can be precipitated by heightened emotional states, most often laughter but also anger, surprise, or fright. These episodes last less than 30 seconds. Initially they occur about 9 times weekly and eventually more than 28 times weekly. In cataplexy's most dramatic but rare form, the entire body musculature becomes limp, and patients slump to the floor. Unless there is a simultaneous sleep attack, patients remain alert. Most often, patients have brief periods of weakness limited to certain muscles, which could easily be dismissed or misinterpreted by the patient, relatives, or physician. For example, the knees may buckle, the jaw drop open, or the head node once or twice. Affected muscles also lose their tone and DTRs.

The flaccid, areflexic paresis of cataplexy with normal ocular movement, breathing, and other vital functions recreates the muscular state characteristic of REM sleep. Moreover, a PSG obtained during cataplexy would demonstrate REM activity with absent EMG activity.

The other disturbances accompanying narcolepsy, namely sleep paralysis and sleep hallucinations, affect only about 10 percent of patients, i.e., only 10 percent of narcolepsy patients have the full narcoleptic tetrad. The paralysis and hallucinations, which can each occur independent of narcolepsy, may be present on awakening (hypnopompic) or falling asleep (hypnagogic). Each has physical, psychologic, and PSG manifestations of REM sleep that have intruded into people's alert state. Like cataplexy, they begin several years after the onset of narcolepsy, but they each occur only about six times weekly.

Patients with sleep paralysis are unable to move for several seconds on awakening or when falling asleep. As in cataplexy and normal REM sleep, they can breathe and move their eyes, but otherwise they are virtually paralyzed. Similarly, patients with sleep hallucinations have vivid, dream-like sensations on awakening or falling asleep: they qualify as an organic cause of visual hallucinations (Table 9-3). During both of these phenomena, PSGs reveal REM activity.

Medical treatment for narcolepsy and its associated disturbances relies on the use of stimulants in combination with medications that suppress REM sleep. Medicines suggested for daytime sleep attacks are pemoline (Cylert), methylphenidate (Ritalin), or amphetamines; for cataplexy, chlorimipramine, imipramine, or protriptyline (Vivactil); for nighttime sleep disturbances, imipramine or triazolam (Halcion).

Sleep Apnea Syndrome

The most common disorder of excessive sleepiness is sleep apnea or the *sleep apnea-hypersomnia syndrome*. This disorder is characterized by multiple 10-second to 2-minute interruptions in breathing (apnea) that partially awaken the patient from nighttime sleep. In the *obstructive variety*, apnea is caused by blockages within the oropharyngeal portion of the respiratory pathway. The most common airway obstacles result from congenital deformities, hypertrophied tonsils or adenoids, trauma, and other structural lesions. The *nonobstructive*, or *central*, *variety* of apnea, which is rare, results from cessation of diaphragmatic movements because of inconsistent CNS respiratory effort. A *mixed* variety also can be found.

Whichever the mechanism, apnea causes awakenings that are too brief and incomplete to be recognized by the patient or the patient's bed partner. The result is the clinical hallmark of profound daytime sleepiness, *daytime hypersomnia*, that forces patients to succumb to multiple, relatively long, unrefreshing daytime naps. The naps, like those in narcolepsy, occur under a variety of inappropriate conditions, such as when driving a car.

The apnea also leads to intermittent profound hypoxia (with oxygen saturation typically falling to 40 percent), cardiac arrhythmias, and pulmonary and systemic hypertension. Directly or indirectly, the apneic episodes also lead to morning headaches, confusion on awakening, and intellectual and emotional impairments.

During sleep, a patient's breathing intermittently seems to cease. Then periods of loud, irregular snoring start as breathing resumes. The snoring is a manifestation of the heavy breathing that acts as a resuscitative mechanism at the end of an apneic episode. The snoring is so characteristic that, in the presence of daytime sleepiness and an irresistible tendency to nap throughout the day, it is virtually diagnostic of sleep apnea.

Patients characteristically tend to be middle-aged, hypertensive, and overweight men; however, older children, adolescents, and young adults can be affected. Even young children who have enlarged tonsils may have sleep apnea. In all age ranges, males are affected much more than females.

The diagnosis of sleep apnea can be confirmed by a PSG that shows periods of apnea, hypoxia, arousals, and respiratory abnormalities (Fig. 17-5). In the obstructive variety, nasal airflow is absent despite chest and diaphragmatic respiratory movements. Because of REM sleep deprivation, REM latency is short. During the night, the episodes of sleep apnea occur in either phase of sleep, but they are more pronounced in REM sleep.

The initial management of this condition, in almost all cases, is to lose weight, stop smoking, and stop using sedatives, hypnotics, and especially alcohol. Also, if patients refrain from sleeping on their back, the airway tends to remain patent. Insertion of a tongue-retaining device or a small nasopharyngeal tube each night can provide relief. If these simple devices are insufficient, ventilation by nasal continuous positive airway pressure (CPAP) will alleviate respiratory impairments. In the past, tracheostomies were performed to bypass the pharynx, but now surgeons can perform simpler procedures, such as a uvulopalatopharyngoplasty, jaw abnormality correction, or, in children, tonsillectomy.

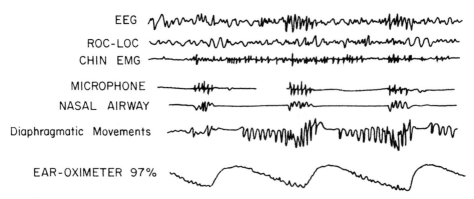

EEG

ROC-LOC

CHIN EMG

MICROPHONE

NASAL AIRWAY

Diaphragmatic Movements

EAR-OXIMETER 97%

FIGURE 17–5. A PSG during sleep apnea shows that, during a period of NREM sleep, the oxygen saturation falls. Then, as diaphragmatic movements reach a crescendo, loud snoring begins. After strenuous diaphragmatic movements, air moves through the nasal airway and oxygen saturation improves. During the hypoxic phase, the EEG became faster and had higher voltage, which indicated a partial arousal.

When there is an element of central sleep apnea, a variety of medications, including protriptyline or medroxyprogesterone, have been reported to be useful. With effective treatment, patients have a dramatic reversal of their daytime sleepiness and cardiovascular abnormalities.

Myoclonus and Restless Legs

A group of nighttime dysfunctions associated with daytime sleepiness are *periodic movements*. They are characterized by regular, episodic movements of the legs or, less often, the arms or trunk that awaken patients and their bed partners, and lead to insomnia of both people. Like narcolepsy and sleep apnea, this disturbance is not confined to a particular sleep phase.

Nocturnal myoclonus are stereotyped, brief (1 to 3 second), bilateral dorsiflexion movements of the foot and toes. They take place at 20- to 40-second intervals, for periods of 10 minutes to several hours, primarily but not exclusively during NREM sleep (Fig. 17-6). They can occur alone or in association with other sleep disorders, use of antidepressants, or withdrawal from various medications. They may be reduced with clonazepam (Klonipin).

Restless leg syndrome is a related but less well-defined condition in which people

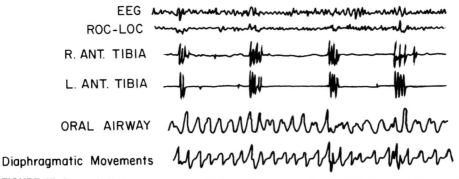

EEG

ROC-LOC

R. ANT. TIBIA

L. ANT. TIBIA

ORAL AIRWAY

Diaphragmatic Movements

FIGURE 17–6. Periodic leg movements, which usually occur during NREM sleep, are illustrated in this PSG. At about 30-second intervals, both anterior tibialis muscles contract synchronously— dorsiflexing the patient's ankles. Despite the movements, *this* patient remains asleep.

have an uncontrollable urge to move their legs. Their legs have abnormal sensations that compel patients to move about. Even after patients fall asleep, their legs continue to move.

All these disorders are different than the generalized bodily jerk preceded by a sensation of falling that affects virtually all people at some time as they "fall" asleep. These movements, called *sleep starts, hypnic jerks,* or *somnolescent starts,* occur in the twilight of sleep and are not associated with periodic movements, other sleep disorders, or any illness.

Other Disorders

The Kleine-Levin syndrome, *periodic hypersomnia,* is a rare sleep disorder. Patients, who are predominantly adolescent males, have lengthy but otherwise normal sleep. Sleep lasts for periods of several days to 2 weeks, three or four times yearly. Patients awaken during these periods to eat great quantities of food and display unusual behavior, including sexual disinhibition. At the same time they are slow, withdrawn, and apathetic. Some authors suggest that the hyperphagia and hypersomnia are akin to a burst of depression, an atypical depression, or the mirror image of anorexia nervosa. Others suggest that they are the result of encephalitis or a manifestation of thalamic or hypothalamic damage. However, no consistent laboratory abnormality has been found that would determine that the disorder is clearly "organic."

In contrast, clearcut cases of encephalitis, brain tumors, and hypothalamic injuries are often cited as causes of daytime sleepiness. Although these disorders might cause the appearance of sleep, in most cases patients are actually stuporous and have other signs of CNS dysfunction, such as intellectual impairment, hemiparesis, and abnormal reflexes. In addition, patients with hypothalamic injuries have endocrinologic disturbances. In virtually all of these cases, EEGs would reveal disorganized cerebral electrical activity, rather than the usual pattern of REM or NREM sleep.

Disorders of the Sleep-Wake Schedule

A variation on the theme of sleep disorders is those conditions in which individuals are able to sleep or remain awake, but only on a schedule that differs from the norm. Since their sleep cycle is displaced, these individuals tend to have alternating periods of insomnia and excessive sleepiness. Without *transient* disruptions, most people adjust their sleep schedule by the end of several days. Some people, however, have a *persistent* scheduling change and tend to adjust their life to their unusual pattern.

Transient Disorders

Periods of several days of a misaligned sleep schedule are commonplace with people who change time zones, usually by east-west jet travel. They have the well-known "jet lag," in which their mind and body adhere to their city-of-origin's day-night schedule. Their individual sleep-wake schedules can best be shifted to their destination's day-night schedule by adopting it before the trip or immediately accepting it on arrival. On long west-to-east flights, taking a hypnotic will advance the sleep schedule to conform immediately to the new time zone. The reverse is easier: stay awake until the normal bedtime.

Another transient schedule disorder follows a *work shift change.* For example, for several days after beginning to work nights rather than days, workers have fatigue and inattention while doing their job at night and inability to fall asleep when they go to bed during the day. Although most workers can make the transition in several days, some may be unsuccessful because their internal schedule is too ingrained or they continue to follow their old schedule on weekends or holidays.

Persistent Disorders

Individuals can have sleep schedules that are almost permanently different from the conventional. Of the several varieties, the most notable is the *delayed sleep phase syndrome*. In this disturbance, which often begins in adolescence, patients cannot fall asleep until the early morning, but once asleep, they have normal sleep phases and, if not awakened, normal sleep length. They would be happy owls if their work or social schedule permitted them to sleep when and as long as necessary, but they feel fatigued being forced to follow a conventional schedule. Unless a detailed evaluation were performed, these individuals might appear to have insomnia or mania at night and excessive sleepiness during the day.

The unique aspect of the delayed sleep phase syndrome is that, although medications are unsuccessful in making the patients fall asleep earlier, patients can *delay* their sleeptime without medication by 30 to 60 minutes successively each night. Thus, using "chronotherapy" to postpone their sleep onset through almost an entire day, eventually they fall asleep at 11 PM and, with effort, maintain that bedtime.

Dysfunction Associated with Sleep, Sleep Stages, or Partial Arousals (Parasomnias)

Parasomnias are behavioral aberrations that disrupt sleep. The most common ones are *night terrors*, *sleepwalking*, and *bedwetting*, which all occur during deep NREM sleep and thus tend to occur during the first 2 hours of sleep when deep NREM sleep predominates. They are believed to be the result of a partial arousal from sleep, rather than manifestations of dreams. Parasomnias usually arise in early childhood, affect boys more often than girls, and cease before puberty. In children, they are not associated with psychiatric disturbances. However, when parasomnias persist or develop in adult life, they are associated with character disorders and even psychosis.

Children are liable to have more than one variety of parasomnia. In these cases, parasomnias might be confused with partial complex seizures (Chapter 10). However, such seizures tend to be stereotyped, undergo secondary generalization, and be followed by (postictal) confusion. A PSG during attacks of either a parasomnia or seizure will be diagnostic.

Night terrors are a type of parasomnia in which young children suddenly awake and behave as though they were in great physical danger. During a night terror, children stare, moan, and sometimes speak a few words with their eyes fully open and their pupils dilated. They sweat, have tachycardia, and hyperventilate. Also, they thrash about and fight attempts to be held, often leaving their parents' arms to walk aimlessly. Parents are neither able to awaken them nor provide comfort. The episode lasts for several minutes and ends abruptly. The children, who are apparently terrified, suddenly return to a deep sleep.

Despite the apparently vivid and awesome features of the episode, children surprisingly have no recollection of it in the morning.

Night terrors can occur several nights a week, but usually take place only a few times a month. They are apt to follow the excessive, deep NREM sleep resulting from sleep deprivation. They may be precipitated by noises or other disruptions that partially rouse children. Unlike dreams, they are not related to frightening events of the day, and during the episode there is no REM activity.

Night terrors can be prevented in some children by enforcing an afternoon nap and by avoiding sleep disruptions, such as preventing loud noises, and not permitting a child more than a few sips of water to drink before sleeping, to avoid urinating. Treatment of an episode is not feasible because of its brevity. When children suffer from night terrors several times a week, prophylactic medical therapy with diazepam (Valium) or imipramine (Tofranil) may be considered. Their impact can be reduced by reassuring the parents that each night terror will cease by itself and that it does not result from pain, parental abuse, or emotional disturbance. Also, most attacks cease by age 8 years, and almost all cease by age 16 years.

In contrast, *nightmares* are essentially dreams that have a frightening content, i.e., "bad dreams." They contain complex imagery that the dreamer is able to recall when awakened during the nightmare or on arising in the morning. Nightmares are unaccompanied by bodily changes or vocalizations other than crying. Often a nightmare ends by itself, but if not, parents can easily interrupt it by awakening the child.

Nightmares can occur throughout the night during any REM period. They may be precipitated by certain medications, such as L-dopa, as well as by psychologic factors. Nightmares often develop when REM activity is increased, as occurs following sleep deprivation, alcohol withdrawal, and discontinuing use of many medications. Therefore, evaluation of frequent nightmares would include exploring not only the circumstances and content of the dreams but also the potential abuse of medications, alcohol, and drugs.

Sleepwalking (somnambulism) usually consists just of sitting or standing during deep NREM sleep. When people walk, they do so slowly with their eyes open, and they travel familiar pathways. Although they seem to be awake, if questioned, they would be confused and inappropriate. Diazepam may be helpful in preventing sleepwalking.

Bedwetting (enuresis) is considered a parasomnia in children older than 5 years and in all adults. In children and also some adults, bedwetting can be treated with imipramine (Tofranil) or with behavior modification therapy devices that complete a low voltage electrical circuit, which "alerts" a child who wets the bed. However, in adults, bedwetting can result not only from a sleep disorder or psychologic disturbance but also from a variety of neurologic illnesses. For example, it can result from degenerative cerebral disease and thus can be associated with dementia. In addition, it can result from seizures and be the only evidence of a nighttime seizure. Also, spinal cord damage, as with multiple sclerosis, or cauda equina injuries can lead to nighttime incontinence. Therefore, when bedwetting develops in older children or adults, a neurologic examination should be included in the evaluation.

Limited, nonperiodic movements can also be parasomnias. *Bruxism*, grinding of the teeth, mainly occurs in the transition from wakefulness to sleep. It can lead to headaches, temporomandibular joint pain, and dental injury. Although daytime bruxism is felt to be psychogenic, the etiology of nocturnal bruxism is unknown. *Head banging*, usually found only in children younger than 5 years, is a rocking head motion unconnected with any particular phase of sleep. In adults, it is associated with psychologic problems.

Neurologic and Medical Conditions Precipitated by Sleep

Many conditions in addition to classical parasomnias are associated with sleep. Some seizures seem to be precipitated by sleep (Chapter 10). For example, about 45 percent of patients with primary generalized epilepsy have seizures predominantly during sleep, and sleep deprivation precipitates seizures in epilepsy patients. Seizures tend to develop in deep NREM sleep, especially following sleep deprivation. The tendency for seizures to develop after sleep deprivation has led to the practice of obtaining an EEG after enforced sleep deprivation. This technique, which is quite harmless yet valuable, elicits sharp waves and a variety of spike-and-sharp wave activity in more than one third of epileptic patients who have no such abnormalities on routine EEGs.

In contrast to seizures that develop during sleep, classic involuntary movement disorders, such as Parkinson's disease and chorea (Chapter 18), are characteristically absent during sleep. Curiously, tics and palatal myoclonus persist during sleep.

Several cardiovascular disorders can occur during sleep. Angina pectoris and myocardial infarctions take place much more often during REM than NREM phases; asthma, congestive heart failure, and gastroesophageal reflux occur with equal frequency in either phase; and thrombotic cerebrovascular infarctions are more frequent during NREM sleep, when pulse and blood pressure are relatively low.

Another disorder clearly associated with sleep is vascular headaches (Chapter 9). Migraines and, even more so, cluster headaches are not only associated with sleep, but they also seem to be precipitated by REM phases. In rare persons, these headaches can occur only during REM periods, but in most people, they begin during early morning intense REM sleep and continue after awakening. Thus, excessive sleep or other conditions that increase REM sleep are associated with headaches. Also, in many cases, medications that suppress REM sleep reduce headaches.

REFERENCES

Anders TF, Carskadon MA, Dement WC: Sleep and sleepiness in children and adolescents. Pediatr Clin North Am 27:29, 1980

Commission on Professional and Hospital Activities: ASDC-APSS Diagnostic Classification of Sleep and Arousal Disorders in Relation to the International Classification of Diseases (ICD-9-CM) Sleep 2:130, 1979

DiMario FJ, Emery ES: The natural history of night terrors. Ann Neurol 20:440, 1986

Guilleminault C (ed): Sleep and Its Disorders in Children. New York, Raven Press, 1987

Guilleminault C, Dement WC: Two hundred thirty-four cases of excessive daytime sleepiness: Diagnosis and tentative classification. J Chron Dis 29:733, 1976

Guilleminault C, Faull KF, Miles L, et al: Posttraumatic excessive daytime sleepiness: A review of 20 patients. Neurology 33:1584, 1983

Hauri P, Olmstead E: Childhood-onset insomnia. Sleep 3:59, 1980

Kales A, Soldatos CR, Kales JD: Sleep disorders: Insomnia, sleepwalking, night terrors, nightmares, and enuresis. Ann Intern Med 106:582, 1987

Kales A, Vela-Bueno A, Kales JD: Sleep disorders: Sleep apnea and narcolepsy. Ann Intern Med *106*:434, 1987

Kramer RE, Dinner DS, Braun WE, et al: HLA-DR2 and narcolepsy. Arch Neurol *44*:853, 1987

Kupfer DJ, Thase ME: The use of the sleep laboratory in the diagnosis of affective disorders. Psychiatr Clin North Am *6*:3, 1983

Moore-Ede MC, Czeisler CA, Richardson GS: Circadian time keeping in health and disease. N Engl J Med *309*:469, 530, 1983

Moran MG, Thompson TL, Nies AS: Sleep disorders in the elderly. Am J Psychiatry *145*:1369, 1988

Neely S, Rosenberg R, Spire J-P, et al: HLA antigens in narcolepsy. Neurology *37*:1858, 1987

Orlosky MJ: The Kleine-Levin syndrome: A review. J Psychosomat *23*:609, 1983

Parkes JD: Sleep and Its Disorders. Philadelphia, W. B. Saunders, 1985

Richman, N: Sleep problems in young children. Arch Dis Child *56*:491, 1981

Weitzman ED: Sleep and aging. In Katzman R, Terry R (eds): The Neurology of Aging. Philadelphia, F. A. Davis, 1983, pp 167–188

Weitzman ED, Czeisler CA, Coleman RM: Delayed sleep phase syndrome. Arch Gen Psychiatry *38*:737, 1981

QUESTIONS: CHAPTER 17

1–15.   Is the statement true or false?

1.   Normal sleep begins in the first stage of NREM sleep and progresses through the four NREM stages before the first period of REM sleep occurs.

2.   REM sleep usually begins about 90 minutes after the onset of sleep.

3.   The bulk of REM sleep occurs in the early evening, whereas the bulk of NREM sleep occurs in the early morning.

4.   The normal sequence of NREM-REM sleep recurs with a periodicity of 90 minutes.

5.   REM sleep is a period of decreased physical and mental activity.

6.   The third and fourth stages of NREM sleep are often called "slow-wave sleep" and can be considered deep sleep, during which there is great restfulness.

7.   Sleep must always begin with the first stage of NREM sleep.

8.   Aside from the artifact caused by eye movement, the EEG obtained in REM sleep is similar to the one found in wakefulness.

9.   The EEG during NREM sleep is characterized by slow activity.

10.   In general, the proportion of REM sleep remains constant from birth to old age.

11.   Most people's sleep-wake schedules are determined by social and occupational factors, rather than by internal, physiologic mechanisms.

12.   Pseudoinsomniacs sleep 4 to 5 hours a night.

13.   Some productive, vigorous, and well-rested people sleep as little as 5 hours nightly.

14.   Fear of having a nightmare may cause insomnia.

15.   Infant boys have penile erections during REM sleep.

16.   In the night after sleep deprivation, which of the following can be expected to occur?

    a.   Sleep may begin with a period of REM activity.
    b.   Epileptiform discharges may emanate from the temporal lobe of patients with partial complex (psychomotor) seizures.
    c.   Total sleep time will increase.
    d.   There will be an increase in time spent in REM sleep.

17–24.   Which of the following characteristics are associated with (a) night terrors, (b) nightmares, (c) both, or (d) neither?

17.   Onset during the first and second stage of NREM sleep

18.   Onset during the third and fourth stage of NREM sleep

19.   Onset during REM sleep

20.   Are a variety of common dreams

21.   Recall for content usual

22.   May be precipitated by loud noises during first NREM period

23.   Patients seem frightened

24.   Are associated with somnambulism

25–42.   Which of the following phenomena typically occur during (a) REM sleep, (b) NREM sleep, (c) either phase, or (d) neither phase?

25.   Sleepwalking (somnambulism)

26.   Asthma

27.   Angina

28.   Bedwetting (enuresis)

29.   Night terrors

30.   Cluster headache

31.   Erections

32.   Migraine headache

33.   Nightmares

34.   Dreams

35.   Seizures

36.   Parkinson tremor

37.   Muscular contraction (tension) headaches

38.   Hemiballismus

39.   Complex motor activity

40.   Tics

41.   Complex intellectual activity

42.   Head banging

43–47.   Is the statement true or false?

43.   Recent studies of the physiology of sleep have confirmed the clinical observation that neurotic or reactive depression is almost always associated with impaired ability to fall asleep, and endogenous depression is almost always associated with early morning awakenings.

44.   Sleep apnea is a disorder only of adults.

45.   Sleep apnea is sometimes associated with narcolepsy.

46.   Sleep apnea leads to cardiovascular disturbances and sometimes to cognitive impairments and poor school performance.

47. Hypnopompic refers to phenomena that occur on awakening, and hypnagogic refers to phenomena that occur on falling asleep.

48. With which of the following is narcolepsy associated?
    a. Cataplexy
    b. Hallucinations
    c. Sleep paralysis
    d. Sleep-onset REM

49. A 27-year-old woman had the onset over 48 hours of lethargy, fever, temporal lobe seizures, and lymphocytic pleocytosis of the CSF. Which of the following illnesses is most likely?
    a. Hypothyroidism
    b. Schizophrenia
    c. Herpes simplex encephalitis
    d. Metastatic carcinoma

50. Which of the following can be causes of shortened REM latency?
    a. Narcolepsy
    b. Barbiturate withdrawal
    c. Depression
    d. Mania
    e. Sleep deprivation
    f. Neuroleptic withdrawal
    g. Sleep apnea
    h. Hypnotic use

51. Which characteristic(s) is (are) common to the sleep patterns seen in depression and following sleep deprivation?
    a. Lengthened sleep latency
    b. Shortened REM latency
    c. Early terminal awakening
    d. Interruptions in sleep

52. Which of the following are found in the night after sleep deprivation?
    a. Increase in total sleep
    b. Short sleep latency
    c. Increase in stage I and II NREM sleep
    d. In children, increased susceptibility for night terrors
    e. Normal REM distribution
    f. Shortened REM latency
    g. Increased deep NREM sleep

53. What is the relationship of seizures to sleep?
    a. Many patients have seizures prominently or exclusively during nighttime sleep.
    b. Seizures occur only in deep NREM sleep.
    c. EEGs obtained after sleep deprivation may reveal electroencephalographic signs even without clinical evidence of seizures.
    d. Sleep deprivation can precipitate a seizure in a previously seizure-free individual.

54. With which physiologic changes is REM sleep associated?
    a. Absent respirations
    b. Lower pulse and blood pressure
    c. Increased intracranial pressure
    d. High voltage, slow EEG activity
    e. Absent limb and chin EMG activity
    f. Penile erections

55. In depressed patients, which of the following are typical?

    a.   Delay in the nighttime body temperature nadir
    b.   Advance of REM activity
    c.   Advance of cortisol excretions
    d.   Delay in MHPG excretion

56. What are the consequences of alcohol withdrawal?
    a.   Hallucinations during the day
    b.   Excessive dreaming
    c.   Increased REM sleep
    d.   Tendency to have seizures
    e.   Decreased NREM sleep
    f.   Agitation
    g.   Insomnia

57. Which of the following conditions usually begin before 25 years of age?
    a.   Delayed sleep phase syndrome
    b.   Head banging
    c.   Kleine-Levin syndrome
    d.   Sleep apnea syndrome
    e.   Narcolepsy
    f.   Cataplexy

58. Which of the following are effective treatments for the delayed sleep phase syndrome?
    a.   Continually advancing the bedtime
    b.   Continually delaying the bedtime
    c.   Hypnotics
    d.   Stimulants

59. Which of the following are accurate statements regarding the sleep of elderly people?
    a.   Their sleep cycle is advanced.
    b.   They have a shortened REM latency.
    c.   REM periods are of equal length and distribution throughout the night.
    d.   Their sleep occurs partly during daytime as irresistible naps.
    e.   They sleep more than young adults.

60. Which factor(s) is (are) the major determinants of most people's sleep schedule?
    a.   Early learning
    b.   Social and occupational demands
    c.   Neuroendocrinic excretion
    d.   Personality type
    e.   Physiologic "clocks"

61. What are the possible effects of withdrawal from medications that have hypnotic effects?
    a.   Insomnia
    b.   Excessive daytime sleepiness
    c.   REM rebound
    d.   Heightened awareness
    e.   Vivid dreams
    f.   Seizures

62. Almost all narcolepsy patients have the major histocompatibility complex antigen HLA DR2. Which one of the following statements regarding this finding is *false*?
    a.   It indicates that narcolepsy has a genetic etiology.
    b.   The short arm of the chromosome 6 is implicated.
    c.   Almost all people with this antigen have narcolepsy.
    d.   Multiple sclerosis patients also have significantly increased proportion of certain HLA antigens.

ANSWERS

1.	True	32.	a.
2.	True	33.	a.
3.	False	34.	a.
4.	True	35.	b.
5.	False	36.	d.
6.	True	37.	d.
7.	False	38.	d.
8.	True	39.	d.
9.	True	40.	c.
10.	False	41.	a.
11.	True	42.	c.
12.	False	43.	False
13.	True	44.	False
14.	True	45.	True
15.	True	46.	True
16.	a, b, c, d, e.	47.	True
17.	d.	48.	a, b, c, d.
18.	a.	49.	c.
19.	b.	50.	a, b, c, d, e, f, g.
20.	b.	51.	b.
21.	b.	52.	a, b, d, f, g.
22.	a.	53.	a, c, d.
23.	c.	54.	c, e, f.
24.	a.	55.	b, c.
25.	b.	56.	a, b, c, d, f, g.
26.	c.	57.	a, b, c, e, f.
27.	a.	58.	b.
28.	b.	59.	a, c, d.
29.	b.	60.	b.
30.	a.	61.	a, b, c, d, e, f.
31.	a.	62.	c.

18

Involuntary Movement Disorders

The involuntary movement disorders* are an important group of conditions, rather than illnesses. For example, neuroleptic-induced disorders are common, and several other movement disorders are associated with mental aberrations, including dementia, depression, or psychosis. These mental changes may precede, accompany, or overshadow the abnormal movements. Similarly, certain movement disorders cause extraordinary physical disabilities but unexpectedly no mental deficits.

This chapter briefly reviews the anatomy, physiology, and neurotransmitters of the basal ganglia, which are considered the anatomic origins of most movement disorders. It then describes the classic disorders that are common and attributable to basal ganglia abnormalities: parkinsonism, athetosis, chorea, hemiballismus, Wilson's disease, and dystonia. Next, it describes disorders that do not conform to classic patterns and where the origin is largely unknown: tremors, tics, Tourette's syndrome, and myoclonus. It concludes with a review of tardive dyskinesia and other neuroleptic-induced conditions. The chapter includes descriptions of several recent studies of these conditions that have been recognized as major medical advances.

THE BASAL GANGLIA

Anatomy and Physiology

Although some texts include additional structures, the basal ganglia are composed of essentially three elements:

- The *corpus striatum* (*striatum*), which includes the *caudate nuclei*, the *putamen*, and the *globus pallidus*
- The *subthalamic nucleus* (*corpus of Luysii*)
- The *substantia nigra* (Fig. 18-1)

Extensive and intricate tracts link the structures of the basal ganglia to each other. Other tracts link the basal ganglia to the cerebral cortex, thalamus, and

---

* Patients with movement disorders may receive assistance from the following organizations: Benign Essential Blepharospasm Research Foundation, P.O. Box 12468, Beaumont, TX 77706, (409) 892-0788; Dystonia Medical Research Foundation, 8383 Wilshire Boulevard, Beverly Hills, CA 90210, (213) 852-1630; National Huntington's Disease Association, (516) 783-9389; Parkinson's Disease Foundation, 650 West 168th Street, New York, New York, NY 10032, (212) 923-4700; Spasmodic Torticollis Association, P.O. Box 873, Royal Oak, MI 48068, (313) 647-2280; Tourette Syndrome Association, 4102 Bell Boulevard, Bayside, NY 11361, (212) 519-6563; United Cerebral Palsy Foundation, 66 East 34th Street, New York, NY 10016, (212) 481-6300.

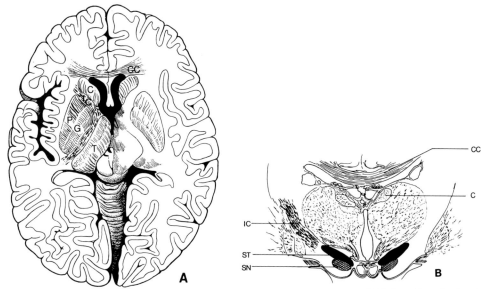

FIGURE 18–1   *A*, In this axial view, which is the plane shown in CT and MRI studies, the basal ganglia can be seen in relation to the brain. The heads of the *caudate nuclei* (C) indent the anterior horns of the lateral ventricles. The *globus pallidus* (G) and *putamen* (P), which together with the caudate are called the *corpus striatum* or *striatum*, are separated from the thalamus (T) by the posterior limb of the internal capsule (IC). *B*, In this coronal view of the midbrain, the *substantia nigra* (SN) and the *subthalamic nuclei* (ST) are below the thalamus. In fresh specimens, the substantia nigra is black and large enough to be readily identified.

other areas of the brain. All these tracts, however, are confined to the brain. They do not descend into the spinal cord.

The projections of the basal ganglia form the *extrapyramidal tract*, which is complementary to the *pyramidal* or corticospinal *tract* (Chapter 2). Although the pyramidal tract regulates voluntary movements, the extrapyramidal tract modulates the movements, maintains appropriate muscle tone, and adjusts posture. The extrapyramidal system consists of delicately balanced excitatory and inhibitory neurons that project to the contralateral corticospinal tract. Thus unilateral injuries of the basal ganglia induce clinical abnormalities in the contralateral limbs.

Neurotransmitters

Although peptide neurotransmitters, such as substance P and the enkephalins, may have an important role, there are three basic basal ganglia neurotransmitters:

- dopamine
- *acetylcholine (ACh)*
- *gamma-aminobutyric acid (GABA)*.

Dopamine

About 80 percent of brain dopamine is concentrated in the striatum and other components of the basal ganalia. Three dopamine tracts have clinical significance. The *nigrostriatal tract*, in which most dopamine is synthesized, projects from the substantia nigra to the striatum. The *mesocortical-mesolimbic tract*, which includes projections from the midbrain to frontal and entorhinal cortex areas, connects the basal ganglia to these areas of the cerebral cortex and the limbic system. The *tubero-infundibular tract* connects the hypothalamic area with the pituitary gland.

Dopamine is also synthesized in sites outside of the brain, particularly in the adrenal medulla. The clinical application of this observation has been studied by transplanting adrenal cells into the brain in attempts to correct the dopamine deficiency in Parkinson's disease.

Dopamine is formed by the decarboxylation of dihydroxyphenylalanine (dopa):

$$HO-\hspace{-0.5em}\bigcirc\hspace{-0.5em}-CH_2-CH-NH_2 \qquad \longrightarrow \qquad HO-\hspace{-0.5em}\bigcirc\hspace{-0.5em}-CH_2-CH_2-NH_2$$

with the HO groups and $HO-C=O$ substituent shown.

| DOPA | *decarboxylation* | Dopamine |

After dopamine is released from the presynaptic neuron, it undergoes either re-uptake or metabolism by *monoamine oxidase* (*MAO*). The main metabolic product is *homovanillic acid* (*HVA*). The concentration of HVA in the CSF corresponds to dopamine activity in the brain. Positron emission tomography (PET) also demonstrates the dopamine activity in the basal ganglia.

On a physiologic level, dopamine activity inhibits caudate activity. On a clinical level, dopamine depletion of the nigrostriatal tract leads to disinhibition of the caudate, causing "parkinsonism," which is characterized by *akinesia* or *bradykinesia* (absent or slow movement). Dopamine blockade also results in an elevated serum prolactin concentration. When dopamine is depleted, its concentration can be restored and the accompanying parkinsonism can be reversed by administering a *dopamine precursor*, such as L-dopa (Fig. 18-2). L-dopa is converted to dopamine as long as enough nigrostriatal (presynaptic) neurons remain intact. When presynaptic neurons have completely degenerated, dopamine effects can be reproduced by a *dopamine agonist*, such as bromocriptine. Even though it is an ergot alkaloid with powerful serotonin effects, bromocriptine has dopamine-like activity.

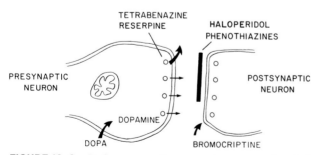

FIGURE 18–2.   In the presynaptic neuron, *precursors*, such as L-dopa, are metabolized to dopamine. Amantadine and amphetamines (not pictured) can enhance dopamine activity by facilitating its release from presynaptic storage sites or by blocking its re-uptake. Dopamine can be depleted from its presynaptic sites by reserpine and tetrabenazine. In the postsynaptic neuron, dopamine effects can be mimicked by *agonists*, such as bromocriptine, which act on dopamine receptors. Dopamine receptors are blocked by neuroleptics.

Dopamine excess leads to *dyskinesias* (abnormal or excessive movements) and physical and mental agitation. In conditions characterized by excess dopamine activity, the presynaptic dopamine concentration may be depleted and dyskinesias reduced by reserpine or by a similar (experimental) drug, *tetrabenazine*. Capitalizing on their dopamine-depleting properties, investigators have been using reserpine and tetrabenazine to treat movement disorders attributable to excessive dopamine activity.

Acetylcholine

Acetylcholine (ACh) is an excitatory neurotransmitter that increases caudate activity and thus opposes dopamine activity (Fig. 18-3). Unlike dopamine, ACh receptors are distributed throughout the entire cerebral cortex. It is formed by the combination of acetyl Coenzyme A and choline utilizing the enzyme choline acetyltransferase (CAT):

$$\text{Acetyl CoA } + \text{ Choline } \xrightarrow{\text{CAT}} \text{ ACh}$$

CAT and ACh concentrations are markedly reduced in certain areas of the brain in Alzheimer's disease (Chapter 7), and a basal ganglia ACh deficiency is postulated in tardive dyskinesia. Increasing ACh activity has been attempted in these conditions by providing precursors, such as choline and lecithin (phosphatidylcholine). A complementary strategy has been to administer physostigmine, an anticholinesterase (a cholinesterase inhibitor), which preserves ACh by retarding its degradation (Fig. 7-5). Although these maneuvers may have increased ACh concentrations, they have not produced the expected benefits.

When decreased ACh activity is desirable, as in the treatment of parkinsonism, anticholinergic medicines are given (Table 18-1). Notably, as might be expected in view of the deficiency of ACh in Alzheimer's disease, anticholinergic medications can cause memory impairment, confusion, and other cognitive dysfunctions.

Gamma-aminobutyric Acid

Gamma-aminobutyric acid (GABA), an inhibitory neurotransmitter found in the striatum, modulates the nigrostriatal system. It is formed from glutamate

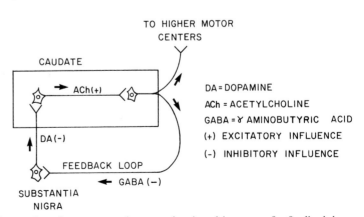

FIGURE 18–3. The interaction of neurotransmitters can be viewed in terms of a feedback loop in which dopamine and gamma-aminobutyric acid (GABA) are inhibitory and acetylcholine (ACh) is excitatory. The physiologic terms "inhibitory" and "excitatory," however, are the opposite of the clinical situation. For example, too much dopamine is associated with dyskinesias and too little with akinesia, and too little GABA is associated with chorea.

by the enzyme glutamate decarboxylase (GAD):

$$\text{Glutamate} \xrightarrow{\text{GAD}} \text{GABA}.$$

In Huntington's disease, GAD and GABA concentrations in the basal ganglia and certain other regions of the brain and in the CSF are reduced. The GABA levels can be increased by the anticonvulsant, valproate (Depakote).

GENERAL CONSIDERATIONS

The involuntary movement disorders have several common clinical features. The movements are increased by anxiety, exertion, fatigue, and stimulants, including caffeine. They can be momentarily suppressed by intense concentration. Also, they are decreased by relaxation and, in some cases, by biofeedback. With the exception of myoclonus and tics, they are absent during sleep.

In many disorders only extrapyramidal damage occurs. Patients with these disorders have neither paresis, spasticity, hyperactive reflexes, nor Babinski signs, which are signs of pyramidal (corticospinal) tract damage, nor dementia or seizures, which are signs of cerebral cortex damage. Patients might be debilitated by uncontrollable movements and inarticulate speech but be fully alert, intelligent, and, by using unconventional means, able to communicate thoughtfully.

Another important consideration is that, at the onset of their illness, patients with movement disorders are liable to be misdiagnosed as having a psychogenic disorder (Chapter 3). The error is usually made because the movements may be bizarre, apparent only during anxiety, and willfully suppressed, but absent during sleep. Thus hypnosis or an amobarbital interview may falsely indicate a psychogenic origin because sedation may abolish or reduce the abnormal movements. Another error in diagnosis occurs when dementia is a component of the illness. In these cases, the dementia may appear to be a psychiatric disturbance and reinforce a misdiagnosis of the abnormal movements.

PARKINSONISM

Clinical Features

The most prominent feature of parkinsonism, whatever its cause, is a tremor. However, for the patient, the most debilitating feature is akinesia. It leads to the classic "masked face" (Fig. 18-4), paucity of trunk and limb movement (Figs. 18-5 and 18-6), and impairment of dressing, bathing, and other "activities of daily living." Akinesia usually begins many months before tremor. In hemipar-

TABLE 18–1. ANTICHOLINERGIC MEDICATIONS

Brand Name	Generic Name	Usual Dosage
Akineton	Biperiden	1–2 mg tid
Artane	Trihexyphenidyl	2–4 mg tid
Cogentin	Benztropine	1–3 mg tid
Kemadrin	Procyclidine	2–5 mg tid

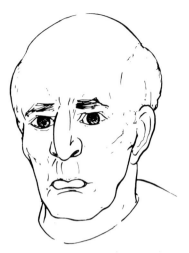

FIGURE 18–4. Since patients with parkinsonism have facial akinesia and rigidity, they have almost no blinking or facial expressions. In addition, their widened palpebral fissures and lack of head motion give them a "stare." This facial appearance has been called a "masked facies," a Latin term for "face" or "countenance," but the term *masked face* is becoming more widely used.

kinsonism, akinesia develops asymmetrically or unilaterally, and despite having normal strength and coordination, patients have difficulty moving one arm and leg.

Akinesia is usually accompanied by "cogwheel" rigidity (Fig. 18-7). This rigidity is not only an important sign of parkinsonism and other extrapyramidal disorders but it is also helpful in distinguishing a parkinson tremor from other varieties of tremor.

A parkinson tremor typically occurs when patients sit with their arms supported, and thus it is called a *resting tremor* (Fig. 18-8). It too can be

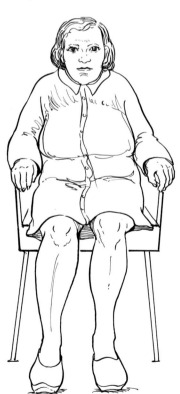

FIGURE 18–5. When patients with parkinsonism sit, they are typically immobile with their legs uncrossed and their feet set flatly on the floor. Their arms remain on the chair or in their lap and are rarely used for gesturing. In contrast to normal people and especially to those with chorea, patients with parkinsonism do not shift their weight from one hip to another or make unnecessary movements of their limbs.

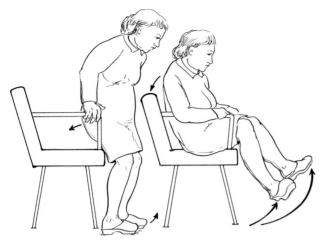

FIGURE 18–6. Patients with akinesia and rigidity cannot rapidly flex their spine, hips, or knees. When sitting, they tend to rock slowly and solidly backward into a chair, and their feet rise several inches off the floor. "Sitting *en bloc*" is an early, reliable manifestation of parkinsonism.

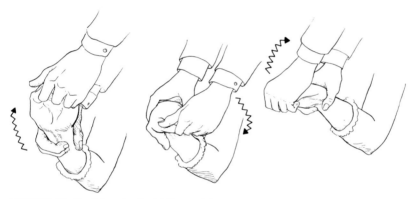

FIGURE 18–7. "Cogwheel rigidity," which can be elicited by rotating the patient's wrist, is characterized by increased tone in all directions of movement and superimposed ratchet-like resistance. In contrast, spasticity, which is the result of corticospinal tract damage, is characterized by sustained resistance up to a point, beyond which it disappears.

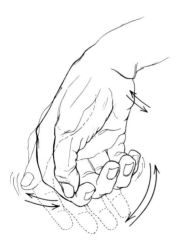

FIGURE 18–8. The *resting tremor* is a relatively slow (4- to 6-Hz) to-and-fro flexion movement of the wrist, hand, thumb, and fingers. Since the cupped hand appears as though it were shaking pills, the movement is commonly known as a "pill-rolling" tremor. The tremor is most apparent when patients sit comfortably. It is exaggerated or sometimes apparent only when patients are anxious. The tremor will be momentarily reduced during the initial phase of many voluntary movements or by intense concentration, and it is absent during sleep.

asymmetric or unilateral; if so, it is more pronounced on the side of akinesia. This tremor differs from cerebellar tremor (Fig. 2-11) and essential tremor (see below). Parkinson tremor isfound at rest and is accompanied by akinesia. It has a regular rate and primarily involves the hands and the feet.

A myriad of other signs, some of which require special examinations, develop in patients who have had parkinsonism for several years. Many are important in their own right, and several may also be found in other illnesses. Patients typically have impairment or loss of *postural reflexes*, which are the mechanisms that alter muscle tone in response to change in position. Their loss, in combination with akinesia and rigidity, leads to a gait impairment, called *marche à petit pas* or *festinating gait*, that is characterized by short steps and a tendency to accelerate (Fig. 18-9). Of the several characteristic gait abnormalities (Table 2-4), the festinating gait is most similar to gait apraxia (Fig. 7-7). Both disorders are characterized by small steps and slowed movements; however, gait apraxia is associated with impairment of voluntary leg motions and the presence of spasticity.

In addition, the voice of parkinson patients often becomes *hypophonic* (low in

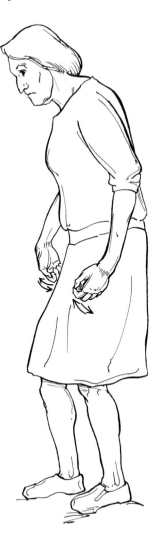

FIGURE 18–9. When parkinsonism patients walk, they are said to have a "festinating gait," in which they take short steps and accelerate their pace. Also, if they take several steps backward, they may have "retropulsion," in which they are unable to stop. When walking, they move "en bloc," in that they do not swing their arms, look about, or have other normal accessory movements. Likewise, when turning en bloc, they simultaneously move their head, trunk, and legs.

volume), tremulous, and devoid of the normal fluctuations in pitch and cadence. Likewise, their handwriting becomes *micrographic* (Fig. 18-10).

Dementia, Depression, and Psychotic Behavior in Parkinson's Disease

Although dementia practically never occurs as an initial symptom of Parkinson's disease, it is found in as many as 40 percent of patients older than 70 years. Dementia most commonly occurs when the illness has had a rapid progression and when antiparkinson medications have had little benefit. Dementia worsens with advancing age and increasing physical impairments, especially more pronounced akinesia.

In some patients with Parkinson's disease, the dementia is associated with impaired attention. These patients have slowed thinking, which is similar to their slowed movements. Their mental slowness, termed "bradyphrenia," has been correlated with abnormalities of norepinephrine, rather than dopamine (Mayeux).

Even though antiparkinson medications improve the physical aspects of the illness, they do not alleviate the dementia. Moreover, they are a frequent cause of confusion, agitation, and hallucinations, e.g., delirium. On the other hand, many patients with Parkinson's disease, who must be carefully identified, are fully lucid and have normal intelligence despite having debilitating physical impairments.

An episodic mental aberration occurs in some patients who have had Parkinson's disease for many years, whether or not they have dementia. It consists of episodes that last for several hours to several days of confusion,

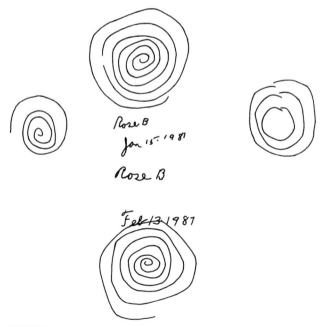

FIGURE 18–10. *Micrographia*, a characteristic feature of parkinsonism, is seen in the patient's upper three spirals, date, and signature. In the lower examples, which were obtained after treatment was initiated, the excursions were larger, bolder, and relatively free of tremor.

vivid dreams, hypersexual behavior (in men), delusions, or hallucinations. These patients have a paranoia that may extend to their physicians. Sometimes the disturbances are precipitated by excessive intake of L-dopa medications, other antiparkinson medications, sedatives, or alcohol. However, these aberrations are usually an unfortunate manifestation of the illness.

Late in the illness, about 10 percent of patients, especially those with dementia, exhibit psychotic behavior that is often abusive. This aberration is typically accompanied by physical manifestations of excessive dopamine activity, such as dyskinesias. The first step in its treatment is to reduce the total dose of the antiparkinson medication, usually by eliminating nighttime doses. Minor tranquilizers might also be tried. Although the concurrent use of L-dopa and dopamine antagonist neuroleptics should generally be avoided, the addition of a neuroleptic, such as thioridazine (Mellaril) 25 mg HS, is frequently necessary to avoid exhaustion, injury, or mental anguish. Even though the physical illness and dementia are burdens, it is the psychotic behavior superimposed on the immobility that usually forces the family to send the patients with Parkinson's disease to a nursing home.

Depression affects 25 to 50 percent of Parkinson's disease patients, and it is associated with dementia and increasing physical disability. Like the dementia associated with Parkinson's disease, the depression does not improve when medications alleviate the physical symptoms. It may result in part from dopamine depletion, but loss of other neurotransmitters, such as serotonin, may be responsible (Mayeux).

Treatment of depression in Parkinson's disease is difficult because of the coexistent physical and cognitive disabilities. Nevertheless, tricyclic antidepressants, trazodone (Desyrel), and fluoxetine (Prozac) are helpful, and their anticholinergic side effects can be beneficial to the physical manifestations of Parkinson's disease. Electroconvulsive therapy has been successful for patients who had been unresponsive to antidepressants. Support groups are popular and helpful.

In contrast to the high prevalence of dementia and depression in Parkinson's disease, manic-depressive illness and schizophrenia are rare but do occur. The infrequent occurrence of Parkinson's disease and schizophrenia is important not only as a clinical point (see below) but also because it belies the classic dopamine hypothesis of schizophrenia: the theory predicts that these two conditions, of decreased and increased dopamine activity, would be mutually exclusive.

Pathology of Parkinson's Disease

In Parkinson's disease, the normally "pigmented nuclei" of the brain (the substantia nigra, locus ceruleus, and the tenth cranial dorsal motor nuclei) are depigmented, and their neurons contain *Lewy bodies*, which are eosinophilic, intracytoplasmic inclusions. As previously mentioned, nigrostriatal neurons are depleted of dopamine, and the CSF concentration of HVA is reduced.

The cerebral cortex in many patients has histologic and biochemical changes also found in Alzheimer's disease. These include numerous senile plaques, abundant neurofibrillary tangles, and loss of neurons. When patients have dementia, the cortex has a proportionately decreased concentration of CAT (Chapter 7).

Causes of Parkinson's Disease and Parkinsonism

Following the landmark discovery that the accidental intravenous injection of a byproduct of illicit narcotic manufacturing, *methyl-phenyl-tetrahydro-pyridine (MPTP)*, caused fulminant and often fatal cases of parkinsonism, the current theory is that toxic substances cause most cases of Parkinson's disease. MPTP is highly toxic to dopamine neurons, and it produces a reliable animal model of Parkinson's disease. Notably, in this model, the development of parkinsonism can be prevented by pretreatment with MAO inhibitors.

In previous decades, Parkinson's disease was attributable to the famous epidemic of encephalitis that followed World War I, and cases due to this unique viral infection were called "postencephalitic Parkinson's disease." Subsequently cerebrovascular disease and genetic influences were suspected but never proved. Pathologic studies have demonstrated that Parkinson's disease does not result from cerebrovascular infarctions. Clinical evaluations have shown that the concordance rate in twins for Parkinson's disease is much too low for the disease to be a genetic condition.

The clinical state of parkinsonism, as is well known, is commonly caused by phenothiazines, haloperidol, and other dopamine antagonist neuroleptics. The similarity between Parkinson's disease and medication-induced parkinsonism is so great that the distinction is almost impossible. There are few reliable guidelines. The history, of course, is crucial. Unlike in neuroleptic-induced parkinsonism, at the onset of Parkinson's disease the rigidity and tremor are asymmetric. As a practical consideration, the coincidence of Parkinson's disease and schizophrenia is so low that, whenever schizophrenic patients appear to have Parkinson's disease, they can be assumed to have either neuroleptic-induced parkinsonism or a neurologic disorder other than Parkinson's disease.

Another newly recognized iatrogenic cause of parkinsonism is the medication metoclopramide (Reglan). Although useful for esophageal reflux and gastric stasis, it antagonizes dopamine and causes parkinsonism, oculogyric crisis, and other signs of dopamine blockade. Other causes of parkinsonism in adults are manganese intoxication, carbon monoxide poisoning, cerebral anoxia (especially from drug overdose), Wilson's disease, acquired immune deficiency syndrome (AIDS), and dementia pugilistica. In most of these conditions, the parkinsonism is only one aspect of the constellation of abnormalities. When parkinsonism develops in older children, causes are medications and drugs, Wilson's disease, and the juvenile form of Huntington's disease (see below)—in these patients, the parkinsonism may be the most prominent or only feature of the illness.

Therapy of Parkinson's Disease

Until the introduction of L-dopa, neurosurgery was the best available treatment. Small lesions were made in the thalamus (thalamotomy). When patients had hemiparkinsonism, lesions were made in the thalamus contralateral to the affected limbs. In most cases, surgery was successful in relieving symptoms for several years. However, it was occasionally complicated by damage to the corticospinal or corticobulbar tracts in the adjacent internal capsule (Fig. 18-1). Similar ablative surgical procedures have also been introduced for other movement disorders, including athetosis and dystonia. They have not been accepted because they also carry grave risks and inconsistent benefits.

Current medical treatment for Parkinson's disease attempts to maintain normal dopamine activity. Since dopamine cannot cross the blood-brain barrier, orally administered L-dopa, "precursor replacement," is the therapeutic mainstay in the first 3 to 5 years of the illness. In this initial phase, sufficient (greater than 20 percent) nigrostriatal neurons must be intact to convert L-dopa to dopamine. Carbidopa, a decarboxylase inhibitor, is usually given in combination with L-dopa, such as in *Sinemet,* to raise the L-dopa brain concentration and minimize systemic side effects (Fig. 18-11). The antiparkinson effects of L-dopa can be supplemented with dopamine agonists, such as bromocriptine (*Parlodel*).

Dopamine toxicity is manifested by dyskinesias and, as described previously, mental aberrations. It limits treatment, especially late in the illness or when dementia is present. The dyskinesias consist of buccolingual movements, chorea of the limbs, and rocking trunk movements that are similar to those of tardive dyskinesia. Despite the apparent problems with dyskinesias—embarrassment, exhaustion, and discomfort—parkinson patients usually choose to bear with them, rather than to reduce the drug dosage. Another characteristic of current L-dopa treatment is that patients are usually so keenly aware of the short effective period of the medicines, which is about 2 to 4 hours, that they may become preoccupied or actually obsessed with taking their medications at the prescribed times.

Anticholinergics are effective, at least in some measure, in treating Parkinson's disease and neuroleptic-induced parkinsonism, and in preventing dystonic reactions from neuroleptics. They are effective presumably because dopamine depletion results in excess ACh activity that can be reversed by anticholinergics (Fig. 18-12). The usual side effects of anticholinergics are dry mouth, consti-

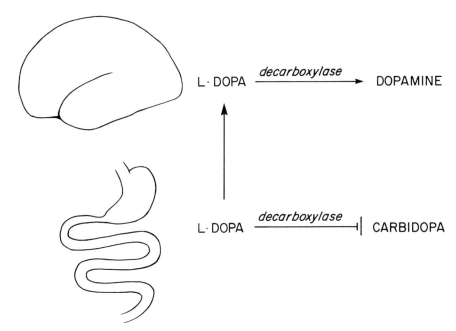

FIGURE 18–11. Sinemet and similar antiparkinson preparations contain the combination of L-dopa and carbidopa, which is a dopa decarboxylase inhibitor that does not cross the blood-brain barrier. By using carbidopa, L-dopa is converted to dopamine almost exclusively in the brain, and systemic side effects are minimal.

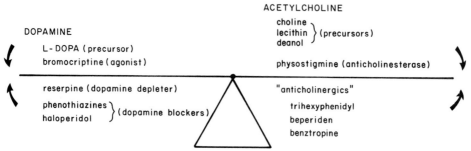

FIGURE 18–12. The countervaling effects of dopamine and acetylcholine can be pictured as a balanced scale. In this model, the left side of the scale would be pulled upward when there is dopamine depletion, as in Parkinson's disease; however, it would be realigned by dopamine precursors, dopamine agonists, or anticholinergics. In cases where excessive dopamine activity is postulated, the left side would be pushed downward; however, it could be realigned by dopamine antagonists, dopamine depleters, or acetylcholine precursors.

pation, and urinary retention. Most important, they may cause memory impairment, confusion, and agitation. Three theoretical problems must be acknowledged: anticholinergics given to patients with parkinsonism or under treatment with neuroleptics might exacerbate the cholinergic deficit in an undiagnosed case of Alzheimer's disease, they might worsen or hasten the development of tardive dyskinesia, and they may contribute to a patient's mental aberrations.

Amantidine (*Symmetrel*) facilitates dopamine and norepinephrine release from presynaptic neurons. This response requires the presence of sufficient presynaptic dopamine, and in treating Parkinson's disease, it may require the simultaneous administration of L-dopa. However, amantidine may be helpful in neuroleptic-induced parkinsonism without administration of L-dopa. Since amantidine is basically an adjunct to other medicines, it rarely produces confusion or hallucinations unless the patient has an underlying psychiatric disorder or is also being given anticholinergics.

Experimental treatments of parkinsonism attempt to preserve dopamine. Deprenyl, the antidepressant, is an antioxidant that retards dopamine metabolism. Unlike most other MAO inhibitors, deprenyl does not leave patients vulnerable to hypertensive crises. Alpha tocopherol (vitamin E), a free radical scavenger, protects dopamine from destruction by intrinsic and extrinsic toxins, including MPTP and free radicals. Trial combinations of deprenyl and Vitamin E in patients in the early stages of Parkinson's disease are in progress in an attempt to halt its progression by preserving dopamine.

A more dramatic experiment is the transplantation of a patient's own adrenal medulla cells, which are capable of synthesizing dopamine, into the basal ganglia or ventricular system of the brain. A related technique is transplanting fetal adrenal cells. Since the brain is an immunologically "privileged site," transplanted fetal cells are not rejected. Despite the rationale, these experiments have been unsuccessful.

ATHETOSIS

Athetosis is a slow, regular, continual twisting of muscles. It is at one end of a spectrum, with hemiballismus at the other, where movements are progressively

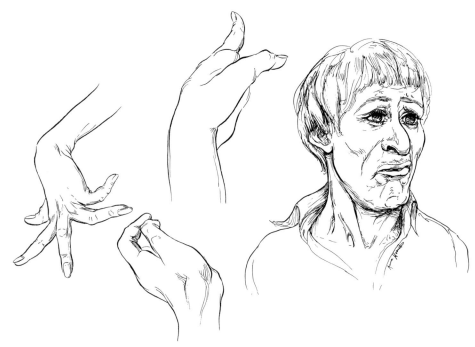

FIGURE 18–13. In athetosis, the face has incessant grimacing and fractions of smiles that alternate with frowns. Neck muscles contract and rotate the head. Laryngeal contraction and irregular chest and diaphragmatic muscle movements cause dysarthria that has an irregular cadence and nasal pitch. Fingers writhe constantly and tend to assume hyperextension postures while the wrists rotate, flex, and extend. These movements prevent writing, buttoning, and other fine hand movements, but they usually permit gross shoulder, trunk, and hip movements.

greater in amplitude and irregularity. Athetosis predominantly affects the distal parts of the limbs and is usually bilateral and symmetric (Fig. 18-13). It is often combined with chorea, *choreoathetosis*.

Athetosis, which almost always becomes apparent in early childhood, results from perinatal hyperbilirubinemia (kernicterus), hypoxia, or prematurity, i.e., choreoathetotic cerebral palsy (Chapter 13). Although athetosis is closely associated with mental retardation, when the perinatal damage is confined to the basal ganglia, some patients have relatively normal intelligence. This may be overlooked in patients with disabling movement disorders and a garbled voice. Neurosurgeons have made thalamic lesions to treat choreoathetotic cerebral palsy in an attempt at recreating their initial success with Parkinson's disease. However, this procedure is hazardous and has been helpful in few patients. Dopamine antagonists suppress the movements, but their long-term use may lead to complications.

HUNTINGTON'S DISEASE

The defect in Huntington's disease, previously called Huntington's chorea, has now been localized to chromosome 4. It is expressed in an autosomal dominant pattern and characterized by chorea and dementia that do not become apparent, except in a juvenile variety, until age 35 to 42 years. Patients succumb one to two decades later to aspiration and inanition. Between 2 and 6 per

100,000 persons suffer from Huntington's disease, making it a relatively common disorder and a frequent cause of dementia in middle-aged adults (Chapter 7). Although families of all races and ethnic backgrounds have been diagnosed as having Huntington's chorea, most cases in the United States have been traced to several 17th-century English immigrants.

A tragic but interesting cohort has recently been found in a small village in Venezuela. This group consists of more than 65 individuals with the illness who have shared the same genetic pool, environment, and lack of neuroleptic treatment. Extensive studies have described affected children, heterozygous individuals in the presymptomatic state (carriers), and several homozygous patients. (The homozygous and heterozygous patients were phenotypically similar.)

Biochemical abnormalities in the basal ganglia are probably responsible for the chorea if not the dementia. In the caudate nuclei, which are characteristically atrophied, the GABA and GAD concentrations are reduced to less than 50 percent of normal. PET studies demonstrate caudate hypometabolism that occurs even before computed tomography (CT) scans show the characteristic atrophy of the caudate (Fig. 20-12). The cerebral cortex, especially in the frontal lobes, is also atrophied, but the GABA and GAD concentrations are normal. In contrast to Parkinson's disease and Alzheimer's disease, cerebral cortex CAT concentrations are normal.

Clinical Features

Whereas athetosis consists of continual, slow, writhing movements, chorea consists of frequent discrete and brisk movements that cause jerks of the pelvis, trunk, and limbs (Fig. 18-14). Likewise, the face has intermittent and random frowns, grimaces, and smirks (Fig. 18-15). Pelvic thrusts and other abnormal movements give the gait a "herky-jerky" pattern (Fig. 18-16) that was the origin of the term *chorea*, which is Greek for "dance."

When Huntington's disease is fully developed, the presence of an involuntary movement disorder, if not chorea itself, is easy to recognize. However, in its earliest stages, chorea is often so subtle that it mimics the nonspecific movements that result from anxiety, restlessness, discomfort, or clumsiness. In this stage, chorea may consist of only excessive face or hand gestures, frequent weight shifting, continual leg crossing, or twitching fingers (Fig. 18-17).

In 3 percent of Huntington's disease cases, symptoms appear before patients are 15 years old. This variety, *juvenile Huntington's disease*, is characterized not by chorea, but by *dystonia* (continual generalized muscle contractions), rigidity, and akinesia—giving these children the appearance of having parkinsonism. In addition, seizures are also common. The juvenile variety is usually transmitted from the patient's father and leads to a demise that is twice as rapid as in the adult variety.

The dementia in adults typically begins 1 year either before or after the chorea; however, some authors have claimed that mental symptoms can precede the chorea by a decade. In the beginning, inattentiveness, erratic behavior, or depression are usually the primary mental symptoms. Mental symptoms, however, are not specific enough for diagnostic purposes. Patients with flagrant chorea almost always have impaired judgment, and later in the illness patients

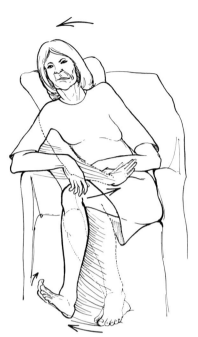

FIGURE 18–14. Patients with chorea, such as this woman who has Huntington's disease, have intermittent and brisk pelvic, trunk, and limb movements that are most often a wrist flick, a forward jutting of the leg, or a shrugging of the shoulder.

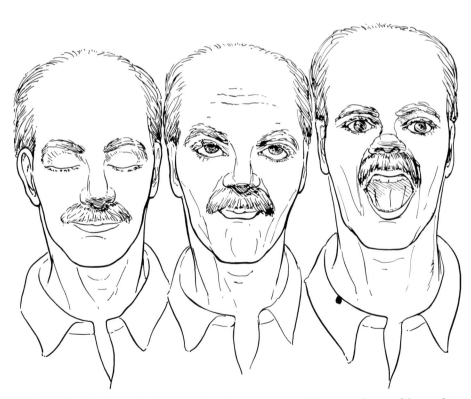

FIGURE 18–15. Huntington's disease patients have unexpected, inappropriate, and incomplete facial expressions, including frowns, eyebrow raisings, and smirks.

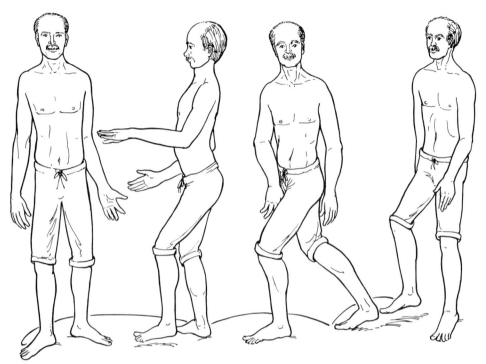

FIGURE 18–16.   The gait in Huntington's disease is not rhythmic or graceful, but lurching and contorted. The abnormalities result from intermittent trunk and pelvic motions, spontaneous knee flexion, lateral swaying, and a variable cadence.

develop profound dementia. At any stage, victims are prone to become alcoholics or commit suicide.

The initial diagnosis still rests on finding chorea and dementia and also on establishing that a relative had been afflicted with a similar disorder. Finding a low GABA concentration in the CSF will support the clinical diagnosis. The electroencephalogram (EEG) shows only nonspecific, low voltage activity with a poorly organized background (Chapter 10). CT and MRI scans reveal atrophy of the cerebral cortex and the caudate nuclei, and a compensatory outward expansion of the anterior horns of the third ventricle (Fig. 20-12). Although

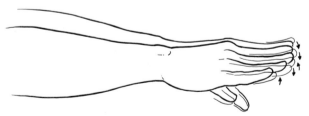

FIGURE 18–17.   The hands of Huntington's disease patients make fidgety movements that could reasonably be mistaken for manifestations of anxiety or restlessness. Their true nature, however, can be demonstrated by having patients stretch out or raise their hands and arms for 30 seconds. These maneuvers precipitate characteristic, momentary flexion or extension finger movements and continuous hyperextension of the wrists. Chorea can also be demonstrated when a patient has intermittent squeezing if asked to grasp two of the examiner's fingers (milkmaid's sign). Likewise, patients with chorea have intermittent withdrawal of their tongue when they attempt to protrude it for 30 seconds.

EEG and scan abnormalities appear late in the illness and usually after the diagnosis can be reached on clinical grounds, DNA analysis is available to detect the abnormal chromosome, even in amniotic fluid cells.

When chorea is mild, it may be suppressed by dopamine antagonists or dopamine depletors, such as tetrabenazine. Attempts have been made to enhance GABA and ACh activity, but these strategies have resulted in little or no reduction in chorea. The dementia is unaffected by any treatment.

Other Varieties of Chorea

Sydenham's chorea (St. Vitus' dance or chorea minor) is a "major diagnostic criterion" of rheumatic fever that begins 2 to 6 months after the carditis and has an average duration of 2 months. It almost exclusively affects children between the ages of 5 and 15 years. Of those children older than 10 years, girls are affected twice as frequently as boys. With the decreasing incidence of rheumatic fever, Sydenham's chorea has become rare except for small outbreaks.

Nevertheless, Sydenham's chorea remains an important condition. It is sometimes the only sign of a serious illness. Since chorea develops months after the carditis, the movements often surprisingly strike otherwise healthy children. Undiagnosed cases may be referred to psychiatrists because children may seem suddenly to have developed irritability and strange behavior. Also, at the onset of uncontrollable movements, children understandably develop anxiety that may be overwhelming. Child psychiatrists may have to distinguish Sydenham's chorea from the onset of tics, dystonia, withdrawal-emergent dyskinesia, and other forms of chorea.

Children who develop Sydenham's chorea have an insidious onset of grimacing, limb movements, and other stigmata of chorea (Fig. 18-18). As during any illness, children may have listlessness, irritability, and emotional lability. They do not develop frank cognitive impairments or major psychiatric disorders, but detailed testing reveals that about 50 percent of them have permanent minor psychologic disturbances. The brains of severely affected patients that have been inspected at postmortem examination have had extensive microscopic hemorrhages.

Chorea recurs in about 20 percent of patients following subsequent attacks of rheumatic fever. Also, women who had Sydenham's chorea in childhood, who start to take oral contraceptives or conceive, may have a recurrence of chorea (see below). In addition, close relatives of Sydenham's chorea patients are liable to develop chorea under any of those same circumstances.

The etiology of Sydenham's chorea is probably cerebrovascular inflammation that can be triggered by streptococcal infections. The movements are thought to recur because of a permanent increased sensitivity to dopamine when estrogen levels are elevated during female puberty, use of oral contraceptives, and pregnancy. Dopamine antagonists suppress the movements and also usually provide much needed sedation, which in turn further suppresses the movements.

Oral contraceptive-induced chorea is a rare reaction to oral contraceptives. In women who are younger than 20 years old, it occurs several months after starting a contraceptive containing estrogen and resolves after contraceptives are stopped. This variety of chorea is not associated with mental abnormalities.

Chorea gravidarum, another rarely occurring variety, almost always develops

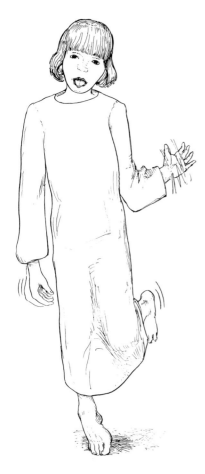

FIGURE 18–18.   Children with Sydenham's chorea may appear to have coy smiles and brief grimaces. They walk with a playful sashay. However, the chorea can be made obvious if the children attempt to hold a fixed position, such as standing at attention or standing on the ball of one foot.

TABLE 18–2.   CAUSES OF CHOREA

Basal ganglia lesions
   Perinatal injury, e.g., anoxia, kernicterus
   Cerebrovascular accidents
   Tumors, abscesses, toxoplasmosis*
Genetic disorders
   Huntington's chorea
   Wilson's disease
Metabolic derangements
   Hypocalcemia, hypothyroidism
   Hepatic encephalopathy
Drugs
   Oral contraceptives†
   L-dopa compounds, precursors, and agonists
   Amphetamines, methylphenidate (Ritalin)
   Neuroleptics
Inflammatory conditions
   Sydenham's chorea
   Pertussis, diphtheria, and other encephalitides
   Systemic lupus erythematosus (SLE)
Miscellaneous
   Carbon monoxide poisoning
   Senile chorea

* AIDS causes chorea when toxoplasmosis involves the basal ganglia.
† Estrogens from contraceptives or pregnancy (chorea gravidarum) cause chorea.

in young primigravidas during their first trimester of pregnancy. Many patients or their close relatives have had Sydenham's chorea, oral contraceptive-induced chorea, or chorea gravidarum. Patients with this condition often become so exhausted, frightened, and irrational that it frequently precipitates a spontaneous abortion or necessitates a therapeutic one. In either case, all symptoms resolve several days after the pregnancy is terminated.

Many other causes of chorea have been described (Table 18-2). In most of these conditions, structural lesions or metabolic derangements injure the basal ganglia. In some, dopamine activity is believed to be selectively increased.

HEMIBALLISMUS

Hemiballismus is manifested by intermittent, gross movements of one side of the body that are similar to those found in chorea, except that they are unilateral and more of a flinging (ballistic) motion (Fig. 18-19). Since the lesion that causes hemiballismus is almost always a small, cerebrovascular infarction in the (contralateral) subthalamic nucleus, hemiballismus is not accompanied

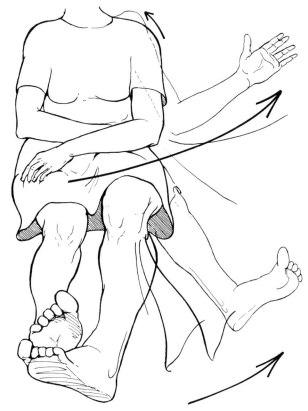

FIGURE 18–19. Hemiballismus is defined as sudden and large-scale movements of the limbs on one side of the body. Patients attempt to suppress the movements by pressing their body or unaffected limbs against the involuntarily moving ones. They also attempt to camouflage the involuntary movements by converting them into apparently purposeful movements. For example, if a patient's arm were to fly upward, he or she might incorporate the movement into a gesture, such as waving to someone.

by mental abnormalities, paresis, or other corticospinal tract signs. It is associated with increased CSF concentration of HVA, which indicates overactivity of the dopamine system.

Patients, who are almost always older than 65 years, have hemiballismus for several days to several weeks, but sometimes a residual movement persists for years. Hemiballismus can be suppressed with neuroleptics that block dopamine activity and induce sedation.

WILSON'S DISEASE

Wilson's disease (*hepatolenticular degeneration*) is an autosomal recessive genetic illness, localized to chromosome 13. It is characterized by dementia, a variety of involuntary movements, and hepatic insufficiency. The cause is an abnormality of copper metabolism that leads to destructive copper deposits in many organs, including the brain.

Symptoms usually become evident between the ages of 16 to 26 years, but many cases develop in younger children. The dementia may begin before the movements. In any case, cognitive impairments can be overshadowed by personality changes, mood alterations, or thought disorders. As with Huntington's disease, no particular pattern or psychologic test is sufficiently reliable to distinguish Wilson's disease dementia from the dementia of other neurologic illnesses. The movements, which are likewise highly variable, may consist of rigidity, akinesia, dystonia, or a *wing-beating* tremor (Fig. 18-20). They tend to occur in combination, be accompanied by corticospinal and corticobulbar tract signs, and mimic other conditions. In particular, Wilson's disease as well as Huntington's disease may induce parkinsonism in young adults, and it can cause dystonia that is indistinguishable from neuroleptic-induced tardive dystonia.

Non-neurologic signs are often as obvious as neurologic ones. Liver involvement leads to cirrhosis, and copper deposition in the cornea leads to a Kayser-Fleischer ring (Fig. 18-21).

The protean manifestations of Wilson's disease require that physicians test for this illness, despite its infrequent occurrence (1 per 100,000 persons), in young adults who develop a wide variety of conditions, including tremor, parkinsonism, dystonia, atypical psychosis, dementia, dysarthria, or chronic

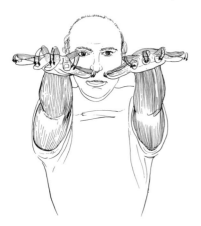

FIGURE 18–20. Wilson's disease may induce parkinsonism, dystonia, or tremors. The characteristic tremor, called *wing-beating*, is coarse and centered on the shoulders. Patients with this tremor, as its name implies, move their arms as though they were attempting to fly.

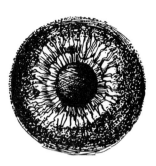

FIGURE 18–21. The Kayser-Fleischer ring, which is pathognomonic of Wilson's disease affecting the brain, is a green-brown pigment in the periphery of the cornea. Typically, it is most obvious at the superior and inferior margins of the cornea where it obscures the fine structure of the iris. In the early stages of Wilson's disease, when the ring is forming, it can be seen only with an ophthalmologist's slit-lamp.

hepatitis. Since the Kayser-Fleischer ring can be observed in virtually all patients with neurologic symptoms, any suspected neurologic patient should undergo a slit-lamp examination. A test that is diagnostic, even when the illness does not affect the brain, is the determination of the concentration of serum ceruloplasmin (the serum protein to which copper adheres): in cases of Wilson's disease, ceruloplasmin concentration is very low. Penicillamine, when given early enough, can reverse the mental deterioration, movement disorder, and non-neurologic manifestations in about 50% of cases.

DYSTONIA

Dystonia Musculorum Deformans

Dystonia musculorum deformans, or *torsion dystonia*, is a group of conditions that are characterized by dystonia, in which slow, powerful twisting or turning (torsion) of limb (appendicular) and neck, trunkal, and pelvic (axial) muscles contorts the body and creates *dystonic postures*. Although the patients become physically incapacitated, their mental abilities remain intact. It is another illness, like choreoathetosis, in which children have terrible movement disorders that may mask a normal intellect.

In about 30 percent of cases, the cause is an autosomal recessive genetic trait. In these cases, symptoms develop in children, who are predominantly Askenazi Jewish, between ages 8 and 14 years. The initial symptom of the childhood-onset variety is usually appendicular dystonia, such as torsion of one foot (Fig. 18-22). Over the next several years, affected children develop torsion of other limbs, the pelvis (tortipelvis), trunk, and neck (torticollis) (Fig. 18-23).

In an adult-onset variety, patients who are mostly non-Jewish and have an autosomal dominant inheritance develop axial muscle involvement as young or middle-aged adults. Their dystonia subsequently spreads slowly or stops when involvement is limited to only one muscle group.

The diagnosis of dystonia musculorum deformans is entirely clinical, since there is no diagnostic abnormality of the blood, EEG, MRI or CT, or brain tissue. Inconsistently effective medications have included anticholinergics, in high doses, and carbamazepine (Tegretol). Thalamotomy is a last resort. Spinal cord stimulation, which was initially described as being curative, has not been shown to be significantly beneficial in long-term studies. Unlike other movement disorders, studies of CSF and autopsy material have implicated norepinephrine abnormalities as a possible cause: CSF obtained from the ventricles shows

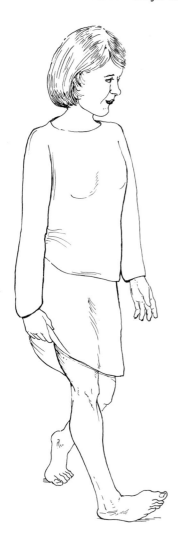

FIGURE 18–22. Patients with dystonia musculorum deformans typically first have involuntary inturning (torsion) of one foot. In this case, because of torsion of the right ankle and hip, the girl's foot twists inward and onto its side.

decreased concentration of the major norepinephrine metabolite, 3-methoxy-4- hydroxyphenylglycol (*MHGP*), in childhood-onset cases. Also, in autopsy cases the norepinephrine content was significantly reduced in several brainstem structures, including the locus ceruleus, which contains the cell bodies of several major noradrenergic tracts.

Other varieties of dystonia musculorum deformans include sporadic cases that do not fit a genetic pattern. As mentioned previously, dystonia can also be a prominent symptom of Wilson's disease, the juvenile form of Huntington's disease, tardive dystonia, and several rare degenerative neurologic diseases. Of this last group, *Lesch-Nyhan syndrome* is most notable. It is a sex-linked recessive genetic illness in which dystonia and other movements develop in children aged 2 to 6 years. Patients also develop self-mutilation, bizarre behavior, mental retardation, corticospinal tract signs, seizures, and hyperuricemia. Although brain concentrations of dopamine, HVA, and CAT are low, the basic abnormality is a deficiency of hypoxanthine-guanine phosphoribosyl transferase (HGPRT), which is an enzyme that is crucial to urea metabolism.

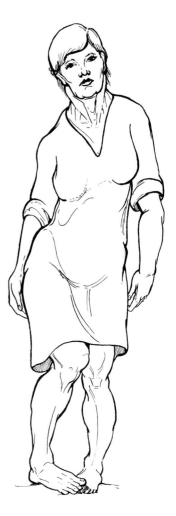

FIGURE 18–23. As dystonia musculorum deformans or torsion dystonia progresses to encompass other portions of the appendicular and axial musculature, patients develop grotesque dystonic postures. Because of continuous exertion, muscles become hypertrophied, and almost all subcutaneous fat is lost. The dystonic postures in this condition are virtually identical to those in Wilson's disease and tardive dystonia.

Focal Dystonia

Several conditions, called the *focal*, *segmental*, or *partial dystonias*, usually begin in adults and consist of dystonia of a single muscle group. As in dystonia musculorum deformans, focal dystonias are unaccompanied by mental impairment, and no confirmatory laboratory test is available. There is usually no preceding neuroleptic treatment or family history of a movement disorder. Patients are particularly apt to be misdiagnosed as having psychogenic disturbances.

A dramatic new therapy that harnesses the paralytic power of *botulinum A toxin* has been successful in each of these conditions (Fig. 18-24). Previously, dopamine and ACh manipulations were attempted but were rarely effective. Although insight-oriented psychotherapy was not effective, claims had been made that biofeedback was helpful.

Spasmodic torticollis is a focal dystonia in which the sternocleidomastoid and other neck muscles undergo involuntary contractions that rotate the patient's head for several seconds to several minutes (Fig. 18-25). Spasmodic torticollis is occasionally a component of dystonia musculorum deformans, but it usually occurs alone. Similar neck muscle contractions can develop as a side effect of

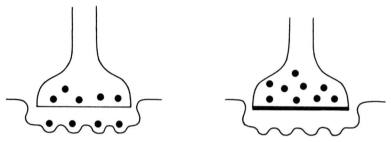

FIGURE 18–24. *Left,* At the normal neuromuscular junction, acetylcholine (ACh) vesicles (*the black dots*) are released from the presynaptic membrane, bind to postsynaptic membrane receptors, and trigger muscle contractions. In focal dystonias, which are characterized by strong prolonged muscle contractions, the neuromuscular system seems to be hyperactive. *Right,* Botulinum A toxin injected into muscles binds irreversibly onto the presynaptic membrane of the neuromuscular junction, prohibits the release of the ACh packets, and thereby weakens the neuromuscular system. The injections reduce dystonic contractions for about 6 months but permit normal muscle function. Afterward, if necessary, botulinum A toxin treatment can be repeated.

neuroleptics or L-dopa, or they can result from cervical nerve root irritation ("wry neck"). Treatment by transection of the neck muscles or their nerves has resulted in unacceptable loss of head control without a reduction in the involuntary movements caused by remaining muscles.

Occupational spasms or *cramps* are painful hand muscle contractions that begin shortly after engaging in a particular activity that is often the basis of the patient's livelihood. Nevertheless, patients can use the same hand muscles in performing similar functions. The most commonly occurring varieties are the writer's, pianist's, and violinist's cramp. For example, an author with a writer's cramp would develop painful hand spasms shortly after starting to write with a pen but not when using the same hand to type, eat, or button clothing.

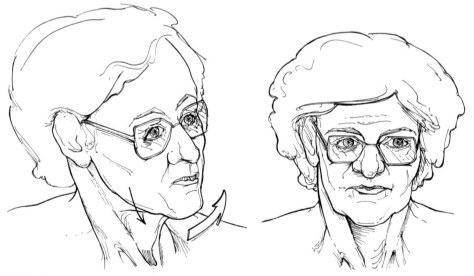

FIGURE 18–25. In spasmodic torticollis, patients have a rotation of their head in a downward and contralateral sweep because of continuous contraction of the sternocleidomastoid muscle. The continuous contractions also lead to muscle hypertrophy. The involuntary rotation can be overcome with a great deal of voluntary effort, which induces a tremor. Alternatively, patients instinctively learn the "trick" that a slight counter-rotational pressure exerted by a finger placed against the chin temporarily stops the movement.

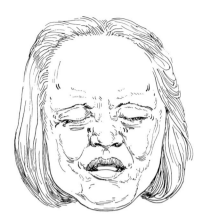

FIGURE 18–26. Patients with Meige's syndrome have forced, dystonic eyelid closure (blepharospasm) and often also lower face and jaw contractions. Meige's syndrome movements differ from the buccolingual movements of tardive dyskinesia in their symmetry, predominant involvement of the upper face, and absence of tongue protrusions.

Spastic dysphonia, which some neurologists consider a manifestation of pseudobulbar palsy or buccofacial apraxia (Chapter 8) rather than a dystonia, is an involuntary contraction of the larynx that occurs only when patients speak. It restricts them to an odd high-pitched whisper. In an apparent paradox, patients can usually shout, sing, and swallow.

Patients with *Meige's syndrome*, a similar condition, have repetitive shutting of their eyelids (blepharospasm), grimacing movements of their lower facial muscles, and, to a lesser extent, jaw closure (Fig. 18-26). Since Meige's syndrome mimics buccolingual dyskinesia, it is usually considered in the differential diagnosis of tardive dyskinesia.

Blepharospasm usually occurs independent of neuroleptic treatment, Meige's syndrome, and the other dystonias (Fig. 18-27). It is probably the most frequently occurring focal dystonia and the one most amenable to botulinum treatment.

Another condition that causes abnormal facial movements and that is not associated with neuroleptic exposure is *hemifacial spasm* (Fig. 18-28). This unique disorder consists of spasms of the muscles on one side of the face that are supplied by the ipsilateral facial nerve (the seventh cranial nerve). The spasms occur 1 to 10 times-per-minute and intermittently disfigure the face. Hemifacial spasm is usually associated with an aberrant vessel or other structural lesion compressing the facial nerve at its origin from the pons (Fig. 4-13). Inserting a cushion between the vessel and the nerve, or removing the lesion with microvascular decompression (Fig. 9-5), alleviates the spasms. [Similar surgery is used in trigeminal neuralgia where dramatic relief is produced by microvas-

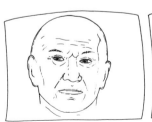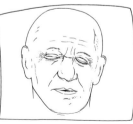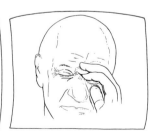

FIGURE 18–27. This elderly gentleman has blepharospasm in which his orbicularis oculi (eyelid) muscles have prolonged (average duration 5 sec.) symmetric contractions. During spasms, his vision is blocked and he resorts to prying open his eyelids. A trick that these patients have is pressing against the eyebrows to alleviate blepharospasm.

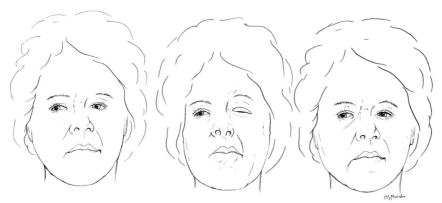

FIGURE 18–28. This 53-year-old woman with hemifacial spasm has left-sided facial muscle contractions that have a long duration (average duration 7 sec.) and variable forcefulness. They repetitively squeeze shut her left eyelids and pull her mouth to her left side.

cular decompression of the trigeminal nerve (the fifth cranial nerve) (Chapter 9).]

The following conditions are often included in discussions of involuntary movement disorders. However, their clinical characteristics are different from those of the conditions discussed so far. Moreover, investigations have failed to find structural abnormalities of the basal ganglia, neurotransmitter imbalances, or, with the exception of Tourette's syndrome, a beneficial response to dopamine or ACh manipulation.

ESSENTIAL TREMOR

Patients with essential tremor, which is sometimes called an "action" or "postural tremor," have a fine tremor of their wrists, hands, and fingers that is elicited by certain hand actions or positions. Patients with severe cases will also have either a "yes" or "no" shaking (titubation) and a quavering voice. The hand tremor is fine and has a frequency that ranges from 4- to 12-Hz. As in other varieties of tremor, the oscillations are in a single plane.

Essential tremor usually develops in young and middle-aged adults and affects about 400 per 100,000 people who are older than 40 years. In some persons, who are said to have *benign familial tremor,* the tremor is inherited in an autosomal dominant genetic pattern. Other cases may develop in elderly people, who are said to have *senile tremor.*

The most characteristic feature of the tremor is that it appears when patients hold their hands against gravity in fixed positions or perform delicate tasks. For example, the tremor is provoked when patients write, hold out their hands, or bring cups or cigarettes toward their mouth (Fig. 18-29). Its conspicuous nature is embarrassing.

Another important feature is that the amplitude of the tremor is suppressed, often to the point of complete elimination, by beverages containing alcohol or treatment with beta adrenergic blockers, such as propranolol (Inderal). Its response to propranolol, which competes with catecholamines (including norepinephrine), indicates that essential tremor probably does not result from

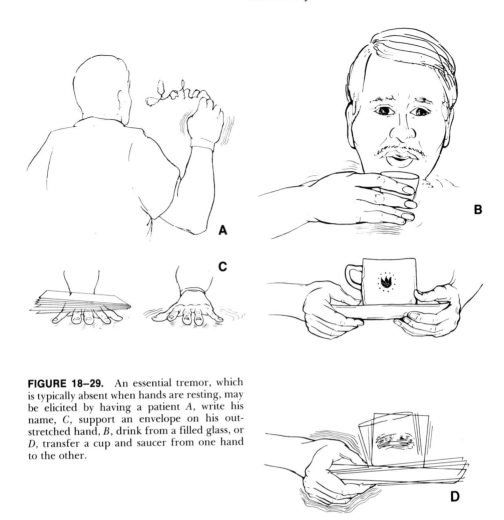

FIGURE 18–29. An essential tremor, which is typically absent when hands are resting, may be elicited by having a patient *A*, write his name, *C*, support an envelope on his outstretched hand, *B*, drink from a filled glass, or *D*, transfer a cup and saucer from one hand to the other.

extrapyramidal dysfunction, but from excessive beta adrenergic sympathetic nervous system activity.*

Several other tremor varieties have a similar appearance, probable origin in excessive adrenergic system activity, and suppression with propranolol. These tremors result from anxiety, hyperthyroidism, or use of steroids or beta adrenergic stimulating agents, such as isoproterenol (Isuprel). Similarly appearing tremors, which also respond to propranolol, are found in patients who take amitriptyline or lithium (see below).

An interesting aspect of anxiety is that it can not only elicit or exacerbate essential tremor but it can also create an identical tremor in the hands and elsewhere. Thus beta blocking medications are used in treatment of anxiety-induced tremors, and they are effective in suppressing the tremulousnessness,

---

* Stimulation of alpha adrenergic receptor sites leads to peripheral artery vasoconstriction. Stimulation of $beta_1$ adrenergic sites leads to cardiac acceleration and lipolysis. Stimulation of $beta_2$ adrenergic sites leads to bronchodilation and vasodilation of coronary, peripheral, and possibly meningeal arteries. Propranolol blocks both $beta_1$ and $beta_2$ adrenergic sites, and metoprolol (Lopressor), which also suppresses essential tremor, is a relatively selective $beta_1$ adrenergic blocker.

quavering voice, and the anxiety of stagefright. In addition, an entirely different psychogenic tremor is rare but recognizable (see below).

To review, tremors discussed in this chapter and previously are clinically different: The parkinson pill rolling tremor occurs at rest, is diminished by the initiation of movements, and is relatively slow (Fig. 18-8). It is usually accompanied by rigidity and akinesia. The intention tremor that results from cerebellar dysfunction is coarse, irregular, and elicited by gross actions (Fig. 2-11). A tremor associated with AIDS also has a variable combination of parkinson and cerebellar features that depend on the presence of the viral encephalitis or toxoplasmosis lesions (Chapter 7). The wing-beating tremor of Wilson's disease remains difficult to categorize, but it too appears to be a combination of a parkinsonian and cerebellar tremor.

TICS

Tics, which are described in the *Diagnostic and Statistical Manual of Mental Disorders, Third Edition, Revised* (*DSM-III-R*), are rapid, repetitive, nonrhythmic, stereotyped movements of functionally related muscle groups. As the DSM-III-R states, tics may be *simple* or *complex* and *motor* or *vocal*. Frequently observed simple motor tics are a head toss, prolonged eye blink, shoulder jerk, and asymmetric smile. Complex motor tics are complicated movements, such as touching or hitting oneself, jumping, stamping, or skipping. Simple vocal tics are short, inarticulate sounds, such as throat clearing, grunting, and sniffing. Complex vocal tics are words or at least fractions of words. Other complex tics or tic-like movements typically involve the patient mimicking words (echolalia), mimicking movements (echopraxia or echokinesis), or touching themselves or others in a furtive, compulsive, and often sexual manner.

The frequency and intensity of tics, as in the classic movement disorders, are increased by excitement, anxiety, and fatigue. In contrast to those disorders, tics are not only defined in the DSM-III-R but they are also decreased or abolished for minutes to hours by voluntary suppression withintense concentration. Also, they vary in intensity over periods of weeks or months, often appearing to remit entirely or respond to treatment. Moreover, tics persist during sleep, when they are apt to be accompanied by night terrors and sleepwalking (Chapter 17).

As described in the DSM-III, three patterns of *Tic Disorders* are recognized by both the neurologic and psychiatric community: *Transient Tic Disorder* (307.21), *Chronic Motor or Vocal Tic Disorder* (307.22), and *Tourette's Disorder* or syndrome (307.23). Although these disorders are probably points on a continuum, they are differentiated by the presence of tics for shorter or longer than 1 year and the presence or absence of the combination of motor and vocal tics.

Transient tics are common in childhood. They are usually simple motor tics that develop in at least 5 percent of all children between the ages of 5 and 10 years in most Western countries. The DSM-III-R stipulates that single or multiple motor or vocal tics must begin before age 21 years and have a duration of less than 1 year. Boys are affected three times more often than girls. A disproportionate number of children with tics have a close relative with one or more tics. Although tics have sometimes been assumed to be a manifestation of anxiety, affected children have no consistent emotional, intellectual, or neurologic abnormalities, and their tics do not respond to psychotherapy or minor tranquilizers. Fortunately, by the end of adolescence, all but 6 percent of children who develop a tic will have a spontaneous remission.

Chronic tics, as described in the DSM-III-R, are either motor or vocal but not both, last longer than 1 year, and are indistinguishable from single tics at their onset. Although the DSM-III-R also specifies that the tics have an onset before age 21 years, neurologists find that chronic tics may occur in adults as a manifestation of encephalitis, myoclonus, Parkinson's disease, or psychoactive substance intoxication. Also, otherwise healthy adults, usually between ages 40 and 60 years, develop tics that might be transient or chronic.

Tics that persist or develop spontaneously in adults are different from those in children. Although tics in children usually involve only the head or neck, those in adults also involve the chest, diaphram, entire trunk, and limbs, i.e., the more caudal structures. Tics in adults tend to be longer in duration, more complex, and more likely to occur in a combination of several tics.

TOURETTE'S SYNDROME

Gilles de la Tourette's (Tourette's) syndrome or disorder is a condition in which children develop *combinations* of vocal and multiple motor tics that last longer than 1 year (Fig. 18-30). Like simple tics, it affects boys three times more frequently than girls, and 90 percent of cases develop by age 13 years. DSM-III-R requires that the onset occur before age 21 years. Tourette's syndrome is usually a life-long illness during which, over periods of 2 to 6 months, tics change in distribution, vary in intensity, and undergo transient remissions. However, recent studies have described complete remissions or permanent substantial reductions in up to one sixth of cases. In affected children, the illness is often greatest at the beginning of the school year and during holiday seasons, and least during the summer months.

Important studies have recently shown the probability of a single autosomal dominant genetic basis for Tourette's syndrome, and also of chronic tics and Tourette's syndrome being aspects of the same condition. For example, Price found that the concordance for Tourette's syndrome was 53 percent in monozygotic twins and 8 percent for dizygotic twins, and when all tics were considered, the concordance rate was 77 percent for monozygotic twins and 23 percent for dizygotic twins. Nevertheless, since not all monozygotic twins had Tourette's, nongenetic factors must be important.

Another recent finding is that 10 to 50 percent of Tourette's patients have a prominent obsessive-compulsive disorder that appears to be caused by an autosomal dominant sex-influenced genetic trait. Older studies had shown that, although children with Tourette's have normal intelligence and no propensity to develop psychosis, almost 50 percent have the DSM-III-R criteria for attention-deficit hyperactivity disorder (ADHD). In view of the association of Tourette's syndrome with ADHD, it is important to note that, in as many as one third of cases, Tourette's syndrome may have developed or been exacerbated in children who received methylphenidate (Ritalin), amphetamines, pemoline (Cylert), or cocaine—CNS stimulants that block the re-uptake of norepinephrine and dopamine. Despite normal intelligence in these children, the combination of social stigmata, ADHD, obsessive thinking, and medications

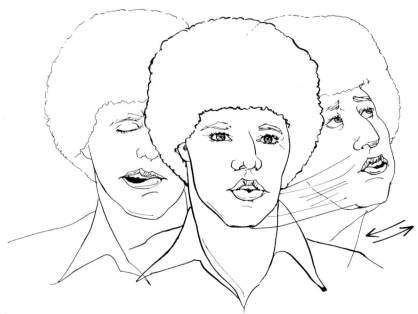

FIGURE 18–30. In a typical Tourette's syndrome case, a young man has multiple motor tics, including head jerking ("head toss"), grimacing of the right side of his mouth ("half-smile"), and depression of his forehead (frowning). The motor tics are accompanied by vocal tics of throat clearing and a short blowing sound. All tics continue throughout the day, being only slightly affected by conversation, eating, and social situations. After several months, each tic may recede or be replaced by another tic.

Motor tics are forceful, and the more rapid, sudden part of the movement is away from the midline. For example, in the head toss, patients seem to fling their head laterally, and patients with the half-smile seem to smirk: patients do not seem to bring their head suddenly forward or rapidly purse one side of their lips. Tics, which often occur in rapid repetition or combination, have lightning-like rapidity. A single head toss has a duration of about 1.0 to 1.5 sec and a half-smile 0.2 to 0.9 sec. However, various tic repetitions and combinations can persist for several seconds and generate complex movements.

probably prevents the majority of Tourette's patients from advancing normally in school.

The cardinal feature of Tourette's syndrome is vocal tics, which are repetitive, stereotyped sounds that the patients blurt out rapidly, irresistibly, and compulsively. Throughout the course of the illness, vocal tics of most patients are simple. They usually consist of inarticulate sounds, such as sniffing, throat clearing, or clicks; however, many patients eventually make loud and disconcerting noises, such as grunting, snorting, or honking. When vocal tics become complex, they can culminate in unprovoked outbursts of obscene words, *coprolalia.* Although most such explosions contain only fractions of obscene words, such as "shi," "fu," or "cun," some are shouted strings of distinct obscenities. Moreover, coprolalia is often accompanied by performing obscene movements or gestures, *copropraxia,* and having intrusions of obscene thoughts, *mental coprolalia.*

Since the original description of the illness, however, many reports have overemphasized coprolalia. Now the DSM-III-R omits it as a criterion. Current studies show that only 60 percent of patients have coprolalia, and in these cases its onset is about 6 years after the recognition of the tics. Astute clinicians should be able to diagnose Tourette's syndrome when tics are subtle and do not include coprolalia.

About 50 percent of patients have soft neurologic signs, and 13 to 50 percent have minor, nonspecific EEG abnormalities. CT and MRI scans are normal. PET scans show decreased glucose utilization in the inferior frontal and cingulate cortex, but this pattern is not distinctive.

An interesting new technique has demonstrated that, unlike the normal situation with voluntary head and neck movement, Tourette's patients have no premovement EEG potential (Obeso) (Fig. 18-31): this finding suggests a subcortical origin of the tics. Another recent study demonstrated low concentration of HVA in the CSF of several untreated patients but a rise after treatment was instituted. Other studies have suggested abnormalities in brain ACh activity, platelet monoamine oxidase concentration, and serotonin metabolism.

Medications are usually not indicated for children with single tics, and guidelines are not established for adults with either single or multiple motor tics without verbal tics. Treatment of Tourette's syndrome with haloperidol suppresses the vocalizations, most motor tics, and many of the other symptoms in about 80 percent of patients. Although haloperidol often causes gynecomastia in young men, it rarely if ever induces tardive dyskinesia in these patients. Other dopamine antagonists, such as fluphenazine (Prolixin) and pimozide (Orap), are reported to be effective. Likewise, tetrabenazine, which depletes dopamine, has been effective. An alpha adrenergic agonist, clonidine (Catapres), has been a popular treatment with little side effects, but its purported usefulness has been challenged.

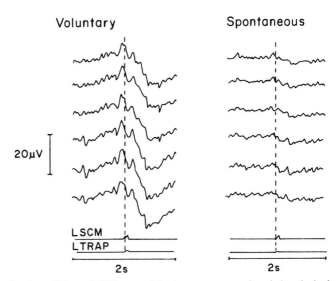

FIGURE 18–31. This is an idealized rendition of EEG potentials that are averaged and time-locked (back-averaged) to movements of the left sternocleidomastoid and trapezius muscles. *Left,* Relatively large amplitude EEG potentials are detectable about 0.5 sec before normal voluntary movements. These are premovement potentials that precede not only conscious voluntary movement but also psychogenic movements. In partial seizures, EEG potentials, but ones of a different pattern, also precede movements. *Right,* In involuntary (spontaneous) movements, including tics, chorea, and myoclonus, premovement potentials are absent. Their absence indicates that these movements have a subcortical origin.

Related Conditions

Several disorders are associated with movements and vocalizations that mimic tics. As defined in DSM-III-R, *Stereotypy/Habit Disorder (307.30)* is a condition in which individuals intentionally perform simple activities in a repetitive, rhythmic, and apparently purposeless manner. Other DSM-III-R criteria are that the movements either harm the person or interfere with normal activity and that they are not a manifestation of a pervasive developmental disorder (autism). Commonly cited examples are hand shaking, body rocking, and face slapping. Although these activities may be habits or mannerisms in normal people, they are closely associated with mental retardation, blindness, Lesch-Nyhan syndrome, and, in fact, autism. Also, to a certain extent, they may have a purpose. The activity enhances sensory input, which is especially valuable to individuals who are blind or who have other sensory losses.

Unexpected vocalizations are another condition that might reasonably be mistaken for Tourette's syndrome. Possibly the most common is the "chronic cough of adolescence." This familiar condition, which is almost always psychogenic, consists of an incessant coughing sound that interrupts conversations and classroom work. It differs from tics in its monosymptomatic quality, relatively late onset, and its tendency to interrupt activities.

Dramatic bursts of speech that contain coprolalia or simple cursing may be found in neurologic conditions that cause motor or vocal tics, such as postencephalitic Parkinson's disease, tardive dyskinesia, and Huntington's chorea. In addition, cursing may be a manifestation of nondominant hemisphere injury (Chapter 8), a method of communicating for someone with aphasia (Chapter 7), or a feature of a poorly defined condition, klazomania.

MYOCLONUS

Myoclonus is defined as asynchronous, irregular, brief, and usually generalized muscle contractions. Unlike the classic movement disorders, it persists when patients are asleep or comatose and can be elicited by either voluntary movement on the part of the patient (action myoclonus) or by the examiner stimulating the patient with noise, touch, or light (stimulus-sensitive myoclonus). Myoclonus probably originates from abnormalities of the motor neurons in the cerebral cortex, brainstem, or spinal cord, rather than the basal ganglia.

Generalized myoclonus usually results from extensive damage to the cerebral cortex and, thus, is associated with dementia, delirium, or seizures. For example, myoclonus is often found in the AIDS-dementia complex and occasionally in Alzheimer's disease. Also, as mentioned in discussions of dementia and EEGs (Chapters 7 and 10), generalized myoclonus is the most prominent physical manifestation of both subacute sclerosing panencephalitis (SSPE) and Creutzfeldt-Jakob disease—two conditions in which patients have myoclonus, dementia, and periodic EEG complexes (Fig. 10-6). Myoclonus also commonly results from metabolic derangements, such as anoxia, uremia, penicillin intoxication, and excessive meperidine (Demerol). In most of these conditions, 5-hydroxytryptophan (5-HTP) or clonazepam (Klonopin) can suppress the myoclonus.

Palatal myoclonus is defined as symmetric contractions of the soft palate. Unlike other movement disorders, they occur regularly (120 to 140 times-per-minute) and are present during sleep, as well as wakefulness. Despite its name, palatal myoclonus has little relationship to generalized myoclonus. In particular, it usually results from small brainstem infarctions that affect the inferior olivary nucleus, and it is not associated with dementia.

MEDICATION-INDUCED MOVEMENT DISORDERS

Dopamine Antagonist Neuroleptics

In addition to neuroleptics occasionally causing the neuroleptic-malignant syndrome (Chapter 6)—lowering the seizure threshhold, altering the EEG (Chapter 10), and causing retinal abnormalities (Chapter 12)—they can cause a variety of striking involuntary movement disorders. These disorders, like classic ones, are usually intensified by anxiety, reduced by concentration, and abolished by sleep.

Acute and Tardive Dystonia

The most dramatic neuroleptic-induced movement disorder is *acute dystonia*. It consists of suddenly developing limb or trunk dystonic postures, repetitive jaw and face contractions, torticollis, or *oculogyric crisis* (Fig. 18-32). Most cases develop in young adults and occur within 1 week of the beginning of neuroleptics or the dose being raised. Acute dystonia may be prevented by giving oral anticholinergics, and it can be aborted by intravenous anticholinergic or antihistamine. It can occur along with all the other complications of dopamine antagonists, including haloperidol, phenothiazines, prochlorperazine (Compazine), and metoclopramide (Reglan), that are used to treat nausea, vomiting, and psychiatric and nonpsychiatric conditions.

A related condition, *tardive dystonia*, which develops up to 3 months after initiation of neuroleptic treatment, has recently been highlighted because it is a chronic complication of neuroleptic therapy in 2 to 20 percent of cases. Although often mild in severity, the dystonia consists of posturing that, as noted previously, is similar to that found in Wilson's disease, torsion dystonia, and, in children, Huntington's disease (Fig. 18-33). Unlike these conditions, tardive dystonia is often accompanied by other movements associated with

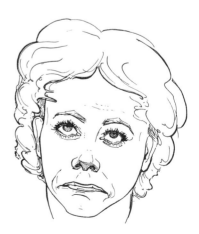

FIGURE 18–32. During an oculogyric crisis, the patient's eyes roll upward or sideward, and the face is forced into a grimace or other abnormal expression. The ocular movements may be related to similar ones in schizophrenic patients (Chapter 12) because both conditions may be caused by dopamine neurotransmission abnormalities in the basal ganglia. If oculogyric crisis and other acute dystonic reactions can be prevented, usually by prophylactic treatment with anticholinergics, patient compliance with a neuroleptic regimen will probably be improved.

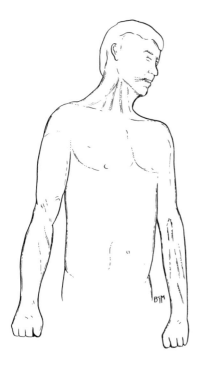

FIGURE 18–33.   Tardive dystonia in a 35-year-old man who has been receiving neuroleptic treatment for several years consists of prolonged twisting postures of his arms and neck (torticollis) and arching of his back. Other cases may have blepharospasm, Meige-like facial grimacing, or backward thrusting of the neck (retrocollis). As in torsion dystonia, the muscles are hypertrophied and there is little body fat.

neuroleptic treatment, such as buccolingual dyskinesia and akathisia. Tardive dystonia partially responds to dopamine depletion with tetrabenazine or reserpine or to dopamine receptor blockade with neuroleptics. Therefore, it is believed to originate from dopamine hypersensitivity. Tardive dystonia, unlike tardive dyskinesia, also reportedly responds to anticholinergics alone or in combination with dopamine depletors.

Akathisia

Akathisia is a continual leg movement that causes patients to move their feet continuously while lying, sitting, or standing (Fig. 18-34). It typically compels them to pace. Unlike other movement disorders, except for tics, patients have a compulsion to move. They have a need to walk and intense feelings of restlessness. The movements in akathisia mimic those of chorea and of the dyskinesias induced by excessive L-dopa treatment, but they are confined to the legs and are accompanied by the prominent subjective symptoms. Also, they may be distinguished by the absence of dysesthesias from the restless leg syndrome and the leg movements in polyneuropathy. Perhaps most commonly, akathisia is mistaken for agitation because the subjective restlessness may exceed the actual leg movements. Akathisia commonly recedes as neuroleptic treatment continues, but it can be alleviated more rapidly by reducing the neuroleptic dosage. A variety of medications, including propranolol, reportedly reduce akathisia.

Tardive akathisia, which develops long after initiation of neuroleptic therapy, persists after neuroleptics have been discontinued (Barnes, Weiner). It may mimic agitated depression, mania, or anxiety. Recent studies have claimed that tardive akathisia as well as common akathisia can be alleviated by propoxyphene (Darvon), which is an opioid analgesic that affects the enkephalin system

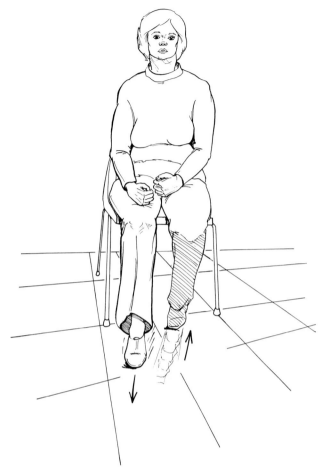

FIGURE 18–34. Akathisia usually consists of continual to-and-fro sliding leg movements, repeated leg crossings, or lateral knee movements. The leg movements are made prominent by the akinesia of the upper trunk, arms, and face.

(Chapter 14) (Walters). Reports of benefits from reserpine, tetrabenazine, amantadine, anticholinergics, and other medications have not been substantiated.

Withdrawal-emergent dyskinesia consists of the transient appearance of transient choreoathetosis, myoclonus, and other movements accompanied by systemic symptoms, such as nausea and diaphoresis, immediately after completing a course of neuroleptic therapy. It usually affects children, lasting less than 6 weeks. Cases lasting longer than 6 months are probably ones of tardive dyskinesia.

Parkinsonism

In contrast to these disorders that involve excessive movement, *neuroleptic-induced parkinsonism* produces akinesia and related symptoms. The akinesia is the most important symptom because, even when still mild and subtle, it can create impediments to normal daily activities. Although the parkinsonism resolves spontaneously, it can be ameliorated by decreasing the dosage of the neuroleptic or by administering amantadine. However, giving anticholinergics to prevent or treat neuroleptic-induced parkinsonism remains controversial because, especially in the elderly, they may induce memory impairment and other cognitive dysfunction. L-dopa should be avoided because it can stimulate cerebral mesolimbic dopamine receptors and precipitate a toxic psychosis.

Tardive Dyskinesia

Tardive dyskinesia, or the *buccolinguomasticatory, choreic,* or *orofacial syndrome* (Fig. 18-35), clearly the most troublesome neuroleptic-induced movement disorder, has been repeatedly postulated to result from dopamine receptor hypersensitivity (Fig. 18-36). Despite the limitations of this theory, it is consistent with several major clinical features of tardive dyskinesia. For example, tardive dyskinesia results from virtually all classes of antipsychotic agents that block dopamine receptors. It begins only a relatively long time (months) after neuroleptics are instituted, when denervation hypersensitivity is expected to develop. It is worsened by reducing the dosage of the neuroleptic or by adding L-dopa, presumably since these changes expose the postsynaptic neuron to more dopamine. The facial movements are in fact similar, although not identical, to those in L-dopa dyskinesia (Karson). Likewise, tardive dyskinesia is somewhat alleviated by increasing the dosage of the neuroleptic. Also, many months after the neuroleptics are discontinued, some cases spontaneously remit, suggesting that dopamine sensitivity can revert to normal.

Unlike other antipsychotic medications, clozapine (Clozaril) reportedly does not induce tardive dyskinesias or similar complications: it might actually suppress tardive dyskinesia. Clozapine is relatively free of side effects because, although it probably affects the cortical and limbic projections, it probably does not block nigrostriatal dopamine receptors. Also, unlike classic neuroleptics, clozapine

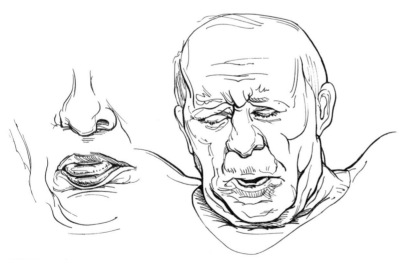

FIGURE 18–35. The most prominent feature of tardive dyskinesia is stereotyped tongue movements accompanied by continual jaw and facial muscle contractions, i.e., chorea that is repetitive and confined to the tongue and lower face. The movements typically include tongue darting, lip smacking, kissing, lip puckering, chewing, and sometimes blepharospasm. In addition, patients often also have dystonia or chorea of the trunk and limbs. They may also have respiratory dyskinesia that leads to grunts or loud, irregular breathing—disturbances reminiscent of Tourette's syndrome.

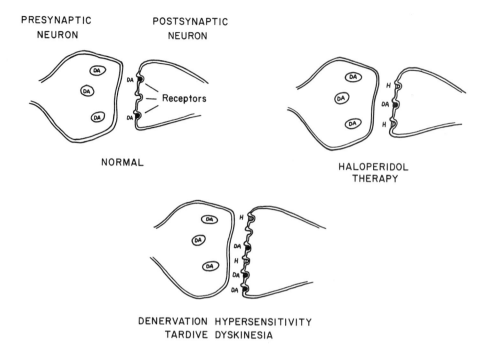

FIGURE 18–36. The denervation hypersensitivity theory proposes that, when postsynaptic dopamine receptors are occupied by neuroleptics, such as haloperidol, dopamine receptor blockade causes physiologic denervation. Postsynaptic receptor sites become more numerous and hypersensitive. Then, after withdrawal of haloperidol, minute quantities of dopamine (or other neurotransmitters), released from the presynaptic neuron or present in the ambient fluid, trigger receptor-mediated responses.

does not raise the serum prolactin level, which suggests that it may not act on the tubero-infundibular tract.

Treatment of tardive dyskinesia seeks to reduce dopamine activity. Simple approaches are to increase the dosage of a dopamine blocking neuroleptic, to substitute a more potent neuroleptic, or to reinstate a neuroleptic if it had been discontinued; however, these plans may create a vicious cycle. Alternatively, reserpine and tetrabenazine, which deplete dopamine, have been helpful in some cases. One method is to give reserpine 0.25 mg per day with a gradual increase to 5.0 mg per day until a clear benefit or a complication, such as hypertension, appears. Of course, reserpine and tetrabenazine might precipitate depression.

Some investigators have achieved success with anticholinergics. However, others claim that, although anticholinergics may prevent neuroleptic-induced parkinsonism and acute dystonia and may treat tardive dystonia, they worsen tardive dyskinesia. Also, they may cause confusion.

Some treatments attempt to balance excessive dopamine receptor sensitivity with enhanced ACh activity. Physostigmine, which prolongs ACh activity, and ACh precursors, such as deanol (Deaner), lecithin, or choline, have all been administered; however, except for brief periods, they have not been helpful. Various other medications, including GABA agonists, such as valproate (Depakote) and baclofen (Lioresal); a calcium channel blocker, diltiazem (Cardizem); lithium; and clonazepam (Klonopin), are not consistently helpful.

DEPARTMENT OF HEALTH AND HUMAN SERVICES PUBLIC HEALTH SERVICE Alcohol, Drug Abuse, and Mental Health Administration NIMH Treatment Strategies in Schizophrenia Study	PATIENT NUMBER	DATA GROUP	EVALUATION DATE

**ABNORMAL INVOLUNTARY
MOVEMENT SCALE
(AIMS)**

PATIENT NUMBER __ __ __ __ __   **aims**   DATA GROUP   EVALUATION DATE __ __ – __ __ – __ __
M M   D D   Y Y

PATIENT NAME

RATER NAME

RATER NUMBER __ __ __

EVALUATION TYPE *(Circle)*

1 Baseline	4 Start double-blind	7 Start open meds	10 Early termination
2 2-week minor	5 Major evaluation	8 During open meds	11 Study completion
3	6 Other	9 Stop open meds	

INSTRUCTIONS: Complete Examination Procedure (reverse side) before making ratings.
MOVEMENT RATINGS: Rate highest severity observed.

Code: 1 = None
2 = Minimal, may be extreme normal
3 = Mild
4 = Moderate
5 = Severe

			(Circle One)				
FACIAL AND ORAL MOVEMENTS:	1.	**Muscles of Facial Expression** e.g., movements of forehead, eyebrows, periorbital area, cheeks; include frowning, blinking, smiling, grimacing	1	2	3	4	5
	2.	**Lips and Perioral Area** e.g., puckering, pouting, smacking	1	2	3	4	5
	3.	**Jaw** e.g., biting, clenching, chewing, mouth opening, lateral movement	1	2	3	4	5
	4.	**Tongue** Rate only increase in movement both in and out of mouth, NOT inability to sustain movement	1	2	3	4	5
EXTREMITY MOVEMENTS:	5.	**Upper** *(arms, wrists, hands, fingers)* Include choreic movements, (i.e., rapid, objectively purposeless, irregular, spontaneous), athetoid movements (i.e., slow, irregular, complex, serpentine). Do NOT include tremor (i.e., repetitive, regular, rhythmic)	1	2	3	4	5
	6.	**Lower** *(legs, knees, ankles, toes)* e.g., lateral knee movement, foot tapping, heel dropping, foot squirming, inversion and eversion of foot	1	2	3	4	5
TRUNK MOVEMENTS:	7.	**Neck, shoulders, hips** e.g., rocking, twisting, squirming, pelvic gyrations	1	2	3	4	5
GLOBAL JUDGMENTS:	8.	**Severity of abnormal movements**	None, normal 1 Minimal 2 Mild 3 Moderate 4 Severe 5				
	9.	**Incapacitation due to abnormal movements**	None, normal 1 Minimal 2 Mild 3 Moderate 4 Severe 5				
	10.	**Patient's awareness of abnormal movements** Rate only patient's report	No awareness 1 Aware, no distress 2 Aware, mild distress 3 Aware, moderate distress 4 Aware, severe distress 5				
DENTAL STATUS:	11.	**Current problems with teeth and/or dentures**	No 1 Yes 2				
	12.	**Does patient usually wear dentures?**	No 1 Yes 2				

ADM 117
Rev. 11-85

FIGURE 18–37. The current Abnormal Involuntary Movement Scale (AIMS) guides the examiner through inspection for dyskinesias of the face, jaw, tongue, trunk, and limbs. The physician is asked to record observations when the patient is at rest, extending the tongue or limbs, or performing certain activities, such as finger tapping, standing, or walking. In addition, the examiner is asked to check for rigidity. This revision of the original (Guy, see references), requests that patients remove their shoes and socks, and it does not rate as less severe those movements that are activated. However, there is omission of tests for akinesia, tremor, and dysarthria.

EXAMINATION PROCEDURE

Either before or after completing the Examination Procedure observe the patient unobtrusively, at rest (e.g., in waiting room).

The chair to be used in this examination should be a hard, firm one without arms.

1. Ask patient to remove shoes and socks.

2. Ask patient whether there is anything in his/her mouth (i.e., gum, candy, etc.) and if there is, to remove it.

3. Ask patient about the <u>current</u> condition of his/her teeth. Ask patient if he/she wears dentures. Do teeth or dentures bother patient <u>now</u>?

4. Ask patient whether he/she notices any movements in mouth, face, hands, or feet. If yes, ask to describe and to what extent they <u>currently</u> bother patient or interfere with his/her activities.

5. Have patient sit in chair with hands on knees, legs slightly apart, and feet flat on floor. (Look at entire body for movements while in this position.)

6. Ask patient to sit with hands hanging unsupported. If male, between legs, if female and wearing a dress, hanging over knees. (Observe hands and other body areas.)

7. Ask patient to open mouth. (Observe tongue at rest within mouth.) Do this twice.

8. Ask patient to protrude tongue. (Observe abnormalities of tongue movement.) Do this twice.

9. Ask patient to tap thumb, with each finger, as rapidly as possible for 10-15 seconds; separately with right hand, then with left hand. (Observe facial and leg movements.)

10. Flex and extend patient's left and right arms (one at a time). (Note any rigidity.)

11. Ask patient to stand up. (Observe in profile. Observe all body areas again, hips included.)

12. Ask patient to extend both arms outstretched in front with palms down. (Observe trunk, legs, and mouth.)

13. Have patient walk a few paces, turn, and walk back to chair. (Observe hands and gait.) Do this twice.

Non-Neuroleptic Facial Dyskinesias

Prominent or exclusive tongue, jaw, and facial movements are of course not peculiar to tardive dyskinesia. They are observable in elderly people who are said to have *buccolingual dyskinesia of the elderly*. In this case, the dyskinesia is often associated with dementia. Also, *stereotyped movements* of the face, mouth, or tongue can be seen in schizophrenic patients who have never received neuroleptics. They may also be found in patients who take L-dopa, antidepressants, and other medications and in those who have chorea, Meige's syndrome, blepharospasm, and tics. In addition, edentulous persons may have *edentulous orofacial dyskinesia*. This condition is characterized by lower facial dyskinesias and minimal tongue movement that is correctable with properly fitting dentures.

The *rabbit syndrome* is fine rhythmic movements of the lips without tongue movements. It is found in patients who are given neuroleptics; however, it is also found in many other individuals. Unlike tardive dyskinesia, it responds to anticholinergics (Yassa). Therefore, the rabbit syndrome should be considered a manifestation of parkinsonism, rather than a variety of tardive dyskinesia.

Before initiating neuroleptic treatment, the psychiatrist should note the presence or absence of abnormal movements and distinguish buccolingual dyskinesia from the non-neuroleptic facial dyskinesias. The Abnormal Involuntary Movement Scale (AIMS), which has been widely used within the psychiatric, although not neurologic, community, is a suitable device (Fig. 18-37). Some limitations, however, are that it measures dyskinesias that fluctuate in intensity during the day; the measurements are gross; akinesia, which is an important sign, is not recognized; and the test does not distinguish among chorea, dystonia, tics, and other dyskinesias.

Other Medications

Antidepressants, because of their anticholinergic properties, cause ocular accommodation impairment (Fig. 12-4), rare cases of narrow-angle glaucoma (Fig. 12-7), and bladder dysfunction (Fig. 15-4). In addition, about 10 percent of patients taking tricyclic antidepressants develop a fine tremor that appears similar to essential tremor and also responds to propranolol. Otherwise, although some antidepressants, such as amoxapine (Ascendin), have dopamine antagonist properties, they rarely cause movement disorders or other signs of extrapyramidal dysfunction.

In contrast, even at therapeutic concentrations, lithium routinely causes a tremor and subtle extrapyramidal dysfunction. At higher concentrations, lithium causes a coarse tremor, but it can be suppressed by propranolol. At excessive concentrations, lithium also causes akinesia, cogwheel rigidity, and dysarthria.

PSYCHOGENIC MOVEMENTS

As discussed previously (Chapters 3 and 18, General Considerations), despite bizarre appearances and other characteristics that suggest a psychogenic disorder, movement disorders are almost always the result of neurologic dysfunction. However, *Conversion Disorder*, *Factitious Disorder*, or *Malingering* have been diagnosed when the movements are relieved by psychotherapy, physical therapy, or use of placebo, or they disappear when the patient is covertly observed (Fahn). These criteria may be valid in certain situations, but they are perilous. In the following disorders, which can be diagnosed as psychogenic using those criteria, movements are self-limited, can be suppressed, or fluctuate widely: acute dystonic reactions, Sydenham's chorea, tardive dyskinesia, tics, and Tourette's syndrome. Moreover, most of these disorders would naturally respond to reduced anxiety that the various interventions, including solitude, might provide. Also, in psychiatric patients with unusual movements, their medications rather than their illness may be responsible.

Nevertheless psychogenic movement disorders do occur. The most common psychogenic movement disorder is probably a dystonia-like posturing. In this case, movements are bizarre, inconsistent in location and intensity ("incongruent"), intermittent ("paroxysmal"), and associated with psychogenic weakness and sensory loss. Tremor is the only other relatively common disorder that often has a psychogenic basis. Psychogenic tremor, in contrast to the anxiety-induced fine tremor, is characterized by tremor in two planes and a variable frequency and intensity that tend to diminish, because of fatigue, during long examinations. In addition, when psychogenic tremors affect one arm, they often switch sides when the affected arm is restrained, and they tend to interfere with some activities but not others that require use of the same muscles.

Some motor activities appear to originate in culturally determined behavior, rather than either neurologic or psychiatric disease. For example, the "Jumping Frenchmen of Maine," a group of otherwise healthy French-Canadian descendants, and the related Cajuns in Louisiana, respond to unexpected loud noises by leaping upward, screaming, or throwing any object that they might be holding.

SUMMARY

The involuntary movement disorders are diagnosed almost exclusively on the basis of the appearance of the movements and possibly other clinical features, such as a history indicative of genetic transmission, an onset in childhood or adolescence (Table 18-3), or the presence or absence of mental abnormalities (Table 18-4). The illnesses for which confirmatory laboratory tests are available are Wilson's disease, SSPE, Lesch-Nyhan syndrome, and Huntington's disease. Major medical advances have been the discovery of MPTP-induced parkinsonism, determination of the affected chromosome in Huntington's disease, study of twins and possibly obsessive-compulsive traits with Tourette's syndrome, use of botulinum toxin in facial dyskinesias, and recognition of tardive dystonia. Unfortunately, treatment of tardive dyskinesia, the most troublesome condition, remains based on the dopamine hypersensitivity theory, which has not led to effective medications.

TABLE 18–3. COMMONLY CITED MOVEMENT DISORDERS THAT BEGIN IN CHILDHOOD OR ADOLESCENCE

Early childhood
    Athetosis or choreoathetosis
    Lesch-Nyhan syndrome*
Childhood
    Dystonia musculorum deformans (childhood-onset variety)*
    Myoclonus from subacute sclerosing panencephalitis (SSPE)
    Tourette's syndrome*
Adolescence
    Wilson's disease*
    Huntington's chorea (juvenile form)*
    Essential tremor*
    Medication and drug-induced movements

* Genetic transmission established.

TABLE 18–4. COMMONLY CITED MOVEMENT DISORDERS THAT ARE ASSOCIATED WITH MENTAL ABNORMALITIES*

Young children
  Athetosis or choreoathetosis†
  Lesch-Nyhan syndrome
Older children and adolescents
  Myoclonus from SSPE
  Wilson's disease
  Huntington's chorea‡
Adults
  AIDS§
  Parkinson's disease
  Myoclonus from Creutzfeldt-Jakob disease, rarely
    Alzheimer's disease

---

* Dementia, depression, or psychotic behavior.
† Despite severe movement disorders, many choreoathetosis patients do not have mental abnormalities (Chapter 13).
‡ Sydenham's chorea may cause persistent but only minor abnormalities.
§ Depending on the presence of encephalitis or toxoplasmosis, AIDS can cause parkinsonism, chorea, tremor, or myoclonus.

REFERENCES

Parkinsonism

Abramowicz M: Drugs for parkinsonism. Med Letter 30:113, 1988

Andersen J, Aabro E, Gulmann N, et al: Anti-depressive treatment in Parkinson's disease. Acta Neurol Scand 62:210, 1980

Cash R, Dennis T, L'Heureux R, et al: Parkinson's disease and dementia: Norepinephrine and dopamine in locus ceruleus. Neurology 37:42, 1987

Dubois B, Danze F, Pillon B, et al: Cholinergic-dependent cognitive deficits in Parkinson's disease. Ann Neurol 22:26, 1987

Duvoisin RC: Parkinson's Disease: A Guide for Patient and Family, 2nd ed. New York, Raven Press, 1984

Glantz RH, Bieliauskas L, Paleologos N: Behavioral indicators of hallucinosis in levodopa-treated Parkinson's disease. Adv Neurol 45:417, 1986

Growdon JH, Corkin S: Cognitive impairments in Parkinson's disease. Adv Neurol 45:383, 1986

Harvey NS: Psychiatric disorders in parkinsonism: 1. Functional illnesses and personality. Psychosomatics 27:91, 1986

Harvey NS: Psychiatric disorders in parkinsonism: 2. Organic cerebral states and drug reactions. Psychosomatics 27:175, 1986

Hietanen M, Teravainen H: Dementia and treatment with L-dopa in Parkinson's disease. Movement Disorders 3:263, 1988

Kidron D, Melamed E: Forms of dystonia in patients with Parkinson's disease. Neurology 37:1009, 1987

Koller WC (ed): Handbook of Parkinson's Disease. New York, Marcel Dekker, Inc., 1987

Koller W, O'Hara R, Nutt J, et al: Monozygotic twins with Parkinson's disease. Ann Neurol 19:402, 1986

Lieberman A, DziatolowskR, Nutt J, et al: Monozygotic twins with Parkinson's disease. Ann Neurol 19:402, 1986

Lieberman A, Dziatolowski M, Kupersmith M, et al: Dementia in Parkinson's disease. Ann Neurol 6:355, 1979

Madrazo I, Drucker-Colin R, Diaz V, et al: Open microsurgical autograft of adrenal medulla to the right caudate nucleus in two patients with intractable Parkinson's disease. N Engl J Med 316:831, 1987

Marttila RJ, Kaprio J, Koskenuo M, et al: Parkinson's disease in a nationwide twin cohort. Neurology 38:1217, 1988

Mayeux R, Stern Y, Rosenstein R, et al: An estimate of the prevalence of dementia in idiopathic Parkinson's disease. Arch Neurol 45:260, 1988

Mayeux R, Stern Y, Sano M, et al: Clinical and biochemical correlates of bradyphrenia in Parkinson's disease. Neurology *37*:1130, 1987

Mayeux R, Stern Y, Sano M, et al: The relationship of serotonin to depression in Parkinson's disease. Movement Disorders *3*:237, 1988

Mayeux R, Stern Y, Williams JBW, et al: Depression and Parkinson's disease. Adv Neurol *45*:451, 1986

Snyder SH, D'Amato RJ: MPTP: A neurotoxin relevant to the pathophysiology of Parkinson's disease. Neurology *36*:250, 1986

Stern Y, Mayeux R: Intellectual impairment in Parkinson's disease. Adv Neurol *45*:405, 1986

Chorea and Hemiballismus

Agrawal BL, Foa RP: Collagen vascular disease appearing as chorea gravidarum. Arch Neurol *39*:192, 1982

Bittenbender JB, Quadfasel FA: Rigid and akinetic forms of Huntington's chorea. Arch Neurol *2*:275, 1962

Folstein SE, Abbott MH, Chase GA, et al: The association of affective didsorder with Huntington's disease in a case series and in families. Psychol Med *13*:537, 1983

Folstein SE, Franz ML, Jensen BA, et al: Conduct disorder and affective disorder among offspring of patients with Huntington's disease. Psychol Med *13*:45, 1983

Goldblatt D, Markesbery W, Reeves AG: Recurrent hemichorea following striatal lesions. Arch Neurol *31*:51, 1974

Ichikawa K, Kim RC, Givelber H, et al: Chorea gravidarum. Arch Neurol *37*:429, 1980

Klawans HL, Moses S, Nausieda PA, et al: Treatment and prognosis of hemiballismus. N Engl J Med *295*:1348, 1976

Koller WC, Trimble J: The gait abnormality of Huntington's disease. Neurology *35*:1450, 1985

Markham CH, Knox JW: Observations on Huntington's chorea in childhood. Pediatrics *67*:47, 1965

Martin JB, Gusella JF: Huntington's Disease: Pathogenesis and management. N Engl J Med *315*:1267, 1986

Nausieda PA, Bieliauskas LA, Bacon LD, et al: Chronic dopaminergic sensitivity after Sydenham's chorea. Neurology *33*:750, 1983

Nausieda PA, Grossman BJ, Koller WC, et al: Sydenham chorea: An update. Neurology *30*:331, 1980

Nausieda PA, Koller WC, Weiner WJ, et al: Chorea induced by oral contraceptives. Neurology *29*:1605, 1979

Prentice PA: Huntington's Disease: A Manual for Care. Toronto, Huntington Society of Canada, 1986

Veasy LG, Wiedmeier SE, Orsmond GS, et al: Resurgence of acute rheumatic fever in the intermountain area of the United States. N Engl J Med *316*:421, 1987

Young AB, Penney JB, Starosta-Rubinstein S, et al: PET scan investigations of Huntington's disease. Ann Neurol *20*:296, 1986

Young AB, Shoulson I, Penney JB, et al: Huntington's disease in Venezuela. Neurology *36*:244, 1986

Wilson's disease

Chung YS, Ravi SD, Borge, GF: Psychosis in Wilson's disease. Psychosomatics *27*:65, 1986

Medalia A, Isaacs-Glaberman K, Scheinberg IH: Neuropsychological impairment in Wilson's disease. Arch Neurol *45*:502, 1988

Rubinstein SS, Young AB, Kluin K, et al: Clinical assessment of 31 patients with Wilson's disease. Arch Neurol *44*:365, 1987

Saito T: Presenting symptoms and natural history of Wilson disease. Eur J Pediatr *146*:261, 1987

Dystonia (Non-Neuroleptic)

Brin MF, Fahn S, Moskowitz C, et al: Localized injections of botulinum toxin for the treatment of focal dystonia and hemifacial spasm. Movement Disorders *2*:237, 1987

Burke RE, Fahn S, Marsden CD: Torsion dystonia: A double- blind, prospective trial of high-dosage trihexyphenidyl. Neurology *36*:160, 1986

Cohen LG, Hallett M: Hand cramps: Clinical features and electromyographic patterns in a focal dystonia. Neurology *38*:1005, 1988

Harrington RC, Wieck A, Marks IM, et al: Writer's cramp: Not associated with anxiety. Movement Disorders *3*:195, 1988

Hornykiewicz O, Kish SJ, Becker LE, et al: Brain neurotransmitters in dystonia musculorum deformans. N Engl J Med *315*:347, 1986

Kaufman DM: Facial dyskinesias. Psychosomatics (in press).

Ludlow CL, Naunton RF, Sedory SE, et al: Effects of botulinum toxin injections on speech in adductor spasmodic dysphonia. Neurology *38*:1220, 1988

Sheehy MP, Marsden CD: Writer's cramp—A focal dystonia. Brain *105*:461, 1982

Wolfson N, Sharpless NS, Thal LJ, et al: Decreased ventricular fluid norepinephrine metabolite in childhood-onset dystonia. Neurology *33*:369, 1983

Essential Tremor

Findley LJ, Koller WC: Essential tremor: A review. Neurology *37*:1194, 1987

Koller WC: Propranolol therapy for essential tremor of the head. Neurology *34*:1077, 1984

Martinelli P, Gabellini AS, Gulli MR, et al: Different clinical features of essential tremor: A 200-patient study. Acta Neurol Scand *75*:106, 1987

Tics and Tourette's Syndrome

Barabas G, Matthews WS, Ferrari M: Disorders of arousal in Gilles de la Tourette's syndrome. Neurology *34*:815, 1984

Frankel M, Cummings JL, Robertson MM, et al: Obsessions and compulsions in Gilles de la Tourette's syndrome. Neurology *36*:378, 1986

Friedhoff AJ, Case TN (eds): Gilles de la Tourette's Syndrome. Advances in Neurology. New York, Raven Press, 1982

Golden GS: Psychologic and neuropsychologic aspect of Tourette's syndrome. In Symposium on the Borderland Between Neurology and Psychiatry. Neurol Clin *2*:91, 1984

Jankovic J, Fahn S: The phenomenology of tics. Movement Disorders *1*:17, 1986

Obeso JA, Rothwell JC, Marsden CD: Simple tics in Gilles de la Tourette's syndrome are not prefaced by a normal premovement EEG potential. J Neurol Neurosurg Psychiatry *44*:735, 1981

Pauls DL, Leckman JF: The inheritance of Gilles de la Tourette's syndrome and associated behaviors. N Engl J Med *315*:993, 1986

Price RA, Kidd KK, Cohen DJ, et al: A twin study of Tourette syndrome. Arch Gen Psychiatry *42*:815, 1985

Regeur L, Pakkenberg B, Fog R, et al: Clinical features and long-term treatment with pimozide in 65 patients with Gilles de la Tourette's syndrome. J Neurol Neurosurg Psychiatry *49*:791, 1986

Shapiro AK, Shapiro ES, Young JG, et al (eds): Gilles de la Tourette's Syndrome. New York, Raven Press, 1988

Singer HS, Tune LE, Butler IJ, et al: Clinical symptomatology, CSF neurotransmitter metabolites, and serum haloperidol levels in Tourette syndrome. In Friedhoff AJ, Chase TN (eds): Gilles de la Tourette's Syndrome. New York, Raven Press, 1982, pp 177–197

Wohfart G, Inguar DH, Hellberg AM: Compulsory shouting (Benedek's "klazomania") associated with oculogyric spasm in chronic epidemic encephalitis. Acta Psychiatr Scand *36*:369, 1961

Medication-Induced and Related Movement Disorders

Beauclair L, Fontaine R: Tardive dyskinesia associated with metoclopramide. Can Med Assoc J *134*:613, 1986

Burke RE, Fahn S, Jankovic J, et al: Tardive dystonia: Late-onset and persistent dystonia caused by antipsychotic drugs. Neurology *32*:1335, 1982

Burke RE, Kang UJ, Jankovic J, et al: Tardive akathisia: An analysis of clinical features and response to open therapeutic trials. Movement Disorders *4*:157, 1989

D'Alessandro R, Benassi G, Cristina E, et al: The prevalence of lingual-facial-buccal dyskinesias in the elderly. Neurology *36*:1350, 1986

Dutton JJ, Buckley EG: Botulinum toxin in the management of blepharospasm. Arch Neurol *43*:380, 1986

Gibb WRG, Lees AJ: The clinical phenomenon of akathisia. J Neurol Neurosurg Psychiatry *49*:861, 1986

Gualtieri CT, Barnhill J, McGimsey J, et al: Tardive dyskinesia and other movement disorders in children treated with psychotropic drugs. J Am Acad Child Psychiatry *19*:491, 1980

Guy W: Abnormal Involuntary Movement Scale (AIMS). In ECDEU Assessment Manual for Psychopharmacology. U.S. Department of Health, Education, and Welfare, pp. 534–37, 1976

Hardie RJ, Lees AJ: Neuroleptic-induced Parkinson's syndrome. J Neurol Neurosurg Psychiatry *51*:850, 1988

Jankovic J. Ford J: Blepharospasm and orofacial-cervical dystonia: Clinical and pharmacological findings in 100 patients. Ann Neurol *13*:402, 1983

Jankovic J, Orman J: Botulinum A toxin for cranial-cervical dystonia: A double-blind, placebo-controlled study. Neurology *37*:616, 1987

Jankovic J, Orman J: Tetrabenazine therapy of dystonia, chorea, tics, and other dyskinesias. Neurology *38*:391, 1988

Jankovic J, Tolosa E (eds): Facial dyskinesias. In Advances in Neurology. New York, Raven Press, 1988

Kang UJ, Burke RE, Fahn S: Natural history and treatment of tardive dystonia. Movement Disorders *1*:193, 1986

Karson CN, Teste CV, LeWitt PA: A comparison of two iatrogenic dyskinesias. Am J Psychiatry *140*:1504, 1983

Walters A, Hening W, Chokroverty S, et al: Opioid responsiveness in patients with neuroleptic-induced akathisia. Movement Disorders *1*:119, 1986

Weiner WJ, Luby ED: Persistent akathisia following neuroleptic withdrawal. Ann Neurol *13*:466, 1983

Yassa R, Lal S: Prevalence of the rabbit syndrome. Am J Psychiatry *143*:656, 1986

Yassa R, Nair V, Dimitry R: Prevalence of tardive dystonia. Acta Psychiatr Scand *73*:629, 1986

Psychogenic Movement Disorders

Batshaw ML, Wachtel RC, Deckel AW, et al: Munchausen's syndrome simulating torsion dystonia. N Engl J Med *312*:1437, 1985

Fahn S, Williams DT: Psychogenic dystonia. Adv Neurol *50*:431, 1988

Saint-Hilaire MH, Saint-Hilaire JM, Granger Luc: Jumping Frenchmen of Maine. Neurology *36*:1269, 1986

QUESTIONS: CHAPTER 18

1–5. Pick the correct answer(s).

1. In general, movement disorders:
   a. Are present intermittently 24 hours a day
   b. Are absent during sleep
   c. May be suppressed for periods of up to 5 seconds by voluntary effort
   d. Are made worse by anxiety

2. Gilles de la Tourette's (Tourette's) syndrome is characterized by:
   a. Multiple motor tics
   b. Single motor tics
   c. Vocal tics
   d. Variation of the pattern of tics
   e. Constant pattern of verbal and motor tics
   f. Frequent obsessive-compulsive traits
   g. Frequent attention deficit disorders

3. Obscenities in Tourette's syndrome are:
   a. Present in all cases
   b. Clearly present in less than one half the cases
   c. Usually develop as an initial symptom
   d. A late manifestation when they occur
   e. May be accompanied by echolalia

4. Tourette's syndrome develops:
   a. Usually before 5 years of age
   b. Usually before 13 years of age
   c. Predominantly in white Anglo-Saxon Protestants
   d. In girls more than boys
   e. In children with family members with either tics or Tourette's

5. Tourette's syndrome is associated with:
   a. Soft neurologic signs
   b. Nonspecific EEG abnormalities
   c. Intellectual impairment
   d. A tendency toward psychoses
   e. MRI abnormalities
   f. Close concordance in twins
   g. Attention deficits

6–9. Match the tremor with the examination that will elicit it.

6. Essential tremor

7. Cerebellar tremor

8. Parkinsonian tremor

9. Lithium-induced tremor

   a. Finger-nose test
   b. Psychologic stress
   c. Extending arms and hands

10–15. Match the tremor with an effective therapy.

10. Essential tremor

11. Cerebellar tremor

12. Parkinsonian tremor

13. Stagefright tremor

14. Hyperthyroidism tremor

15. Delirium tremens

   a. L-dopa
   b. Propranolol (Inderal)
   c. Amantadine (Symmetrel)
   d. Trihexyphenidyl (Artane)
   e. None of the above

16–20. Pick the correct answer(s).

16. Spasmotic torticollis is:
   a. Confined to the muscles of the neck and shoulders
   b. May be the first manifestation of dystonia musculorum deformans
   c. May be a manifestation of tardive dystonia
   d. May be resisted by slight pressure applied to the chin

17. In the recessively inherited form of dystonia musculorum deformans:
   a. Low levels of MHGP indicate a norepinephrine abnormality.
   b. Patients are usually muscular and rarely obese.
   c. The symptoms first appear between ages 8 and 14 years.
   d. Mental abilities are preserved.
   e. The disorder may be confused with Wilson's disease, which can cause dystonia as well as tremor.

18. In the dominantly inherited form of dystonia musculorum deformans:
   a. Patients tend to have involvement of the trunk and neck muscles first.
   b. The symptoms begin in adult life.
   c. Patients may present with tortipelvis.
   d. MRI studies reveal brainstem abnormalities.

19. Dystonia musculorum deformans may be effectively treated with:
   a. L-dopa
   b. Neuroleptics
   c. Spinal cord stimulation
   d. Stereotactic ablation of portions of the thalamus

20. Chronic dystonia of the head and neck muscles in young adults may result from:
   a. Dystonia musculorum deformans
   b. Wilson's disease
   c. Huntington's disease
   d. Neuroleptic medications, i.e., tardive dystonia

21–31.   Match the movement disorder with its symptoms.

21.   Unilateral involvement

22.   Bilateral involvement

a.   Athetosis
b.   Chorea
c.   Hemiballismus

23.   Most often associated with dementia

24.   Associated with mental retardation and seizures

25.   Continual movements

26.   Intermittent movements

27.   Greatest movement in distal portions of the extremities

28.   Prominent involvement of facial muscles

29.   Exacerbated by anxiety

30.   Dance-like quality to gait

31.   Patients suppress movements by pressurefrom the rest of their body

32–40.   Match the illness with its description.

32.   Recessive sex-linked inheritance

33.   Autosomal recessive inheritance

34.   Autosomal dominant inheritance

a.   Huntington's chorea
b.   Sydenham's chorea
c.   Wilson's disease
d.   None of the above

35.   May develop in children

36.   *Not* associated with progressive mental deterioration

37.   Mental changes may precede involuntary movements

38.   Movements may be ameliorated by neuroleptics

39.   Presence of Kayser-Fleischer ring

40.   Associated with rheumatic fever

41–49.   Match the illness with the underlying abnormality.

41.   Cerebral cortical anoxia

42.   Increased CSF measles antibodies

a.   Huntington's chorea
b.   Wilson's disease
c.   Hemiballismus
d.   Creutzfeldt-Jakob
e.   Choreoathetotic cerebral palsy
f.   Parkinsonism
g.   Myoclonus
h.   SSPE

43.   Perinatal kernicterus

44.   Low serum ceruloplasmin

45.   Infarction of the subthalamic nucleus

46.   Movement disorders seen in AIDS dementia

47. Probably caused by an infectious agent

48. Atrophy of the caudate heads

49. Cavitary lesions of the globus pallidus and putamen

50–53. Is the statement true or false?

50. Only one neuroleptic-induced movement disorder may occur at a time.

51. Tetrabenazine and reserpine both deplete dopamine from the presynaptic neurons.

52. Phenothiazines induce oculogyric crises and other acute dystonias only when used as an antipsychotic medication.

53. Tardive dyskinesia rarely develops when haloperidol (Haldol) is used for Tourette's syndrome.

54–58. Match the description with the condition.

54. Akathisia

55. Oculogyric crisis

56. Acute dystonic reactions

57. Tardive dystonia

58. Tardive (oral choreic) dyskinesia
    a. Occurs early in course of treatment
    b. Improves when the medication is reduced
    c. Responds to anticholinergic medications, such as diphenhydramine (Benadryl)
    d. May be briefly suppressed by voluntary effort
    e. Improves as patient remains on medication
    f. Occurs late in course of treatment

59. Which disorders that may develop in adolescence are associated with mental impairments and involuntary movements?
    a. Creutzfeldt-Jakob disease
    b. Wilson's disease
    c. Choreoathetotic cerebral palsy
    d. Huntington's chorea
    e. SSPE
    f. Essential tremor

60. In which ways does the childhood variety of Huntington's chorea differ from its adult variety?
    a. Patients have marked rigidity.
    b. Dementia does not develop.
    c. The outcome is not fatal.
    d. Patients may appear to have parkinsonism.
    e. Seizures are frequent.
    f. Chorea is absent or minimal.
    g. Patients may have dystonia posturing.

61–65. Match the disturbances, which are often felt to be psychogenic, with their neurologic description:

61. A 70-year-old man develops a high-pitched squeaky voice that forces him to speak in a whisper. Nevertheless, he can sing in a normal volume and pitch.

62. An actor begins to have a (stagefright) high-pitched voice and hand tremor while on stage.

63. Continual forced bilateral eyelid closure prevents a 70-year-old man from seeing.

64. A middle-aged woman develops continual face, eyelid, and jaw contractions.

65. An author develops hand cramps when writing with a pen, but he can type, play tennis, and button his shirts.
- a. Blepharospasm
- b. Writer's cramp
- c. Spasmodic dysphonia
- d. Meige's syndrome
- e. Oromandibular dystonia
- f. Anxiety-induced tremor (stagefright)
- g. Aphasia

66. Which of the following structures are usually considered to be portions of the corpus striatum?
- a. Substantia nigra
- b. Caudate nuclei
- c. Putamen
- d. Subthalamic nuclei
- e. Globus pallidus

67. What are the characteristics of the nigrostriatal tract?
- a. It links the substantia nigra to the corpus striatum.
- b. The substantia nigra are normally black, but in Parkinson's disease they are discolored.
- c. It produces about 80 percent of the dopamine of the brain.
- d. Its stimulation inhibits caudate activity.
- e. It cannot be seen under the microscope.
- f. Its major metabolic product is HVA.

68. Sinemet is a combination of L-dopa and which other substance?
- a. Carbidopa, a dopa decarboxylase inhibitor
- b. Bromocriptine (Parlodel)
- c. Anticholinergics

69. About 50 percent of Parkinson's disease patients have depression, dementia, or both. In these patients, which clinical, histologic, or chemical abnormalities are present?
- a. Senile plaques, neurofibrillary tangles, and neuron loss
- b. Physical incapacity
- c. Long duration of illness
- d. A reduction in choline acetyltransferase (CAT) in proportion to the dementia

70. Which of the following statements describe the Lesch-Nyhan syndrome?
- a. It is characterized by the onset of dystonia and other movements in children aged 2 to 6 years.
- b. It is an autosomal dominant genetic illness.
- c. Brain HVA and CAT concentrations are low.
- d. The basic deficit is a deficiency of HGPRT.
- e. Hyperuricemia is present.

71. In which conditions is myoclonus found?
- a. Cerebral anoxia
- b. SSPE
- c. Creutzfeldt-Jakob disease
- d. Alzheimer's disease
- e. Meperidine (Demerol) use
- f. Psychogenic disturbances
- g. AIDS dementia

72. Which of the following are characteristics of palatal myoclonus?
- a. A frequency of 1- to 3-Hz
- b. A frequency of 120 to 140 per minute

    c.   Disappearance during sleep
    d.   Underlying brainstem infarction
    e.   Association with dementia

73. Which of the following is *not* a characteristic of MPTP-induced parkinsonism?
    a.   It has provided a laboratory model of Parkinson's disease.
    b.   Pretreatment with monoamine oxidase inhibitors protects animals.
    c.   Patients respond, at least temporarily, to L-dopa replacement.
    d.   It leads to other manifestations of neuroleptic-induced movement disorders.

74. When botulinum A toxin is used to treat blepharospasm, Meige's syndrome, and other orofacial dyskinesias, which principles are involved?
    a.   Botulinum, like tetrobenazine, depletes dopamine.
    b.   Botulinum binds to the postsynaptic neuron.
    c.   Botulinum prevents release of ACh from the presynaptic neuromuscular junction neuron.

75–77. Match the neurotransmitter with its metabolic product(s).

75. Norepinephrine   a.   HVA

                                  b.   5-HIAA

76. Dopamine   c.   VMA

77. Serotonin   d.   MHPG

78. Which of the following statements regarding back-averaged premovement EEG potentials is true?
    a.   They are present in focal motor seizures.
    b.   They are present in voluntary movements.
    c.   They indicate a cortical origin of motor activity.
    d.   Their absence indicates a subcortical origin of movements.
    e.   They are present in chorea, myoclonus, and tics.

ANSWERS

1.	b, c, d.	**17.**	a, b, c, d, e.
2.	a, c, d, f, g.	**18.**	a, b, c.
3.	b, d, e.	**19.**	d.
4.	b, e.	**20.**	a, b, c, d.
5.	a, b,g.	**21.**	c.
6.	c.	**22.**	a, b.
7.	a.	**23.**	b.
8.	b.	**24.**	a.
9.	c.	**25.**	a.
10.	b.	**26.**	b, c.
11.	e.	**27.**	a.
12.	c, d.	**28.**	a, b.
13.	b.	**29.**	a, b, c.
14.	b.	**30.**	b.
15.	e.	**31.**	c.
16.	a, b, c, d.	**32.**	d.

33.	c.	**56.**	a, c.
34.	a.	**57.**	a, c, f.
35.	a, b, c.	**58.**	d, f.
36.	b.	**59.**	b, d, e.
37.	a, c.	**60.**	a, d, e, f, g.
38.	a, b, c.	**61.**	c.
39.	c.	**62.**	f.
40.	b.	**63.**	a.
41.	g.	**64.**	d.
42.	h.	**65.**	b.
43.	e.	**66.**	b, c, e.
44.	b.	**67.**	a, b, c, d, f.
45.	c.	**68.**	a.
46.	f, g.	**69.**	a, b, c, d.
47.	d, h.	**70.**	a, d, e.
48.	a.	**71.**	a, b, c, d (rarely), e,g.
49.	b.	**72.**	b, d.
50.	False	**73.**	d.
51.	True	**74.**	c.
52.	False	**75.**	c, d.
53.	True	**76.**	a.
54.	a, b, d, e.	**77.**	b.
55.	a, c.	**78.**	a, b, c, d.

19

Neurologic Manifestations of Brain Tumors and Metastatic Cancer

Tumors that arise within the brain or its coverings, the meninges, are called *primary brain tumors*. Even in older people, in whom their incidence is greatest, primary brain tumors occur less than 5 percent as frequently as cerebrovascular accidents (CVAs) (Chapter 11). Nevertheless, brain tumors command unique attention because of their unpredictable onset and tragic consequences, and because a common symptom, headache (Chapter 9), is a well-known manifestation of a brain tumor. For psychiatrists too, brain tumors are unique. Tumors typically develop insidiously and often produce mental impairments months before physical deficits. Thus, tumor symptoms may initially be mistaken for depression or Alzheimer's disease. Lastly, brain tumors are the epitome of "organicity" causing psychiatric symptoms.

*Metastatic tumors** that have spread to the brain or spinal cord by hematogenous dissemination from underlying cancers occur about as frequently as primary brain tumors. However, they present even more complex problems. These patients have debilitating neurologic symptoms as a result of brain or spinal cord metastases, as well as many neurologic symptoms produced by non-neurologic metastases and many forms of treatment.

VARIETIES

Primary brain tumors include the *astrocytoma* and *glioblastoma multiforme*, which are both considered *gliomas*. Astrocytomas affect children as well as adults, are relatively benign, and develop in the cerebrum, optic nerves, and the structures of the posterior fossa (cerebellum, pons, and medulla). Astrocytomas are the most common brain tumor in children, and they tend to be cystic and located in the cerebellum. These tumors may be totally removed, and the cure rate is about 90 percent. In contrast, astrocytomas in adults usually occur in the cerebrum, infiltrate extensively, and evolve into malignant tumors. Total surgical removal is rarely practical, and thus cure rates are low. However,

---

* Patients with brain tumors may receive assistance from the American Cancer Society, 261 Madison Avenue, New York, New York 10016, (212) 736-3030.

combined surgery and radiotherapy can prolong life expectancy for as long as 10 years.

Glioblastomas are highly malignant and infiltrative, occur almost only in adults, develop in the cerebrum, and grow rapidly, typically infiltrating through the corpus callosum (Figs. 19-1 and 20-6). Surgical excision is often attempted, but cure is rarely achieved. Radiotherapy, steroids, and chemotherapy reduce the size and subsequent regrowth of the tumor. These treatments can provide a brief (6 month to 1 year) physically comfortable survival. However, progressive mental deterioration, due to radiotherapy, other treatments (see below), or persistence of the tumor, is expectable.

Meningiomas, tumors that arise from the meninges of the brain or spinal cord, are another frequently occurring primary brain tumor (Fig. 20-5). They grow slowly and develop exclusively in adults. Often meningiomas are small and innocuous, and do not necessarily need to be removed. Since meningiomas grow slowly, and slowly growing lesions in certain regions tend to be asymptomatic, meningiomas over the frontal lobes can grow to extraordinary sizes, e.g., 400 cc, before they cause symptoms. They are usually accessible to surgery and can be totally removed. Radiation rarely has a role in their treatment.

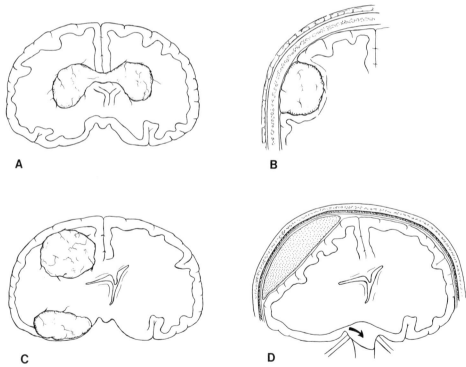

A   **B**

C   **D**

FIGURE 19–1. *A*, A *glioblastoma* typically infiltrates in a "butterfly pattern" from one cerebral hemisphere through the corpus callosum to the other, disrupting both frontal lobes (Fig. 20-6A). *B*, *Meningiomas* arise from the meninges overlying the surface of the brain. Since they grow slowly, meningiomas cause relatively little brain displacement or destruction (Fig. 20-5). *C*, *Metastatic tumors* are often multiple and surrounded by edema. Thus, large areas of brain are damaged (Fig. 20-6B). *D*, A *subdural hematoma*, typically over the cerebral hemisphere (Figs. 20-10 and 20-11), can compress the underlying brain and push it through the tentorial notch below, i.e., cause *transtentorial herniation*. In this usually fatal condition, the brainstem and ipsilateral oculomotor (third cranial) nerve are compressed.

toxoplasmosis (Figs. 20-7 and 20-8) and cytomegalic inclusion disease because the clinical and CT signs of these conditions are similar (Chapter 7). Treatment of the lymphoma, whatever its cause, includes radiotherapy and chemotherapy.

Metastatic tumors tend to be multiple, surrounded by edema, and rapidly growing. Their multiplicity, combined volume, and their surrounding edema (Fig. 20-6) together impose a burdensome mass. The most common metastatic

Another variety of primary brain tumor is the *primary cerebral lymphoma*. Although lymphomas commonly involve the brain as part of systemic lymphoma disorders, the primary cerebral lymphoma is a neoplasm of only the brain. It is often a consequence of an impaired immunologic system and is thus seen in patients with the acquired immune deficiency syndrome (AIDS) and in patients receiving immunosuppressive therapy for renal and cardiac transplants. In AIDS patients, cerebral lymphomas are difficult to distinguish from cerebral brain tumors originate from primary tumors of the lung, breast, or kidney or from malignant melanomas. On the other hand, gastrointestinal, pelvic, and prostatic cancers metastasize to the brain rarely or only late in their course.

Several cancers routinely spread to the brain. For example, 30 percent of lung cancer patients, 50 percent of testicular cancer patients, and 75 percent of malignant melanoma patients have metastases to the brain. Overall, about 20 percent of cancer patients develop cerebral metastases, and occasionally the discovery of a metastatic brain tumor is the first indication that a person has cancer. Whatever the origin of the metastatic cancer, steroids, which dramatically reduce the edema, and radiotherapy are palliative; however, cure of cancer once brain metastases have occurred is rare.

INITIAL PHYSICAL MANIFESTATIONS

The most frequent initial physical manifestations of primary or metastatic brain tumors are seizures, headaches, and physical deficits. Although mental symptoms occur in almost about 75 percent of cases (see below), physical symptoms, even though they are present in only about 25 to 50 percent of cases, are more reliable indicators of the presence of a tumor.

Seizures do not result from tumors of the brainstem or cerebellum, but they are the initial symptom of brain tumors affecting the cerebrum in approximately one half of cases. In people older than 50 years, seizures are caused about as often by brain tumors as by CVAs. Since seizures from brain tumors are a manifestation of cerebral cortex irritation, they are partial elementary or partial complex seizures, rather than absences (petit mal) or other primary generalized seizures (Chapter 10). When a tumor-induced partial seizure occurs, it often undergoes secondary generalization and thereby mimics a primary generalized seizure.

Brain tumor headaches occur frequently as an initial manifestation, but their characteristics are not distinctive. Even the presence of headaches is misleading because fewer than 1 out of 1,000 people with headaches have a tumor. Brain tumor headaches are most often initially generalized, dull, and responsive to mild analgesics, such as aspirin. In most cases, headaches at their onset appear to result from muscle contraction or tension. As with migraine headaches, with which they are also apt to be confused, brain tumor headaches tend to be worse in the early morning hours, when they often awaken a patient from sleep.

Only in advanced cases, when intracranial pressure is markedly raised, are

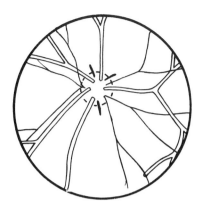

FIGURE 19–2. Papilledema is characterized by reddening of the optic disk, which loses its distinct margin, and also by distention of the retinal veins. With acute papilledema, the disk is elevated and hemorrhages appear at its edge. (Compare with the normal disk in Figure 4-3.)

tumor headaches severe and associated with nausea and vomiting. Then the increased intracranial pressure also causes generalized physical and mental dysfunction. Pressure transmitted along the optic nerve to the optic disks causes *papilledema* (Fig. 19-2). The physician should bear in mind that, since the notorious syndrome of headache, nausea and vomiting, and papilledema occurs relatively late in the course of brain tumors, only a minority of patients have it during an initial examination. Its absence should not be taken as evidence against the presence of a brain tumor.

Tumors of the cerebellar or cerebral hemispheres can cause common physical neurologic deficits, such as hemiparesis, that follow the usual clinical correlations (Chapters 2–6). In more than one half of cases at the first medical evaluation, however, tumors do not cause these deficits because they are small, slowly growing, or located in "silent areas" of the brain, namely the right frontal or anterior temporal lobes.

Tumors that arise from cranial nerves lead to readily recognizable distinct deficits. For example, optic nerve gliomas cause optic atrophy with blindness. Acoustic neuromas, which develop in the cerebellopontine angle and are associated with neurofibromatosis, cause unilateral tinnitus and progressive hearing loss.

Meningiomas are a special case. As discussed previously, small meningiomas are frequent, and either small or large ones can be asymptomatic. However, meningiomas tend to develop in certain locations and produce characteristic signs. A meningioma arising from the falx, a *parasagittal meningioma*, can compress the medial motor cortex and cause spastic paresis of one or both legs. Meningiomas can also arise from the meninges over the sphenoid wing (Fig. 20-5). These *sphenoid wing meningiomas* cause paresis of eye movement, proptosis, and compression and irritation of the adjacent temporal lobe. Likewise, *olfactory groove meningiomas* compress the immediately adjacent olfactory and optic nerves and the overlying frontal lobe (Foster-Kennedy Syndrome, Chapter 4). They cause anosmia, unilateral blindness, and, when large, signs of frontal lobe dysfunction (see below and Chapter 7).

INITIAL MENTAL MANIFESTATIONS

The major mental manifestations of brain tumors, especially when they involve the frontal lobe, are emotional dulling, loss of initiative, and reduced capacity to execute complex mental tasks. These impairments, which evolve over several weeks, are not necessarily accompanied by intellectual (cognitive) decline. Despite having developed mood changes and apathy, for example, patients might satisfactorily recall six digits or perform simple calculations. Slowness, bewilderment, and apathy, but not any actual loss of cognitive ability, retard intellectual function.

Another important consequence of frontal lobe tumors is impairment of normal inhibitory systems. In these cases, patients quickly react to any irritation, tend to use profane language, cry with little provocation, but rarely laugh. In advanced stages, these tumors cause urinary incontinence.

Mental changes from tumors differ in subtle ways from those in the early stages of Alzheimer's disease (Chapter 7). In the tumor patients, personality changes tend to be prominent while cognitive capacity is preserved. In Alzheimer's disease patients, memory loss or impaired judgment tend to develop before the personality changes. Moreover, their cognitive changes develop insidiously and are initially unaccompanied by physical deficits.

An even more difficult distinction is that between tumor-induced mental changes and depression or pseudodementia. Consummate clinical acumen is required to discern signs of a primary or metastatic brain tumor. Guidelines, which are admittedly not fully reliable, are that the presence of cognitive or language impairment, or certainly the presence of specific physical and neurologic symptoms, requires consideration of a tumor in a patient who otherwise seems depressed.

On the other hand, in a patient with a known brain tumor, a psychiatrist should attempt to determine how much of the patient's abnormal mental state is psychogenic, situational, neurologic, or iatrogenic, and, most important, whether it is reversible (Table 19-1). Being able to achieve an overview, a psychiatrist might help cancer patients, their families, and other physicians weigh the benefits against the side effects of various treatments.

Causes of Mental Changes

Mental changes are caused not only by primary or metastatic brain tumors but they are also often caused or precipitated by pain, insomnia, or side effects of treatment. Brain tumors themselves, the most common and obvious etiology, cause mental changes in the absence of overt hemiparesis or other physical deficits in over 50 percent of cases at the time of diagnosis. Tumors affecting the frontal or temporal lobes, especially on the nondominant side of the brain, frequently produce personality changes with few physical deficits. In later stages, as cerebral tumors grow, accumulate surrounding edema, infiltrate, or, in the case of metastases, increase in number, the severity of physical and mental impairments progresses in parallel.

Not only do tumors injure one or more areas of the brain but their volume (mass) also raises intracranial pressure. The extra mass is particularly burdensome because the brain is encased within the rigid skull and, unlike the liver with metastases, has little room to expand. With increased intracranial pressure, patients develop lethargy, impaired concentration, slowness of thought, headache, nausea, vomiting, and papilledema.

Increased intracranial pressure and the same symptoms can occur when metastases block the normal flow of cerebrospinal fluid (CSF). Metastases in the cerebellum sometimes expand to obstruct CSF flow through the fourth ventricle and precipitate obstructive *hydrocephalus*. A similar situation occurs

TABLE 19–1. IMPORTANT ITEMS IN THE NEUROLOGIC EVALUATION OF CANCER PATIENTS WITH MENTAL ABERRATIONS

What is the primary tumor?
    Lung, breast, kidney, malignant melanoma*
Where are metastases known to be present?
    Brain, liver, lung, spine
Does the patient have symptoms or signs of a cerebral lesion?
    Headache, seizures, hemiparesis, papilledema
What treatments have been given?
    Radiation: total dose and schedule
    Chemotherapy: medications and complications
    Analgesics: daily dose, route, indication
    Psychotropics: antidepressants, sedatives, tranquilizers
    Others: steroids, antiemetics, cimetidine
What is the patient's general status?
    Pain control
    Sleep schedule and restfulness
    Nutrition, weight change, and appetite
    Temperature, sweats
What are the results of important laboratory tests?
    Complete blood count
    Liver and renal function tests
    Serum calcium concentration
    CT or MRI scan
    CSF analysis (lumber puncture)†
    EEG†

* Cancers that tend to metastasize.
† Limited indications.

when cancer cells coat the meninges at the base of the brain. In this condition, *carcinomatous meningitis*, various cranial nerves are compressed, and more important, since reabsorption of CSF at the base of the brain is retarded, communicating hydrocephalus develops.

Whether or not brain tumors are present, many medications routinely used in cancer patients can create mental aberrations. The most important group of these medications are narcotic analgesics. Too large a dosage of narcotics causes confusion, lethargy, or stupor. In particular, the metabolic products of meperidine (Demerol) can lead to a toxic psychosis. On the other hand, too little or otherwise improperly prescribed narcotics can lead to unrelieved suffering, restless sleep, and obsessive drug-seeking behavior.

Other medications likely to induce mental changes in cancer patients are sedatives, antiemetics that contain antihistamines or phenothiazines, cimetidine (Tagamet), anticonvulsants, steroids, and psychotropics. Although the side effects of common medications are usually predictable, sometimes their mental side effects in cancer patients are unexpected. For example, patients might have undiagnosed liver metastases that slow the metabolism of drugs. Patients whose body mass is reduced might be given a relatively large dose of medicine. Interactions among several potent medicines might also cause drug-induced mental changes.

The usual cancer chemotherapy regimens cannot penetrate the blood-brain barrier and do not cause mental status changes unless they are administered in extraordinarily high doses or for prolonged periods. A notable and unfortunate exception is methotrexate. When administered with craniospinal radiotherapy for childhood leukemia, it often injures the brain. Although methotrexate protects the CNS from leukemia invasion, its use may be complicated by confusional states, learning disabilities, and permanent intellectual impairment.

Another cause of mental aberrations is cranial or "whole brain" radiotherapy. High-dose radiation, especially when administered over a short time period, can cause necrosis of small cerebral arteries, which leads to numerous small stroke-like cerebral infarctions termed *radiation necrosis* or *radiation arteritis*. Characteristically, the physical and mental deficits begin about 6 to 18 months after completion of a course of radiotherapy, and they often accumulate over several more months to result in irreversible dementia and multiple physical impairments. A comparable iatrogenic complication, which can occur when the spine or mediastinum is radiated, is radiation necrosis of the spinal cord, or *radiation myelitis*.

Medications or metastases can also cause renal, pulmonary, or hepatic failure. The organ failure, usually in the late stages of cancer, can lead to a toxic-metabolic encephalopathy (Chapter 7). Ectopic hormone production is another complication of cancer. Excess parathyroid hormone production causes hypercalcemia, and inappropriate antidiuretic hormone (ADH) secretion causes marked electrolyte abnormalities—conditions that lead to mental changes.

Finally, infection is one of the most common and difficult to diagnose, but potentially correctable, causes of mental aberrations. Brain tumor patients, as well as other cancer patients, are susceptible to infection because they are debilitated, may have indwelling intravenous lines and urinary catheters, and, most important, have radiotherapy- and chemotherapy-induced immunosuppression. These patients routinely develop pneumonia, sepsis, and bacterial infections that often manifest as only apathy or delirium without the common indicators of infection, such as fever and leukocytosis. Sometimes fungi, particularly *Cryptococcus*, and other unusual organisms cause opportunistic infections of the brain or meninges.

Similarly, viruses can affect patients who have received intensive chemotherapy. Several can cause a patchy loss of myelin in the brain. For example, *progressive multifocal leukoencephalopathy* (*PML*), which is probably caused by a papovavirus, results in diffuse mental and physical impairments. When memory impairment predominates, the condition is sometimes called *limbic encephalitis*. In an apparently related group of conditions, the *paraneoplastic syndromes* or *remote effects of carcinoma*, patients have diffuse neurologic impairments but no direct evidence of viral or other type of infection.

DIAGNOSTIC TESTS FOR BRAIN TUMORS

Computed tomography (CT) and magnetic resonance imaging (MRI) scans are the most readily available, reliable, cost-effective* diagnostic procedures (Chapter 20). Either scan will reveal the size, location, and, in many cases, the variety of a tumor. They usually can identify other intracranial lesions, including CVAs and subdural hematomas. They can also demonstrate hydrocephalus, PML, and many other complications of tumors. Equally important, a normal scan will virtually eliminate the possibility of tumors and most of these other conditions.

---

* The cost of a CT scan is about $250 and an MRI scan about $750 in 1989.

In comparison, EEGs are simply not useful for detecting tumors, hydrocephalus, or other structural lesions (Chapter 10). Even with some large but slowly growing tumors, such as meningiomas, EEGs may show few or only nonspecific abnormalities. However, the EEG remains a good test for detecting toxic-metabolic encephalopathy. Since CT and MRI are so accurate, arteriography is rarely required.

With rare exceptions, a lumbar puncture to analyze CSF should not be performed when a brain tumor or other intracranial mass lesion is suspected. In these cases, the CSF is usually not diagnostic because it is usually either normal or only nonspecifically abnormal (Chapter 20). Moreover, a lumbar puncture can precipitate transtentorial herniation (Fig. 19-3). A lumbar punc-

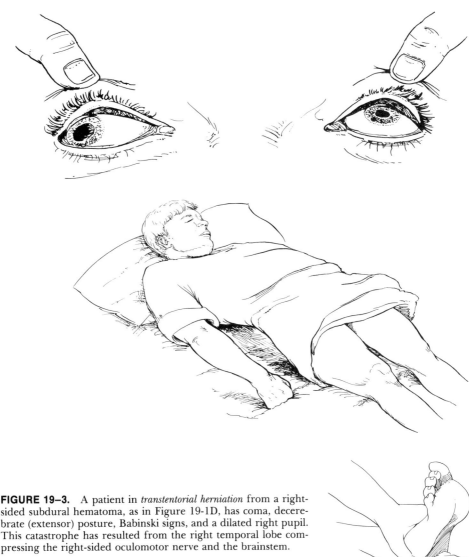

FIGURE 19–3. A patient in *transtentorial herniation* from a right-sided subdural hematoma, as in Figure 19-1D, has coma, decerebrate (extensor) posture, Babinski signs, and a dilated right pupil. This catastrophe has resulted from the right temporal lobe compressing the right-sided oculomotor nerve and the brainstem.

ture is, however, indicated when patients are suspected of having carcinomatous meningitis or a chronic, usually fungal, infectious meningitis. In those cases, the CSF must be examined for carcinoma cells, cultured for fungi, and tested for cryptococcal antigens.

RELATED CONDITIONS

Pituitary Adenomas

Although pituitary adenomas are also considered tumors of the brain, their clinical manifestions, histology, and treatment are entirely different from the brain tumors that have been discussed so far. Classic studies described major mental and physical abnormalities as common manifestations of pituitary adenomas; however, those symptoms arose from massive pituitary tumors that produced extraordinary secretions of hormones, expanded out of the sella to encroach on the adjacent temporal lobes, or obstructed the flow of CSF through the third ventricle. These adenomas, even when they are "microscopic," are now detected early in their course by using readily available sophisticated diagnostic tests that include CT and MRI scans and hormone radioimmuno-assay—practical applications of two recent Nobel Prize-winning concepts.

The majority of pituitary adenomas are either *prolactinomas,* which secrete prolactin, or *chromophobe adenomas*, which are nonsecretory. Pituitary adenomas occur almost only in adults, are histologically benign, and rarely grow beyond the pituitary gland. They can be microscopic in size; however, chromophobe adenomas typically grow large enough to exert pressure on surrounding structures (Fig. 19-4). Upward pressure on the diaphragm sella causes bitemporal or generalized headache, and pressure on the optic chiasm, which is above the diaphragm, causes a characteristic bitemporal hemianopsia or bitemporal superior quadrantanopsia (Chapter 12).

The earliest symptoms are referable to hormone irregularities, but they may be subtle and initially attributable to psychologic problems, old age, or minor medical illnesses. Most often the symptoms consist of decreased libido, menstrual irregularities, galactorrhea, or infertility. Later, pituitary hormone insufficiency results in lack of energy, apathy, and listlessness. Patients may appear to be depressed, but their cognitive capacity is usually normal.

A sagittal MRI scan or coronal CT scan will reveal almost all pituitary adenomas. In patients with prolactinomas and most chromophobe adenomas, the serum prolactin level is elevated. Treatment varies with the tumor type and institutional expertise but usually consists of radiation, transphenoidal micro-surgery, or, with prolactin-secreting tumors, bromocriptine. Treatment with radiation or craniotomy, which risks damaging the temporal lobes, can lead to memory impairment and partial complex seizures.

Less common pituitary growths secrete *growth hormone*, which can cause *acromegaly,* or *adrenocorticotropin hormone (ACTH)*, which can cause *Cushing's syndrome.* These growths are not really adenomas but are mostly collections of hyperplastic cells of insufficient mass to cause visual impairment or severe headache. Their hormones do alter the patient's body habitus and reduce vigor. In the past, various psychologic symptoms varying from depression to psychosis were attributed to the growths; however, they do not affect mental function

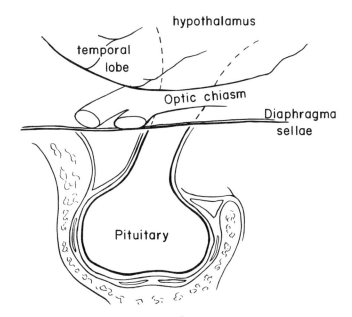

FIGURE 19-4. Pituitary adenomas grow laterally and inferiorly against the walls of the sella turcica and upward against the *diaphragm sella*. Large adenomas compress the optic chiasm, causing a distinctive bitemporal hemianopsia or bitemporal superior quadrantanopsia (Fig. 12-9). Continuouspressure on the chiasm leads to optic atrophy.

When lesions in this area are extraordinarily large, they may compress and damage the adjacent medial inferior surface of the temporal lobe. A craniotomy or radiotherapy directed at a pituitary tumor may also damage the adjacent temporal lobe.

The suprasellar region of the brain, which is above the diaphragm sella, contains the hypothalamus. Lesions in this area, such as craniopharyngiomas, compress the optic chiasm and cause diabetes insipidus as well as pituitary insufficiency.

unless they secrete a marked excess of hormones. Radioimmunoassays can readily detect hormone concentrations. Treatment usually requires individualized courses of radiation, surgery, or medications including bromocriptine.

In contrast to these relatively benign conditions, the *craniopharyngioma*, a tumor that occurs in children as well as in adults, is frequently fatal. It is a calcified cystic congenital lesion derived from Rathke's pouch. Unlike pituitary adenomas, it grows within the hypothalamus, which is located above the diaphragm sella (Fig. 9-4). Since it disrupts endocrine function, affected children have retarded physical and mental growth; adults develop impaired libido, amenorrhea, and apathy; and children and adults develop diabetes insipidus. When craniopharyngiomas are large, they press downward on the optic chiasm and cause optic atrophy and visual field defects similar to those found with large pituitary adenomas. When the third ventricle is compressed, patients develop hydrocephalus, which causes papilledema with headache, nausea and vomiting—the classic signs of increased intracranial pressure. Treatment relies on surgery, at least to drain the cyst if not to remove the tumor.

An important non-neoplastic pituitary condition is *postpartum pituitary necrosis*, better known as *Sheehan's syndrome*. It is pituitary insufficiency that classically results from obstetric deliveries complicated by hypotension. One month to several years postpartum, affected women have scant menses, absent lactation, and constant fatigue with diminished libido. In severe cases patients have weight loss, receding secondary sexual characteristics, and hypotension. Similar symptoms may develop because of postpartum autoimmune hypothyroidism. In both conditions, patients are liable to be misdiagnosed as having psychogenic postpartum depression.

Spine Metastases

Although primary brain tumors, such as glioblastomas, do not metastasize, lung, breast, and other forms of cancer are liable to metastasize to a vertebral body of the spine as well as the brain. Metastatic tumors often grow into the epidural space of the spinal canal to compress the spinal cord (Fig. 19-5). At the onset, these *epidural tumors* cause severe pain not only in the affected region (local pain) but also along the path of the affected nerve roots (radiating pain). For example, patients with thoracic spine metastases typically have interscapular spine pain that radiates around the chest in a band-like pattern, and patients with lumbar spine metastases have lower back pain that radiates down the legs. If the metastatic tumor continues to grow, it will cause quadriplegia when the cervical spinal cord is compressed or paraplegia when the thoracic spinal cord is compressed (Chapter 2). Spinal cord compression at any level will also cause loss of sensation and incontinence of urine and feces. Of course, even with complete spinal cord compression, mental functions are preserved.

In short, spinal cord compression by epidural tumors, a dreadful complication of cancer, causes pain, paraplegia or quadriplegia, and incontinence. Early diagnosis can prevent spinal cord compression, but once compression is complete, which might occur in 48 hours after the onset of weakness, the deficits

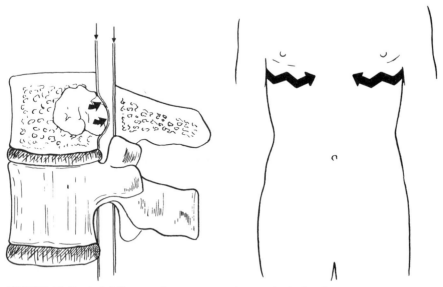

FIGURE 19–5. *Left,* When carcinoma metastasizes to the body of a vertebra, it typically grows posteriorly to encroach on the spinal *epidural space* (*thin arrows*), which contains the spinal cord and its nerve roots. This common situation, called an *epidural metastasis,* causes spinal cord compression, which leads to paraplegia or quadriplegia, loss of sensation (hypalgesia) below the level of the lesion, and usually fecal and urinary incontinence. *Right,* Patients have "local pain" from destruction of the vertebrae and a characteristic band-like "radiating pain," which follows the course of the nerves. The location of the pain, which is usually severe, and the level of the hypalgesia reliably indicate the site of an epidural metastatic tumor (Fig. 2-15).

are usually permanent. Myelography is still the definitive diagnostic test; however, in the near future, when it has better resolution, MRI of the spine will be preferable. Therapy usually consists of steroids, radiation, and, sometimes, decompressive laminectomy.

Other Causes of Limb Weakness

Several conditions characterized by weakness result from cancer-related muscle or peripheral nerve damage. Many are mild and reversible, but some cause the worst symptoms of the malignancy.

Patients are commonly weak because of cachexia. They have muscle weakness and atrophy with systemic symptoms, such as anorexia, weight loss, and diffuse pain. Patients and clinicians alike recognize this situation and know that it indicates extensive spread of cancer. Experienced physicians can acknowledge failure of their primary medical treatments, but can continue to provide realistic symptomatic therapy based on analgesics, sedatives, and antiemetics.

Some other causes of weakness in cancer patients are not associated with cachexia or muscle atrophy, and can be reversed. They include an inflammatory muscle disorder (polymyositis), side effects of medications (hypokalemic and steroid myopathies), and a condition similar to myasthenia gravis (Lambert-Eaton syndrome).

An iatrogenic and frequent cause of limb weakness is chemotherapy-induced polyneuropathy (neuropathy). For example, vincristine and related compounds routinely cause weakness and sensory loss in all four limbs. Paraparesis from chemotherapy can be so sudden that it mimics an epidural spinal cord compression; however, its typical clinical picture of distal sensory loss and weakness, areflexia, and the absence of back pain indicates the neuropathy (Chapter 5). Although permanent neuropathy also occasionally develops as a remote effect of cancer, most cases of chemotherapy-induced neuropathy resolve over several months.

Nerve injuries (mononeuropathies) can result from anorexia with loss of muscle bulk and subcutaneous fat. Peripheral nerves, deprived of their protective cushion, are then vulnerable to pressure even as light as the patient's own weight. The sciatic, peroneal, and radial nerves are most often injured when patients are bedridden, moved carelessly in stretchers, or secured too firmly in wheelchairs. These injuries cause paresis of hand, wrist, or ankle movement (Table 5-1). They can be prevented by providing foam rubber cushions for elbows, hips, and ankles; gently moving the patient; and repositioning weak patients every 2 hours.

The worst cancer complication affecting the peripheral nerves is tumor infiltration of a nerve plexus. When lung and breast cancers invade the brachial plexus, or pelvic cancers invade the lumbosacral plexus, patients develop excruciating pain, as well as paresis of the entire limb. Since the nerves themselves are invaded, the pain is poorly responsive to radiotherapy and analgesics (Chapter 14).

DISORDERS THAT MIMIC BRAIN TUMORS

Cerebrovascular accidents as well as tumors occur predominantly in older people and cause similar mental impairments and physical deficits, including seizures. The major clinical difference between these two illnesses is generally in their onset. Whereas cerebrovascular accidents usually occur immediately or develop over several days, often being discovered first when the patient awakens in the morning, brain tumors usually evolve over several weeks. Another difference is that, even when patients develop extensive physical and intellectual deficits following a CVA, they usually remain alert and free of headaches. For example, a patient with a CVA may be fully alert despite having a homonymous hemianopsia, hemiparesis, and hemisensory loss. To produce a comparable deficit, a tumor would have to extend through an entire cerebral hemisphere. It would then be large enough to cause signs of increased intracranial pressure. Finally, whereas seizures from CVAs develop about 6 months after the CVA, they develop at the onset or early in the course of a tumor.

A *subdural hematoma* is another important disorder that mimics tumors. Intracranial venous bleeding, usually initiated by head trauma, causes a hematoma in the potential space between the dura (the thick layer of the meninges) and the underlying brain (Fig. 19-1; and Figs. 20-10 and 20-11). Over a period of several weeks, the subdural hematoma, which may be either unilateral or bilateral, accumulates fluid and progressively enlarges. As it grows, the subdural hematoma compresses one or both cerebral hemispheres, causing generalized cerebral dysfunction.

Older people are especially prone to subdural hematomas because they bleed intracranially after minor or even no obvious head injury. Also, the bleeding continues unchecked after its onset because their atrophic brains do not compress the bleeding veins.

Subdural hematomas probably occur as often as primary brain tumors. They cause headaches and seizures, but sometimes their only symptoms are personality and intellectual impairments. Fortunately, subdural hematomas may be easily evacuated through small "twist-drill" holes. When promptly treated, cerebral function is fully restored. In other words, subdural hematomas are a relatively common and correctable form of dementia.

Uncommon cerebral mass lesions—that also begin with mental changes, physical deficits, or seizures—are brain abscesses and arteriovenous malformations (AVMs). Although life-threatening conditions, they need not be considered individually by the nonspecialist. Not only are they rare but they will also be visualized by CT or MRI scans even when they are not suggested by the clinical evaluation.

Pseudotumor cerebri is an interesting metabolic disorder characterized by fluid retention in the brain. As its name suggests, pseudotumor mimics real tumor because the fluid retention causes increased intracranial pressure and thus leads to headaches and papilledema (Chapter 9). Although pseudotumor is found almost exclusively in obese young women who have menstrual irregularities, its etiology is unknown. A scan will indicate cerebral swelling, and a lumbar puncture will show markedly elevated CSF pressure (300 to 600 mm H_2O).

INDICATIONS FOR EVALUATION FOR BRAIN TUMORS

Brain tumors and related conditions should be evaluated without waiting for florid physical or mental deficits to appear. Physicians should not rely exclusively on the mental status examination to distinguish between psychologic disorders and brain tumors. In addition to surveillance for common symptoms of brain tumors, careful attention to common complaints of fatigue, weight loss, menstrual irregularity, or infertility should prompt evaluation for pituitary insufficiency and hypothyroidism.

Neurologists generally order a CT or MRI scan, admittedly quite liberally, for any patient who has intellectual decline, those over 50 years who develop substantial emotional changes, and most adults with headaches that are not clearly caused by vascular imbalance or muscle contraction (Chapter 9). They often also suggest a scan and other tests (Chapter 7) for patients who develop any new mental illness severe enough to warrant psychiatric hospitalization for the first time. In particular, they suggest a CT or MRI scan before depressed patients undergo electroshock therapy (ECT). A tumor or other mass lesion, in addition to possibly causing the depression, during ECT might either precipitate status epilepticus or swell and cause transtentorial herniation. Finally, whenever the patient is worried about a brain tumor, no matter how groundlessly, a scan might be performed to settle the issue and permit appropriate therapy to begin.

REFERENCES

Amino N, Mori H, Iwatani Y, et al: High prevalence of transient post-partum thyrotoxicosis and hypothyroidism. N Engl J Med *306*:849, 1982

Ch'ien LT, Aur RJA, Stagner S, et al: Long-term neurological implications of somnolence syndrome in children with acute lymphocytic leukemia. Ann Neurol *8*:273, 1980

Corsellis JAN, Goldberg GJ, Norton AR: "Limbic encephalitis" and its association with carcinoma. Brain *91*:481, 1968

Duffner PK, Cohen ME, Myers MH, et al: Survival of children with brain tumors. Neurology *36*:597, 1986

Kornblith PL, Walker MD, Cassady JR: Neurologic Oncology. Philadelphia, J. B. Lippincott Company, 1987

QUESTIONS: CHAPTER 19

1. An 8-year-old boy, who had a 6-week history of progressively greater difficulty with athletic activities, develops a severe headache, papilledema, and ataxia. Of the following, which is the most likely illness?

    a.   Meningioma of the cerebellum
    b.   Glioblastoma of the cerebrum
    c.   Metastatic carcinoma
    d.   Astrocytoma of the cerebellum

2. A 60-year-old man who has smoked two packs of cigarettes daily since age 20 develops psychomotor seizures. He has headaches, a left superior quadrantanopsia, and mild left hemiparesis. In addition, he has right-sided dysmetria and intention tremor. Of the following conditions, which is the most likely illness?

    a.   Subdural hematomas
    b.   Metastatic carcinoma: right temporal lobe and right cerebellar hemisphere
    c.   Glioblastoma of the left temporal lobe
    d.   Cerebrovascular accidents in the right temporal lobe and right cerebellar hemisphere

3. A 60-year-old woman has apathy and impaired ability to concentrate. Otherwise her history is unremarkable and neurologic examination is unrevealing. From a neurologic point of view, what should be the next step in her evaluation?

    a.   CT or MRI scan
    b.   EEG
    c.   Neuropsychologic testing
    d.   Additional preliminary assessment

4. A 30-year-old woman with neurofibromatosis has impaired ability to hear while listening with the telephone receiver next to her right ear. She also has tinnitus on the right and mild loss of auditory acuity on the right, but otherwise her neurologic examination is normal. Of the following, which is the most likely illness?

    a.   Left temporal lobe meningioma
    b.   Hysteria
    c.   Otitis media
    d.   Cerebellopontine angle tumor

5. A 55-year-old woman developed mild paresis of the left leg, where hyperactive DTRs and a Babinski sign were found. She refused further evaluation until 11 months later, when she had a seizure that began with clonic movements of the left foot, then leg, and finally the arm. On examination, there is left hemiparesis, hyperactive DTRs, and a Babinski sign. Of the following, which is the most likely illness?

    a.   Right cerebral glioblastoma
    b.   Right cerebral meningioma
    c.   Left cerebral glioblastoma
    d.   Left cerebral meningioma

6. Which of the following are apt to cause headaches in the elderly?

    a.   Subdural hematomas
    b.   Open-angle glaucoma
    c.   Brain tumors
    d.   Pseudotumor cerebri
    e.   Temporal arteritis
    f.   Nitroglycerin and other vasodilator medications

7. Brain tumor headaches often begin with headaches that are worse in the early morning, waking patients from sleep. Which of the following headaches typically also begin in the early morning?

    a.   Muscle contraction (tension) headache
    b.   Pseudotumor cerebri
    c.   Migraine
    d.   Trigeminal neuralgia
    e.   Postconcussive syndrome
    f.   Cluster headache

8. An obese 22-year-old woman with moderately severe, generalized headaches has papilledema and a right sixth cranial nerve palsy. She is alert and otherwise her neurologic and general medical examination is normal. After routine blood and chemistry tests are found to be normal, a CT scan shows small ventricles, but no indication of an intracranial mass lesion. What would be the most appropriate next step?

    a.   Arteriography to look for a brainstem glioma or cerebrovascular accident
    b.   EEG
    c.   Lumbar puncture to measure the pressure and withdraw CSF

9. A 45-year-old policeman with various emotional difficulties has become obsessed in thinking that he has a brain tumor. Careful medical and neurologic examinations are normal. What would most neurologists do next?

    a.   Offer reassurance.
    b.   Suggest psychotherapy.
    c.   Give an antidepressant.
    d.   Treat him for tension headaches.
    e.   Take other steps.

10. A 60-year-old man with pulmonary carcinoma develops confusion and agitation. He refuses a full neurologic examination, but physicians find that he has no obvious hemiparesis or nuchal rigidity. The CT of his head is normal. Which of the following are frequent causes of an alteration in mental state in such a patient?

    a. Seizures
    b. Pneumonia
    c. Liver metastases
    d. Increased intracranial pressure
    e. Inappropriate ADH secretion
    f. Hypercalcemia
    g. Hyperkalemia

11. Two months later in the above case, a CT scan reveals two ring-shaped lesions with surrounding lucency. The patient becomes combative during the evaluation. Which medication should be given?

    a. Haloperidol or another neuroleptic
    b. Antidepressants
    c. Steroids
    d. Hypnotics

12. A 65-year-old woman with an onset of dementia has no physical or neurologic abnormalities, aside from frontal release reflexes and hyperactive DTRs. A full laboratory and EEG evaluation reveals no specific abnormality. A CT scan shows atrophy and a small meningioma in the right parietal convexity. What would be the most appropriate next step?

    a. Have the tumor removed.
    b. Diagnose Alzheimer's disease tentatively and repeat the clinical evaluation and the CT scan in 6 to 12 months.

13. A 75-year-old man, who has longstanding dementia, suddenly develops increased irritability and behavioral disturbances. His cognitive impairments are pronounced, but not much more than usual. He has no change in his functional physical capacity, and a brief neurologic examination reveals no lateralized signs or indication of increased intracranial pressure. He is treated with a major tranquilizer. One week later, the patient became somnolent. Medication is stopped, but the patient does not return to his former behavior.

The next day, the patient has a seizure and subsequently is found to be comatose with a left hemiparesis. No abnormalities are found on a general medical examination, routine laboratory tests, or a CT scan (with and without contrast) of the head. The patient suddenly dies. Autopsy discloses cerebral atrophy and moderately large, chronic bilateral subdural hematomas. Which aspects of chronic subdural hematomas does this case illustrate?

    a. Subdural hematomas are apt to occur in the elderly, especially if there is a history of dementia and cerebral atrophy.
    b. Chronic subdural hematomas are often bilateral.
    c. Early in their course, chronic bilateral subdural hematomas often do not cause lateralized physical signs.
    d. Subdural hematomas may be undetected on CT scans because at some time they are isodense to the adjacent brain. They may be then manifested only by compression of the cerebral hemispheres and obliteration of the normal gyri and sulci pattern.
    e. Elderly people may develop subdural hematomas with little or no head trauma.

14. Which structure is *not* located in the posterior fossa?

    a. Sphenoid wing
    b. Bulb
    c. Basilar artery
    d. Cerebellum

15. Match the brain lesion with the group at risk:

    1. Chronic subdural hematoma

2. Cerebellar astrocytoma
3. Cerebral lymphoma
a. Drug addicts
b. Elderly individuals
c. Homosexuals
d. Children

16. Which of the following is *not* indicative of a pituitary adenoma?
a. Increased serum prolactin level
b. Cognitive impairment
c. Galactorrhea
d. Bitemporal hemianopsia
e. Decreased libido
f. Menstrual irregularity
g. Headaches
h. Bitemporal superior quadrantanopsia

17. Which of the following pituitary conditions is most likely to become apparent in a 14-year-old child and cause delayed puberty and social and academic decline?
a. Chromophobe adenoma
b. Prolactinoma
c. Cushing's syndrome
d. Craniopharyngioma

18. Which of the following conditions are usually manifest by papilledema when they are first detected?
a. Chromophobe adenoma   f. Pseudotumor cerebri
b. Obstructive hydrocephalus   g. Cerebral glioblastoma
c. Normal pressure hydrocephalus   h. Optic glioma
d. Cerebellar astrocytoma   i. Acoustic neuroma
e. Cerebral astrocytoma   j. Parasagittal meningioma

19. A 65-year-old man with metastatic prostate carcinoma has been in agony from bone metastases. He is agitated, demanding, and obsessed with acquiring narcotics. He has become a major management problem, and his family is also becoming disruptive. What should be a psychiatry consultant's initial response to this situation after being assured that the patient has no cerebral metastases, hypercalcemia, or other metabolic aberrations?
a. Help the primary physician control the patient's pain. Once the pain is controlled, the situation can be studied in detail.
b. Stop all medications because they can be the cause of the behavioral disorder.
c. Use major tranquilizers.
d. Before treating further, check with an MRI scan and a lumbar puncture for signs of cerebral metastases or opportunistic infections.

20. A 55-year-old man, who had had a "total resection" of a right frontal astrocytoma followed by whole brain radiotherapy 7 months before a psychiatry consultation, describes himself as "depressed." He has emotional dulling, anorexia, anxiety, insomnia, and a tendency to cry. Examination reveals a mild left-sided hemiparesis and a left homonymous hemianopsia, which were present since surgery, but no anosognosia or somatopagnosia. What are some of the likely neurologic causes of this patient's apparent depression?

ANSWERS

1. d. Since there is ataxia, the lesion is probably in the cerebellum. The papilledema indicates hydrocephalus. Astrocytomas, the most common variety of brain tumors occurring in childhood, typically develop in the cerebellum, and, in children, are curable.

2. b. The patient has partial complex seizures, visual field loss, and hemiparesis from a right temporal lobe lesion. He also has right-sided coordination impairments from a right cerebellar lesion. These two lesions are probably manifestations of multiple metastatic tumors, but multiple embolic CVAs are possible. Subdural hematomas rarely cause seizures or cerebellar dysfunction, although they also often occur bilaterally. He is too old to have developed multiple sclerosis, and headaches are not a symptom of this illness.

3. d. Patients who may have either psychologic or medical (including neurologic) illness should have a complete physical examination. They usually should have routine medical tests that include CBC, SMA 6 and 12, thyroid function, and serology tests. Of those tests aimed at detecting a brain tumor, a CT or MRI scan is the most efficient. An EEG may be helpful because of the possibility of Creutzfeldt-Jakob disease and metabolic abnormalities associated with dementia. Of course, at the conclusion of the evaluation, the patient might be diagnosed as having pseudodementia.

4. d. Neurofibromatosis or von Recklinghausen's disease is associated with neuromas of the acoustic nerve, optic nerve gliomas, and meningiomas. Acoustic neuromas, the most common cerebellopontine angle tumor, typically cause speech discrimination impairment, tinnitus, and gradual loss of auditory acuity. Lesions of the cerebral hemispheres or the brainstem do not cause such auditory disturbances (Chapter 4).

5. b. The evolution of a hemiparesis over a relatively long (11-month) time, especially when it is accompanied by a partial (motor) seizure, suggests a cerebral tumor. In view of the chronicity, a meningioma is more likely than a glioblastoma.

6. a, c, e, f. Open-angle glaucoma (b) is not associated with headaches. Pseudotumor (d), although it causes headaches, occurs almost exclusively in young adults.

7. c, f. Migraine and cluster headaches characteristically develop during REM sleep, which occurs predominantly in the early morning.

8. c. A lumbar puncture for diagnostic and therapeutic reasons should be performed as soon as possible. The patient has pseudotumor cerebri with stretching of the sixth cranial nerves. (Sixth or third cranial nerve dysfunction because of increased intracranial pressure is called a "false localizing sign.") In pseudotumor, the CSF pressure will usually be above 300 mm—markedly elevated. Prolonged papilledema, because of untreated increased intracranial pressure, will lead to optic atrophy and then blindness. Pseudotumor is one of the rare exceptions when lumbar puncture is done in the presence of papilledema.

9. e. Even though brain tumors are rare in people at that age, most neurologists would, of course, order a CT or MRI scan for several reasons. At the onset, about 50 percent of the patients with tumors have no overt physical neurologic deficits referable to a tumor. Other structural lesions, such as an arteriovenous malformation or subdural hematoma, could be responsible for the patient's symptoms. Furthermore, with a normal scan, a neurologist can give more secure reassurance, feel protected in the event of a medical-legal problem, and refer the patient to a psychiatrist who will feel more confidence in accepting the patient.

10. a, b, c, d, e, f.

11. a, c. A neuroleptic should be given at least until the patient's behavioral disturbances subside. Since steroids, such as dexamethasone (Decadron, Hexadrol, and others), will reduce the edema and thus the volume of the lesion, they will bring about a rapid and dramatic, although short-lived, improvement in most cases. Some neurologists would also prophylactically give an anticonvulsant because cerebral metastases often cause seizures.

12. b. The meningioma is probably irrelevant to the dementia. These tumors grow so slowly that they can be followed with periodic scans. They should be removed, of course, if they are large enough to compress brain tissue or become symptomatic. An MRI scan might be more helpful than a CT scan in demonstrating that the lesion is a meningioma but not whether the patient has Alzheimer's disease.

13. a, b, c, d, e.

14. a.

15. 1-b; 2-d; 3-a and c.

16. b.

17. d. Unlike other tumors that cause pituitary insufficiency, craniopharyngiomas are congenital lesions that are typically located in the suprasellar region. Also, since they develop in children as well as adults, these tumors can cause delayed puberty and poor school performance. When craniopharyngiomas are large, they cause the visual impairments characteristic of pituitary tumors, e.g., bitemporal hemianopsia or superior quadrantanopsia and optic atrophy. They also tend to cause diabetes insipidus, because they develop in the hypothalamus, and obstructive hydrocephalus whenthey grow to occlude the third ventricle. They are cystic and have calcium on CT, MRI, and histologic studies.

18. b, d, f. Tumors and other conditions that lead to hydrocephalus usually cause papilledema early in the course of the illness. In contrast, small and infiltrating tumors usually do not produce enough mass effect to cause papilledema before they come to medical attention. Other symptoms, such as seizures, are the first manifestations. In other words, it is a mistake to exclude a tumor as a diagnostic consideration just because a patient does not have papilledema.

19. a and possibly c. Metastases to the brain from prostatic cancer are very rare, but ones to bone are common, and they are very painful. Usually bone pain from metastatic prostate cancer is controlled with hormonal manipulation, radiotherapy, and narcotic analgesics that are administered on an "as needed (PRN)" basis. If the pain persists, drug-seeking behavior is expectable. Then pain must be controlled with long-acting narcotics, such as methadone, or narcotics given by continuous intravenous infusion. The narcotics, which act on the CNS, may be enhanced by steroids and nonsteroidal anti-inflammatory agents, which act on the sites of bone metastases. Additional analgesia, and also mood improvement and sleep restfulness, may be gained if amitriptyline is administered. Until these changes are implemented, major tranquilizers may be required.

20. Despite a surgeon's reassurance that he was able to remove a tumor "entirely," the nature of astrocytomas when they occur in the cerebral hemispheres is that they are infiltrating and that total removal of all tumor cells is rarely accomplished. Sometimes, however, total removal is possible when the large region of surrounding brain is removed. Such surgery is possible only with the nondominant frontal lobe or sometimes with the tip of either frontal, temporal, or occipital lobe.

If the tumor persists, it probably has grown through the corpus callosum to invade the other frontal lobe. This patient would then be displaying signs of bilateral frontal lobe injury, which is manifested by personality changes and pseudobulbar palsy.

Some investigators claim that depression and similar changes in affect are especially common with nondominant cerebral hemisphere damage. However, to the extent that patients have anosognosia, left-sided neglect, and other aspects of the nondominant parietal lobe syndrome, they would be indifferent to a left-sided hemiparesis and other deficits. Another possibility is that the cerebral radiation has caused radiation necrosis. This side effect, in which cerebral arteries become occluded, usually causes diffuse cerebral dysfunction and often motor as well as mental impairments. It typically begins between 6 and 18 months after the completion of radiotherapy. Since most brain tumor patients are usually treated with anticonvulsants and steroids, all the indications, interactions, and serum concentrations of the medications should be evaluated. The side effects of anticonvulsants include liver dysfunction, apathy, confusion, and sedation. Steroids may induce anxiety, insomnia, and, in high doses, marked mental aberrations, i.e., steroid psychosis.

This patient might benefit from antidepressant medications. Even though the problem is likely to be mostly neurologic and uncorrectable, antidepressants might elevate the patient's mood, help his sleeplessness, and reduce the pathologic crying.

20

Lumbar Puncture, Computed Tomography, and Magnetic Resonance Imaging

LUMBAR PUNCTURE

Examining a sample of CSF (cerebrospinal fluid), usually obtained by a lumbar puncture (LP)* is most often required to evaluate signs of meningitis (headache, fever, and nuchal rigidity) or symptoms of a subarachnoid hemorrhage (the sudden development of a severe headache, especially if described as the worst of the patient's life). In evaluating patients with dementia, a lumbar puncture is indicated, but only for those who may have a systemic illness, syphilis, acquired immunodeficiency syndrome (AIDS), or other illness that causes immunosuppression: these patients might have neurosyphilis or cryptococcal or tuberculous meningitis. In children who develop dementia, an LP is indicated because they could have subacute sclerosing panencephalitis (SSPE), which is diagnosed by the presence of antimeasles antibodies in the CSF. On the otherhand, a lumbar puncture is not necessary in cases of dementia attributable to Alzheimer's disease or multiple infarctions.

In several neurologic illnesses, the CSF can reveal characteristic abnormalities. For example, in Guillain-Barré syndrome (Chapter 5), the CSF has a high protein concentration in contrast to only a slight increase in cell concent. In multiple sclerosis (Chapter 15), the CSF often contains oligoclonal bands and myelin basic protein.

Only a few guidelines are available for correlating neurologic illnesses with abnormalities in the CSF color, white blood cell count, and concentration of protein and glucose (the "CSF profile"). With most infectious or inflammatory illnesses, but with the notable exception of Guilllain-Barré syndrome, the CSF has an increase in the white blood cell count (a "CSF pleocytosis") that is parallelled by a rise in protein concentration and a decrease in the glucose concentration. In bacterial meningitis this trend is accentuated, and CSF pleocytosis is polymorphonuclear instead of lymphocytic. With the exception of several infective agents for which antigen testing is immediately available, reliable identification of virus, fungus, and mycobacterium often requires 1 to 3 weeks of culture. Therefore, the patient's initial diagnosis and first several

---

* The cost of a lumbar puncture in 1989 is about $250.

TABLE 20–1.   CEREBROSPINAL FLUID (CSF) PROFILES*

	Color	WBC/mm	Protein (mg/100 ml)	Glucose (mg/100 ml)	Miscellaneous
Normal	Clear	0–4†	30–45	60–100	
Bacterial meningitis	*Turbid*	*100–500°*	*75–200*	*0–40*	Gram-stain may reveal organisms
Viral meningitis	*Turbid*	*50–100†*	50–100	40–60	
TB and fungal meningitis‡	*Turbid*	*100–500†*	100–500	40–60	Cryptococcal antigen should be ordered
Neurosyphilis	Clear	5–200†	*45–100*	40–80	VDRL positive§
Guillain-Barré syndrome	Clear	5–20†	*80–200*	60–100	
Subarachnoid hemorrhage	*Bloody*	#	45–80	60–100	Supernatant usually xanthochromic

* Characteristic abnormalities in italics.
° Mostly polymorphonuclear cells.
† Mostly lymphocytes.
‡ In carcinomatous meningitis, the CSF profile is similar to fungal meningitis, but malignant cells may be detected.
§ About 40 percent of neurosyphilis cases have a false-negative VDRL CSF test (see Chapter 7).
# White and red cells are in same proportion as in blood (1:1,000).

days of treatment are usually based on the clinical evaluation and the CSF profile (Table 20-1).

In some circumstances, despite the potential value of the CSF examination, a lumbar puncture is sometimes contraindicated. It should not be performed when patients have an extensive sacral decubitus ulcer because the lumbar puncture needle may drive bacteria into the spinal canal. It should not be performed above the first lumbar vertebra, the lower boundary of the spinal cord, so that the spinal cord will not be struck by the needle.

The most common contraindication to a lumbar puncture is the presence of an intracranial mass lesion. This prohibition is based on the fear that a lumbar puncture could suddenly reduce pressure in the spinal canal and lead to transtentorial herniation caused by the unopposed force of a cerebral mass (Fig. 19-3). Moreover, CSF examination is not helpful in diagnosing most mass lesions, such as brain tumors, cerebrovascular accidents (CVAs), subdural hematomas, and toxoplasmosis abscesses, because their CSF profile is not distinctive. Therefore, unless physicians suspect acute bacterial meningitis or subarachnoid hemorrhage, where rapid diagnosis is crucial, they usually do not perform a lumbar puncture or they postpone it until after an intracranial lesion has been excluded by computed tomography (CT) or magnetic resonance imaging (MRI).

COMPUTED TOMOGRAPHY

Computed tomography displays the brain, skull, other tissues, and various abnormalities in a black to white scale, with the normal brain being gray. Structures that are increasingly more radiodense than brain, such as tumors, blood, and calcifications, are increasingly closer to white. Structures that are increasingly less radiodense than the brain, particularly the ventricles, which are filled with CSF, are increasingly closer to black. Common lesions that are virtually black are cerebral infarctions, chronic subdural hematomas, and the edema surrounding tumors.

When iodine-containing "contrast" solutions are administered, blood-filled structures become more radiodense. This phenomenon, "contrast enhancement," highlights vascular structures, such as arteriovenous malformations, glioblastomas, and the membranes of chronic subdural hematomas.

In several situations CT should be avoided or modified. Since CT exposes the patient to a dose of ionizing radiation that is slightly greater than that of a conventional x-ray skull series, even though the radiation dose is still relatively small and is confined to the head, CT examinations must be limited in number and avoided in pregnant women. Also, since the contrast solution can provoke a reaction in individuals who are allergic to iodine-containing substances, including shellfish, contrast solutions should be selectively administered. Also, contrast solution administration should be avoided in patients with diabetes, dehydration, or other hyperviscosity states because, since they are hyperosmolar, contrast solutions might precipitate renal failure.

CT and MRI scans, which are generally cost-effective,* are far more reliable than the electroencephalogram (EEG), conventional x-ray skull series, or isotopic brain scan. They are indicated for numerous neurologic conditions, including dementia, delirium, aphasia, other neuropsychologic deficits, headaches in elderly individuals, partial seizures, and clinical or EEG evidence of structural lesions (Figs. 20-1 to 20-12). These scans are usually not particularly indicated, however, in cases of chronic pain, sleep disturbances, absence (petit mal) seizures, cluster and migraine headaches, Parkinson's disease, tics, and essential tremor. They are clearly not indicated in evaluation of muscle and peripheral nerve diseases, including myasthenia gravis, amyotrophic lateral sclerosis (ALS), polyneuropathy, and muscular dystrophy—diseases of the peripheral nervous system or muscles.

Although specific criteria are not yet established for ordering CT or MRI scans for individuals who appear to have psychiatric illness, their use has become commonplace in the evaluation of patients who have developed atypical psychosis, profound depression, episodic behavioral disturbances, or clinical or EEG signs that a structural lesion is present. These scans can exclude structural lesions that could account for the psychiatric symptoms; however, relationships remain problematic between psychiatric symptoms and cerebral atrophy, small cerebral lesions, and congenital abnormalities.

Although CT and MRI scans generally show no differences between most psychiatric patients and controls, several studies have shown that about 20 percent of chronic schizophrenic patients, compared to those with affective disorders and to control groups, have large CSF-filled lateral ventricles and a small brain volume. This hydrocephalus, called "hydrocephalus ex vacuo" or "increased ventricular-brain ratio," is most pronounced in the temporal horns of the lateral ventricles. Another difference is that some schizophrenic patients lack the normal cerebral asymmetry, in which the cortex of the dominant (usually left) hemisphere is normally more convoluted than that of the non-dominant (Chapter 8). The abnormal ventricular enlargement in schizophrenic

---

* In 1989, the approximate cost of a CT scan is $250 and an MRI scan $750.

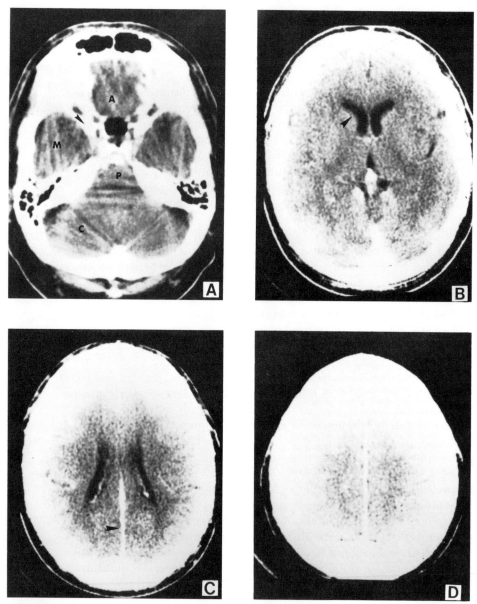

FIGURE 20–1. Four representative, progressively higher *transaxial*, or *axial*, view CT scans of a normal brain. *A*, The anterior fossae *A*, contain the anterior frontal lobes and the olfactory nerves. Immediately posterior is a circular black area, which represents the sella turcica. However, artifacts from bone and relatively poor resolution prevent visualization of its pituitary gland. The middle fossae (*M*) contain the anterior temporal lobes, which are situated behind the sphenoid wing (*arrowhead*). The posterior fossa contains the cerebellum. (*C*), and the medulla and pons (*P*), which are called the bulb. The black streaks that seem to cut across the posterior fossa are artifacts from the skull. *B*, The anterior horns of the lateral ventricles are concave because of indentation by the heads of the caudate nuclei (*arrowhead*). A calcified pineal gland is the small white structure in the center. The third ventricle is the small triangular black area anterior to the pineal gland. *C*, The lateral ventricles spread lengthwise in the hemispheres, which are separated by the white, straight sagittal sinus (*arrowhead*). *D*, The cerebral cortex is adjacent to the inner table of the skull. Since the normal gyri are separated by thin sulci, individual gyri are not discernible.

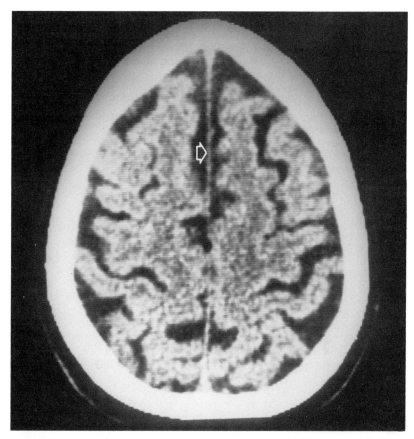

FIGURE 20–2. This CT scan shows cerebral atrophy. The gyri are thin and distinct, and the sulci are prominent and wide. Because of the atrophy, the cerebral cortex is retracted from the inner table of the skull and from the sagittal sinus (*open arrow*)—in contrast to the normal situation (Fig. 20-1D) in which the gyri are indistinguishable, sulci are not discernible, and the cortex seems to blend into the skull. Cerebral atrophy, as pictured in this CT scan, is a normal concomitant of old age, and it is not necessarily associated with intellectual deterioration. However, it is closely associated with Alzheimer's disease, Down's syndrome, AIDS-dementia complex, alcoholism, degenerative neurologic illnesses, some varieties of schizophrenia, and numerous other conditions. See Figure 20-16 for the MRI appearance of cerebral atrophy.

patients is associated with severe psychiatric illness and is not attributable to age, medication, or electroshock therapy. Compared to patients without the ventricular enlargement, these patients more frequently have a history of perinatal complications, a preponderance of negative symptoms (in most studies), greater resistance to neuroleptics, more cognitive impairments, and worse outcomes.

Loss of cerebral asymmetry, other dominant hemisphere abnormalities, and also relatively small cerebellar hemispheres have been described in children with autism. However, these cerebral abnormalities have been found inconsistently and were present mostly in children who also had mental retardation or congenital physical neurologic impairments.

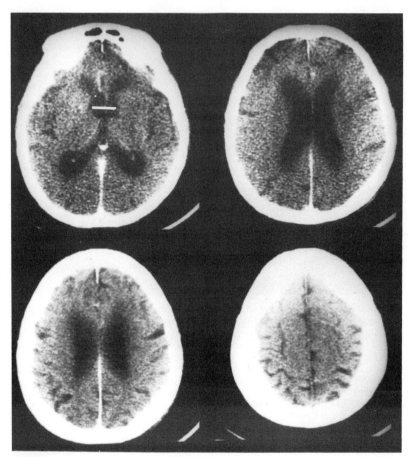

FIGURE 20–3.   This CT scan illustrates that cerebral atrophy also leads to expansion of the lateral ventricles, "hydrocephalus ex vacuo" or an "increased ventricular-brain ratio," and widening of the third ventricle (*line*).

FIGURE 20–4. *Top two scans*, In normal pressure hydrocephalus (NPH), CT scans show ventricular dilation, including widening of the ventricular horns of the lateral ventricles (Fig. 20-15), but little or no cerebral atrophy. *Bottom two scans*, Following instillation of a shunt (*open arrow*), the size of the ventricles decreases. In this pair of scans, notice the linear artifacts emanating from the shunt. Unfortunately, the distinction between NPH and hydrocephalus ex vacuo, based exclusively on CT and MRI scans, is unreliable.

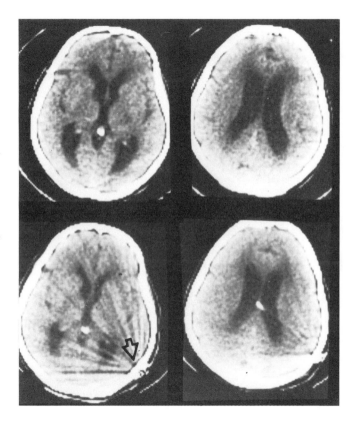

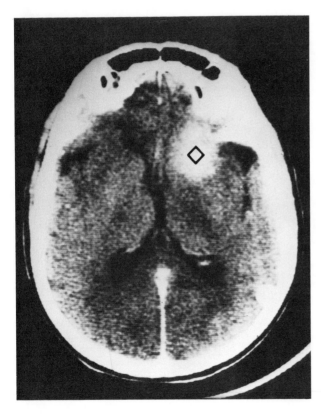

FIGURE 20–5. This CT scan shows a radiodense lesion (*diamond*), typical of a meningioma, arising from the right sphenoid wing. These lesions can irritate the temporal lobe posteriorly, triggering partial complex seizures, or they can grow anteriorly and compress the frontal lobe and the olfactory (first cranial) nerve, i.e., cause the Foster-Kennedy syndrome (Chapter 4). In contrast to glioblastomas (Fig. 20-6A), large infarctions (Fig. 20-8A), and subdural hematomas (Fig. 20-10), meningiomas are slowly developing and exert little mass effect. Moreover, small meningiomas are commonplace and do not produce mental changes. Because of their radiodense calcium composition, which contains virtually no water, meningiomas are one of the few structural lesions that are more readily visualized on CT than MRI scans.

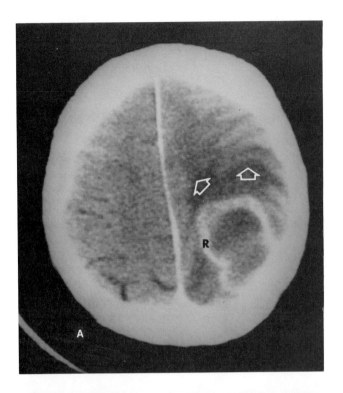

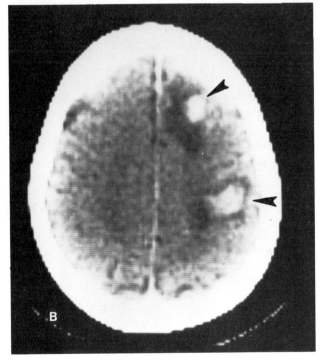

FIGURE 20–6.   *A*, This contrast-enhanced CT scan illustrates a glioblastoma. A dark region of the tumor is surrounded by the characteristic white, contrast enhancing ring (*R*) and a large border of black brain edema (*open arrows*). The mass effect of the lesion compresses the adjacent brain and shifts midline structures, such as the sagittal sinus, contralaterally. *B*, This CT scan, which is also contrast-enhanced, shows two metastatic tumors (*arrows*) in the right cerebral hemisphere. Each metastatic tumor is radiodense because of the contrast administration, relatively solid, and surrounded by edema. Distinguishing between a glioblastoma and a single metastatic lesion is often difficult.

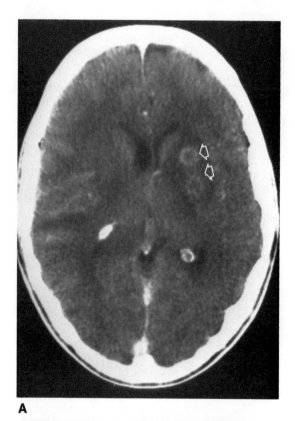

A

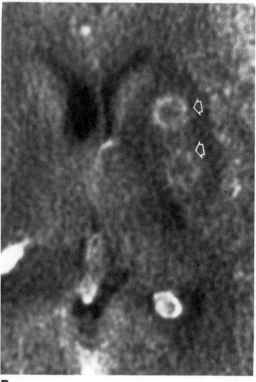

B

FIGURE 20–7. A contrast-enhanced CT scan (*A*) and an enlargement of a section (*B*) of two toxoplasmosis lesions (*open arrows*) in an AIDS patient. Both lesions are circular, white, and surrounded by dark areas that indicate cerebral edema. The adjacent anterior horn of the lateral ventricle is compressed, and the normally calcified choroid plexus, which is large, white, and circular, is pushed posteriorly—signs of swelling of the cerebral hemisphere. See Figure 20-18 for toxoplasmosis detected by MRI.

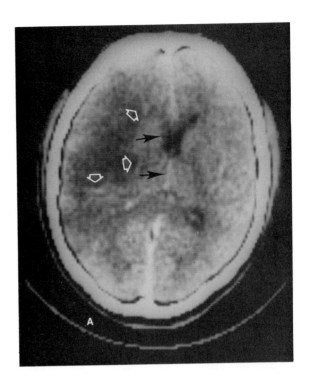

FIGURE 20–8. *A*, This CT scan of a left middle cerebral artery infarction (*open arrows*) is typically radiolucent. The infarction is so large that it has a mass effect that compresses the adjacent lateral ventricle and shifts midline structures contralaterally (*solid arrows*). *B*, This CT scan shows a right parietal cerebral hemorrhage. Since blood is relatively radiodense, the hemorrhage is seen as a white globular area (*arrows*). It has a mass effect that obliterates the occipital horn of the ipsilateral lateral ventricle. The three small white areas are the normally calcified choroid plexus of the third and lateral ventricles.

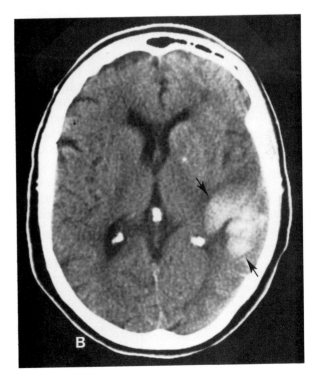

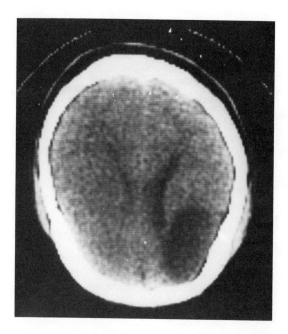

FIGURE 20–9. A porencephaly is a common congenital cerebral injury that is often responsible for seizures, spastic contralateral hemiparesis, and mental retardation. Since it is less dense than brain, the porencephaly is radiolucent, and it has an effect opposite to that of a mass lesion: its absence of brain tissue leads to expansion of the adjacent lateral ventricle and ipsilateral shift of midline structures.

MAGNETIC RESONANCE IMAGING

When nuclei are placed in a strong magnetic field and exposed to radiofrequency stimulation, their own magnetic field is altered, and they "vibrate" (resonate). After the stimulation, the nuclei emit energy as they resume their usual states. In the brain, the energy is emitted mostly from hydrogen nuclei (protons) in water-containing tissue. The 20 percent greater water content of gray matter compared to white matter and the differences in water content among various tissues result in *signals* of different *intensity*. These signals eventually generate the MRI scans.

MRI scans offer extraordinary resolution and several other advantages over CT (Table 20-2). By simple manipulations in the software, rather than by having to contort the patient, MRI scans of the brain can be generated in the three major planes: transaxial (conventional top-down view), coronal (front-to-back view), and sagittal (side view). Another advantage of MRI is that, since most of the skull is comprised of cortical bone, which contains no water, images of the brain are free of interference from the skull. Thus, MRI can generate

TABLE 20–2.   ADVANTAGES OF MRI OVER CT

Greater imaging ability
  Has greater resolution: can detect smaller objects
  Distinguishes white from gray matter
  Displays images routinely in three planes
Absence of interference from bone
  Can display posterior fossa structures, pituitary gland, eyeballs
  Can image the spinal cord
Nonutilization of ionizing radiation
Ability to indicate certain illnesses
  Reveals plaques of multiple sclerosis

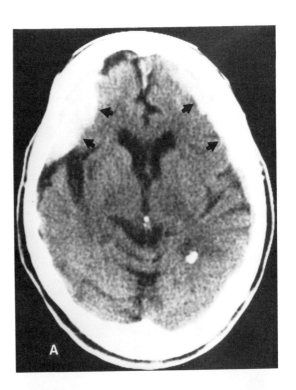

FIGURE 20–10. *A*, Since *acute* subdural hematomas (*arrows*) contain fresh blood, which is radiodense compared to brain, they are white on a CT scan. Large ones compress the underlying brain and cause headaches, stupor, and lateralized neurologic signs, such as hemiparesis. If these acute subdural hematomas are not removed by neurosurgery, they can cause transtentorial herniation (Figs. 19-1 and 19-3). Large acute subdural hematomas cause a rapidly evolving neurologic picture that is not likely to be confused with dementia, a thought disorder, or an emotional disturbance. *B*, In contrast, small and slowly evolving, *chronic* subdural hematomas (*arrows*) contain aged, liquefied blood, which is less radiodense than brain. Chronic subdural hematomas are black on a CT scan and are usually bordered by a radiodense, contrast-enhancing membrane. They compress the underlying brain, although to a lesser extent than do acute subdural hematomas. Chronic subdural hematomas cause weeks of headache, cognitive impairments, and personality change, but little or no hemiparesis or other lateralized neurologic sign. Thus, a chronic subdural hematoma might initially be mistaken for a psychiatric disorder.

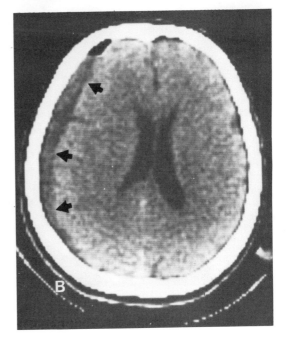

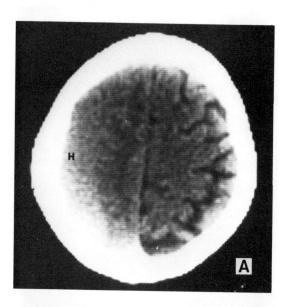

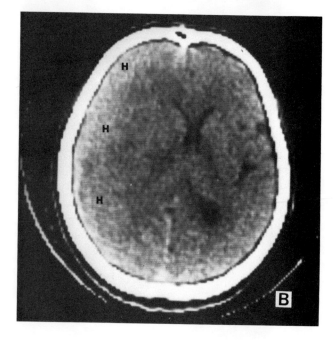

FIGURE 20–11. Between the time that subdural hematomas are acute and chronic, their density is equal, *isodense,* to brain. Isodense subdural hematomas, which may cause the clinical features of chronic subdural hematomas, are almost indistinguishable from the underlying brain on the CT scan because the interior of the hematoma (*H*), like the brain, is gray; however, their presence is suggested by a unilateral "loss" by compression of the gyri-sulci pattern (*A*), and signs of a mass, such as shift of midline structures (*B*).

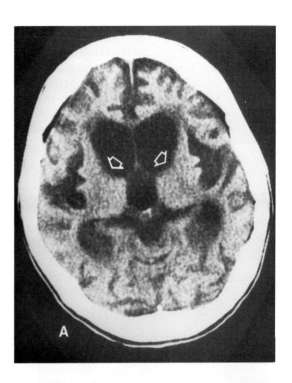

FIGURE 20–12. *A*, This CT scan shows the brain of a patient with Huntington's disease. The characteristic abnormality is that the anterior horns of the lateral ventricles are convex because of atrophy of the caudate nuclei (*arrows*). Contrast the shape of the ventricles in Huntington's disease to the normal shape (Fig. 20-1B) and that seen in hydrocephalus ex vacuo (Fig. 20-3)—in both of these conditions, the ventricles are concave. In addition, in Huntington's disease, as in many other illnesses, the brain is atrophied, sulci are copious, and ventricles are massively enlarged. *B*, This *coronal* view of the MRI scan of the same patient also shows the convex expansion of the ventricles, gigantic sulci and sylvian fissures (*S*), and cerebral atrophy. Compare this scan to the coronal view of the normal brain (Fig. 20-13B). These changes, as dramatic as they may be, occur long after the disease can be diagnosed on clinical grounds. However, positron emission tomography may show changes earlier than the CT or MRI scan in Huntington's disease.

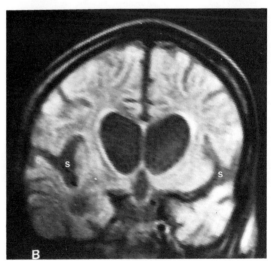

detailed images of the cerebellum and other posterior fossa contents, pituitary gland, spinal cord, eyes, and other structures that are shielded from ionizing radiation by bony casings (Figs. 20-13 to 20-18). On the other hand, MRI poorly detects lesions with little or no water content, such as some meningiomas.

Although administration of contrast solutions is not necessary, newly available "paramagnetic" agents, such as gadopentetate, enhance intracranial abnormalities. In addition to detecting small intracranial and intraspinal structures, MRI can assist the diagnosis of illnesses in which the composition of the brain tissue is altered. For example, MRI can reveal the characteristic white matter plaques of multiple sclerosis and the subtle white matter changes of progressive multifocal leukoencephalopathy (PML).

However, MRI is no more effective than CT in diagnosing several major illnesses—Alzheimer's disease, AIDS-dementia complex, and psychiatric illnesses. Also, compared to CT, MRI has some notable disadvantages (Table 20-3). The MRI procedure, which takes 30 to 40 minutes, requires that patients be placed entirely within the bore of the magnet, which is an awesome long and narrow tunnel with an opening that is just slightly wider than their body and a length of about 9 feet. Even excluding individuals known to be vulnerable to claustrophobia, at least 10 percent of other patients, sometimes in a state of

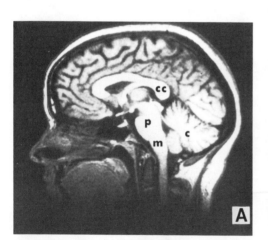
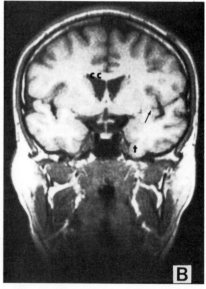

FIGURE 20–13. *A,* An MRI *sagittal* view of a normal brain reveals exquisitely detailed cerebral gyri and sulci, the corpus callosum (*cc*), and the three main structures of the posterior fossa—the pons (*p*), medulla (*m*), and cerebellum (*c*). In addition, the cervicomedullary junction and various non-neurologic soft tissue structures are apparent. *B,* This MRI coronal view illustrates the corpus callosum (*cc*), the "great commissure," bridging the cerebral hemispheres. The white matter of the corpus callosum and subcortical cerebral hemispheres is distinct from the ribbon of gray matter of the cerebral cortex. The anterior horns of the lateral ventricles, with their concave lateral borders, are beneath the corpus callosum and anterior and medial to the caudate nuclei and internal capsule (Figs. 7-6 and 18-1A). The cerebral cortex around the left sylvian fissure (*arrow*) is usually more convoluted than that around the right, conferring greater cortical area for language function on the dominant hemisphere. The frontal lobe is above the sylvian fissure and the temporal lobe is below. The medial-inferior surface of the temporal lobe (*t*), which is the origin of most partial complex seizures, is sequestered by the bulk of the temporal lobe above and the sphenoid wing anteriorly. It is far from the sites of conventional scalp EEG electrodes.

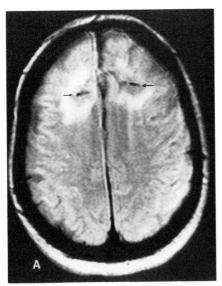
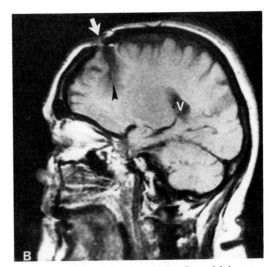

FIGURE 20–14. This MRI scan was performed on a patient who had had a frontal lobotomy about 40 years previously. As in this case, this surgical procedure did not involve removing the frontal lobes, but rather drilling a hole through the skull above each frontal lobe and passing a sharp instrument down into the brain immediately anterior to the motor cortex. The surgeon would attempt to sever the white matter tracts that are connections to the anterior frontal lobe; however, the incision would usually only interrupt the superior connections. *A,* The axial view shows black horizontal slits, the incisions (*arrows*), which are surrounded by scar tissue. *B,* This sagittal view through the right cerebral hemisphere shows the skull defect (*white arrow*), where the incision starts, and the lowermost extent of the incision (*black arrow*), which is only about halfway down through the frontal lobe. The frontal lobe anterior to the incision is atrophied. A posterior portion of the lateral ventricle may be seen (*V*).

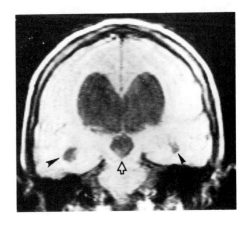

FIGURE 20–15. This MRI scan shows a coronal view of the brain of a patient with normal pressure hydrocephalus. It demonstrates the classic findings: in the absence of cerebral atrophy, dilation of the lateral ventricles, their temporal horns (*black arrows*), and the third ventricle (*open arrow*).

TABLE 20–3. DISADVANTAGES OF MRI OVER CT

Cost is approximately three times greater than CT.

Scan requires about 40 minutes, more than twice as long as CT.

Being in the magnet tunnel often precipitates a claustrophobic reaction.

Ferrous metal devices cannot be placed near the MRI magnet.

    Patients cannot have a pacemaker, intracranial aneurysm "clip," or many other implanted ferrous metal devices.

    Respirators and most other life-supporting machinery cannot be placed near the magnet.

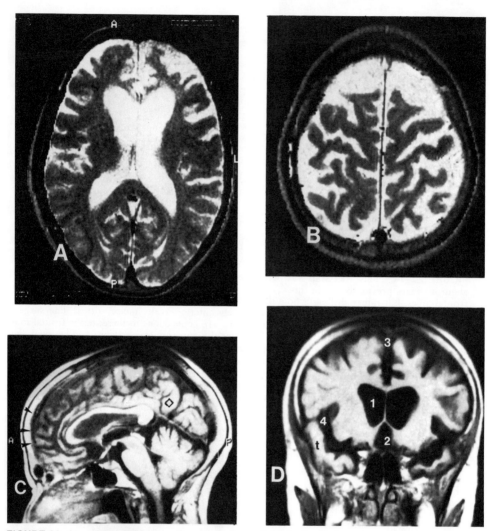

FIGURE 20–16. These MRI scans show four views of cerebral atrophy, which can be contrasted to the normal brain (Fig. 20-13). MRI emphasizes cerebral atrophy because it does not detect the cortical bone of the skull, which contains virtually no water. The head is visualized because the scalp, blood, fat, and other soft tissue contain water. MRI provides exquisite detail, multiple views, and little artifact, but no indication of the etiology of cerebral atrophy. *A,* In an axial view through the cerebral hemispheres, the CSF is white and fills the dilated lateral ventricles and sulci. Since the frontal lobe gyri are more atrophied than those of the other lobes, the CSF fills the frontal sulci and the anterior interhemispheric fissure. *B,* In a higher axial view, the surface of the brain has thin gyri and copious amounts of CSF in the sulci and over the cortex, occupying the void left by the atrophied brain. *C,* In a sagittal view, where the MRI is programmed not to detect a signal from CSF, it shows thin, ribbon-like frontal lobe gyri (*arrowheads*) and less atrophied parietal lobe gyri (*diamond*). The corpus callosum, pons, and cerebellum are easily visualized. *D,* In a coronal view through the frontal lobes, also where the CSF is not portrayed, the typical manifestations of cerebral atrophy include (*1*) dilated lateral ventricles, (*2*) an enlarged third ventricle, (*3*) enlargement of the anterior interhemispheric fissure because of separation of the medial surfaces of the frontal lobes, and (*4*) massively dilated Sylvian fissures with the atrophic temporal lobe (t) below and the atrophic frontal lobe above.

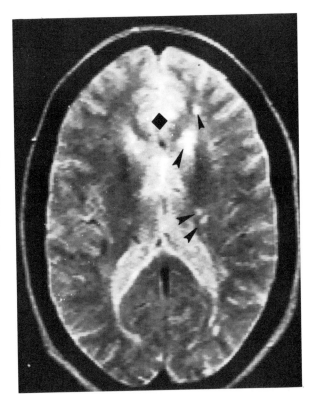

FIGURE 20–17. This MRI scan shows multiple cerebral plaques in a patient with multiple sclerosis. As is typical, the lesions are white and are clustered in the white matter deep in the cerebral hemispheres, particularly in the periventricular regions (*arrowheads*) and the frontal lobe (*diamond*).

panic, will abort the procedure. Wearing a sleep mask or prophylactically taking minor tranquilizers might ameliorate fear, but heavy sedation is inadvisable because a patient's respiratory rate cannot be easily monitored during the procedure.

A potentially life-threatening problem with MRI is that all nearby ferrous metals are attracted or adversely affected by the MRI magnet. Pacemakers, implanted hearing devices, intracranial aneurysm clips, and other implanted

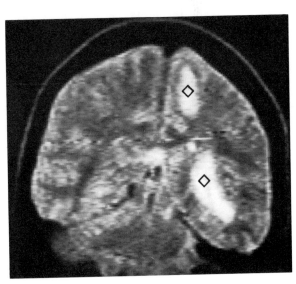

FIGURE 20–18. This MRI scan shows a coronal view of two toxoplasmosis lesions with surrounding edema (*diamonds*). Although MRI is more capable of detecting small and multiple toxoplasmosis lesions, CT is better able to portray their characteristic ring-like structure.

medical devices might be dislodged or ruined if the patient were exposed to the intense magnetic field of an MRI study. Likewise, patients who require respirators, electrocardiograph monitors, and other life-supporting machinery cannot undergo an MRI study because the magnet would pull the devices away from the patient.

Positron Emission Tomography

In contrast to CT and MRI, which provide detailed images of the brain, spinal cord, and structural abnormalities, positron emission tomography (PET) roughly maps the relative metabolic activity of various brain regions. This technique is currently based on detecting energy, in the form of positrons, released during metabolism of fluorine-18 labeled fluorodeoxyglucose (FDG). Since FDG is absorbed into the brain and metabolized as though it were endogenous glucose, the rate of positron emission is directly proportional to the rate of glucose metabolism. In the future, PET will utilize other metabolic substrates, such as phosphate and dopamine.

PET has analyzed cerebral metabolism during normal activities, following administration of medications, and in a limited number of neurologic illnesses. It has shown that, in partial complex epilepsy, the affected temporal lobe is generally hypoactive in the interictal period but hyperactive during seizures. Deciding which temporal lobe is epileptogenic by this method, which is complementary to electroencephalography, is one step in determining whether surgical excision of temporal lobe tissue would benefit patients with intractable epilepsy. PET is also helpful in studying individuals who may be in the early stages of Parkinson's disease and Huntington's disease. In patients with Alzheimer's disease, but only in severe cases, PET shows decreased cerebral metabolism, especially in the frontal lobes. In patients with schizophrenia, most studies portray general cerebral hypometabolism, but some indicate that the frontal lobes are most affected. In patients with depressive illness, although unipolar and bipolar varieties may differ, patients also have cerebral hypometabolism.

In its current form, PET will probably not attain practical usefulness in most medical centers because it is prohibitively expensive. Moreover, logistical problems prevent use of the equipment: the FDG and other substrates must be produced in a cyclotron, and because of their rapid decay, the cyclotron must be near the PET facility.

A positive alternative is a similar but less sophisticated procedure, *single photon emission computed tomography (SPECT)*. Without requiring elaborate preparation of metabolic substrates, SPECT can provide useful maps of metabolic activity in the brain in Alzheimer's disease, Parkinson's disease, and structural lesions.

REFERENCES

Andreasen NC (ed): Brain Imaging: Applications in Psychiatry. Washington, American Psychiatric Press, 1989

Bondareff W, Raval J, Colletti PM, et al: Quantitative magnetic resonance imaging and the severity of dementia in Alzheimer's disease. Am J Psychiatry *145*:853, 1988

Brant-Zawadzki M, Norman D (eds): Magnetic Resonance Imaging of the Central Nervous System. New York, Raven Press, 1987

Cohen BM, Buonanno F, Keck PE, et al: Comparison of MRI and CT scans in a group of psychiatric patients. Am J Psychiatry *145*:1085, 1988

Damasio H, Maurer RG, Damasio AR, et al: Computerized tomographic scan findings in patients with autistic behavior. Arch Neurol *37*:504, 1980

Duara R, Grady C, Haxby J, et al: Positron emission tomography in Alzheimer's disease. Neurology *36*:879, 1986

Farkas T, Wolf AP, Jaeger J, et al: Regional brain glucose metabolism in chronic schizophrenia: A positron emission transaxial tomographic study. Arch Gen Psychiatry *41*:293, 1984

Gaffney GR, Isai LY, Kuperman S, et al: Cerebellar structure in autism. Am J Dis Child *141*:1330, 1987

Garber HJ, Weilburg JB, Buonanno FS, et al: Use of magnetic resonance imaging in psychiatry. Am J Psychiatry *145*:164, 1988

Gonzalez CF, Grossman CB, Masdeu JC: Head and Spine Imaging. New York, Wiley Medical, 1984

Hayden MR, Martin WRW, Stoessl AJ, et al: Positron emission tomography in the early diagnosis of Huntington's disease. Neurology *36*:888, 1986

Jacobson HG (ed): Instrumentation in positron emission tomography. JAMA *259*:1531, 1988

Jagust WJ, Budinger TF, Reed BR: The diagnosis of dementia with single photon emission computed tomography. Arch Neurol *44*:258, 1987

Johnson KA, Davis KR, Buonanno FS, et al: Comparison of magnetic resonance and roentgen ray computed tomography in dementia. Arch Neurol *44*:1075, 1987

Johnson KA, Holman BL, Mueller SP, et al: Single photon emission computed tomography in Alzheimer's disease. Arch Neurol *45*:392, 1988

Luchins DJ, Weinberger DR, Wyatt RJ: Schizophrenia and cerebral asymmetry detected by computed tomography. Am J Psychiatry *136*:753, 1982

Pandurangi AK, Bilder RM, Rieder RO, et al: Schizophrenic symptoms and deterioration: Relation to computed tomographic findings. J Nerv Ment Dis *176*:200, 1988

Prior MR, Tress B, Hoffman WL, et al: Computed tomography study of children with classic autism. Arch Neurol *41*:482, 1984

Schwartz JM, Baxter LR, Mazziotta JC, et al: The differential diagnosis of depression: Relevance of positron emission tomography studies of cerebral glucose metabolism to the bipolar-unipolar dichotomy. JAMA *258*:1368, 1987

Weinberger DR, Delisi LE, Perman GP, et al: Computed tomography in schizophreniform disorder and other acute psychiatric disorders. Arch Gen Psychiatry *39*:778, 1982

ADDITIONAL REVIEW QUESTIONS

Q1: A 60-year-old man is brought for evaluation of dementia. On mental status testing he performs poorly on questions that require memory. In contrast, he satisfactorily completes questions that require judgement, language, and other relatively sophisticated intellectual functions. How does this clinical picture differ from typical Alzheimer's disease dementia?

A1: The patient has a chronic *amnestic syndrome*, in which memory is impaired to a much greater degree than other intellectual functions. In typical Alzheimer's disease and multiple infarct dementia, memory is lost typically in proportion to judgment, insight, and other intellectual function. Although Alzheimer's disease patients can have an amnestic syndrome, it would be more typical of patients who have Wernicke-Korsakoff syndrome, partial complex status epilepticus, or temporal lobe injury, as can occur in head trauma, *Herpes simplex* encephalitis, and cerebrovascular accidents (CVAs). In some of these conditions, memory impairments are accompanied by features of the Klúver-Bucy syndrome.

Q2: A 22-year-old man with tonic-clonic seizures has about one seizure a week. Which of the following are likely causes of this high frequency of seizure activity?
    a. He does not comply with medication(s).
    b. There is the presence of hysteric as well as genuine seizures.
    c. He suffers from neurofibromatosis.
    d. He suffers from Jakob-Creutzfeldt disease.
    e. He suffers from tuberous sclerosis.
    f. He takes drugs, alcohol, or medications other than anticonvulsants.
    g. The wrong anticonvulsant or the incorrect dose has been prescribed.

A2: a, b, e, f, g.
    a. Noncompliance is a frequently occurring cause of "uncontrollable" or refractory seizures.
    b. Hysteric seizures are often found in patients with genuine seizure disorders.
    e. Tuberous sclerosis is a neurocutaneous disorder characterized by facial adenomata, dementia, and refractory seizures.
    f. Use of many medications interferes with anticonvulsant activity, although most often they potentiate anticonvulsant activity, precipitating toxicity.
    g. The physician should always consider the possibility that he or she erred in the diagnosis or treatment plan.

Q3: The patient is found to have a phenytoin (Dilantin) level of 8 mg/dL (the therapeutic level is 10 to 20 mg/dL). Of the possibilities listed above, which is the single most commonly occurring?

A3: a.

Q4: When therapeutic concentrations of phenytoin (Dilantin) are achieved, genuine seizures persist. Which of the plans should the physician follow?
    a.   Increase the phenytoin dose.
    b.   Stop the phenytoin.
    c.   Add a second anticonvulsant, such as phenobarbital, to phenytoin.
    d.   Reconsider the diagnosis and treatment.

A4: c, d.
    c.   Adding a second anticonvulsant, now that therapeutic levels of one anticonvulsant are achieved, is the best plan.
    d.   Reconsideration should always be performed when therapies do not achieve the expected result. Ideally, the patient would have EEG and videotape monitoring with frequent determinations of the anticonvulsant levels. However, little additional benefit will result and toxicity will ensue at greater than therapeutic levels. Abrupt cessation of any anticonvulsant may precipitate status epilepticus.

Q5: A 19-year-old Marine recruit has status epilepticus, fever, stupor, and nuchal rigidity. Which therapies or diagnostic tests should be performed as soon as possible?
    a.   Parenteral anticonvulsants
    b.   Oral anticonvulsants
    c.   Thiamine (50 mg IV)
    d.   Lumbar puncture
    e.   Penicillin or penicillin in combination with chloramphenicol

A5: a, d, e. The presumptive diagnosis is meningitis-induced seizures.

Q6: A 30-year-old man with a long history of aggressive behavior and other antisocial actions has an EEG that shows an isolated, phase-reversed spike focus intermittently over the left frontal lobe. Which statements are appropriate?
    a.   In retrospect, the behavioral disturbances were the result of partial complex (psychomotor) seizures.
    b.   The EEG has absolutely no bearing on the case.
    c.   Certain EEG abnormalities are characteristically found in antisocial people.
    d.   Both the EEG and the behavior may reflect cerebral damage.

A6: d. The EEG indicates the presence of a structural lesion in the left frontal lobe that could be a source of seizures. Lesions in the frontal lobe as well as those in the temporal lobe can cause the partial complex seizures. However, since there are no stereotyped behavioral disturbances and the EEG shows no paroxysmal activity, most neurologists would not make the diagnosis of seizures with the information at hand.

Q7: A 16-year-old woman who has had both absence (petit mal) and generalized tonic-clonic seizures, which require high doses of two anticonvulsants, has confusion, disorientation, agitation, and dysarthria. Otherwise her medical and neurologic examination reveals no abnormality. Which conditions may be the cause of her mental abnormalities?
    a.   Anticonvulsant intoxication
    b.   Postictal psychosis following an absence (petit mal)
    c.   Postictal psychosis following a tonic-clonic seizure
    d.   Petit mal status
    e.   Oral contraceptive-induced seizures

A7: a, c, d.
    a.   Anticonvulsant intoxication is common, and it is the most likely cause.
    c.   Postictal confusion is often accompanied by agitation and behavior abnormalities.
    d.   Petit mal status is rare but possible.
Incorrect answers:
    b.   There are no postictal symptoms with petit mal seizures.
    e.   There is no such entity.

Q8: In the case just described, what would be the best therapeutic plan after routine evaluation reveals no other abnormalities?
    a. Obtain blood for anticonvulsant determination.
    b. Obtain a CT or MRI scan to exclude a new structural lesion, such as a subdural hematoma.
    c. Give diazepam intravenously.
    d. Obtain an EEG.

A8: a, b, d.

Q9: An 8-year-old boy begins to have 10- to 20-second episodes of repetitive lip smacking, eyelid fluttering, and finger rubbing. During these episodes he is incoherent. Afterward he is confused and sleepy. What is the most likely diagnosis?
    a. Absence (petit mal) seizures
    b. Partial complex (psychomotor) seizures
    c. Attention deficit disorder
    d. Psychologic aberrations

A9: b This child is having typical partial complex seizures; he has incoherence, not loss of consciousness; stereotyped, simple, repetitive movements and sounds; and subsequent (postictal) confusion and somnolence. Such attacks have different manifestations, etiology, and treatment from absences (a).

Q10: If the EEG in the case just described shows an intraictal pattern that supports the diagnosis, which medicine would be the most appropriate?
    a. Valproate (Depakene)
    b. Carbamazepine (Tegretol)
    c. Phenytoin (Dilantin)
    d. Ethosuximide (Zarontin)

A10: b. Carbamazepine (Tegretol), although some authors might suggest phenytoin (Dilantin) or primidone (Mysoline).

Q11: During the course of evaluation for dementia, a patient's CT scan reveals a small, dense lesion without surrounding edema arising from the right parietal convexity. The brain is not compressed by the lesion, which is felt to be a meningioma. What symptoms might such a lesion likely cause?
    a. Dementia
    b. Partial complex seizures
    c. Absence seizures
    d. Partial seizures without secondary generalization
    e. Partial seizures with secondary generalization

A11: d, e. Small meningiomas that do not have edema and do not compress the underlying brain are commonplace and are rarely of medical consequence. Although they are considered "brain tumors," such meningiomas are usually innocuous, incidental findings. They might, however, cause seizures by irritating the underlying cortex. In this case, partial seizures might arise from the underlying parietal cortex, causing sensory symptoms on the left side of the body. Although the seizure activity might remain limited to sensory phenomena, it also might undergo generalization to cause generalized tonic-clonic activity. Such a small meningioma, however, would not cause dementia because its small size and lack of cerebral compression would not damage enough cerebral tissue to interfere with intellectual function. Small asymptomatic meningiomas, especially in the elderly, need not be removed.

Q12: An 18-year-old woman has had 2 years of premenstrual episodes, lasting 1 to 3 days, consisting of malaise, "depression," nausea, and a dull, throbbing headache behind her left eye. An EEG during an episode reveals some theta (slow) activity diffusely and intermittently. What is the single most likely diagnosis?
    a. Partial complex seizure(s)
    b. Cyclic depression
    c. Premenstrual tension

    d.   An arteriovenous malformation (AVM)
    e.   None of the above

A12: e. Most likely, the woman has premenstrual common migraine headaches. Partial complex seizures are not usually accompanied by a headache, usually do not last more than 20 minutes, and do not have merely scattered theta activity on an intraictal EEG. An AVM would not cause multiple headaches, autonomic symptoms, or mood changes.

Q13: Which of the following patients is most likely to have a seizure?
    a.   A 65-year-old man with left Bell's palsy
    b.   A 70-year-old woman with a right third cranial nerve palsy and left hemiparesis
    c.   A 55-year-old woman with rapidly progressive paresis and sensory loss of her left arm and more so her left leg, which has hyperactive DTRs and a Babinski sign
    d.   A 40-year-old man who, following an upper respiratory tract infection, develops ascending flaccid, areflexic weakness of the legs

A13: c. This patient probably has a right parasagittal (parafalcine) meningioma, a right frontal glioblastoma, or another mass lesion in this location. Whatever its nature, any cerebral mass lesion routinely causes seizures. Only lesions of the cerebral cortex itself or of the meninges that press on the cortex are likely to cause seizures. Thus, the patient with the left seventh cranial nerve palsy (a), right midbrain infarction (b), or Guillain-Barré syndrome (d) would not be expected to have seizures.

Q14: Many phenomena, conditions, tests, and illnesses have been named after two neurologists, i.e., paired eponyms. Match the eponyms with one or more of the associated findings:

1.	Kayser-Fleischer	a.	None of the ones below
2.	Brown-Séquard	b.	Peripheral neuropathy and mental changes
3.	Watson-Schwartz	c.	An opacity in the cornea indicative of an illness characterized by dementia and involuntary movement
4.	Wernicke-Korsakoff		
5.	Creutzfeldt-Jakob		
6.	Niemann-Pick		
7.	Niemann-Marcus		
		d.	Disassociation of pain and temperature in the legs
		e.	Disassociation of paresis and position sense loss in the legs
		f.	Disassociation of paresis and hypalgesia in the legs
		g.	Dementia with myoclonus in an elderly man
		h.	Fatal illness of infancy
		i.	Detectable in utero or prenatally

A14: Correct answers: 1-c Wilson's disease; 2-f spinal cord transection; 3-b acute intermittent porphyria; 4-b; 5-g; 6-h, i; 7-a.

Q15: Changes in deep tendon, plantar, and gag reflexes are a salient feature of many neurologic illnesses. Match the illnesses with one or more of the expected reflex alterations.

1.	Guillain-Barré syndrome	a.	Hyperactive deep tendon reflexes
2.	Multiple sclerosis	b.	Hypoactive deep tendon reflexes
3.	Acute intermittent porphyria		
4.	Myasthenia gravis	c.	Extensor plantar reflexes (Babinski signs)
5.	Wernicke-Korsakoff syndrome		
6.	Amyotrophic lateral sclerosis	d.	Unresponsive or flexor plantar reflexes
7.	Brachial plexus injury		
8.	Herniated lumbar intervertebral disk	e.	Hyperactive gag reflex
9.	Parasagittal meningioma	f.	Hypoactive gag reflex

10. Multiple cerebral infarctions
11. Spastic hemiparesis
12. Brainstem infarctions
13. Myotonic dystrophy
14. Duchenne's muscular dystrophy
15. Chronic nitrous oxide abuse
16. Diabetes mellitus neuropathy
17. Cauda equina syndrome
18. Lupus cerebritis
19. Lupus neuropathy
20. Ascending polyneuropathy
21. Poliomyelitis
22. Pseudobulbar palsy
23. Bulbar palsy
24. "Sciatica"
25. Brown-Séquard syndrome
26. Tabes dorsalis
27. Optic neuritis
28. Combined-system disease
29. Anxiety
30. Multi-infarction dementia

A15:

1. b, d, f.	16. b, d.
2. a, c, e.	17. b, d.
3. b, d, f.	18. a, c, e.
4. d, f.	19. b, d.
5. b, d.	20. b, d (i.e., Guillain-Barré).
6. a, c, e.	21. b, d (f in bulbar form).
7. b, d.	22. e (reflexes variable).
8. b, d.	23. f (reflexes variable).
9. a, c.	24. b, d.
10. a, c, e.	25. a, c.
11. a, c.	26. b, d.
12. a, c, e or f (depending on site of lesion.	27. d.
	28. a, c.
13. b, d.	29. a, e.
14. b, d.	30. a, c, e.

Q16: Which conditions in question 15 involve upper motor neuron injury?

A16: 2, 6, 9, 10, 11, 12, 18, 22, 25, 28, 30.

Q17: Which conditions in question 15 involve lower motor neuron injury?

A17: 1, 3, 4 (neuromuscular junction), 5, 6, 7, 8, 15, 16, 17, 19, 20, 21, 23, 24.

Q18: Match the most appropriate diagnostic or confirmatory procedure with the condition:

1. Multiple sclerosis	a. CT or MRI
2. Cerebellar infarction	b. Electroencephalography (EEG)
3. Subdural hematoma	c. Electromyography (EMG) and nerve conduction velocity (NCV)
4. Bacterial meningitis	
5. Hydrocephalus	
6. Myotonic dystrophy	d. Lumbar puncture (LP)
7. Myasthenia gravis	e. Myelography
8. Muscular dystrophy	f. Pneumoencephalography
9. Diabetic neuropathy	g. Slit-lamp examination
10. Alzheimer's disease	h. Tensilon test
11. Wilson's disease	i. None of the above
12. Spinal cord compression	
13. Absence (petit mal) seizures	
14. Combined-system disease (pernicious anemia)	

15. Hepatic encephalopathy
16. Radial nerve palsy
17. Meningioma of sphenoid ridge
18. Subacute sclerosing panenceph-
    alitis (SSPE)
19. Down's syndrome
20. Brain abscess
21. Creutzfeldt-Jakob disease
22. Meningioma of spinal cord
23. Partial complex seizures
24. Carpal tunnel syndrome
25. Mental retardation
26. Cerebral arteriovenous malfor-
    mation
27. "Cerebral palsy"
28. Cryptococcal meningitis
29. Optic neuritis
30. Lumbar herniated interverte-
    bral disk
31. Huntington's chorea
32. Wernicke's encephalopathy
33. Amaurosis fugax
34. Frontal lobe tumor
35. Lithium toxicity
36. Parkinsonism
37. Postictal *v* psychogenic seizures
38. Herpes encephalitis
39. Normal pressure hydrocephalus
40. Porphyria with mental changes
41. Pseudotumor cerebri
42. Postconcussive syndrome
43. Wallenberg's syndrome
44. Sydenham's chorea

A18: 1. i. The diagnosis of multiple sclerosis is predominantly a clinical one, although the CSF might be helpful if it reveals myelin basic protein or oligoclonal bands. Visual evoked responses (VER) are helpful but not diagnostic. MRI might reveal characteristic but not diagnostic lesions.
2. a.
3. a.
4. d.
5. a.
6. c. (EMG)
7. h.
8. i. Muscular dystrophy is predominantly a clinical diagnosis, but CPK and other serum enzyme determinations and a muscle biopsy would be helpful confirmatory information.
9. c. (NCV)
10. i. The CT, MRI, and EEG may be normal in early Alzheimer's disease.
11. g. Alternatively a serum ceruloplasmin determination would be an appropriate test.
12. e.
13. b.
14. i. A serum B_{12} determination or a Schilling test would be the appropriate tests.
15. b. The EEG will have slow and disorganized background activity. In classic cases, it will have triphasic waves.
16. c. (EMG and NCV)
17. a.
18. b, d. The EEG will often show periodic complexes, and the CSF will have elevated measles antibody titers.

19. i. A chromosome test would reveal trisomy or translocation of chromosome 21.
20. a.
21. b. A brain biopsy, however, would be definitive.
22. e. In the future, a CT or MRI scan of the spinal cord will be the procedure of choice.
23. b. Ideally, EEG and videotape telemetry would be performed.
24. c.
25. i.
26. a.
27. i.
28. d. The CSF must be analyzed for cryptococcal antigen, an India ink preparation must be made, and fluid should be cultured for fungus.
29. i. VER would be abnormal.
30. e. In the near future, a CT or MRI scan of the spine will be the procedure of choice.
31. i. Although a scan might show atrophy of the caudate nuclei, such a finding would be present only in advanced cases.
32. i. Mamillary body hemorrhages and other pathologic changes are too small to be seen on CT.
33. i. Carotid arteriography might reveal atherosclerotic stenosis and ulcerations, which might form a nidus for platelet emboli.
34. a.
35. i. A test of the blood level would be the most appropriate, but the EEG would be abnormal early in toxicity. It would show slowing and disorganization of the background.
36. i.
37. b. Postictally, EEGs are depressed and serum prolactins elevated.
38. a, b, d.
39. a. A CT scan would be helpful but there is no one specific diagnostic test.
40. i. When porphyria is associated with mental changes, it is of the "acute intermittent" variety. During an attack, examination of the urine will show excessive porphyrins. A Watson-Schwartz test will be positive.
41. d and a. A lumbar puncture will reveal elevated pressures (usually in excess of 300 mm). Since the differential diagnosis of pseudotumor is tumor, a CT or MRI scan must be performed. In addition to showing absence of a tumor or other mass lesions, it will show small ventricles.
42. i. Minor, inconsistent EEG abnormalities are often but not necessarily found in this admittedly nebulous condition.
43. a. Infarctions of the lateral medulla (Wallenberg syndrome) can now be detected with these tests.
44. i. The CT scan is normal in cases of Sydenham's chorea. However, the CT and MRI scans are abnormal in Huntington's chorea and Wilson's disease, at least in their advanced stages.

Q19–21: A 67-year-old man has had 3 weeks of progressively more severe, dull, bifrontal headaches, which are worse in the morning and relieved partially by aspirin. The patient is apathetic and inattentive, but allowing for his age, there is no cognitive impairment. He is unsteady, but the housestaff find no other physical deficit.

Q19: Which of the following causes of headaches might be seriously considered in this case?

    a. Glioblastoma or metastatic carcinoma
    b. Migraine headaches
    c. Carbon dioxide retention
    d. Cryptococcal meningitis
    e. Subdural hematoma, despite lack of trauma
    f. Meningococcal meningitis
    g. Cluster headaches
    h. Trigeminal neuralgia
    i. Brain abscess

A19: a, c, d, e, i.

Q20: What should the order be of the immediate diagnostic steps?
  a. EEG
  b. Lumbar puncture
  c. Routine laboratory evaluation, including a chest x-ray
  d. Arterial blood gas analysis
  e. Complete history and physical
  f. CT or MRI

A20: e, c, f. If these are normal, a, b, and possibly d.

Q21: Before any tests could be performed, the attending neurologist finds that the patient does have papilledema, paresis of the left leg, and a left Babinski sign. Where would he or she expect that a CT scan would show a lesion?
  a. Left side of the spinal cord
  b. Right side of the brainstem
  c. Right internal capsule
  d. Right frontal lobe

A21: d. Tumors in this location typically produce only subtle physical signs.

Q22–23: A 29-year-old woman has a 19-year history of monthly, almost exclusively left frontal and periorbital dull, throbbing, aching headaches. They begin in the early morning and are associated with slight nausea, photophobia, and, despite the nausea, hunger. Her mother has had similar headaches. The patient's physical examination and routine laboratory tests are normal.

Q22: Which would be the best initial management plan?
  a. Obtain a CT or MRI scan.
  b. Obtain an EEG.
  c. Give a therapeutic trial of a vasoconstrictor medication, e.g., Cafergot.
  d. Give a therapeutic trial of a mild analgesic-sedative combination (e.g., Fiorinal), including trials of medication at bedtime.
  e. If possible, eliminate skipped meals, excessive as well as insufficient sleep, and all food and beverages containing alcohol.

A22: e or either c or d (this author suggests d). If the patient responds to simple measures, further evaluation may not be necessary. In general, with cases of common migraine headache, such as this, extensive evaluation is not warranted if patients respond. In any case, an EEG would not be very helpful, and CT scan should be avoided in young people, especially women in their child-bearing years.

Q23: The woman, however, begins to have more frequent, intense, and incapacitating headaches. Plans c, e, and e do not help. An MRI scan is done and shows no abnormalities. What should the next therapeutic plan be?
  a. Prophylactic treatment with beta blockers, e.g., propranolol (Inderal)
  b. Prophylactic treatment with methysergide (Sansert)
  c. Daily use of vasoconstrictor medications

A23: a. When common or classic migraine headaches occur more than once a week, prophylactic therapy is indicated. In this case, a beta blocker medication would probably be effective and not subject the patient to the risks of retroperitoneal fibrosis, which may be a complication of (improper) use of methysergide (Sansert). Tricyclic antidepressants are often used with success in prevention of migraines.

Q24–29: Match the clinical features of the headache with the diagnosis:

Q24: Severe, prostrating headache occurring during coitus

Q25: Generalized dull headache in an obese young woman with papilledema and sixth cranial nerve

Q26: Frontal headaches in a 70-year-old man

Q27: A series of 30-minute periorbital headaches in a 40-year-old man that are often precipitated by wine

Q28: If untreated, may be complicated by blindness

Q29: Brief periods (less than 5 seconds) of sharp pains in the right lower jaw that may be precipitated by brushing teeth

    a. Pseudotumor cerebri
    b. Subarachnoid hemorrhage
    c. Trigeminal neuralgia
    d. Temporal arteritis
    e. Open-angle glaucoma
    f. Closed-angle glaucoma
    g. Cluster

A24–29:

24: b.

25: a.

26: d.

27: g.

28: a, d, e, f.

29: c.

Q30: A 65-year-old man, who has nonfluent aphasia, understands and complies with most simple verbal requests. However, when asked to pretend to show how he would use a comb, he runs his hand and fingers through his hair. What is the name of this phenomenon?

    a. Dementia
    b. Ideational apraxia
    c. Limb apraxia
    d. Finger agnosia

A30: c. The patient used his body part as the object he should have imagined and pretended to employ. Another example would be if he had been asked to show how he would use a toothbrush and he actually brushed his teeth with his finger. He probably would have been successful, nevertheless, if he had been handed either a comb or a toothbrush. He also would have been able to mimic the examiner's actions.

Limb apraxia, and more so buccofacial apraxia, is associated with aphasia. The importance of limb apraxia is that the disorder is one of language-motor integration rather than a manifestation of dementia.

In contrast, patients with ideational apraxia are unable to perform a series or sequence of simple motor activities, such as pretending to fold, stamp, and mail an envelope. Inability to perform such a sequence might also be overcome by using actual objects or by mimicking the examiner. Nevertheless, if the patient is unable to perform this sequence of activities in the abstract, he is said to have ideational apraxia. Unlike limb apraxia, ideational apraxia is closely associated with Alzheimer's disease, multi-infarct dementia, and other forms of dementia.

Q31: For which studies is MRI clearly superior to CT?
    a. Diagnosis of pituitary adenomas
    b. Diagnosis of multiple sclerosis
    c. Use in patients who are allergic to fish or iodine
    d. Diagnosis of Alzheimer's disease

A31: a, b, c. MRI is an excellent test for visualizing tissues that are surrounded by bone, such as the pituitary gland and spinal cord. CT cannot visualize these tissues because the surrounding bone creates artifact. Multiple sclerosis is much more apparent on MRI than CT because MRI can detect the changes in water content in multiple sclerosis plaques. It can show plaques that are small or located in the cerebrum, cerebellum, brainstem, or spinal cord. Since no contrast solutions are infused for MRI, there is no problem with a patient who is allergic to iodine or fish (which has a high iodine content) as there is in CT when iodine infusion is indicated—as for AVMs, tumors, and chronic subdural hematomas.

Although the MRI study will illustrate cerebral atrophy more vividly than the CT scan, neither test will be able to indicate that the atrophy is due to Alzheimer's disease rather than being, as is more often the case, due to the normal atrophy of older age.

Q32: Following a successful cardiac arrest resuscitation, a 70-year-old man has apathy and psychomotor retardation. He says only a few simple words. However, he repeats many long, complex phrases and accompanies singers on the radio. During these times, his articulation is good. He does not have a hemiparesis or homonymous hemianopsia. What is the nature of this patient's language impairment?

     a.   Nonfluent aphasia
     b.   Fluent aphasia
     c.   Frontal lobe dysfunction
     d.   Transcortical aphasia

A32: d. Transcortical aphasia results from isolation of the arc of Broca's area, the arcuate fasciculus, and Wernicke's area from the remainder of the cerebral cortex. Since this crucial arc of language function remains intact, patients are able to repeat words, phrases, and songs. However, since this area is isolated, they are not able to integrate language with other intellectual functions.

Transcortical aphasia usually results from cerebral anoxia and has been recently recognized as an important, but admittedly uncommon, variety of aphasia. It is often accompanied by intellectual and personality changes because the cerebral anoxia still affects extensive areas of the cerebral cortex.

Although this patient may have been difficult to examine, the physician should attempt to evaluate patients with simple, verbal bedside testing for aphasia.

TESTS FOR APHASIA

> Observation of Spontaneous Speech
>
> Three Formal Tests
>
>   Comprehension
>
>   Naming
>
>   Repeating

Q33: Two 70-year-old hypertensive men are admitted to the hospital. Both have been in good health aside from hypertension. Which patient is more likely to have aphasia?

     a.   The patient with right hemiparesis, deviation of the eyes to the left, and a right homonymous henianopsia
     b.   The patient with right hemiparesis and eyes deviated to the right

A33: a. This patient has an infarction in the left cerebral hemisphere that has caused damage to the visual tracts, which has resulted in a right homonymous hemianopsia, and also damage to the left frontal conjugate gaze center (Fig. 12-11), forcing his eyes to deviate to the left. Since such an extensive area of the left cerebral cortex is damaged, he is likely to have aphasia.

The patient in *b* probably has a brainstem infarction because the eyes are deviated toward the side of the hemiparesis (Fig. 12-12). Patients with brainstem lesions, provided they are alert, usually do not have aphasia or other intellectual impairments.

Q34–35: An 80-year-old man, who has had a cardiac arrest, remains comatose for 2 weeks. Then he occasionally opens his eyes and appears to move his limbs. One month after the cardiac arrest, he is evaluated for his mental competence.

The patient stares at the examiner but does not answer questions, follow verbal requests, or cooperate with other aspects of the examination. The patient tends to assume a flexion posture, and all of his muscles have increased tone. The patient breathes spontaneously and has roving eye movements. His pupils are equal and reactive to light. He has palmomental, snout, and extensor plantar reflexes. An EEG shows no organized background activity.

Q34: Where is the site of the brain damage?
    a. The entire brain
    b. The brainstem
    c. The entire cerebrum
    d. The cerebral cortex

A34: d. The cerebral cortex is the area of the brain that is most susceptible to anoxia. The patient's flexed posture, which is similar to a fetal position, frontal release signs, and absence of organized EEG background activity all indicate severe cerebral cortex damage. Since the patient's pupillary, extraocular, and respiratory muscles all function, the brainstem can be assumed to be intact. Although terminology may vary, the diagnosis of patients with extensive cerebral cortical damage and intact brainstem function, which is a common condition, is usually called the *persistent vegetative state.*

Q35: Which is the best description of the patient's mental capacity?
    a. He probably has profound and permanent cognitive impairment.
    b. He has the ability to understand but not express thoughts.
    c. A determination cannot be made for at least 6 more months.
    d. In the presence of global aphasia, an estimate of cognitive capacity cannot be accurate.

A35: a. In most individuals, and especially in the aged, maximal functional recovery from cerebral anoxia occurs within the first 2 weeks.

Q36: Which of the following conditions does *not* tend to cause cerebral cortex damage and result in the persistent vegetative state?
    a. Suicide attempts with carbon monoxide
    b. Occlusion of the left carotid artery
    c. Embolus to the basilar artery
    d. Drug overdose
    e. Cardiopulmonary arrest
    f. Strangulation

A36: b,c. The persistent vegetative state almost always results from bilateral extensive cerebral cortex damage. It does not usually result from damage to a single hemisphere, no matter how severe or extensive. Damage to the brainstem may initially cause coma, but afterward if there is recovery of consciousness, the patient should not have cognitive impairment. Thus, patients with the Weber (midbrain) and Wallenberg (lateral medulla) infarctions do not have intellectual impairments.

Q37–49: Match the headaches with precipitating causes:

37: Menses	a.	Common or classic migraine
38: Red wine	b.	Cluster headache
39: REM sleep	c.	Tic douloureux
40: Touching affected area	d.	None of the above
41: Too much sleep		
42: Cool breeze		

43: Genetic factors

44: A vascular loop pressing on the trigeminal nerve

45: Histamine

46: Type A personality

47: Exclusively high socioeconomic background

48: (May occur in) childhood

49: Almost only above age 55

A37–49:

37: a.

38: a, b.

39: a, b.

40: c.

41: a.

42: c.

43: a.

44: c.

45: d.

46: d.

47: d.

48: a.

49: c.

Q50: A 29-year-old woman has had several headaches every week for 10 years. They are usually present on awakening in the morning, although she may develop them if she misses her 10:00 AM coffee break. Her headaches also occur in the afternoon, while driving her car for several hours, or during psychologically stressful episodes. Most headaches are bitemporal, more on the left than the right. After several hours, her headaches become generalized and dull. Sometimes, however, they begin as a dull ache in the upper neck and then seem to gravitate to behind the left eye. Rest, aspirin compound products, and coffee often relieve the headaches. She rarely has to leave work early because of the pain. Afternoon naps relieve most headaches completely. The patient's mother, maternal grandmother, and ll-year-old daughter have had headaches, but she is unaware of the details of their headaches. The remaining medical history, physical and neurologic examinations, and routine laboratory work are unremarkable. Formulate a diagnosis and suggest initial management.

A50: This patient probably has the most frequently occurring headache problem that neurologists encounter: a combination of muscle contraction (tension) and common migraine headaches. There is no indication that the patient suffers from a structural lesion in view of the chronicity of the headaches and lack of accompanying neurologic physical signs.

The components of the headaches that suggest that they are partly migrainous are the following: the headaches begin in the early morning and may be averted by taking coffee (caffeine). They are located unilaterally, especially in the periorbital or retro-orbital area. They are relieved by sleep, not merely resting, and they are alleviated by aspirin-caffeine compounds. Finally, although muscle contraction headaches may have a familial occurrence (on a psychogenic basis), a female-family incidence, as in this case, is indicative of genetically inherited susceptibility.

The headaches are also partly the result of muscle contractions. Those headaches located in the neck and dull bitemporal headaches are from muscle contractions as are those that occur after difficult work, long drives, and psychologically stressful episodes.

An important, typical feature of this case is that the two types of headaches alternate, vary, and blend because prolonged muscle contraction headaches lead to migraine headaches and mild, prolonged common migraine leads to muscle contraction headaches. Either or both, of course, cause anxiety, which exacerbates the pain and discomfort.

Opinion might differ over the appropriate initial management. Some physicians would perform CT or MRI to alleviate their own as well as the patient's concern about a structural lesion, such as a brain tumor or arteriovenous malformation. Other physicians, including the author, would postpone such tests while attempting to eliminate the headaches by simple medical means.

Therapy would start by having the patient record the various headaches and potential precipitating factors on a calendar. Menses, excessive work days, vacations, use of wine, and other factors would be considered as possible provoking factors that then could be avoided.

Meanwhile therapy would be directed first toward the common migraine headache, by this author at least, because these headaches are more readily treated. When they occur once a week or less, a mild analgesic-sedative compound, such as Fiorinal, might be given. When they occur more frequently, prophylactic therapy with a beta blocker might be given. Depending on the psychologic circumstances, treatment of the muscle contraction headaches might begin with aspirin. Then a mild sedative or even an antidepressant, which would provide analgesic as well as psychologic benefit, could be added.

Q51–56: Below are six sketches of spinal cords stained such that normal myelin is stained black, gray areas are crosshatched, and demyelinated areas are white (unstained). Match the sketches (Q51–56) with the descriptions of the clinical associations (a-f).

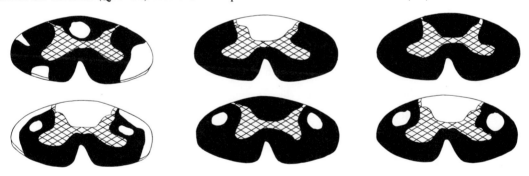

    a. A 45-year-old man with progressively severe intellectual and personality impairment for 4 years has loss of vibration and position sensation, absent reflexes in the legs, and a floppy-foot gait. His pupils are miotic. They constrict to closely regarded objects but not to light.

    b. A 65-year-old man, who had a complete gastectomy 4 years ago, now has dementia, hyperactive DTRs, bilateral Babinski signs, and loss of vibration sensation in the legs.

    c. A 70-year-old woman has weakness of the left leg, right arm, and neck muscles. She has atrophy of many limb muscles and fasciculations of the tongue and most of the atrophic muscles.

    d. A 35-year-old man has optic neuritis, internuclear ophthalmoplegia, and gait impairment because of ataxia, weakness, and spasticity.

    e. A 40-year-old woman and her sister have pes cavus, intention tremor of the limbs, and loss of position and vibration sensation.

    f. A 70-year-old man who has schizophrenia sustains a frontal lobe gunshot wound. He takes Dilantin, which leads to cerebellar dysfunction. He becomes so distraught that he becomes an alcoholic and suffers an episode of severe confusion, nystagmus, and bilateral abducens nerve palsy.

A51–56:

51: d. The spinal cord shows multiple areas (plaques) of demyelination (sclerosis). The patient has signs of optic nerve, brainstem, and spinal cord dysfunction. Both the clinical and pathologic material indicate multiple sclerosis.

52: a. The spinal cord shows demyelination of the posterior columns. Loss of these tracts causes loss of position sensation, which makes patients walk with high, uncertain, and awkward steps. This patient is described as having Argyll-Robertson pupils and mental abnormalities. This is a case of syphilis of the brain and spinal cord (tabes dorsalis).

53: f. The spinal cord remains normal despite the cerebral injury, drug-induced cerebellar dysfunction, and Wernicke's encephalopathy.

54: e. There is degeneration of the spinocerebellar, posterior column, and cortico-spinal tracts. Loss of the spinocerebellar and posterior column tracts, which indicates a spinocerebellar degenerative illness, such as Friedreich's ataxia, causes intention tremor, position and vibration sense loss, and a foot deformity (pes cavus).

55: c. The spinal cord shows demyelination of the corticospinal tracts and loss of the anterior horns, which contain the motor neurons. This is the picture of motor neuron disease when, typically, both the upper and lower motor neuron systems degenerate. The patient has the clinical features of amyotrophic lateral sclerosis (ALS), the most common form of motor neuron disease.

56: b. The spinal cord shows demyelination of the posterior columns and the corticospinal tracts. This combination, termed "combined system disease," is associated with B_{12} deficiency from pernicious anemia or surgical removal of the stomach. It is associated with dementia, paraparesis, hyperactive DTRs, and position and vibration sense loss. These findings are similar to those of tabes dorsalis with dementia; however, combined-system disease causes hyperactive DTRs and Babinski signs, whereas tabes dorsalis causes hypoactive DTRs and Argyll-Robertson pupils, but neither paraparesis nor Babinski signs.

Q57–61:   Match the disease with the associated abnormality:

57: Idiopathic Parkinson's disease	a.	Dopamine depletion
58: Hemiballismus	b.	Dopamine block
	c.	Contralateral subthalamic nucleus infarction
59: Wilson's disease		
	d.	Caudate atrophy
60: Huntington's chorea	e.	Copper metabolism abnormality
61: Haloperidol-induced		

A57–61:

57: a. **58:** c. **59:** e. **60:** d.   **61:** b.

Q62–66:   Match the medication with its potential side effects:

62: L-dopa

63: Anticholinergics

64: Sinemet

65: Oral contraceptives

66: Choline

    a. Constipation
    b. Anhidrosis
    c. Buccolingual dyskinesias
    d. Agitation
    e. Fishy smell

     f.   Sexual hyperactivity
     c.   Buccolingual dyskinesias
     d.   Agitation
     e.   Fishy smell
     f.   Sexual hyperactivity
     h.   Somnolence
     i.   Hallucinations
     j.   Dry mouth
     k.   May hasten development of tardive dyskinesia
     l.   Pupillary dilatation

A62–66:

62: c, d, f, g, i.

63: a, b, d (unusual), h (unusual), j,k, and l (minimal).

64: Same as 62.

65: g. (Oral-contraceptive-induced chorea is a rare complication found in young nulliparous women who usually themselves or their relatives have had Sydenham's chorea.)

66: e.

Q67–72: How does the tremor of parkinsonism differ from that of essential tremor? (True/False)

67: Only Parkinson's tremor is absent during sleep.

68: Only Parkinson's tremor is sometimes found in many family members.

69: Only essential tremor often begins in the third or fourth decade of life.

70: Only essential tremor is fine and rapid.

71: Only Parkinson's tremor is associated with rigidity or bradykinesia.

72: Only essential tremor may be reduced by alcoholic drinks and propranolol.

A67–72:

67: False: both are absent during sleep.

68: False: a common variety of essential tremor is called "benign familial tremor."

69: True, with rare exceptions

70: True

71: True

72: True

Q73–79: Which conditions induce tremor? (Yes/No)

73: Excessive coffee consumption

74: Lithium usage

75: Amantadine (Symmetrel)

76: Steroids

77: Amitriptyline (Elavil)

78: Hypothyroidism

79: Hyperthyroidism

A73–79:

73: Yes.

74: Yes. Fine tremor is often associated with mild lithium intoxication. Gross tremor is a sign of intoxication.

75: No. This antiviral medication suppresses Parkinson's tremor.

76: Yes, although high doses are required.

77: Yes. Mild tremor with amitriptyline use is not clearly a sign of toxicity.

78: No.

79: Yes.

Q80: A 71-year-old man has been receiving numerous psychotropic medications for many years. Funduscopy reveals flecks of dark pigment scattered about the retina. Which of the following medications is (are) most likely responsible?
    a.   Chlorpromazine (Thorazine)
    b.   Imipramine (Tofranil)
    c.   Thioridazine (Mellaril)
    d.   Amitriptyline (Elavil)

A80:   a, c.

Q81–86:   Match the visual field loss associated with each condition:

81: Left homonymous hemianopsia with macular sparing	a. Retinal injury, e.g., embolus or detachment
82: Fortification scotoma	b. Hysteria c. Migraine
83: Central scotoma, lasting for 2 weeks	d. Diabetes insipidus e. Loss of libido
84: Bitemporal hemianopsia	f. Optic atrophy g. Amaurosis fugax
85: Unilateral superior quadrantanopsia	h. Internal capsule infarction i. Aphasia j. Occipital infarction
86: Enlarged blind spot	k. Optic or retrobulbar neuritis l. Pseudotumor cerebri

A81–86:

81: j.

82: c.

83: k.

84: d, e, f (all associated with pituitary tumors).

85: a.

86: l.

Q87–89: A 29-year-old woman awakens one morning with pain in and around her right eye. She can see only large objects using the right eye, but the vision in the left eye remains 20/30 corrected (using glasses). The pain in the right eye increases on any eye movement, but there is no diplopia. The pupils are round and equal. The optic discs and fundi appear normal. The condition lasts for at least 48 hours.

Q87: What is the most likely condition that has caused this problem?
    a.   Hysteria
    b.   Left occipital infarction
    c.   Optic or retrobulbar neuritis
    d.   Multiple sclerosis
    e.   Classic migraine
    f.   None of the above

A87: c. Inflammation of the optic nerve (optic neuritis), typically in its portion behind the eyeball (retrobulbar neuritis), is the single most likely cause. Although this condition is often a harbinger or complication of multiple sclerosis, in about two thirds of cases, optic neuritis patients never develop other indications of multiple sclerosis.

Q88: A skeptical physician believes that this patient has a conversion reaction. Which observations or positive tests would probably be present that would indicate that the patient does have optic neuritis?

    a.   Constriction of the right pupil as light is shown into it
    b.   Dilation of the right pupil as light is rapidly moved from the left to the right eye
    c.   Finding abnormal visual evoked responses (VERs) in the right eye
    d.   Abnormal CT scan
    e.   Abnormal electroencephalogram (EEG)
    f.   Oligoclonal bands and myelin basic protein in the CSF

A88: b, c, f.

Q89: Which of the following medications or techniques have been said to be effective treatment for multiple sclerosis?

    a.   ACTH
    b.   Phenytoin (Dilantin)
    c.   Plasmapheresis
    d.   Cyclophosphamide

A89: a, d.

Q90: An 80-year-old man, who is being treated for depression, complains of right-sided frontotemporal headaches. His vision in the right eye is impaired. Temporal arteries are prominent, but not especially tender. There is no papilledema, hemiparesis, or other neurologic sign. Which conditions must be considered immediately?

    a.   Open-angle glaucoma
    b.   Metastases to the skull
    c.   Meningioma
    d.   Optic neuritis
    e.   Temporal arteritis
    f.   Narrow-angle glaucoma

A90: e, f.

Q91–102: Differences between Horner's syndrome and oculomotor (third cranial nerve) palsy are important. Indicate which features are associated with either one, both, or neither:

91: Pupillary dilation

92: Ptosis

93: Miosis (pupillary constriction)

94: Associated with diabetes

95: Found in cluster headache

96: Found with Pancoast's tumors

97: Associated with medullary lesions

98: Associated with pontine lesions

99: Associated with midbrain lesions

100: Causes diplopia

101: Associated with syringomyelia

102: Found occasionally in migraine

    a.   Horner's syndrome
    b.   Oculomotor nerve palsy
    c.   Both
    d.   Neither

A91–102:

91:	b.	**97.**	a.
92:	c.	**98:**	d.
93:	a.	**99:**	b.
94:	b.	**100:**	b.
95:	a.	**101:**	a.
96:	a.	**102:**	b.

Q103: Which factors may precipitate angle-closure glaucoma? (Yes/No)
  a. Topically applied agents that cause pupillary dilation, e.g., phenylephrine (Neosynephrine)
  b. Atropine, scopolamine, and other atropine-like medications
  c. Sympathomimetic drugs
  d. Drugs that interfere with parasympathetic activity
  e. Tricyclic antidepressants because of their atropine-like effects
  f. Anticholinergic medications
  g. Propranolol and topically applied beta blockers
  h. Ephedrine and neosynephrine
  i. Any medication that retards re-uptake or metabolism of norepinephrine
  j. Any drug that acts like norepinephrine

A103:
  a. Yes. Such medications, which are often instilled during funduscopy, sometimes precipitate angle-closure glaucoma.
  b. Yes
  c. Yes. Topically administered sympathomimetics, but not (for practical purposes) systemically administered ones, may precipitate glaucoma.
  d. Yes. Only predisposed people, however, are at risk.
  e. Yes. Phenothiazines too may cause glaucoma, although such a complication occurs very rarely.
  f. Yes. Only predisposed people are at risk.
  g. No. In fact, topically applied beta blockers are used in treatment of glaucoma.
  h. Yes
  i. Yes
  j. Yes

Q104: A 40-year-old alcoholic man who has mild, chronic cirrhosis is brought to the Emergency Room because he suddenly became confused. Examination reveals disorientation, slurred speech, and asterixis. There is no nystagmus, extraocular paresis, or pupillary abormality. Laboratory data include the following: mildly abnormal liver function tests, 26% hematocrit, and blood in the stool. Which conditions ought to be considered?
  a. Wernicke's encephalopathy
  b. Alcohol-induced hypoglycemia
  c. Hepatic encephalopathy
  d. Subdural hematoma
  e. Delirium tremens (DTs)

A104: c. Hepatic encephalopathy is the most likely cause. People with cirrhosis or other causes of hepatic insufficiency will develop encephalopathy when gastrointestinal bleeding occurs from esophageal varices or gastric ulceration.

In this case, the anemia and bloody stool indicate gastrointestinal bleeding. Sometimes encephalopathy will occur merely following a meal of high protein content. Most important, mental changes and asterixis often occur, as in this case, before liver function test abnormalities become pronounced.

Wernicke's encephalopathy, alcohol-induced hypoglycemia, and subdural hematoma should always be considered in alcoholics with mental changes. Although no neurologic signs indicate any of these diagnoses, all such patients routinely should receive intravenous thiamine and, after blood tests are drawn, intravenous glucose.

Q105–113: Match the ocular abnormality with the most probable site of the lesion:

105: Right third cranial nerve paresis and left hemiparesis

106: Left sixth cranial nerve paresis and right hemiparesis

107: Right Horner's syndrome, right facial hypalgesia, right limb ataxia, and left limb and trunk hypalgesia

108: Internuclear ophthalmoplegia

109: Right sixth and seventh cranial nerve paresis and left hemiparesis

110: Ophthalmoplegia with normally reactive pupils, ptosis, and facial paresis

111: Small, irregular pupils that accommodate but do not react

112: Fever, agitated confusion, and dilated pupils

113: Stupor, miosis, and pulmonary edema
    a. Myasthenia gravis
    b. Scopolamine intoxication
    c. Right pontine lesion
    d. Left pontine lesion
    e. Left pontine lesion
    f. Right midbrain lesion
    g. Midline brainstem lesion
    h. Left lateral medullary lesion
    i. Right lateral medullary lesion
    j. Syphilis
    k. Heroin or methadone overdose

A105–113:

105: f.	**110.** a.
106: e.	**111:** j.
107: i.	**112:** b.
108: g.	**113:** k.
109: c.	

Q114: Which of the following are found in the brains of people with Alzheimer's disease but not in brains of normal elderly persons?
    a. Loss of weight
    b. Increase in sulci width
    c. Expansion of the lateral ventricles
    d. Major loss of large cortical neurons
    e. *Marked* reduction of choline acetyltransferase in the hippocampus
    f. Mild memory impairment
    g. *Multiple* neurofibrillary tangles
    h. Similarity to brains of Down's syndrome patients and retired boxers
    i. Presence of senile plaques

A114: d, e, g, h. Cerebral atrophy (a, b, c) and the presence of some plaques (i), neurofibrillary tangles, and granulovacuolar degeneration are found in normal brains but are only quantitatively more pronounced in the brain with Alzheimer's disease. Likewise, mild memory impairment in people with early Alzheimer's disease is similar to that found in the normal elderly.

Q115–122: Mental changes are often accompanied by physical abnormalities. Match the associated signs:

115: Parkinson's disease patient with agitation, hallucinations, and _____

116: Dementia, gait apraxia, and _____

117: Delirium, sixth cranial nerve palsy, ataxia, peripheral neuropathy, and _____

118: Dementia, chronic hepatic insufficiency, corneal discoloration, and _____

119: Dementia, position sense loss, positive VDRL, and miotic _____

120: Seizure patient with lethargy, confusion, dysarthria, ataxia, and _____

121: Child with rapidly progressive mental and personality impairment, high measles antibody titre in the CSF, and _____

122. Elderly man with rapid development of dementia, periodic EEG, and _____

A115–122:

 a. Seventh cranial nerve palsy
 b. Incontinence
 c. Tremor and/or rigidity and bradykinesia
 d. Nystagmus
 e. Myoclonus
 f. Pupils that do not react
 g. Pupils that do not accommodate
 h. Seizures
 i. Dyskinesias

A115–122:

115: i.	**119:** f.
116: b.	**120:** d.
117: d.	**121:** e.
118: c.	**122:** e.

Q123–132: Match the illness with the findings in Q115–122 or note "none of the above":

123: Wernicke-Korsakoff syndrome

124: Normal pressure hydrocephalus

125: Wilson's disease

126: Creutzfeldt-Jakob disease

127: Tertiary syphilis

128: Anticonvulsant intoxication

129: Subacute sclerosing panencephalitis (SSPE)

130: Alzheimer's disease

131: Multiple sclerosis

132: Parkinson's disease with L-dopa intoxication

A123–132:

123: 117	**126:** 122
124: 116	**127:** 119
125: 118	**128:** 120

129: 121

130: None of the above, but rarely 122

131: None of the above

Q133: If patients use topical pilocarpine because they have narrow-angle glaucoma, can they use tricyclic antidepressants and phenothiazine medications?

A133: Yes, as a general rule.

Q134: Which features indicate amyotrophic lateral sclerosis (ALS), peripheral neuropathy, both, or neither:

a.	Muscle atrophy	d.	Hypoactive DTRs
b.	Fasciculations	e.	Atrophy of tongue muscles
c.	Babinski signs	f.	Stocking-glove hypalgesia

A134:

a.	Both	d.	Peripheral neuropathy
b.	ALS	e.	ALS
c.	ALS	f.	Peripheral neuropathy

Q135: Which of the following illnesses may cause peripheral neuropathy and mental changes?

a.	Cervical spondylosis	e.	Heavy metal intoxication
b.	Wernicke-Korsakoff syndrome	f.	Syphilis
c.	Porphyria (acute intermittent)	g.	Uremia
d.	ALS	h.	Nitrous oxide abuse

A135: b, c, e, f, g, h.

Q136: An elderly gentleman with dementia has a gait abnormality in which he excessively raises his legs, so that he seems to be climbing as he walks. His pupils are small, poorly reactive, and irregular. What is the gait abnormality?

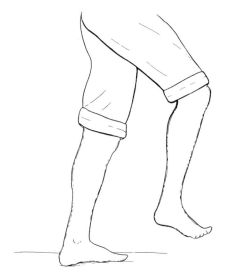

a. Gait apraxia
b. Congenital spastic paraparesis
c. Steppage gait from posterior spinal cord degeneration

A136: c. The patient has tertiary syphilis with tabes dorsalis and Argyll-Robertson pupils. Since he has lost proprioception, he raises his legs so that his feet clear the floor.

Q137–139:   Match the confabulation with the lesion that might produce it:

137:   The patient, who is blind, "describes" clothing that an examiner is wearing. His pupils are round and reactive to light.

138:   A patient with recent onset of left hemiparesis says that he cannot move his left arm and leg because he is too tired.

139.   An agitated, diaphoretic middle-aged man describes bizarre occurrences and experiences visual hallucinations. When asked to repeat six digits, he says a random selection of numbers.

    a.   Nondominant parietal lobe infarction
    b.   Bilateral occipital lobe infarctions
    c.   Hemorrhage into the limbic system

A137–139:

137:   b. In cortical blindness, in which the pupillary reactions are characteristically normal, patients tend to confabulate (Anton's syndrome). It occurs after sudden injury of both occipital lobes, usually from infarction or trauma.

138.   a. Patients with hemiparesis from a nondominant hemisphere infarct often confabulate, deny, and use other typical defense mechanisms in discussing their hemiparesis. The parietal lobe is almost always damaged, and the hemiparesis is almost always on the left.

139.   c. Patients with alcohol withdrawal can have confabulations, alone or as part of delirium tremens. However, the frequency of confabulations in Wernicke-Korsakoff syndrome is usually overestimated.

Q140:   Which of the following substances cause cerebellar dysfunction?
    a.   Ethanol
    b.   Dilantin
    c.   INH
    d.   Elavil
    e.   Mercury

A140:   a, b, e. (Elavil causes tremor, but not because of cerebellar damage.)

Q141:   A 35-year-old man staggers into the Emergency Room. He is lethargic and disoriented. There is nystagmus, gait ataxia, and finger-to-nose dysmetria. Which illness is he most likely to have? What is the *specific* therapy?
    a.   Subdural hematoma
    b.   Cerebral infarction
    c.   Wernicke-Korsakoff syndrome
    d.   Hysteria

A141:   c. Thiamine 50 mg IV

Q142:   An 11-year-old boy is admitted because of headache, nausea, and vomiting. He has had clumsiness for the 2 weeks before admission. His optic disks are edematous. He has ataxia and bilateral hyperactive DTRs and Babinski signs. Which is the most likely diagnosis?
    a.   Multiple sclerosis
    b.   Drug abuse
    c.   Cerebellar tumor
    d.   Spinocerebellar degeneration

A142:   c. Cerebellar astrocytomas, which are relatively common in youngsters, block the aqueduct of Sylvius, creating hydrocephalus (manifested by headaches, nausea, vomiting, and papilledema).

Q143:   An 18-year-old soldier sustained a mild head injury in basic training. Examination revealed striking tremors and ataxia of gait (although no falls occurred), but no dysarthria, nystagmus, or dysmetria. The best course to pursue would be:

    a.   Do immediate CT.
    b.   Give thiamine IV.
    c.   Do lumbar puncture.
    d.   Observe.

A143: d, a. The signs of cerebellar disease are incomplete and inconsistent. Failing to fall when the person is apparently severely ataxic is *astasia abasia* and usually a sign of psychogenic difficulty. The best course would be to observe (d) or, for reassurance, obtain a CT scan (a), although this need not be performed immediately.

Q144: A 30-year-old man is brought to the Emergency Room of Elsewhere Hospital describing his new digital watch as a "timer for destruction of the world." He speaks in circumlocutions and tangents and he often repeats phrases and sentences, but he does not use jargon, neologisms, or paraphasias. Physicians are not able to obtain any additional history or to perform any physical or neurologic examinations.
    What conditions must be given immediate consideration?
    a.   Aphasia
    b.   Acute organic mental syndrome (delerium)
    c.   Psychiatric disturbances
    d.   The impending destruction of the world, i.e., the man is correct.

A144: a, b, c.

Q145: With calming and a small dose of phenothiazine, the man in the previous question is able to cooperate. He then carefully describes the "powers" of his new watch. The physicians demonstrate that the man is oriented, has good memory, and his judgment is otherwise intact. Nevertheless, one physician insists that the patient is aphasic.
    Which tests of language function must the skeptical physician perform?

A145: Metaphor is a linguistic device used by orators, poets, humorists, and sports-casters among other people. Psychotic patients may actually believe that objects have been transformed, but these people, when calm, will be able to identify the object. Even schizophrenics with true jargon speech, as well as this man, *will be able to follow the three routine tests of language function*:

- Following requests
- Naming common objects
- Repeating phrases

Q146: Which of the following symptoms might constitute a "narcoleptic tetrad"?
    a.   Inability to move on awakening (sleep paralysis)
    b.   Hunger or anorexia
    c.   Vivid dreams when falling asleep (hypnagogic hallucinations)
    d.   Daytime sleepiness (narcolepsy)
    e.   Night terrors (pavor nocturnus)
    f.   Episodic loss of muscle tone (cataplexy)

A146: a, c, d, f.

Q147: Which of the following are characteristic of an attack of narcolepsy?
    a.   Preceded by a boring situation
    b.   Preceded by a feeling of fatigue
    c.   Duration of 15 minutes or less
    d.   Immediate onset of REM sleep
    e.   Absent deep tendon reflexes (DTRs)
    f.   Average age of onset before 25 years of age
    g.   About a dozen episodes weekly
    h.   Usually accompanied by total paralysis
    i.   Narcoleptic attacks begin several years before attacks of cataplexy
    j.   Attacks are usually refreshing

A147:   a, b, c, d, e, f, g, i, j. (h is incorrect because patients more often have loss of tone (cataplexy) in a limited area of musculature, such as the legs or jaw, than in their entire body.)

Q148:   Which of the following conditions are associated with excessive daytime sleepiness?
    a. Night terrors
    b. Obstructive sleep apnea
    c. Jactatio capitis nocturnus (nighttime head banging)
    d. Use of "sleeping pills" at bedtime
    e. Enuresis
    f. Narcolepsy
    g. Nonobstructive sleep apnea

A148:   b, d, f, g.

Q149:   In addition to excessive daytime sleepiness, which of the following are complications of obstructive sleep apnea?
    a. Systemic hypertension
    b. Cardiac arrhythmias
    c. Pulmonary hypertension

A149:   a, b, c.

Q150:   How do night terrors differ from nightmares? (True/False)
    a. Night terrors, one of the "parasomnias," occur in stage 3 or 4 of NREM sleep, but nightmares occur in REM sleep.
    b. Both night terrors and nightmares are vivid, frightening dreams that might be analyzed.
    c. Night terrors usually occur early in the night during the long stretches of stage 3 and 4 NREM sleep, often occurring when the child is abruptly stimulated. Nightmares occur mixed with other dreams, all of which the child may recall.
    d. The child with a nightmare typically awakens fully from the dream and may be able to recount many vivid details, but the child with a night terror usually returns to sleep.
    e. Frequent night terrors or nightmares are both indications for diazepam (Valium) or imipramine (Tofranil) at bedtime.

A150:   a, true; b, false (night terrors are brief episodes of fear similar to a startle response); c, true; d, true; e, false (these and similar medications are indicated only for night terrors and then only when under certain circumstances).

Q151:   Which of the following sleep-related phenomena occur during REM sleep, stage 3 or 4 of NREM sleep, or either?
    a. Sleepwalking somnambulism
    b. Bedwetting (enuresis)
    c. Night terrors
    d. Nightmares
    e. Penile erections
    f. Cluster headaches
    g. Dreams
    h. Teeth mashing (bruxism)
    i. 1 to 3-Hz EEG activity
    j. High frequency asynchronous EEG activity
    k. Flaccid muscles and absent DTRs
    l. Increase in cerebral blood flow

A151:

a.	NREM	g.	NREM
b.	NREM	h.	Either
c.	NREM	i.	NREM
d.	REM	j.	REM
e.	REM	k.	REM
f.	REM	l.	REM

Q152:   As close as possible, match the developmental milestone with the month/year in which 50 percent of infants or children achieve it, according to the Denver Developmental Screening Test:

1.	Stands alone well	a.	1 month
2.	Pedals tricycle	b.	2 months
3.	Smiles responsively	c.	4 months
4.	Plays ball with examiner	d.	6 months
5.	Walks well	e.	8 months
6.	Stacks two blocks	f.	10 months
7.	Separates from mother easily	g.	12 months
8.	Draws a man in three parts	h.	14 months
9.	Sits without support	i.	18 months
10.	Three words other than mama, dada	j.	24 months
11.	Pulls self to stand	k.	30 months
12.	Laughs	l.	3 years

A152:

1.	g.	7.	l.
2.	j.	8.	m.
3.	a.	9.	d.
4.	g.	10.	h.
5.	g.	11.	e.
6.	h.	12.	b.

Q153:   What is the sequence in which a child learns to copy the cross, circle, diamond, and square?

A153:   circle, cross (or x), square, diamond

Q154:   Children may have an acute confusional state. In children, which groups of substances are well-known causes of mental changes?

a. Phenytoin (Dilantin), phenothiazines, haloperidol, oral hypoglycemics
b. Sedatives, e.g., phenobarbital
c. "Cold" medications, especially those containing antihistamine
d. Bronchodilators for treatment of asthma, especially those containing sympathomimetics
e. Alcohol or drug intoxication

A154:   All of the above. Most notable is the paradoxical reaction in which a sedating substance causes agitation, hyperactivity, and insomnia in children. Other relatively common causes of acute confusional state would include (viral) encephalitis, head trauma, postictal confusion, and any bacterial infection, e.g., pneumonia, otitis media.

Q155:   Two days after an 11-year-old boy seems to have recovered from an upper respiratory tract viral illness, he has a series of seizures followed by coma. His temperature is 101°F and his liver is enlarged, but otherwise there are no abnormal physical abnormalities. Laboratory tests show an elevated serum transaminase (SGOT) and prolonged prothrombin time (PT).
Which conditions are likely to be the cause of the rapid onset of fever, coma with seizures, and such laboratory abnormalities following an upper respiratory tract infection?

a. Guillain-Barré syndrome
b. Multiple sclerosis
c. Mononucleosis
d. Wilson's disease
e. Wernicke-Korsakoff syndrome
f. Reye's syndrome

A155:   c, f.

Q156:   An adolescent with a chronic, major psychiatric disorder begins to drink excessive quantities of tap water and other fluids and to urinate large volumes. After 1 week, he develops a seizure and then coma. Which of the following conditions might have caused such voluminous fluid intake and excretion?

a.	The psychiatric condition	c.	Diabetes mellitus
b.	Diabetes insipidus	d.	Excessive salt intake

A156: a, b, c, d. Polyuria and polydipsia may be caused by psychogenic factors; an excessive serum solute load, such as from glucose or sodium; or absence of antidiuretic hormone, such as found in pituitary tumors.

Q157: In the previous question, assuming the patient did not have excessive salt intake, what might be the cause of the seizure?
  a. A hypothalamic or pituitary tumor that compresses the hypothalamus or grows into the temporal lobe
  b. Hyperglycemia/hyperosmolarity from diabetes mellitus
  c. Hyponatremia (serum sodium of 120 or below) from compulsive water ingestion

A157: a, b, c.

Q158: Which conditions can amniocentesis detect?
  a. Down's syndrome
  b. Cerebral palsy
  c. Galactosemia
  d. Wilson's disease
  e. Tay-Sachs' disease
  f. Mental retardation
  g. Phenylketonuria (PKU)
  h. Midline closure defects, e.g., meningomyelocele

A158: a, c, e, g, h.

Q159: Which conditions can fetal prenatal ultrasound scanning determine?
  a. Twins
  b. Placental placement
  c. Fetal sex
  d. Limb size
  e. Hydrocephalus
  f. Urinary tract abnormalities
  g. Fetal uterine placement
  h. Midline closure defects

A159: a, b, c, d, e, f, g, h.

Q160: What side effects of antipsychotic drugs are caused by blockade of the tubero-infundibular dopamine tract?

A160: Blockade of the tubero-infundibular or hypothalamic-pituitary dopamine tract leads to an increase in prolactin, leading some patients to gain weight, and in women sometimes to lactation and amenorrhea.

Q161: Sinemet (L-dopa plus carbidopa) will potentially increase levels of which biogenic amines?

A161: Since L-dopa is a precursor of dopamine, norepinephrine, and epinephrine, it will potentially increase levels of all three of these catecholamines.

Q162: What distinguishes neurotransmission of acetylcholine (ACh) from dopamine and norepinephrine?

A162: Acetylcholine is a neurotransmitter in the peripheral nervous system as well as in the CNS. More important, it is rapidly and entirely metabolized (by cholinesterases) rather than undergoing re-uptake into the presynaptic neuron.

Q163: Botulinum toxin A injection into affected muscles is coming into wide use as a treatment for blepharospasm, Meige's syndrome, and other orofacial dystonias. Which mechanism best explains its actions?
  a. It interferes with dopamine metabolism and causes parkinsonism.
  b. It causes paresis through CNS blockade.
  c. It induces a myasthenia-like state.
  d. It prevents release of presynaptic neuromuscular junction ACh.

A163: d. Botulinum toxin causes paresis of muscles by preventing their stimulation with ACh. Myasthenia is associated with postsynaptic ACh abnormalities. When used in treatment of facial muscle disorders, botulinum toxin provides remarkable reduction of movements for about 6 months. If the toxin were to escape from the site of injection, it could cause respiratory muscle paralysis.

Q164: A 29-year-old woman presents to a hospital with a history of *2 years* of generalized muscle contractions. On inspection the muscles are apparently well developed, and she appears to have an athletic build. She moves her limbs, trunk, and neck in continuous, writhing, and grotesque postures. What are common causes of this condition?

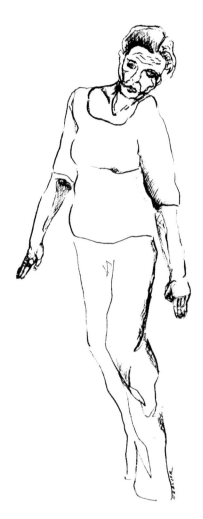

A164: This person has chronic dystonia. The organic nature and chronicity are indicated by muscle hypertrophy and lack of bodily fat. In young adults, dystonic postures may be caused by Wilson's disease, Huntington's disease, neuroleptics (tardive dystonia), and dystonia musculorum deformans.

Q165: Which of the following are characteristic of Tourette's syndrome?
    a.   Tendency toward obsessive-compulsive traits
    b.   Close concordance in twins
    c.   Close concordance in twins only if any tic disorder is included
    d.   Association with attention deficit disorder
    e.   Premovement potentials on back-averaged movement-locked EEGs

A165: a, c, d.

Q166: A 20-year-old sailor, who has a history of "glue sniffing," develops paresthesias and mild weakness in his hands and toes. What part of the nervous system is damaged?

A166: One of the major components of glue is N-hexane and other volatile solvents that have a great potential for abuse. Chronic exposure to these substances causes a neuropathy because they are lipophilic and damage the lipid-rich myelin cover of peripheral nerves.

Q167: A 25-year-old man, who has 2 weeks of premature ejaculation, develops spastic paresis and paresthesias below his waist. Routine history and physical examinations are otherwise unremarkable. A myelogram and CT scan of the head show no abnormalities. Of the following tests, which will be diagnostically helpful?

    a.   Visual evoked responses (VERs)
    b.   CSF oligoclonal band studies
    c.   CSF myelin basic protein
    d.   Antistriational antibody studies
    e.   Anti-ACh receptor antibodies
    f.   EEG

A167: a, b, c. These tests can indicate multiple sclerosis (MS), and VERs, in particular, can indicate optic nerve involvement (optic or retrobulbar neuritis). In contrast, antistriational antibodies indicate that a thymoma is present in a patient with *myasthenia gravis*. Anti-ACh receptor antibodies indicate general myasthenia gravis. An EEG is not diagnostically helpful for MS, myasthenia, or related conditions. Even though a CT scan was normal, an MRI scan might reveal cerebral MS plaques.

Q168: Which of the tests listed in the above question is generally positive in MS in exacerbation but negative in MS in remission?

A168: c. Myelin basic protein is found in exacerbation of MS but not when it is in remission. CSF oligoclonal bands are found in all stages of multiple sclerosis. When the optic nerves are involved even asymptomatically, the VERs are abnormal. However, each of these studies may be abnormal in conditions other than multiple sclerosis. Both CSF studies may be positive in chronic CNS inflammatory conditions, such as neurosyphilis, AIDS, and chronic fungal meningitis. VERs may be positive in optic nerve gliomas or other conditions affecting the optic pathways.

Q169: Which of the following results have *not* been shown by epidemiologic studies of MS patients?

    a.   The incidence of MS is roughly proportional to the distance from the equator in the Southern as well as in the Northern Hemisphere.
    b.   The incidence of MS is remarkably low in Orientals, black Africans, native Israelis, and Latin Americans.
    c.   Spouses have an increased incidence.
    d.   Blood relatives have an increased incidence.

A160: c.

Q170: Which findings usually accompany MS-induced sexual impairment?
    a.   Optic neuritis
    b.   Urinary impairment
    c.   Internuclear ophthalmoplegia
    d.   Leg spasticity

A170: b, d. These are symptoms of spinal cord involvement, which is usually the cause of MS-induced sexual impairment.

Q171: What do prolonged VER latencies indicate?
    a.   Optic or retrobulbar neuritis
    b.   Optic or retrobulbar neuritis, despite no clinically demonstrable visual impairment
    c.   Internuclear ophthalmoplegia (INO)
    d.   Psychogenic blindness rather than Anton's syndrome
    e.   Optic neuritis that is not a manifestation of multiple sclerosis

A171: a, b, e. Prolonged VER latencies are abnormal. They suggest a lesion of the visual system including the eye, optic nerve, and cerebral cortex. Only about one third of optic neuritis cases later develop multiple sclerosis.

Q172: Following surgery on the anterior communicating artery, a patient is found to be apathetic, mute, incontinent, and paraparetic. Which of the following complications probably has developed?

    a.   The spinal cord and brain have been damaged.

    b.   Depression has developed.

    c.   Both anterior cerebral arteries were occluded.

    d.   The patient developed normal pressure hydrocephalus (NPH), i.e., dementia, gait apraxia, and incontinence.

A172: c. The anterior communicating arteries supply a large portion of the frontal lobes, including the medial surface of the motor strips. These regions control the voluntary function of the legs and bladder. Infarction of these arteries creates marked personality impairments along with weakness of both legs and loss of bladder control. NPH sometimes develops following subarachnoid hemorrhages, but NPH patients have gait apraxia rather than paraparesis.

Q173: Which of the following conditions might lead to a patient's having "putrid smells" that the physician cannot detect?

    a.   Seizures that originate in the uncus

    b.   Sinusitis

    c.   Migraine aura

    d.   Seizures that originate in the parietal lobe

    e.   Phenytoin

A173: a, b. Migraine headaches, curiously, often have visual but rarely olfactory auras.

Q174: Which of the following conditions cause Horner's syndrome?

    a.   Lateral medullary infarctions

    b.   Cluster headaches

    c.   Lung carcinoma

    d.   Migraine headaches

    e.   Occlusion of the posterior inferior cerebellar artery

    f.   Cervical spinal cord lesions

    g.   Cerebral infarctions

    h.   Injury to C-8 and T-1 nerve roots

A174: a, b, c, e, f, h.

Q175: An elderly man falls down a flight of stairs, fracturing his right femoral neck and right humerus. After the hip is "pinned" and the arm is set, he is noted to be confused, agitated, and unintelligible. Which of the following possibilities must be considered?

    a.   Fat emboli

    b.   Neurologic illness precipitating the fall

    c.   A left cerebral infarction

    d.   Development of a subdural hematoma

    e.   An electrolyte disturbance

    f.   A medication causing an adverse reaction

    g.   Aspiration pneumonia

    h.   Alcohol or other substance withdrawal

A175: a, b, c, d, e, f, g, h.

Q176: Which of the following would be helpful in the case described in the preceding question?

    a.   CBC, electrolytes, BUN determinations

    b.   EEG

    c.   CT scan

    d.   Review of medications

    e.   Chest x-ray

    f.   Review of history

    g.   Lumbar puncture

h.   Urine for fat analysis
i.   Sedating the patient until the situation is clarified
j.   Echoencephalogram

A176: a, c, d, e, f, h, i.

Q177: In which conditions might lumbar puncture be indicated?
a.   Subdural hematoma
b.   Brain abscess
c.   Brain tumor
d.   Unruptured arteriovenous malformation
e.   Pseudotumor cerebri
f.   Multiple sclerosis
g.   Bacterial meningitis
h.   Subacute sclerosing panencephalitis (SSPE)
i.   Viral encephalitis
j.   Sexual impairment

A177:   e, f, g, h, i. Lumbar punctures should not be done when intracranial mass lesions are suspected because CSF analysis will not be helpful and the procedure might precipitate transtentorial herniation.

Q178:   Which of the following are complications of alcoholism?
a.   Mammillary body hemorrhage
b.   Peripheral neuropathy
c.   Neurofibrillary tangles
d.   Central pontine myelinolysis
e.   Corpus callosum degeneration (Marchiafava-Bignami syndrome)
f.   Cerebellar degeneration
g.   Granulovacuolar changes
h.   Sclerotic plaques

A178: a, b, d, e, f.

Q179:   Which of the following illness(es) is (are) characterized by a normal mental state despite quadriparesis and respiratory distress?
a.   Guillain-Barré syndrome
b.   Locked-in syndrome
c.   Persistent vegetative state
d.   Myasthenia gravis
e.   Porphyria

A179: a, b, d.

Q180:   An emaciated 13-year-old girl has weakness, sensory loss, and areflexia of her distal lower extremities. She then develops eversion and dorsiflexion weakness of her left ankle. How can both a peripheral neuropathy and a left superficial peroneal nerve injury be explained?
a.   Her polyneuropathy is nutritional.
b.   The mononeuropathy is a compression injury.
c.   She has a vasculitis (e.g., lupus), which causes both polyneuropathy and mononeuropathy multiplex.
d.   They cannot be explained.

A180:   a, b, c (rare). A systemic illness, such as lupus, is possible, but patients rarely present with neurologic signs. Anorexia nervosa can lead to a nutritional neuropathy when the patients fail to take vitamins or high protein, fat-soluble foods. Whatever the cause of the weight loss, nerves lose their overlying subcutaneous fatty tissue. The nerves' protection then is lost and they are vulnerable to compression, even as slight as crossing one leg over the other.

Q181:   An adolescent girl has twitchy, restless movements. Aside from irritability, her mental and emotional status is normal. Which tests would be most appropriate?

a. VDRL
b. Inquiries about oral contraceptives
c. Antistreptolysin O Titer (ALSO)
d. Pregnancy test
e. Lupus preparation

A181: b, c, d, e. Chorea in adolescence can be a manifestation of pregnancy (chorea gravidarum), an idiosyncratic reaction to oral contraceptives, rheumatic fever (Sydenham's chorea), lupus, or various metabolic derangements. In adolescence, it may be indistinguishable from myoclonus (as seen in SSPE) or tremors (as seen in Wilson's disease). Curiously, in adolescents Huntington's chorea does not usually cause chorea, but rather rigidity that appears like parkinsonism.

Q182: Which area of the brain is larger on one side than the other?
a. The uncus
b. The motor strip
c. The planum temporale
d. The basal ganglia
e. One cerebral hemisphere if the other is damaged by an in utero vascular accident
f. The frontal lobe

A182: c, e. The planum temporale, the superior surface of the temporal lobe that contains Heschl's and Wernicke's areas, is almost always larger in the dominant than the nondominant hemisphere. This normal asymmetry is lost in brain damage, some schizophrenic patients, and many autistic children. When a cerebral hemisphere is damaged in utero, that hemisphere fails to grow fully. The contralateral limbs, in such cases, will be foreshortened. Also, focal seizures may originate from the damaged hemisphere.

Q183: A 70-year-old man has the abrupt onset of confusion, amnesia, and personality changes. A neurologist makes a diagnosis of transient global amnesia (TGA). Most neurologists believe TGA is the result of ischemia of both posterior cerebral arteries. Although that theory may be true, which test might be performed to diagnose other conditions that might mimic TGA?
a. Serum phenobarbital concentrations
b. EEG
c. Serum potassium
d. Blood glucose
e. Blood alcohol level

A183: a, b, d, e. Some individuals develop mental aberrations, "a paradoxical reaction," if they take hypnotic medications, including phenobarbital and alcohol. Partial complex seizures and hypoglycemia should also always be considered in acute confusional states. Although low serum potassium (hypokalemia) causes weakness, it does not cause mental disturbances.

Q184: Which of the following tumors is most likely to cause partial complex seizures?
a. Olfactory groove meningioma
b. Sphenoid wing meningioma
c. Parasagittal meningioma

A184: a, b. Sphenoid wing meningiomas can typically irritate the temporal lobe and cause partial complex seizures. Also, olfactory groove meningiomas irritate the frontal lobe, which is the origin of 10 to 20 percent of partial complex seizures.

Q185: Which of the following neoplasms are AIDS victims likely to develop?
a. Cerebellar astrocytoma
b. Cerebral lymphoma
c. Glioblastoma multiforme
d. Kaposi's sarcoma

A185: b, d.

Q186: Which conditions may be complicated by fever, muscle necrosis, and renal impairment?
  a. Malignant hyperthermia
  b. DTs
  c. Catatonia
  d. Hallucinogen intoxication
  e. Duchenne's dystrophy
  f. Neuroleptic-malignant syndrome

A186: a, b, c, d, f.

Q187: In the preceding question, how does neuroleptic-malignant syndrome differ from the other choices?

A187: Neuroleptic-malignant syndrome follows use of neuroleptic medications that block dopamine transmission. Malignant hyperthermia, which is usually an inherited condition, follows administration of general anesthesia. Neuroleptic-malignant syndrome causes much greater muscle rigidity and fever than catatonia, DTs, or hallucinogens.

Q188: What is the purpose of combining carbidopa with L-dopa, as in Sinemet?
  a. Carbidopa is a peripheral dopamine decarboxylase inhibitor, which raises CNS levels of L-dopa.
  b. Carbidopa is a dopamine antagonist.
  c. Carbidopa is a dopamine agonist.
  d. Carbidopa is anticholinergic.
  e. Carbidopa acts on the postsynaptic neuron.

A188: a.

Q189: What is the purpose of using bromocriptine (Parlodel) in the treatment of Parkinson's disease?
  a. It is a dopamine precursor.
  b. It is a dopamine agonist.
  c. It has anticholinergic properties.
  d. It affects the presynaptic neuron.
  e. It affects the postsynaptic neuron.

A189: b, e.

Q190: A 32-year-old man who suffers from partial complex epilepsy has developed increasing confusion, irritability, and lethargy. His current regimen is phenytoin 300 mg/day and primidone 750 mg/day. Blood anticonvulsant levels, MRI, lumbar puncture, EEG, and routine tests disclose no significant abnormality. Of the following, which would be the best management plan?
  a. Increase both anticonvulsants.
  b. Substitute carbamazepine for the primidone.
  c. Stop both anticonvulsants.
  d. Add carbamazepine (Tegretol) to the two current anticonvulsants.

A190: b. Primidone is the most likely offender. Although the patient may be intoxicated with anticonvulsants despite normal levels, completely withdrawing anticonvulsants might precipitate status epilepticus.

Q191: Which anticonvulsant is metabolized into phenobarbital?
  a. Primidone (Mysoline)
  b. Phenytoin (Dilantin)
  c. Carbamazepine (Tegretol)
  d. Valproic acid (Depakote)

A191: a.

Q192: Which procedures might be helpful in determining the dominant hemisphere?
  a. Positron emission tomography (PET)
  b. Computed tomography (CT)

    c. EEG with sphenoidal electrodes
    d. Magnetic resonance imaging (MRI)
    e. Intracarotid sodium amobarbital injection
    f. Wada test
    g. Visual evoked responses (VER)
    h. Brainstem auditory evoked responses (BAER)

A192: a, e, f. The Wada test is based on intracarotid amobarbital injections.

Q193: Which of the following may be found in a right-handed patient who undergoes a complete commissurotomy?
    a. Stimulation of either hemisphere can provoke various emotions.
    b. The patient will not be able to describe what the right hand is doing.
    c. Seizures will be confined to a single hemisphere.
    d. The left hand will be able to copy a figure seen in the left visual field, but the patient will not be able either to write or say the name of the figure.
    e. The patient will be able to copy with the right hand what he or she sees in the right visual field, but will not be able to say or write the name of that figure.

A193: a, c, d.

Q194: What is false about serotonin?
    a. It is an indoleamine.
    b. 5-Hydroxyindoleacetic acid is its metabolic product.
    c. It is found in high concentrations in the dorsal raphe nucleus.
    d. It is an endogenous opiate.
    e. When it or its precursors are injected into the ventricles, sleep is induced.

A194: d.

Q195: Which analgesics does naloxone antagonize?
    a. Heroin
    b. Morphine
    c. Stimulation-produced analgesia
    d. Hypnosis

A195: a, b, c.

Q196: When nonsteroidal anti-inflammatory agents are given for menstrual cramps, with which substances do they interfere?
    a. Enkephalins
    b. Endorphins
    c. Prostaglandins
    d. Serotonin
    e. Dopamine

A196: c.

Q197: Which statements are true regarding the dorsal raphe nucleus?
    a. It contains high concentrations of endorphins.
    b. Stimulating it causes pain.
    c. Stimulating it produces analgesia.
    d. Stimulating it produces behavioral changes.
    e. Its destruction causes analgesia.
    f. It contains high serotonin concentrations.
    g. Microinjections of procaine (Novacaine) cause analgesia.
    h. Microinjections of morphine cause analgesia.

A197: c, f.

Q198: A 14-year-old boy is brought to the Emergency Room in stupor. He is apneic and his pupils are miotic. Which one of the following conditions is most likely to be the cause of this constellation of findings?

     a.   Brainstem stroke
     b.   Heroin or other narcotic overdose
     c.   Hypoglycemia
     d.   Postictal stupor
     e.   Psychogenic disturbance

A198: b. Pontine strokes may cause this constellation, but they rarely occur in this age group. The other conditions generally cause dilated pupils and do not cause apnea.

Q199: Which of the following are complications of intravenous heroin use?
     a.   Pulmonary edema
     b.   Cerebrovascular accidents
     c.   Tetanus
     d.   Malaria
     e.   Acquired immune deficiency syndrome (AIDS)

A199: a, b, c, d, e.

Q200: Which of the following are common to endogenous opiates and morphine?
     a.   Euphoria
     b.   Polypeptide structure
     c.   Respiratory depression
     d.   Reversal with naloxone

A200: a, c, d.

Q201: In which CNS areas are opiate receptors located?
     a.   The basal ganglia
     b.   A delta fibers
     c.   The spinal dorsal horn
     d.   The amygdala
     e.   Unmyelinated C fibers

A201: a, c, and d. The A delta and C fibers are parts of the peripheral nervous system. Although they carry pain sensation, they do not use endogenous opiates for neurotransmission.

Q202: Which of the following roles have been ascribed to serotonin?
     a.   It is concentrated in the raphe nuclei where it modulates the sleep cycle.
     b.   It is found in the dorsal horn of the spinal cord where it has a role in analgesia.
     c.   It is found in the periaqueductal gray matter where it has a role in pain perception and modification.
     d.   It is found in the nucleus raphe magnus, where it has a role in pain interpretation and reduction.
     e.   Serotonin itself is an endogenous opiate.
     f.   Some tricyclic antidepressants inhibit the uptake of serotonin.

A202: a, b, c, d, f.

Q203: Three family members brought to the Emergency Room are each suffering from respiratory distress and weakness of the head, neck, and shoulders. They also have dilated and poorly reactive pupils. Ocular motility impairments that seem like internuclear ophthalmoplegia are present. One patient had optic neuritis as a young woman. Which of the following conditions is the most likely diagnosis?
     a.   Multiple sclerosis
     b.   Atropine intoxication
     c.   Insecticide poisoning
     d.   Botulism
     e.   Myasthenia gravis

A203: d. Botulism, which typically strikes groups of people, can produce bulbar palsy and ocular motility impairments that mimic internuclear ophthalmoplegia. Insecticide poisoning also produces respiratory distress, but in such cases the pupils are almost always miotic and fasciculations are prominent.

Q204–206:   This 29-year-old woman has developed a tremor that is most pronounced when she writes, drinks coffee, and lights a cigarette.

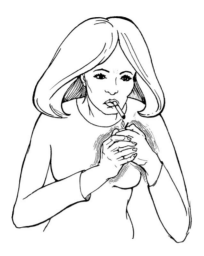

Q204:   Which of the following conditions can lead to such a tremor?
   a.   Essential tremor
   b.   Wilson's disease
   c.   Anxiety
   d.   Huntington's chorea
   e.   Athetosis
   f.   Benign familial tremor

A204:   a, b, c, and f. Essential tremor and benign familial tremor are probably varieties of the same condition. Wilson's disease is a rare but important condition that might be considered in young adults who develop tremor. Anxiety can produce a tremor that is indistinguishable from essential tremor and that may have a similar etiology and positive response to beta adrenergic blockers.

Q205:   Which tests should be performed to exclude Wilson's disease when only mild tremors were evident?
   a.   CT
   b.   EEG
   c.   Lumbar puncture
   d.   Serum ceruloplasmin
   e.   Serum copper concentration
   f.   Slit-lamp examination

A205:   d, f.

Q206:   If the patient did have an essential tremor, which group of medications are most often effective?
   a.   Anticholinergics
   b.   Dopamine agonists
   c.   Neuroleptics
   d.   Beta-adrenergic blockers
   e.   Antiviral agents
   f.   Alpha-adrenergic blockers

A206:   d.

Q207–213: Match the EEG pattern with the associated conditions.

207: Periodic complexes

208: Triphasic waves

209: Movement artifact

210: Excessive beta activity

211: 3-Hz spike-and-slow wave

212: Focal, phase-reversed delta activity

213: Postictal EEG depression

a. Absences
b. Brain tumor
c. Use of sedatives or tranquilizers
d. Psychogenic seizures
e. Electroshock therapy
f. Tonic-clonic seizure
g. Creutzfeldt-Jakob disease
h. Subacute sclerosing panencephalitis (SSPE)
i. Uremia
j. Hepatic encephalopathy

A207–213:

207: g, h

208: i, j

209: d

210: c

211: a

212: b

213: e, f

Q214: What is the consequence of a deficiency in choline acetyltransferase?
a. Decreased acetylcholine
b. Increased cholinesterases
c. Parkinson's disease
d. Possibly dementia

A214: a, d.

Q215: Which of the following analgesic systems do *not* use the endogenous opiate system?

a. Narcotics
b. Aspirin
c. TENS
d. Periventricular gray matter stimulation
e. Hypnosis
f. Tricyclic antidepressants
g. Nonsteroidal anti-inflammatory agents

A215: b, e, f, g.

Q216: How do neurotransmitters differ from classic endocrine hormones, such as T_4?

a. They or their byproducts circulate in detectable quantitiess in the blood.
b. They are produced and stored at a site adjacent to the target organ.
c. They or their byproducts are present in significant quantity in the cerebrospinal fluid but not in the blood.
d. They are steroids.

A216: b, c.

Q217: A 40-year-old bachelor, who is in psychoanalysis, begins to describe that his knees often weaken whenever he meets a beautiful woman. During these episodes, which are momentary but frequent, he never falls and does not lose his end of the conversation. The loss of strength in his legs seems to occur only in social situations, but it defies psychoanalysis. Which neurologic conditions may be responsible?
a. Petit mal (absence) seizures
b. Basilar artery TIA
c. Cataplexy
d. Orthostatic hypotension
e. Vasovagal attack
f. Hypokalemic paralysis

A217: c. Cataplexy is the brief loss of muscle tone that is often precipitated by overwhelming emotional states, such as anger, fear, and joy. Although in classic cases the entire body muscular tone is lost and people collapse to the floor, more commonly isolated muscle groups lose tone. For example, patients with cataplexy often lose the muscle tone in their jaw or neck muscles, and these patients merely have slackening of the jaw or a brief forward movement of their head.

Cataplexy, by itself, does not cause loss of consciousness or amnesia. It if often found, however, in patients with the narcolepsy-cataplexy syndrome, which includes hallucinations and paralysis on awakening and falling asleep.

Petit mal seizures cause loss of consciousness but no loss of body tone. They usually have an onset in childhood, and in at least two thirds of the cases the absence seizures diminish by the time patients reach adulthood.

Basilar artery TIAs, orthostatic hypotension, and vasovagal attacks all cause lightheadedness or frank loss of consciousness along with generalized muscle weakness. Hypokalemic paralysis causes a gradual onset of generalized bodily weakness that has a duration of at least 15 minutes.

Q218: In what way does Huntington's chorea in adolescents differ from that in adults?
    a.   Prominent rigidity
    b.   No dementia
    c.   Akinesia prominent
    d.   Seizures frequent
    e.   Different course
    f.   Mimics Parkinson's disease

A218: a, c, d, f.

Q219: In which conditions might a lumbar puncture precipitate transtentorial herniation?
    a.   Acute subdural hematoma
    b.   Pseudotumor cerebri
    c.   Chronic subdural hematoma
    d.   Glioblastoma

A219: a, c, d.

Q220: With which findings is the concentration of senile plaques associated?
    a.   Older age
    b.   Schizophrenia
    c.   Poor performance on the Bleeded test
    d.   Depression
    e.   Trisomy 21
    f.   Head trauma

A220: a, c, e, f.

Q221: In depressed people, which of the following neuroendocrine changes are routinely found?
    a.   Advanced shift of MHPG excretion
    b.   Delay in body temperature nadir
    c.   Advanced shift of REM sleep
    d.   Delay in peak cortisol excretion
    e.   Advanced shift of body temperature nadir

A221: a, c, e.

Q222: Which conditions frequently increase REM latency?
    a.   Depression
    b.   Drug withdrawal
    c.   Excessive alcohol use
    d.   Narcolepsy

A222: c.

Q223:   In Huntington's chorea, what is the change in CSF GABA concentration?
     a.   GABA is increased.
     b.   GABA is decreased.
     c.   GABA is unchanged.

A223:   b. Determination of a lowered GABA concentration in the CSF sometimes confirms the clinical impression of Huntington's chorea.

Q224–230:   How are the following medications thought to treat or prevent pain?

224.   Aspirin

225.   Nonsteroidal anti-inflammatory agents

226.   Tricyclic antidepressants

227.   Methysergide

228.   Cafergot

229.   Inderal

230.   Narcotics

     a.   Vasoconstriction
     b.   Activation of the endogenous opiate system
     c.   Beta adrenergic blocking
     d.   Inhibition of prostaglandin synthesis
     e.   Interference with platelet serotonin
     f.   Increase of serotonin levels

A224–230

A224: d.	**A228:** a.
A225: d.	**A229:** c.
A226: f.	**A230:** b.
A227: e.	

Q231:   A 28-year-old woman complains of gait impairment. She has a history of vigorous exercise, taking large quantities of vitamins, and avoiding red meat and alcohol. On examination, she has marked sensory loss in all limbs and absent DTRs, but her strength is normal. Which of the following conditions are most likely to be responsible for her complaints?
     a.   Cervical spondylosis
     b.   Myopathy
     c.   Vitamin toxicity
     d.   Iron deficiency anemia

A231:   c. Pyridoxine (vitamin B_6) in large daily doses creates a neuropathy that impairs sensation and is reversible after the vitamins are withdrawn. Although iron deficiency does not create a neuropathy, thiamine and folate deficiency, often a consequence of alcoholism, can produce a neuropathy.

Q232:   A 68-year-old house painter has weakness, atrophy, and areflexic DTRs in his upper extremities. In addition, he has sensory loss in his right hand, brisk DTRs in his legs, and a right Babinski sign. Which of the features suggest that he has cervical spondylosis rather than ALS?
     a.   Hand atrophy
     b.   Hyperactive DTRs in the legs
     c.   Sensory loss
     d.   The Babinski sign

A232:   c. House painting, which involves prolonged neck hyperextension, leads to cervical spondylosis as an occupational hazard. Whatever the cause, cervical spondylosis leads to sensory and lower motor neuron loss in the upper extremities and upper motor neuron signs in the lower extremities. Cervical spondylosis is a much more frequently occurring condition than ALS.

Q233: What are the potential neurologic side effects of oral contraceptives?
   a. Dementia
   b. Chorea
   c. Multiple sclerosis
   d. Increase in migraine headaches
   e. Peripheral neuropathy
   f. Cerebrovascular accidents in certain women

A233: b, d, f. The tendency toward cerebrovascular accidents, which is associated with high-dose estrogen, is probably restricted to older women who are hypertensive or who smoke.

Q234: In which conditions might a contrast CT scan produce serious complications?
   a. Asthma
   b. Iodine allergy
   c. Encephalitis
   d. Diabetic nephropathy
   e. Dehydration
   f. Seizure disorder

A234: b, d, e. The contrast solution contains iodine, which might precipitate the Stevens-Johnson syndrome, laryngeal edema, or other manifestations of allergy. Patients with diabetes or dehydration might develop acute tubular necrosis. MRI does not require use of a contrast agent.

Q235: What is the most characteristic finding in standard intelligence tests in people with early dementia?
   a. Decreased performance, decreased verbal scales
   b. Decreased performance, relatively normal verbal scales
   c. Decreased verbal, relatively normal performance scales
   d. None of the above

A235: b.

Q236: In contrast to patients with early dementia, what will standard intelligence tests show in patients with depression-induced cognitive changes?
   a. Decreased performance, decreased verbal scales
   b. Decreased performance, relatively normal verbal scales
   c. Decreased verbal, relatively normal performance scales
   d. None of the above

A236: a. Verbal and performance scales are usually both lowered; however, performance scales might be lower because of psychomotor retardation, and they might change as attention and mood fluctuate.

Q237: As people age, what is the most common EEG finding?
   a. Loss of amplitude
   b. Slowing of the background activity
   c. Presence of beta activity
   d. Fragmentation of background

A237: b.

Q238: What are the consequences of alcohol withdrawal?
   a. Increased REM activity
   b. Insomnia
   c. Increased dreaming
   d. Tendency to have seizures

A238: a, b, c, d.

Q239: Which test is the most likely to reveal asymptomatic frontal lobe multiple sclerosis plaques?
    a.   EEG
    b.   CT
    c.   MRI
    d.   Lumbar puncture
    e.   Visual evoked responses

A239: c. MRI is superior to CT for detecting changes in the chemical composition of myelin, as occurs in multiple sclerosis. Moreover, it has better anatomic resolution and no risks of contrast infusion.

Q240: Which findings are more closely associated with aphasia than dementia?
    a.   Right homonymous hemianopsia
    b.   Focal EEG slowing
    c.   Paraphasic errors
    d.   Seizures
    e.   Circumducted or hemiparetic gait

A240: a, b, c, d, e.

Q241: Does use of phenytoin (Dilantin), phenobarbital, or carbamazepine (Tegretol) tend to give false-positive, false-negative, or no different results in the dexamethasone suppression test?

A241: False-positive

Q242: In what ways do hypnagogic hallucinations *differ* from partial complex seizures?
    a.   They are associated with flaccid, areflexic musculature.
    b.   They often have an auditory component.
    c.   They are associated with EEG spikes.
    d.   They have visual, auditory, and emotional aspects.
    e.   They are varied.

A242: a, e.

Q243: Which analgesic properties are found with narcotics that are *not* found with nonsteroidal anti-inflammatory agents?
    a.   Antipyretic activity
    b.   Dependence
    c.   Respiratory depression
    d.   Tolerance
    e.   Euphoria
    f.   Withdrawal symptoms
    g.   Prostaglandin synthesis inhibition

A243: b, c, d, e, f.

Q244: Which structure contains 80 percent of the brain's dopamine content?
    a.   Third ventricle
    b.   Thalamus
    c.   Cerebral cortex
    d.   Corpus striatum

A244: d.

Q245: Which structures will "enhance" during a contrast CT scan?
    a.   Glioblastoma
    b.   Cerebral infarct
    c.   Arteriovenous malformation (AVM)
    d.   Cerebral hemorrhage
    e.   The contents of a subdural hematoma
    f.   The membrane of a subdural hematoma

A245: a, c, f, rarely b.

Q246: A 50-year-old man who has developed a slowly progressive dementia is suspected of having neurosyphilis, The CSF shows protein concentration of 100 mg/100 ml, 10 lymphocytes/mm, and a negative VDRL. Which of the following plans are appropriate?

    a. Repeat the lumbar puncture to determine the CSF cryptococcal antigen titer, culture CSF for TB, and obtain CSF cytology.
    b. Disregard the negative VDRL and treat the patient for neurosyphilis.
    c. Perform a brain biopsy.
    d. Base the diagnosis on a CSF FTA-ABS test.

A246: a, b. A CSF FTA-ABS test on spinal fluid is unreliable. This patient should be treated for neurosyphilis as further evaluation is undertaken. Notably, as many as 40 percent of neurosyphilis patients may have negative CSF VDRL tests because of natural resolution of the serologic variables or partial, possibly inadequate antibiotic treatment. Nevertheless, since the VDRL is negative, other conditions, such as crypto-coccal meningitis, should be considered.

Q247: Which of the following conditions that cause dementia tend to occur in families?

    a. Pick's disease
    b. SSPE
    c. Alzheimer's disease
    d. Creutzfeldt-Jakob disease

A247: a, c. About one third of the patients with Alzheimer's disease have had a similarly affected parent or sibling. In rare families, Alzheimer's disease appears to be transmitted as an autosomal dominant trait. In them, Alzheimer's disease appears at a younger age and follows a fulminant course. Pick's disease, which is rare in the United States, has a familial tendency, but genetic transmission has not been established.

Q248: Which condition is *not* associated with shortened REM latency?

    a. Night terrors
    b. Narcolepsy
    c. Depression
    d. Withdrawal from sedatives
    e. Withdrawal from neuroleptics
    f. Cataplexy

A248: a.

Q249: A person complains of developing a recurrent, vivid dream. His bed partner has noted that, after mumbling, the patient falls asleep and, on two occasions, has had enuresis. What preliminary tests should be done?

    a. He should be monitored in a sleep laboratory.
    b. He should have an EEG with hyperventilation and photic stimulation.
    c. He should undergo an amobarbital interview.
    d. He should have an EEG following sleep deprivation.

A249: b, d.

Q250: The patient in question 249 has an EEG following sleep deprivation that shows a paroxysm of spike and spike-and-wave activity, but further evaluation is unremarkable. What medication is indicated?

    a. Sedatives
    b. Hypnotics
    c. Antidepressants
    d. Neuroleptics
    e. Anticonvulsants
    f. Antabuse

A250: e.

Q251: Which one of the following illnesses is the most likely cause of rapidly progressive intellectual impairment in an 8-year-old girl?
- a. Mental retardation
- b. A glycogen-storage disease
- c. Subacute sclerosing panencephalitis (SSPE)
- d. Duchenne's muscular dystrophy

A251: c. Of these conditions, SSPE is probably the most common degenerative neurologic condition that affects girls. Glycogen-storage diseases are indolent and not necessarily associated with intellectual impairment. Duchenne's muscular dystrophy does not affect females. In males, it causes intellectual impairments that are subtle and slowly progressive.

Q252: Sometimes high-dose steroid treatment is complicated by "steroid psychosis," hypokalemic myopathy, or fungal meningitis—all conditions that initially may be misdiagnosed as psychogenic. Nevertheless, steroids are commonly used in a variety of neurologic illnesses. Which of the following illnesses are commonly treated with steroids?
- a. Metastatic brain tumor
- b. Multiple sclerosis
- c. Lupus cerebritis
- d. Bell's palsy
- e. Uremic encephalopathy
- f. Myasthenia gravis

A252: a, b, c, d, f.

Q253: One week after a right cerebral infarction, a 60-year-old man develops burning pain in the left side of his face, and his left arm, leg, and trunk. There is marked sensory loss to all modalities in these regions and a mild left hemiparesis. What is the origin of the patient's pain?
- a. Parietal lobe injury
- b. Psychogenic impairment
- c. Lateral spinothalamic damage
- d. Thalamic injury

A253: d. The patient has "thalamic pain," which is a distressing consequence of a cerebrovascular accident in the thalamus. The pain can persist for years, but it is usually limited to about 6 months and sometimes responds to treatment with either phenytoin (Dilantin) or carbamazepine (Tegretol).

Q254: Which structures are usually considered to be parts of the basal ganglia?
- a. The corpus striatum
- b. The cerebellum
- c. The putamen
- d. The caudate nuclei
- e. Meynert's nuclei
- f. The globus pallidus
- g. The substantia nigra
- h. The subthalamic nucleus

A254: a, c, d, f, g, h.

Q255: Which of the structures in question 254 are usually considered to be part of the corpus striatum?

A255: c, d, f.

Q256: Which of the following tests *do not* rely on ionizing radiation?
- a. CT
- b. MRI
- c. Isotopic brain scan
- d. EEG

A256: b, d.

Q257: What will the cisternogram show in classic cases of normal pressure hydro-cephalus?

    a. Radioactivity over the cerebral hemispheres
    b. Persistent basilar or intraventricular radioactivity
    c. Radioactivity lingering in the spinal canal
    d. None of the above

A257: b.

Q258: In patients with Alzheimer's disease with cerebral atrophy, what will the cisternogram show?

    a. Radioactivity over the cerebral hemispheres
    b. Persistent intraventricular radioactivity
    c. Lingering of radioactivity in the spinal canal
    d. None of the above

A258: a. Although the cisternogram is somewhat helpful in distinguishing between Alzheimer's disease and normal pressure hydrocephalus, it should not be considered sufficient to make a definite diagnosis.

Q259: In which illnesses are elevated CSF measles antibodies found?

    a. Alzheimer's disease
    b. Creutzfeldt-Jakob disease
    c. SSPE
    d. Multiple sclerosis

A259: c, d.

Q260: Which are characteristic features of sleep patterns following sleep deprivation?

    a. Early terminal awakening
    b. Relatively normal REM distribution
    c. Decreased REM latency
    d. Increased sleep latency
    e. Increased total sleep

A260: b, c, e.

Q261: Which physiologic processes are found in sleeping people when the EEG shows great quantities of high voltage, 1 to 3-Hz activity?

    a. Some limb EMG activity
    b. Relatively low blood perssure and pulse
    c. Penile erections
    d. Rapid eye movement

A261: a, b. Such EEG activity is "slow wave" or deep NREM sleep.

Q262: Which of the following conditions might cause rigidity and akinesia but no tremor in adolescents?

    a. Huntington's chorea
    b. Wilson's disease
    c. Parkinson's disease
    d. Medications
    e. Tourette's syndrome
    f. Sydenham's chorea
    g. Cerebral palsy
    h. Serotonin excess

A262: a, b, c, d, g.

Q263: Which sleep changes are *not* associated with old age?

    a. Multiple brief awakenings
    b. Shift to earlier time of sleep and awakening
    c. Increased amount of stage 4 NREM sleep
    d. Shortening of total sleep time

A263: c.

Q264–266: Match the illness that can cause mental changes with its physical manifestations?

264. Porphyria

265. Hypothyroidism

266. Pellegra

    a. Dermatitis, diarrhea
    b. Abdominal pain
    c. Ataxia, coma

A264–266:

264: b.

265: c.

266: a. Pellegra causes the "3 D's": dermatitis, diarrhea, and dementia.

Q267: In patients with the human variety of the Klúver-Bucy syndrome, which symptom is *least* common?
    a. Oral exploration
    b. Amnesia
    c. Uncontrollable sexual activity
    d. Placidity

A267: c. In humans who develop the Klüver-Bucy syndrome (typically from Herpes encephalitis, contusion of the temporal lobes, or multiple CVAs), sexual activity is limited and generally consists only of minor verbal and behavioral changes, but usually not overt aggression or homosexual activity. Also, although humans have oral exploration, it is less pronounced than in animals.

Q268: Sometimes medical treatments produce neurologic damage as a complication of an otherwise major benefit. Which of the following statements is *false*?
    a. Human growth hormone injections given to correct short stature in children have caused Creutzfeldt-Jakob disease.
    b. Smallpox vaccinations rarely cause an episode of disseminated CNS demyelination.
    c. Measles vaccination causes subacute sclerosing panencephalitis (SSPE).
    d. Artificial insemination with donor semen has induced acquired immunodeficiency syndrome (AIDS).

A268: c. Although elevated measles antibody titers are found in the CSF of patients (who are usually children) with SSPE, measles virus has not been proven to be the cause of this illness, and similar abnormalities have also been found in patients with multiple sclerosis. Studies have shown that the incidence of SSPE has been markedly reduced following the use of measles vaccination programs and that measles vaccinations have not caused SSPE.

The development of Creutzfeldt-Jakob disease in children given growth hormone extracted from human pituitary glands led to the use of growth hormone synthesis from genetically engineered bacteria. Creutzfeldt-Jakob disease has also been transferred by use of depth EEG electrodes and corneal transplantation.

Smallpox vaccinations occasionally cause "postvaccinial demyelination," a condition in which multiple areas of the CNS become demyelinated. Its clinical and histologic features mimic multiple sclerosis; however, postvaccinial symptoms and signs occur in a single episode. This complication has been the major reason that smallpox vaccinations are given sparingly.

AIDS transmission has been documented to have resulted from homosexual, heterosexual, and artificial semen transfer as well as from blood transfusions. Semen used for artificial insemination and blood used for transfusion are usually tested for AIDS, hepatitis, syphilis, and other sexually transmitted illnesses.

Q269: A 30-year-old woman has the sudden onset of "the worst headache of her life." She has nuchal rigidity, but otherwise her neurologic examination is normal. A CT scan shows blood density material in the right Sylvian fissure. What is the best diagnostic procedure to perform?

    a. Lumbar puncture
    b. EEG
    c. Isotopic brain scan
    d. Cerebral arteriography

A269: d. The patient probably has had a subarachnoid hemorrhage from a ruptured "berry" aneurysm. Cerebral arteriography would document the aneurysm, reveal its location and anatomy, and exclude the possibility of other sources of bleeding, such as a mycotic aneurysm or small arteriovenous malformation (AVM). A lumbar puncture would probably be superfluous and possibly dangerous because it could lead to a rerupture of the aneurysm or, if a large hematoma were present, transtentorial herniation.

Q270: In which brain region do patients with Alzheimer's disease have a pronounced neuron loss that results in an acetylcholine deficit?

    a. Frontal lobe
    b. Frontal and temporal lobe
    c. Hippocampus
    d. Nucleus basalis Meynert

A270: d. The most important area is the nucleus basalis Meynert. Although patients also have neuron loss in the hippocampus, that loss is not associated with an acetylcholine deficiency.

Q271: Which conditions can cause akinesia and rigidity (i.e., parkinsonism) in young adults?

    a. MPTP
    b. Beta stimulator medications
    c. Metoclopramide (Reglan)
    d. Huntington's chorea
    e. Dementia pugilistica

A271: a, c, d, e. MPTP is a toxic byproduct of the illicit manufacture of narcotics. It is directly toxic to the nigrostriatal pathway, and it causes parkinsonism almost immediately after it is injected. Beta stimulators, such as asthma medications, cause a fine rapid tremor that is similar to an essential tremor or lithium-induced tremor.

Metoclopramide (Reglan), which has become a widely used medication for treatment of diabetic gastric stasis, esophageal reflux, and other disorders of gastric motility, is a dopamine antagonist. Thus, it causes parkinsonism and also oculogyric crises. As discussed previously, Huntington's chorea that develops in children and young adults often causes rigidity and bradykinesia (i.e., parkinsonism), rather than chorea. Dementia pugilistica, the "punch drunk" syndrome, consists of a combination of dementia and parkinsonism. It is a chronic progressive condition that is related to the amount of head trauma that boxers sustain.

Q272: After a fall, an 80-year-old man who is known to have Alzheimer's disease begins to have the rapid loss of remaining cognitive function and then becomes lethargic. A CT scan shows swelling of the right cerebral hemisphere and shift of midline structures. Which structural lesions are most likely to have developed?

    a. A CVA
    b. A glioblastoma
    c. A subdural hematoma
    d. A pseudotumor cerebri

A272: c. An *isodense* subdural hematoma appears as brain swelling, but infarctions and tumors are discrete lesions. People with cerebral atrophy, especially the elderly, are prone to develop subdural hematomas, which are usually radiodense (white) when acute and radiolucent (black) when chronic. At some time in their course, subdural hematomas are often isodense to the brain. Subdural hematomas are probably as common as primary brain tumors, and they are a correctable cause of dementia.

Q273: In which conditions is the choline acetyltransferase (CAT) concentration of the cerebral cortex markedly reduced?

    a.   Alzheimer's disease
    b.   Trisomy 21
    c.   Parkinson's disease without dementia
    d.   Huntington's chorea
    e.   Parkinson's disease with dementia

A273: a, b, e.

Q274: In Alzheimer's disease, the concentrations of which substances are markedly reduced in the cerebral cortex?

    a.   CAT
    b.   Gamma-aminobutyric acid (GABA)
    c.   Somatostatin
    d.   Dopamine

A274: a.

Q275: A 29-year-old homosexual man has weight loss, lymphadenopathy, change in affect, and two seizures of his left arm. CT scan shows a large circular lesion in the right frontal lobe. Which of the following tests should be performed and what results can be expected?

    a.   Mononucleosis spot test
    b.   Human immunodeficiency virus (HIV) antibody determination
    c.   CSF examination for cryptococcus
    d.   Serum toxoplasmosis titer
    e.   Blood tests for syphilis

A275: b, d, e. This patient probably has acquired immune deficiency syndrome (AIDS). Since HIV antibodies are present in 90 percent of AIDS patients, he will probably have a high antibody titer. When AIDS patients have signs of a cerebral lesion, such as focal seizures, a CT or MRI scan is necessary to look for cerebral toxoplasmosis, lymphoma, or other mass lesions. Until such lesions are excluded, a lumbar puncture should not be performed. Cerebral toxoplasmosis, which typically causes hemiparesis and seizures, is a common neurologic complication of AIDS. With cerebral toxoplasmosis, serum toxoplasmosis titers are usually elevated. Also, since syphilis often develops in male homosexuals, especially those who have AIDS, blood tests may indicate that the patient has neurosyphilis. AIDS dementia from HIV encephalitis, but not the single cerebral lesion, could produce the changes in affect.

Q276: A 15-year-old waitress has episodes that last 3 to 5 minutes during which she feels "dizzy and dreamy" and has paresthesias in her fingertips and around her mouth. Sometimes, she states, during these episodes her wrists bend and her fingers cramp together (see figure, p 497). An EEG during an episode showed slowing of the background activity and bursts of high voltage smooth 3 Hz activity. Of the following conditions, which one is the most likely to be occurring?

    a.   Partial complex seizures
    b.   Panic attacks
    c.   Petit mal (absence) seizures
    d.   None of the above

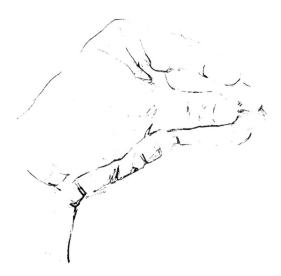

A276: d. She is probably having episodes of hyperventilation with carpopedal spasms and EEG slowing. These episodes might be a part of panic attacks, but they are not a manifestation of seizures. The clinical impression of hyperventilation can be confirmed if patients can reproduce their symptoms by hyperventilating for 2 to 4 minutes.

Q277: The patient in the preceding question is asked to hyperventilate. After 90 seconds, she becomes giddy and then irrational and inappropriate. What is the best way to abort the test?

A277: She probably has developed slight cerebral hypoxia because of reduction in carbon dioxide tension in the blood and consequent reduction in cerebral blood flow. She should be asked to breathe into a paper bag.

Q278: A young man who has been hospitalized for 2 days with the Guilllain-Barré syndrome became agitated and developed paranoid ideation and then hallucinations. He had no history of similar disturbances. Aside from the mental status changes, there were no signs of CNS dysfunction. Porphyria and other causes of peripheral neuropathy with mental status abnormalities were excluded. A psychiatrist is consulted to prescribe a sedative. Which treatment is most desirable?

A278: Guilllain-Barré syndrome is a disease of the peripheral nervous system that does not directly affect the brain. Mental aberrations may, however, complicate the condition. The most important manner in which they may develop is if chest and diaphragm muscle paresis causes hypoxia. Another cause of mental aberrations is treatment with high doses of steroids, i.e., "steroid psychosis." Two rare causes are electrolyte imbalance from inappropriate ADH secretion and hydrocephalus from blockage of the CSF reabsorption pathways by the proteinaceous CSF. Psychologic stress, especially with sleep deprivation, "ICU psychosis," can precipitate mental aberrations, but purely psychogenic explanations are actually infrequent and should be entertained only after life-threatening causes have been considered.

Q279: A 32-year-old woman is referred to a psychiatrist for postpartum depression because, for the 5 months following a difficult delivery of her fifth child, she has been complaining of being "unable to cope" with the family. She claims not to have the energy to do the housework or the inclination to undertake her usual activities. She never resumed her menses or regained her libido. She has anorexia and mild weight loss. She has no headaches, cognitive loss, visual changes, or other neurologic symptoms.

Her obstetrician, internist, and a neurologic consultant all find no physical signs of illness. Nevertheless, which conditions may be responsible?

    a.   Multiple sclerosis
    b.   Lupus
    c.   Sheehan's syndrome
    d.   Pregnancy

A279: c. Postpartum pituitary necrosis (Sheehan's syndrome) is usually caused by deliveries complicated by hypotension. Its symptoms, which may not develop for several months to several years postpartum, include failure of lactation, scanty or no menses, sexual and generalized indifference, and being easily fatigued. Aside from loss of secondary sexual characteristics and, in severe cases, hypotension, patients may have no physical abnormalities. Similar postpartum behavioral disturbances may be caused by autoimmune inflammatory hyper- or hypothyroidism.

By way of contrast, anorexia and weight loss are not typical symptoms of pregnancy unless associated with nausea and vomiting. A conception soon after delivery, of course, can prevent resumption of menses, but the other symptoms would not be present. During pregnancy multiple sclerosis (MS) is usually stable or seems to improve; however, during the postpartum period exacerbations typically occur. This patient is unlikely to have MS because she has no discrete physical neurologic deficits, and the change in menses and failure to lactate are not signs of MS. Lupus and other forms of vasculitis rarely present with CNS involvement. Even when they do affect the CNS, they cause seizures, stroke-like deficits, and florid psychiatric symptoms followed in quick succession by systemic signs.

Q280: A 22-year-old woman with chronic asthma that has a strong psychogenic component is hospitalized for a severe asthma attack. After being vigorously treated in an intensive care unit and failing to respond rapidly, she abruptly demands to sign out of the hospital. A psychiatric consultant finds that she is alert and oriented, but she is agitated and tremulous. Her judgement is flawed and her activity is impetuous. Which of the following plan(s) is (are) medically acceptable?

    a.   Use heavy sedation.
    b.   Administer a tranquilizer.
    c.   Transfer her from the intensive care unit.
    d.   Stop all medications.

A280: b. Until the origin of the mental aberrations can be discovered, the patient's potentially dangerous behavior must be curtailed. Possible explanations in this patient might be cerebral hypoxia, carbon dioxide retention, steroid psychosis, excessive beta adrenergic stimulants (e.g., epinephrine), or delirium tremens. "ICU psychosis" is not an acceptable explanation, and a patient who deteriorates should have a thorough medical and neurologic investigation and close observation. Although medications are often the cause of mental aberrations, abruptly discontinuing all of them may produce worsening of the underlying medical illness and precipitate new problems, such as adrenal crisis if high-dose steroids are stopped. Also, sedating patients with respiratory difficulty will not only mask signs of cerebral hypoxia, but it may also lead to carbon dioxide retention. Overall, the development of confusion in a patient with asthma is a sign of a serious development.

Q281: A 27-year-old man with a history of intractable seizures and violent behavior has had numerous EEGs that have shown only equivocal abnormalities. His serum phenytoin (Dilantin) concentration has always been below the therapeutic range despite a 500 mg/day prescription. He is suspected of abusing phenobarbital and other barbiturates, which he obtains on the basis of his diagnosis of epilepsy.

After seriously injuring a friend during a fistfight in a bar, his lawyer attributes the violence to the seizure disorder. As part of the medical-legal evaluation, an EEG is performed (see below). During the study, the patient becomes rigid and then has symmetric motor activity of his limbs. His face becomes red and afterward he becomes unresponsive.

Please evaluate the case in view of the history and the EEG.

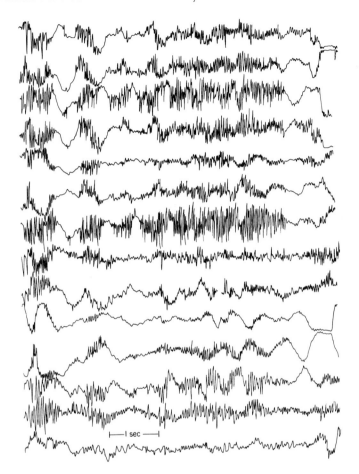

A281: Individuals with sociopathic behavior might convincingly mimic seizures. They can foster a diagnosis of intractable seizures for many reasons, including a desire to evade the legal system and to obtain medications. Likewise, a patient with genuine seizures might let them become intractable by failing to take anticonvulsants. Although anticonvulsants tend to produce slowed thinking, memory impairment, and apathy, a reasonable balance between benefits and side effects usually can be achieved. The most common explanation for a low serum anticonvulsant level is neither impaired absorption nor rapid metabolism but failure to take the prescribed dosage.

Directed purposeful violence (aggression) as a manifestation of a seizure is an extremely rare phenomenon if it exists at all. Moreover, aggression that occurs in bars is obviously more likely to be the result of alcohol consumption.

The most prominent features of this EEG are bursts of high voltage activity in the beginning and middle third of the sample. This activity is *muscle artifact*, which can be caused by either voluntary or involuntary scalp muscle contraction. A more important pattern in this EEG is the alpha and beta activity. This normal activity occurs during a pause in the muscle artifact and can be seen above and below the 1-second marker. Although the presence of muscle artifact cannot distinguish between genuine and psychogenic seizures, the presence of normal EEG activity even in the midst of an apparent generalized tonic-clonic seizure clearly indicates that the episode is psychogenic.

Following genuine generalized tonic-clonic seizures, the EEG becomes low voltage and slow, i.e., it has "postictal depression." Also, the serum prolactin concentration will be markedly elevated compared to its baseline. In contrast, following a psychogenic seizure, the EEG has normal activity and the serum prolactin concentration is normal.

Q282:   A 15-year-old girl complains of severe bitemporal headaches for 1 week. She has been the same height for 2 years, has failed to develop secondary sexual characteristics, and, in retrospect, for the past 2 years has been doing increasingly poorly in school and with friendships. A neurologist finds that she has a bitemporal hemianopsia and pallor of both optic discs. Her urine is persistently dilute. A CT scan reveals a large calcium-containing cystic lesion in the suprasellar region.

Which lesion is most likely responsible for the patient's endocrine deficiency and decline in academic and social skills?

    a.   Chromophobe adenoma
    b.   Craniopharyngioma
    c.   Protactinoma
    d.   Pregnancy

A282:   b. The patient has had an intracranial lesion for at least 2 years, judging by her failure to grow taller or undergo puberty, the duration of the academic and social problems, and the presence of calcium in the lesion. The optic atrophy also suggests chronicity of at least several months. The diabetes insipidus, indicated by the persistently dilute urine, and the CT scan both suggest a lesion in the hypothalamic region. Overall, the data indicate pituitary insufficiency from a slowly enlarging mass lesion in the suprasellar region.

Of all the conditions listed, craniopharyngiomas are the only ones to develop in children as well as adults. They are congenital lesions that have an indolent but progressive course. They cause hypothalamic dysfunction that leads to pituitary insufficiency and signs of a pituitary area mass lesion, e.g., temporal headaches, bitemporal visual field cuts, and optic atrophy.

Q283:   Which of the following are possible causes of mental impairments that occur in patients with metastatic carcinoma *without* brain metastases?

    a.   Meperidine (Demerol)
    b.   Limbic encephalitis
    c.   Progressive multifocal leukoencephalopathy (PML)
    d.   Cryptococcal meningitis
    e.   Hypercalcemia
    f.   Inappropriate ADH secretion
    g.   Liver metastases causing hepatic failure

A283:   All. A wide variety of mental status changes develop in such patients. Sometimes the changes are caused by metabolic derangements from cancer-induced fluid and electrolyte imbalance or from failure of vital organs. Several causes of mental status change are iatrogenic, such as narcotic analgesics, opportunistic infections, and cerebral radiation necrosis.

Q284:   Although the etiology of the narcolepsy-cataplexy syndrome has not been established, the recent finding of a major histocompatibility complex antigen, HLA DR2, in virtually all patients has had many implications. Which of the following statements may be inferred from the finding?

    a.   All people with the HLA antigen have narcolepsy-cataplexy.
    b.   Narcolepsy-cataplexy is caused by a genetic abnormality.
    c.   The short arm of chromosome 6 contains the related gene.
    d.   HLA antigens are related to the body's immune system.

A284:   c and d. Since the HLA DR2 antigen is found in 22 percent of people who did not have the narcolepsy-cataplexy syndrome (i.e., controls), it is not diagnostic. Other HLA antigens have been found to be increased in multiple sclerosis, ankylosing spondylitis, and other conditions; however, their etiologic role is still not established. For example, certain HLA antigens are associated with poliomyelitis, but that illness is clearly due to a viral infection and the HLA profile merely reflects a vulnerability to infectious or inflammatory conditions.

Q285:   What is the etiologic implication of the combination of Parkinson's disease being found rarely in identical (monozygotic) twins and the finding that MPTP can reproduce the disease's clinical and histologic features?

> a. These findings are inconsistent and have no implication.
> b. They indicate a genetic basis.
> c. They indicate a toxic etiology.

A285: c. These recent observations indicate that a toxic substance, possibly an environmental agent, causes Parkinson's disease. If genetic factors were important, the incidence in identical twins would have been increased.

Q286: A 75-year-old woman complains of pain in the right side of her face and her right shoulder, arm, and hand. She is referred to a psychiatrist because she is distraught by the discomfort and spends hours wrapping bandages around her arm and hand to protect the limb. She describes the pain as a burning numbness that becomes like an electric shock whenever it is touched by a person, clothing, light breeze, or, especially, an irritating object. She also has insomnia, anorexia, and weight loss.

The problem began 2 months before when a stroke initially caused her to have only clumsiness and sensory loss on the right side of her body. She never has had aphasia, visual field loss, or seizures. What is the condition from which she now suffers?

> a. Postherpetic neuralgia
> b. The effects of a thalamic infarction
> c. Sensory seizures

A286: b. She has had a thalamic infarction because of the sensory loss and motor impairment (clumsiness) at the onset and the extent of the sensory symptoms. Thalamic infarctions can cause dysesthesias (conversion of benign to painful sensations) and hyperpathia (grossly exaggerated perception of pain) as well as severe spontaneous pain. When these phenomena are present, patients should avoid exposing the sensitive areas. As is often the case, chronic pain has precipitated vegetative signs.

In thalamic pain, anticonvulsants have been reported to have inconsistent benefit in ameliorating the pain. Narcotics have surprisingly little direct benefit. Tricyclic antidepressants may have some benefit. The pain usually recedes spontaneously over 3 to 6 months.

Q287: A 50-year-old woman has metastatic breast carcinoma. She has been maintained on meperidine (Demerol) 50 mg q4h IM, antiemetic suppositories, and intravenous fluids and nutrition. During 4 weeks she improves with treatment, begins to ambulate, and takes food and medication orally. Several days later, however, she begins to feel anxious and fatigued and suffers from pain. A re-evaluation discloses no new metastases, metabolic aberrations, infections, or other complications of cancer. What common iatrogenic problem may have precipitated the pain recurrence and anxiety?

A287: Although the cancer may have continued to spread despite an initially good response, a simpler and more readily correctable problem would be that, as the patient improved, the same dose of a narcotic given parenterally was given orally. The changed routes of administration may have led to undertreatment of pain and narcotic withdrawal symptoms.

Q288: A deer hunter is accidentally shot in his left lower neck. The bullet passed through the brachial plexus and causes arm weakness. During the 2 months after the accident, some strength returned but continual pain developed. He complained of pains and had dysesthesia in the entire arm and especially the hand. The skin had become shiny and was alternately warmer and colder than the other hand. The painful condition, which was not treated in any specific manner, precipitated a depression for which a psychiatric consultation is requested. What is the best treatment for the painful condition?

> a. Non-narcotic analgesics and antidepressants
> b. TENS
> c. Sympathetic blockade (or block)
> d. Physical therapy

A288: c. The patient has causalgia, which is a distinctive painful condition that usually results from a penetrating wound that partly severs a major nerve's trunk or proximal portion. The pain, skin changes, and other symptoms originate from an intermingling of efferent sympathetic fibers with afferent sensory (pain) fibers.

Patients complain of burning pain and also have dysesthesias and hyperpathia. Abnormal sympathetic innervation of the skin and blood vessels causes the skin and temperature changes.

The best treatment is first a temporary block of the brachial plexus and, if successful, a permanent block, by injection into the stellate ganglion. The procedure is so specific that it has diagnostic value. Alternatively, an intravenous infusion of guanethidine into the affected limb, which would create a transient chemical block of the regional sympathetic ganglia, has recently been described as a less invasive diagnostic procedure that has temporary therapeutic value. The other treatments have symptomatic value.

Q289: A 25-year-old female renal transplant patient who has developed a red vesicular rash in her left upper face complains of severe pain and becomes distraught. The rash is diagnosed as a Herpes zoster infection. However, since her psychologic reaction and degree of pain seem disproportionately great, a liaison psychiatrist is consulted. What are the potential neurologic complications of the conditions?

A289: She has an acute Herpes zoster rash in the left VI distribution. Not only is the acute infection painful but the subsequent pain (postherpetic neuralgia) is also excruciating. The severity of the condition is often not appreciated, and thus patients are frequently undertreated. Narcotics are usually indicated.

In addition to causing severe pain, an infection in this region may lead to involvement of the cornea and then loss of the eye. In rare cases, the infection may disseminate to the brain and cause an encephalitis, or to the spinal cord and cause a myelitis. Acyclovir may prevent dissemination of the skin infection to the CNS.

Q290: The 45-year-old woman, in this figure, says that she has developed a habit of blinking frequently and involuntarily with her left eye. The eyelid closure, the physician observes, is forceful, lasts about 4 to 6 seconds, and is intensified by anxiety. She has no ocular abnormality, change in intellectual capacity, prior neurologic conditions, or medical illnesses. With which area is this problem associated?
    a.   Psychologic mechanisms
    b.   Basal ganglia
    c.   Cranial nerves
    d.   Autonomic nervous system
    e.   Unknown regions

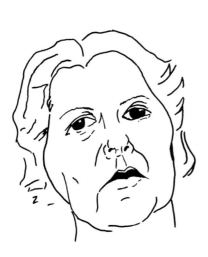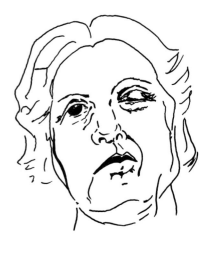

A290: c. The patient has hemifacial spasm. Note that on her left side she has contraction of the muscles around her mouth that pull it laterally, as well as sustained closure of her left upper and lower eyelids. This condition, which is diagnosed primarily by its appearance, consists of frequent, forceful, and prolonged contractions (spasms).

Hemifacial spasm develops in middle-aged and older individuals and is associated with compression of the facial nerve at its origin from the brainstem by an aberrant vessel. This example of a cranial nerve injury causing a movement disorder is unique. Moreover, if the compression can be relieved by neurosurgical placement of a cushion between the nerve and the vessel, hemifacial spasm can be relieved.

In contrast, although tics that involve one eye may develop in people of the same age as this patient, tics are of momentary duration and they affect only one or both eyes. They usually do not affect the lower and upper face on the same side. Also in contrast, tardive dyskinesia may cause facial movements, but it does not cause such unilateral movements. Psychogenic movement disorders are rare and should not be diagnosed without long observation and intensive investigation.

Q291: A teenaged couple attempted suicide by sitting in a car with the engine running in a closed garage. They were discovered in a comatose state but still alive. Three months later the young man was alert but bedridden. He remained in a flexed posture, mute, and unresponsive to stimulation. The young woman could be placed in a chair and had her eyes open. Although she did not follow verbal requests, initiate conversation, or respond purposefully, she would repeat incessantly whatever questions or requests were put to her. Almost as a reflex she would reiterate sentences and long phrases that she heard from visitors, television, and casual conversations near her bed. From what disorders did these young people suffer?

A291: The man probably had complete cerebral cortex destruction from carbon monoxide poisoning manifested by dementia and decorticate posture, i.e., the persistent vegetative state. The woman has incomplete cortex damage from the carbon monoxide. Her injury spared the language arc in the perisylvian region: Wernicke's area, the arcuate fasciculus, and Broca's area. The much larger surrounding "watershed" area of the cerebral cortex is more sensitive to carbon monoxide, hypoxia, and similar insults. Except for the preservation of her ability to repeat, she has lost all of her intellectual functions. She has a rare but classic case of isolation aphasia or mixed transcortical aphasia. Her echolalia, which is indicative of the disorder, should not be mistaken for a psychologic phenomenon.

Q292–294: Match the neurotransmitter with its metabolic product(s):

292: Norepinephrine

293: Dopamine

294: Serotonin

    a. 5-HIAA
    b. VMA
    c. HVA
    d. MHPG
    e. MPTP

A292–294:

292: b, d.

293: c.

294: a.

Q295: Of the following, which is the most common cause of coma in the United States?
    a. Subarachnoid hemorrhage
    b. Psychogenic conditions
    c. Barbiturate overdose
    d. Partial complex seizures

A295: c. Subarachnoid hemorrhage that causes coma and psychogenic coma are relatively rare. Partial complex seizures cause impairment of consciousness but not coma.

Q296: A psychiatric consultation is requested because a 25-year-old man, who has been a drug addict recovering uneventfully from abdominal surgery, became agitated, severely anxious, irrational, and diaphoretic. Immediately before the change in behavior, over his protests that he was allergic, the patient had received pentazocine (Talwin) for incisional pain. While a full investigation is being undertaken, which of the following medications would be most appropriate?

    a. A major tranquilizer
    b. Methadone
    c. Alcohol
    d. Phenobarbital
    e. Steroids
    f. Benadryl

A296: b. Pentazocine, butorphanol (Stadol), and other mixed narcotic agonist-antagonist preparations can precipitate withdrawal in narcotic addicts. Being aware of their vulnerability, narcotic addicts often claim, with some justification, that they are allergic to these preparations. Methadone or other narcotics will abort the withdrawal symptoms and provide at least short-term relief.

Q297: Metachromatic leukodystrophy (MLD) is a rare autosomal recessive genetic illness of young and middle-aged adults, although more commonly it affects children and adolescents. MLD may be diagnosed by finding decreased arylsulfatase activity in serum, white blood cells, fibroblasts, urine, and amniotic fluid cells. This illness causes demyelination in both the peripheral and the central nervous systems that cannot be treated. What are the clinical manifestations of this illness?

    a. Movement disorders
    b. Myopathy
    c. Peripheral neuropathy
    d. CNS and PNS demyelination
    e. Dementia associated with peripheral neuropathy
    f. Dementia that is correctable
    g. Mental changes that can be confused with schizophrenia

A297: c, d, e, g.

Q298: With which pathologic finding is Alzheimer's disease dementia most closely associated?

    a. Enlarged ventricles
    b. Increased concentration of neurofibrillary tangles
    c. Neuron loss
    d. Increased concentration of neuritic plaques

A298: d.

Q299: Which feature is *not* common to Alzheimer's disease and Down's syndrome?

    a. Abnormalities on chromosome 21
    b. Dementia
    c. Increased concentration of plaques and tangles
    d. Decreased cholinergic activity
    e. Abnormalities in the nucleus basalis Meynert
    f. Normal intelligence until the onset of dementia

A299: f.

Q300: Regarding illness that causes dementia, match the cutaneous lesion with the cerebral lesion:

    a. Adenoma sebaceum   1. Spirochetes
    b. Kaposi's sarcoma   2. Cerebrovascular calcifications
    c. Penile chancre   3. Cerebral tubers
    d. Facial angioma   4. HIV encephalitis

A300: a-3; b-4; c-1; d-2.

Q301: Regarding Alzheimer's disease dementia, match the histologic feature with its description.

    a. Neurofibrillary tangles
    b. Neuritic plaques
    c. Substantia innominata
    1. Distinct group of neurons beneath the globus pallidus
    2. Paired helical filaments
    3. Cluster of degenerating nerve terminals with an amyloid core

A301: a-2; b-3; c-1.

Q302: Regarding AIDS dementia, which of the following statements are *true*?
    a. The probable cause is a direct cerebral HIV infection.
    b. Toxoplasmosis is often an additional infection.
    c. The incidence of in utero transmission rate may be as high as 50 percent.
    d. Dementia may be the first symptom of AIDS.
    e. The first associated physical signs are usually slowness of movement and tremulousness; however, parkinsonism and myoclonus—extreme forms of these initial signs—occur later in the illness.

A302: a, b, (*not* c, the in utero rate far exceeds 50 percent when mothers have AIDS), d, e.

Q303: An 28-year-old nurse, who has previously been well, is hospitalized for the sudden onset of generalized muscle weakness that a neurology consultant diagnoses as hypokalemia. What are the causes of hypokalemic myopathy that suddenly develop in young and middle-aged adults?
    a. Adrenal crisis
    b. Renal failure
    c. Diuretic use
    d. Vomiting
    e. Diarrhea from laxative use

A303: c, d, e. Adrenal and renal failure usually cause hyperkalemia and systemic symptoms but not myopathy. The other conditions that cause hypokalemic myopathy in previously healthy young adults may be signs of underlying illness; however, they are often self-induced.

Q304: In which way are dopamine and acetylcholine similar neurotransmitters?
    a. Both act extensively in the PNS and CNS.
    b. Both are distributed evenly throughout the CNS.
    c. Both are conserved by re-uptake by the presynaptic neuron.
    d. They are distributed in separate pathways in the brain.

A304: d.

Q305: A 28-year-old woman, who has a summer home in East Hampton, Long Island, complained in September of malaise and joint pains. When these symptoms seemed to resolve in October, she then felt as though she had a continual low grade temperature, but she was not able to record elevations. After a routine medical evaluation revealed no cause, she considered herself to be a hypochondriac. In November, facial weakness developed on one side and, 6 days later, on the other. A circular rash, with a 6-inch diameter, was found on her lower chest. During the next week, a polyneuropathy developed. What illness has she contracted?

A305: She has Lyme disease, which is an infectious illness caused by a spirochete that is transmitted by a tick. Infected ticks, which bite people when they walk through wooded areas, live on deer in New England, Long Island, the Pacific Northwest, Wisconsin, and Minnesota. The illness typically causes malaise, fatigue, headache, arthralgias or frank arthritis, cardiac conduction disturbances, and a bull's-eye red rash. Neurologic complications are meningitis, facial nerve paresis that might be misdiagnosed as Bell's palsy, and a peripheral neuropathy that can mimic Guillain Barré syndrome. Serologic tests, which are unreliable because they are often negative early in the illness, must be repeated in suspected cases. Since Lyme disease has protean and often nonspecific manifestations, and the serologic test results are often false-negative, it may initially be misdiagnosed. Lyme disease, mononucleosis, chronic Epstein-Barr virus (EBV) infection, AIDS, and various psychiatric disturbances are causes of chronic fatigue.

Q306: Removal of toxic substances, including antibodies, from the blood may be accompanied by plasmapheresis. In which diseases has this technique been an effective treatment?
- a. Schizophrenia
- b. Multiple sclerosis
- c. Guillain-Barré syndrome
- d. Myasthenia gravis

A306: c, d.

Q307: In which ways are CNS and PNS myelin similar?
- a. They are both derived from oligodendroglia.
- b. They are both derived from Schwann cells.
- c. They are both insulators of electrochemical nerve transmission.
- d. They are antigenically similar.
- e. They are usually injured by the same illnesses.

A307: c.

Q308: A 40-year-old man, who had received neuroleptic treatment, began to notice that when he was tired his eyelids would have twitches. The movements would be more pronounced if he drank coffee or was anxious. Over the following year, his eyelids would forcefully contract for 5 to 30 seconds, covering his eyes completely. Which conditions might be present?

A308: On the basis of the initial symptoms, the patient might have been diagnosed as having had fasciculations of the orbicularis oculi, called myokymia. There are common coarse twitches that are typically induced by caffeine, anxiety, and fatigue. Subsequently, his prolonged, forceful contractions of the eyelids should be diagnosed as blepharospasm. This condition is an involuntary movement disorder of the face (a facial dyskinesia) that may be a variety of tardive dyskinesia, an entity unto itself, or the first manifestation of the extensive dystonic facial dyskinesia, Meige's syndrome. Systemic medications, such as anticholinergics, offer little benefit for blepharospasm, but injections of botulinum toxin into the affected muscles may alleviate the spasms. Facial dyskinesias are an important entity in which psychiatrists have to distinguish among movements induced by psychologic factors, neuroleptics, other medications, and various neurologic disorders.

Q309: Match the condition with its cause.
- a. Lyme disease
- b. Tabes dorsalis
- c. N-hexane neuropathy
- d. Toluene-induced CNS and PNS demyelination
- e. Accumulation of metachromatic granules in the brain, peripheral nerves, gallbladder, and other organs
- f. Neuropathy from abusing a dental anesthetic
- g. Neuropathy from megavitamin treatments
- 1. Inhaling glue vapor
- 2. Genetic absence of aryl-sulfatase-A
- 3. Inhaling nitrous oxide
- 4. Spirochete infection
- 5. Pyridoxine (vitamin B_6) intoxication

A309: a-4; b-4; c-1; d-1; e-2; f-3; g-5.

Q310: Match the diagnostic technique with the purpose.
- a. Restriction fragment length polymorphisms (RFLPs)
- b. Tensilon test
- c. Wada test
- d. Arylsulfatase-A determination in leukocytes
- 1. Determination of the dominant hemisphere
- 2. Identification of chromosome abnormalities
- 3. Diagnosis of metachromatic leukodystrophy
- 4. Diagnosis of myasthenia gravis

A310: a-2; b-4; c-1; d-3.

Q311: Carbamazepine (Tegretol) is used in treatment of psychiatric illnesses as well as of seizures. Which are its common side effects?
- a. Liver dysfunction
- b. Gum hypertrophy
- c. Cerebellar impairments in children
- d. Leukopenia
- e. Anemia
- f. Stevens-Johnson syndrome
- g. Mental aberrations if the medication is introduced too rapidly

A311: a, d, e, g.

Q312: Which of the following statements concerning prions are false?
- a. They contain RNA.
- b. They contain reverse transcriptase.
- c. They are infective agents.
- d. They may be the cause of Creutzfeldt-Jakob disease.
- e. They are identifiable in cerebral biopsy tissue of Alzheimer's disease patients.

A312: a, b, e. Prions are protein-containing infective agents that do not have any DNA or RNA. They are believed to cause Creutzfeldt-Jakob disease because they can be identified in cerebral biopsies of the victims. It is the human immunodeficiency virus (HIV) that is an RNA virus that contains reverse transcriptase.

Q313: With which conditions are Duchenne's dystrophy associated?
- a. Absence of dystrophin, a newly discovered muscle protein
- b. Abnormality of the X chromosome
- c. Abnormalities of the structure of dystrophin
- d. Alzheimer's disease

A313: a, b.

Q314: Which are features of neuroleptic-malignant syndrome (NMS), malignant hyperthermia (MH), both, or neither?
1. Precipitated by succinylcholine given before electroshock therapy
2. Muscle rigidity
3. Markedly elevated CPK
4. Hyperpyrexia causes cerebral cortical damage
5. Rhabdomyolysis
6. Inherited tendency
7. Reportedly responds to dantrolene
8. Impaired mental state
- a. NMS
- b. MH
- c. Both
- d. Neither

A314: 1-b; 2-c; 3-c; 4-c; 5-c; 6-b; 7-c; 8-c.

Q315: A 27-year-old man with epilepsy since childhood, characterized by primary generalized tonic-clonic seizures, was being treated with phenytoin (Dilantin) 400 mg daily. When he developed lethargy, confusion, nystagmus, and ataxia, a serum phenytoin level was found to be much greater than the therapeutic range. What will be the effect of stopping the phenytoin until the next office visit, which would be in 1 month?
- a. Partial seizures may begin.
- b. The behavioral and cognitive impairments will probably improve.
- c. Generalized status epilepticus may develop.
- d. If one anticonvulsant cannot suppress seizures, the next step should be to switch to a different one rather than add a second.

A315: b, c, d. The patient has phenytoin intoxication. Virtually all anticonvulsants cause mental aberrations when elevated blood concentrations are reached. The best method to treat anticonvulsant intoxications is to withdraw the medication for several days, during which time the patient should improve and the blood level should reach a therapeutic range. Then, unless a confounding problem has occurred, such as addition of another medication, the anticonvulsant should be restarted at a smaller dose. Abrupt withdrawal of an anticonvulsant may precipitate status epilepticus, which is a life-threatening condition. Likewise, suddenly stopping chronic barbiturate or alcohol use may cause status epilepticus. As a general rule for treatment of epilepsy, use of a single anticonvulsant (monotherapy) with careful monitoring of the clinical status and blood concentrations is preferable to use of two or more anticonvulsants (polypharmacy).

Q316: Match the clinical description of patients with mental status changes with the appropriate CT scan:

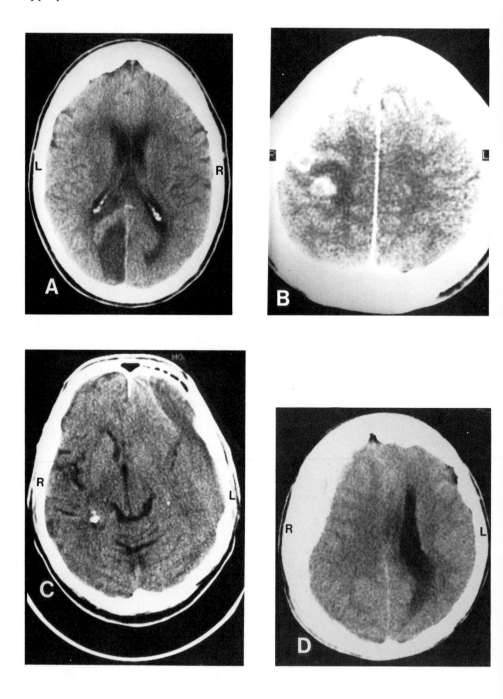

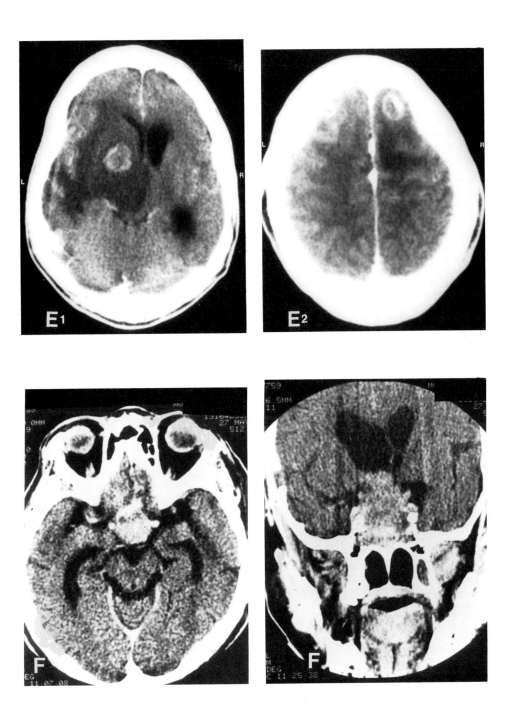

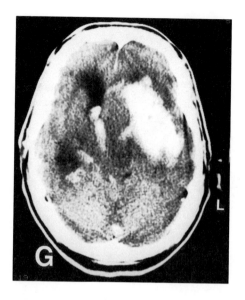

1. A 23-year-old woman, who had just delivered a baby boy 5 days before, had the sequential development of personality changes, agitation, garbled speech, seizures, and finally right hemiparesis. She had had an uneventful pregnancy. She did not use alcohol, tobacco, or drugs, but her boyfriend is a former drug addict.

2. A 45-year-old man was placed in restraints and given neuroleptics for agitated behavior. Later in the night, although the patient is stuporous, he complains loudly of a headache. Examination reveals papilledema and a mild left hemiparesis that the patient, in his obtundation, seems to ignore.

3. A 65-year-old man compains that for several weeks he has had difficulty reading newspapers and books. Although his memory and other aspects of his general intellect are intact, he stumbles, almost incoherently, when reading. Nevertheless, he can repeat phrases, comprehend spoken statements, and even transcribe entire sentences.

4. An 80-year-old man has malaise, mild frontal headaches, and progressively severe cognitive impairments with prominent anomias. Otherwise, he has no abnormalities on neurologic or general medical examination. Routine laboratory tests, including a sedimentation rate, are normal.

5. A 50-year-old man is unable to concentrate on his work, which consists of making architectural drawings. When he relates his history, he seems inattentive, but his cognitive capacity is grossly normal.

6. A 38-year-old woman, who has been infertile, has the onset of headaches and bitemporal hemianopsia.

7. A 55-year-old hypertensive man has the sudden onset of a severe headache, aphasia, and right hemiparesis.

A316:

1-E. The CT scans show two circular lesions that are each enhanced by contrast infusion. In these scans the presence of contrast infusion can be surmised by the falx, a thick vascular structure, being white. Note the standard of placing "L" or "R" notations on the appropriate side of the scan. As is the case with many machines, the CT picture is "reversed." In this case, a large lesion surrounded by extensive edema is deep in the left cerebral hemisphere (Scan E1). Another is in the right frontal lobe (E2). In the lower cut (E1), the anterior and occipital horns of the left lateral ventricle are compressed, and midline structures are shifted to the right. In the higher cut, however, a shift is not possible because the falx acts as a rigid barrier. The lesions, being multiple masses and enhanced by contrast, are indicative of toxoplasmosis, bacterial abscesses, and metastatic tumors. Given the history of the patient being the sexual partner of a drug addict, the most likely diagnosis is cerebral toxoplasmosis as a manifestation of AIDS. In addition, if she has AIDS, the infant will probably have AIDS.

2-D. The CT scan shows a thick white border overlying the right side of the brain. Bone, fresh blood, and calcium are denser than brain and therefore portrayed as white on a CT scan. Also, the right lateral ventricle is obliterated by compression. Note that this machine, like many others, portrays the brain in reverse. The patient has an acute subdural hematoma over the right cerebral hemisphere. The hematoma, which probably resulted from head trauma, has caused stupor, increased intracranial pressure, left hemiparesis, and anosognosia.

3-C. This CT scan shows a relatively large dark semicircular area to the left of the falx, which is the thin white vertical line between the occipital lobes. This abnormality is in the left occipital lobe. Its lucency and distinctive pattern indicate that it is an infarction of the left posterior cerebral artery. The patient has the interesting and important neuropsychologic condition called "alexia without agraphia" or inability to read but preserved ability to write. It results from damage to the left occipital lobe and posterior corpus callosum (Fig. 8-4) usually from an infarction in the distribution of the left posterior cerebral artery. The perisylvian language arc is preserved. Alexia without agraphia and corpus callosum transection are often cited as disconnection syndromes. In these conditions, transfer of information between or within cerebral hemispheres is impaired.

4-C. This CT scan shows an abnormality overlying the left frontal lobe that has a white rim in the most anterior portion. The black to gray intensities indicate that its density is less than the brain. Cerebrospinal fluid, edematous fluid, aged blood, and necrotic brain—all portrayed as black on the CT—are the most common hypodense tissues. The frontal horn of the left lateral ventricle is compressed, and the left frontal lobes are shifted slightly to the right. This CT scan indicates a chronic subdural hematoma. The symptoms of chronic subdural hematomas are usually a dull headache and cognitive impairments, including exacerbations of age-related language impairments, such as anomias. Although the subdural hematomas are typically produced by trauma, patients often do not recall a preceding episode. Sionce chronic subdural hematomas are slowly evolving, they do not cause chronic papilledema or priminent lateralized signs. They are easily evacuated by a neurosurgeon installing burr holes or other methods of drainage. Most important, subdural hematomas are a commonly occurring, correctable cause of dementia.

5-B. The CT scan shows a lesion in the posterior portion of the right cerebral hemisphere, which consists almost entirely of the parietal lobe. The lesion has a white center and fragments of a white ring surrounding it. The white falx indicates that all these structures are enhanced by infusion of contrast material. The lesion is probably a tumor or other mass. Lesions in parietal cortex, whatever their etiology, are associated with constructional apraxia, hemi-inattention, anosognosia, and, according to some neurologists, impaired emotional communication. This patient's presenting symptom is probably a manifestation of constructional apraxia. Since symptoms referable to lesions in the right hemisphere are often accompanied by anosognosia, patients may ignore them or describe them only in imprecise terms.

6-F. *Left,* This is an axial, contrast-enhanced, CT scan through the orbits. It reveals a circular radiodense lesion. *Right,* In this coronal view, the lesion can be seen to be arising from the sella turcica and growing into the hypothalamus and third ventricle. The lateral ventricles are pushed aside and one is dilated, which suggests that blockage of the third ventricle has caused hydrocephalus. The white, wishbone-shaped structure in the axial CT view is the normal venous drainage. Lesions in the pituitary region in adults, which are usually pituitary adenomas, cause endocrinologic disturbances, bitemporal hemianopsia, and headaches. Craniopharyngiomas are uncommon lesions.

7-G. In the left side of the brain (the right side of the picture), the CT reveals a large intracerebral hemorrhage with blood that has extended into the contralateral ventricle. Hypertensive cerebral hemorrhages usually occur in the putamen, thalamus, pons, or cerebellum.

Q317–318: A physician is called to see a colleague, who is known to be hypertensive and seriously depressed, because of severe headache, nausea, vomiting, and diaphoresis. He finds that the colleague is stuporous with nuchal rigidity and bilateral Babinski signs. The blood pressure is 210/130 mm Hg. Bottles of chlorpromazine, isocarboxazid, propranolol, meperidine, and hydrochlorothiazide are in the medicine chest.

Q317:   What is the most likely diagnosis?.
   a.   Medication interaction
   b.   Meningitis
   c.   Intracranial hemorrhage
   d.   None of the above

A317:   c. The patient has classic signs of an intracranial hemorrhage: headache, stupor, nausea, vomiting, nuchal rigidity, and Babinski signs. The origin could have been a common hypertensive cerebral hemorrhage that was not prevented by the antihypertensive medications. Alternatively, the etiology could have been a drug-induced hemorrhage, with the most likely culprit being the isocarboxazid (Marplan). That medication, like tranylcypromine (Parnate), phenelzine (Nardil), and others, is a monamine oxidase (MAO) inhibitor. MAO inhibitors cause acute, severe hypertension if certain foods, such as aged cheese, or medications are ingested. Sometimes depressed people purposefully take prohibited foods in suicide attempts. Drug-induced hypertension can result in subarachnoid or intracerebral hemorrhages.

Q318:   If the problem is caused by an MAO inhibitor, what should be the best antidote? Which of the following medications should be given in the interim?
   a.   Meperidine
   b.   Chlorpromazine
   c.   Propranolol
   d.   Hydrochlorothiazide
   e.   Phentolamine
   f.   Dibenzoxazepine

A318:   The most specific treatment for a MAO inhibitor is the alpha adrenergic blocking agent, phentolamine (Regitine), at a dose of 5 mg given slowly intravenously. Of the medications that are usually readily available, propranolol or chlorpromazine would be most helpful. Although the headache may be agonizingly severe, meperidine (Demerol) is contraindicated.

Q319:   Which of the following substances injected into the penis will induce an erection in a man with erectile dysfunction?
   a.   Epinephrine
   b.   Papaverine
   c.   Phentolamine
   d.   Testosterone
   e.   Prolactin

A319:   b, c. In a newly introduced treatment for erectile dysfunction, papaverine, a smooth muscle relaxant, and phentolamine (Regitine), an alpha adrenergic blocker, injected individually or together induce erections. This treatment is useful in a variety of illnesses, including multiple sclerosis, diabetes, local nerve injury, and even psychogenic conditions. These injections will even permit orgasms to occur. After intercourse, injections of epinephrine will abort the erection. The treatments may be complicated by priapism and ischemia. Testosterone treatments rarely have value, except as a placebo, in men with normal hormones. Serum prolactin concentrations are often elevated in pituitary tumors or adenomas that cause reduced libido.

Q320:   Which chemical process converts dopa to dopamine?
   a.   Oxidation
   b.   Hydroxylation
   c.   Decarboxylation
   d.   Deamination

A320: c. Decarboxylation converts both endogenous dopa and the medicine L-dopa to the neurotransmitter dopamine, which is a monamine. This reaction takes place in the adrenal glands, several other non-CNS tissues, and the nigrostriatal tract. Carbidopa inhibits the enzyme, dopa decarboxylase, in non-CNS tissue; however, since carbidopa does not cross the blood-brain barrier, synthesis of dopamine continues in the brain. Administered with dopa, carbidopa permits use of smaller doses of dopa and reduces the systemic side effects. When L-dopa is administered, monamine oxidase inhibitors usually should not also be given. However, certain monamine oxidase inhibitors retard the metabolism of dopamine and can be given in Parkinson's disease.

Q321: Which structure connects the hippocampus and the hypothalamus?
  a. Corpus callosum
  b. Cingulate gyrus
  c. Fornix
  d. None of the above

A321: c. The fornix connects the hippocampus with the mammillary bodies, which are a section of the hypothalamus. The mammillary bodies communicate through the mammillothalamic tract with the anterior nucleus of the thalamus.

Q322: A college student finds that she develops unilateral throbbing headaches during weekends and vacations. Aside from psychologic considerations, what factors may be precipitating her headaches?

A322: She probably has migraine rather than tension-muscular contraction headaches because her headaches are unilateral and throbbing rather than symmetric, continual, and dull. The pattern of migraine headaches occurring during restful times is commonplace. One theory is that when a continual stress-induced outpouring of vasoconstricting steriod hormones ceases, as during postexamination school breaks, the cerebral and systemic arteries dilate and permit undampened pulsations to strike pain-sensitive cerebral structures. Other factors that can precipitate migraine headaches during school breaks are disrupted sleep schedules and drinking alcoholic beverages.

Index

Note: Page numbers in *italics* refer to illustrations; page numbers followed by t refer to tables.